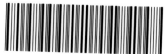
DANA PRESS

THE DANA GUIDE TO BRAIN HEALTH EDITING AND WRITING STAFF

DANA PRESS

Jane Nevins, Editor in Chief
Donna Deaton, Executive Assistant
Kristine Pauls, Production Editor

WRITERS

Sandra J. Ackerman
Sharon Broll
Lynne Lamberg

Ann MacDonald
Steve Nadis
Ann Parson

THE DANA GUIDE TO BRAIN HEALTH ART STAFF

Elizabeth Thompson, Art Researcher
Kathryn Born, Illustrator

Leigh Coriale, Illustrator
Robert Finkbeiner, Illustrator

THE DANA GUIDE TO BRAIN HEALTH CD-ROM

CyberMedia Services, Production and Development

THE DANA GUIDE TO

BRAIN HEALTH

FLOYD E. BLOOM, M.D.

M. FLINT BEAL, M.D.

DAVID J. KUPFER, M.D.

Editors

DANA PRESS / NEW YORK · WASHINGTON

Hardcover published in 2003 by The Free Press, a Division of Simon & Schuster, Inc.

DANA
PRESS

COVER BY OSPREY DESIGN

Manufactured in the United States of America

10 9 8 7 6 5 4 3 2 1

The Library of Congress has catalogued the hardcover edition as follows:

The Dana guide to brain health / Floyd E. Bloom, M. Flint Beal, David J. Kupfer, editors.
    p.   cm.
    Includes bibliographical references and index.
    1. Brain—Popular works.   2. Brain—Diseases—Popular works.   3. Mental illness—
Popular works.   4. Neurology—Popular works.   I. Title: Brain health.
II. Bloom, Floyd E.   III. Beal, M. Flint.   IV. Kupfer, David J.

RC341 .D173   2003
612.8'2—dc21   2002072207

ISBN: 0-7432-0397-6 (Cloth)
ISBN 10: 1-932594-10-8 (Paper)
ISBN 13: 978-1-932594-10-2 (Paper)

This book is dedicated to our friend and colleague, David Mahoney, Chairman and CEO of The Dana Foundation from 1977 until his death, in 2000. He directed the Foundation's work into educating the public about brain research, exemplifying his instinct for the public good and for the Foundation's special ability to nurture a young science on the brink of its potential. While the neuroscience field has formally recognized his great contribution, his personal drive and dedication will always be a vivid model to everyone who met him.

—The Editors

ACKNOWLEDGMENTS

The editors wish to thank our 104 colleagues—physicians, psychiatrists, and neuroscientists, neurologists, and neurosurgeons—who prepared the individual sections of this book and contributed their suggested further resources for the CD-ROM. Their enthusiasm for bringing the latest findings to a general audience is a wonderful example of their insight and commitment and one of the many reasons their peers hold them in such high regard. We also wish to thank The Dana Foundation, especially its chairman, William Safire, and president, Edward F. Rover, for making this book possible and ensuring the logistical support necessary to bring so many pieces together into the coherent whole we envisioned.

In particular, we would like to acknowledge the Dana Press staff who participated in this project: Jane Nevins, editor in chief, who directed it; Kristine Pauls, production editor who has orchestrated this edition and the CD-ROM; Donna Deaton, whose administration of paperwork, deadlines, and contacts kept everything on track; and the Dana Press's fine team of consulting professionals for the hardcover edition—the experienced reference book editor and writer John Bell; the expert medical illustrators Kathryn Born, Leigh Coriale, and Robert Finkbeiner; the inexhaustible hunter-gatherer Betsy Thompson, art researcher; the first-rate science writers whose skill is seen in the opening narrative chapters—

Sandra J. Ackerman, Steve Nadis, Ann MacDonald, Lynne Lamberg, Ann Parson, and Sharon Broll, who helped to edit many of the sections.

We also thank the Dana staff who participated in preparing the hardcover edition as well as the excellent group at The Free Press who published it in 2003.

As editors, we needed and received marvelous support at our respective bases. We thank our administrative coordinators—Greta Strong at Cornell Weill Medical Center, and Donna Donovan at the UPMC Health System in Pittsburgh—for their excellent help in our preparation of this book. And last, but most important, we want to express our gratitude to our wives and children. As medical professionals themselves, our wives keenly appreciated the challenge of such a project, and we are immensely grateful for their enthusiasm and support. Floyd E. Bloom wishes to thank Jody Corey-Bloom, his two children, and four grandchildren; M. Flint Beal thanks Judy and their children, Bradley and Emily; and David J. Kupfer thanks Ellen Frank and their six children and eight grandchildren.

CONTENTS

Using Our Heads: A Foreword by William Safire   xiii

Introduction: Welcome to Your Brain   xvii

How to Read This Book   xxi

Contributors   xxiii

Your Brain: A Primer   follows page xxxii

PART I   Understanding Your Brain

1. How to Think About the Brain   3

2. How We Know: Learning the Secrets of the Brain   14

3. Basic Brain Care: Protecting Your Mental Capital   31

4. The Brain-Body Loop   41

PART II   Your Brain Through Life

5. Prenatal Development   61

6. Brain Development in Childhood   83

7. The Adolescent Brain   102

8. The Brain in Adult Life and Normal Aging   116

PART III   The Healthy Brain

9. The Body Manager   135

     B1 The Major Senses: Sight, Hearing, Taste, Smell, and Touch   136

     B2 Body Regulation   142

     B3 Basic Drives: Eating, Sleeping, and Sex   150

     B4 Movement, Balance, and Coordination   158

     B5 Pain Perception   165

     B6 Consciousness   171

10. Emotions and Social Function   179

   B7 Emotions   180

   B8 Inhibition and Control   185

   B9 Temperament   190

   B10 Attention and Motivation   196

11. Learning, Thinking, and Remembering   200

   B11 Decision Making and Planning   201

   B12 Intelligence   210

   B13 Learning and Memory   217

   B14 Speech, Language, and Reading   226

   B15 Visualization and Navigation   232

   B16 Creativity, Talents, and Skills   236

P A R T I V   Conditions of the Brain and Nervous System

12. Conditions That Appear in Childhood   247

   C1 Dyslexia   248

   C2 Attention Deficit/Hyperactivity Disorder   254

   C3 Mental Retardation   259

   C4 Cerebral Palsy   265

   C5 Autism   270

   C6 Metabolic Diseases   278

   C7 Neurofibromatosis   284

   C8 Hydrocephalus   288

   C9 Spina Bifida   293

   C10 Tumors of Childhood   298

13. Disorders of the Senses and Body Function   306

   C11 Sleep Disorders   307

   C12 Narcolepsy   315

   C13 Epilepsy and Seizures   319

   C14 Dizziness and Vertigo   327

   C15 Seeing Problems   332

   C16 Hearing Problems   341

   C17 Smelling and Tasting Problems   347

   C18 Autonomic Disorders   352

   C19 Chronic Fatigue Syndrome   357

14. Emotional and Control Disorders   362

   C20 Depression   363

   C21 Anxiety and Panic   371

   C22 Social Phobia (Social Anxiety Disorder)   376

   C23 Obsessive-Compulsive Disorder   379

   C24 Bipolar Disorder   385

   C25 Schizophrenia   390

   C26 Borderline Personality Disorder   394

   C27 Eating Disorders   399

   C28 Post-Traumatic Stress Disorder   405

   C29 Substance Abuse and Addiction   409

   C30 Alcoholism   419

   C31 Violence and Aggression   426

   C32 Suicidal Feelings   429

15. Infectious and Autoimmune Disorders   434

   C33 Multiple Sclerosis   435

   C34 Shingles/Herpes Zoster   444

   C35 Neurological Complications of AIDS   448

   C36 Lyme Disease   453

   C37 Meningitis   458

   C38 Viral Encephalitis   462

   C39 Creutzfeldt-Jakob Disease   468

   C40 Systemic Lupus Erythematosus   471

16. Disorders of Movement and Muscles   476

   C41 Parkinson's Disease   477

   C42 Parkinsonism Plus   484

   C43 Tremors   490

   C44 Dystonia, Spasms, and Cramps   494

   C45 Tourette's Syndrome and Tics   497

   C46 Ataxia   501

   C47 Huntington's Disease   505

   C48 Peripheral Neuropathy   511

   C49 Guillain-Barré Syndrome   516

   C50 Bell's Palsy   520

   C51 Myopathies   523

C52 Myasthenia Gravis 530

C53 Amyotrophic Lateral Sclerosis 535

17. Pain 539

C54 Headache 540

C55 Migraines 548

C56 Back Pain and Disk Disease 553

C57 Chronic Pain 559

C58 Trigeminal Neuralgia 565

18. Nervous System Injuries 569

C59 Ischemic Stroke 570

C60 Hemorrhagic Stroke 576

C61 Brain Trauma, Concussion, and Coma 581

C62 Spinal Cord Injury 591

C63 Paraneoplastic Syndromes 600

C64 Brain Tumors 604

C65 Nutritional Disorders 610

C66 Chemicals and the Nervous System 617

19. Disorders of Thinking and Remembering 624

C67 Alzheimer's Disease 625

C68 Amnesias 635

C69 Dementia 639

C70 Trouble with Speech and Language 643

C71 Apraxias 648

C72 Agnosias 651

Glossary 655

Appendix A: Drugs Used to Treat the Brain and Nervous System 661

Appendix B: Suggested Reading 669

Appendix C: Resource Groups 673

The Dana Alliance for Brain Initiatives 687

The European Dana Alliance for the Brain 695

About the Editors 701

Index 703

USING OUR HEADS

A Foreword by William Safire

A decade ago, in a place called Cold Spring Harbor, on Long Island, New York, two quite different men convened a meeting of scientists that was to have a powerful effect on how we explore and treat the most important organ of all—the human brain.

One was James Watson, a Nobel laureate for his codiscovery of the structure of DNA, who was concerned about the public's apparent lack of interest in, and active financial support for, brain research. The other was David Mahoney, a fabled marketing executive turned philanthropist, head of The Dana Foundation, who knew why the United States government's vaunted "Decade of the Brain" was having trouble getting off the ground.

"Your goal of 'understanding the brain' isn't good enough," the former adman told the assembled scientists, many of whom looked askance at exhortation from this outsider that Watson introduced. "People want to know what you can do for them. They don't want to hear about general 'research'; they want to know what you can do to make their lives healthier and better. You have to offer them hope. That means you have to go out on a limb and lay out your specific goals for treatments and cures."

"David scared a lot of us at first," says Steven E. Hyman, M.D., who later became Director of the National Institute of Mental Health and is now Provost at Harvard University. "We were taken aback when asked to make promises. Now I see the extraordinary wisdom of his request."

The scientists at that Cold Spring Harbor meeting debated the need to get specific about what they thought could be done before the end of the twentieth century. Inspired by the practicality and enthusiasm of Watson and Mahoney, and well aware of the fierce competition for private and public funding, they decided to take the plunge into greater public communication. Then and there, the Dana Alliance for Brain Initiatives was formed, setting out achievable goals for research that would lead to the treatment of diseases and disorders. Here is a sampling of its initial goals:

- Identify the genes that are defective in familial Alzheimer's and Huntington's diseases, and the genes responsible for hereditary forms of manic-depressive illness.

- Develop new medications and therapeutic strategies to reduce nerve cell death and enhance recovery of function after strokes and other forms of brain injury.

- Identify new treatments to promote nerve regeneration following spinal cord and peripheral nerve injury.

- Discover, test, and apply agents that will block the action of cocaine and other addictive substances.

- Develop new treatments for pain associated with cancer, arthritis, migraine headaches, and other debilitating illnesses.

- Elucidate the neuronal mechanisms involved in learning and memory.

In the decade since, progress has been dramatic toward these and several other goals; in subsequent meetings, senior scientists made candid self-assessments of work toward clinical treatment and issued realistic "report cards." Through Dana newsletters like *BrainWork,* radio programs like *Gray Matters,* and television documentaries and books published by Dana Press (originator of the book in your hand), news of the exciting potential of brain research has reached millions. As the Dana Alliance, with its European counterpart, has expanded to more than 400 scientists, including 14 Nobelists, around the world (see the member names on pages 687–699 of this book), an international "Brain Awareness Week" has become the focal point for dialogue between scientists and the lay public around the world.

The purpose of focusing attention on neuroscience is to stimulate much stronger research investment and to attract young scientists into the field, thereby to offer even more realistic hope to sufferers of brain disorders and their families. We know that neurological and psychiatric disorders account for more hospital and nursing home admissions in this country than all other diseases and disorders combined. We know, too, that with greater effort, rapid advances in treatment and even in cures are possible. In 2002, many members of the Dana Alliance met in New York to set new goals, building on the successes—and frustrations—of the past decade.

"Our mission as neuroscientists has to go beyond brain research," they agreed. "People not only want to know how and why research is done, they also want to know why it matters to them." And the field of "neuroethics" was born, "to allay the public's concerns that the findings of brain science could be used in ways that might be harmful or ethically questionable." As the study of the brain gains momentum, here are some of the new goals set forward by the Dana Alliance:

1. Combat the devastating impact of Alzheimer's disease.
2. Discover how best to treat Parkinson's disease.
3. Decrease the incidence of stroke and improve post-stroke therapies.
4. Develop more successful treatments for mood disorders such as depression, schizophrenia, obsessive-compulsive disorder, and bipolar disorder.
5. Uncover genetic and neurobiological causes of epilepsy and advance its treatment.
6. Discover new and effective ways to prevent and treat multiple sclerosis.
7. Develop better treatments for brain tumors.
8. Improve recovery from traumatic brain and spinal cord injuries.
9. Create new approaches for pain management.
10. Treat addiction at its origin in the brain.
11. Understand the brain mechanisms underlying the response to stress, anxiety, and depression.

(Why, the reader will wonder, the odd number of 11 goals? Surely it would have been better to edit them down to ten, as in commandments, or add one to make a memorably even dozen. Goes to show, I suppose, that Dana Alliance members still think like neuroscientists and not like marketers.)

New research tools are speeding discoveries. In pursuing their new set of goals, brain scientists and doctors will be able to take advantage of genomic research, which many believe promises to transform neurology and psychiatry by enhancing or blocking the action of specific genes. Advanced imaging techniques that provide real-time examination of the brain in action, or in an abnormal state, are likely to provide understanding that will lead to clinical advances unimagined only a decade ago. As stem cell controversies are resolved, research will make it possible to replace brain cells lost to disease or injury, not only lengthening human lives but also making future centenarians happier and more productive.

Even as clinicians and researchers focus on the practical treatments that give patients hope, they are impelled to address the big question of basic research. What neural circuits allow us to form memories, use language, and foster creativity? How can the brain's interaction with the body's immune systems be improved so that we can better defend ourselves against pathogens, both natural and artificial? And the sort of question that used to be asked only by theoretical physicists: Is a "unified field theory of the brain" achievable in our time to allow us to fulfill some unknown human potential?

A considerably more minor question: What's a newspaper pundit and language maven doing, dealing with this esoteric subject? It happens that David Mahoney enticed me into the field of philanthropy in science and education at Dana in the early 1990s, assigning me to launch the Dana Press. Since his death in 2000, I've been Dana chairman, carrying on the work, getting more deeply involved with the mystery, stimulus, and controversies of supporting brain research. Has it been satisfying? That, as neuroscientists never say, is a no-brainer. Like many nonscientists, I've found nothing more fascinating than the study and the popular explication of the fast-developing astronomy of the mind.

This book is for amateurs like most of us—potential patients without patience for long-winded technical analyses of what goes on, and goes wrong, inside our heads. As a major home health reference on the brain, *The Dana Guide to Brain Health* is the first of its kind. It emphasizes how the latest scientific findings are being translated into actual treatment of people in pain or puzzlement. Because of the need for an up-to-date, authoritative guide to the many brain-related ailments, we found the time ripe for a major book to serve readers as the most trustworthy, understandable source possible—a kind of basic "bible" of the brain.

Virtually every one of us will be touched by brain-related disorder, either as a patient or in caring for an afflicted loved one. That's why a book such as this—providing clear information not only about these disorders but also about ways to keep your brain healthy through a long life—should prove both useful and reassuring.

Many of the more than 100 contributors to this book are members of the Dana Alliance. All are among the foremost doctors and scientists in their fields. Dana is grateful to them, and especially to the three distinguished medical editors—Floyd E. Bloom, M.D., M. Flint Beal, M.D., and David J. Kupfer, M.D. Their individual brilliance, enthusiasm for the potential of the brain, and compassion for victims of brain disorders have produced a remarkable resource for everyone's home library.

At a recent meeting of heart specialists, a visiting neuroscientist rose to hail the importance of their work in cardiology. "The heart is an extremely important organ," he assured them. "It keeps the brain alive."

INTRODUCTION:
WELCOME TO YOUR BRAIN

You may have picked up this book because you suspect that you or someone close to you is experiencing problems connected with the brain. Alternatively, you may have picked it up because you have always been interested in the brain, or because your curiosity has been stimulated by a news report about exciting scientific discoveries. Being able to provide helpful information in all those situations is why we were so excited to participate in creating *The Dana Guide to Brain Health* and why so many excellent scientists and clinicians have contributed their expertise to it. Never before has a book like this been created. In fact, only in recent decades have we learned enough about the brain to assemble this overall guide to its development, health, and disorders.

Whatever your reason for reading these words, the chances are pretty high that *The Dana Guide to Brain Health* will be useful to you in your lifetime. That is because diseases of the brain rank at the top of the list of our most serious health problems. The most common brain disease, stroke, has a lower frequency than cancers and heart diseases, but the total effects of all the brain diseases—including strokes, Alzheimer's disease, depression, schizophrenia, and many more conditions described in this volume—

account for more long-term care and more chronic suffering than all other medical problems *put together.*

The cumulative cost of brain diseases may startle you. It is so high because many of the brain's most devastating diseases begin early in life and can last for a lifetime. But brain-related diseases are also fairly common, even more so when we expand that group to include disorders involving the rest of our nervous system. One survey in the 1990s found that nine out of ten Americans had either an illness involving their brain or nervous system or had a friend or relative experiencing one.

Furthermore, brain health controls our everyday lives. Medical diagnoses like clinical depression, substance abuse, and Alzheimer's disease have become topics of daily conversation. They all relate to the brain, as do less dire conditions like migraine headaches, tics, and dyslexia. How much do we know about these disorders? How much should you be concerned about them in your own life? *The Dana Guide to Brain Health* offers you the essential brain information and, when possible, health-preserving advice.

It has become increasingly apparent in recent decades that, like it or not, the brain and nervous system are involved in every aspect of our health. Conditions of the mind affect those of the body, and vice versa. For centuries people have been able to see the obvious bases for cancer, heart disease, and other physical illnesses, but now we can also see the mechanisms of many nervous-system disorders. Recent advances in the biology of brain function have begun to clarify the brain's physical basis and to reveal the interplay among the many genes on which the brain relies. We are starting to understand how each of us inherits some degree of vulnerability to such complex diseases as epilepsy, stroke, schizophrenia, depression, and alcoholism, which may nor may not emerge in a person's lifetime.

Even if you and your loved ones stay neurologically and psychologically healthy, we believe that you will find great value in this book. Your brain is the basis for who you are: your intellect, your personality, your emotional states. We all depend on our brains for our graceful (or not so graceful) movements, our vocabularies, our capacities to learn and remember, even our ability to sleep soundly. We are also inevitably affected by the brains of our friends, relatives, colleagues, and people we randomly encounter in our lives because their brains help determine their behavior toward us. The human brain is said to be the most complex tissue ever known, and we are a long way from understanding it. Yet the brain is involved in so many aspects of our lives that we will undoubtedly benefit from learning all we can about it.

In the last half-century, technological breakthroughs have let us discover more about the brain than in all the previous millennia. We still know far less than what we do *not* know, but our methods for watching the brain in action (such as functional magnetic resonance imaging, or fMRI, which is explained in chapter 2) are giving us greater insight into which of its complex parts work together to do what and when. With the complete inventory of the human genome now accessible, we are likely to make substantially more progress. Already we know that humans seem to have around 30,000 genes, at least half of which the brain either uses exclusively or shares with just a few of the more complex other organs. Gradually we will learn where to look for the effects of brain-related genes in health and in the early stages of disease. So much progress is being made in understanding the brain that almost every day brings reports of discoveries. This book can help you understand that exciting new science and what it could mean to you and your loved ones.

We hope *The Dana Guide to Brain Health* will prove helpful to you in working with your doctors and other health professionals. Unfortunately, we all know that the time available for medical consultations is limited; physicians feel as much frustration about that situation as patients do. *The Dana Guide to Brain Health* will give you a head start on how to explain to your doctor what you think may be wrong. You can list the pertinent symptoms and their history in a way that will let you and your doctor make the most of your appointment. This book also provides information on diagnostic tests and possible treatments. Use it to assemble your questions about what you should expect and what you'll need to watch out for.

The Dana Guide to Brain Health thus offers not only a ready reference to our latest understandings of brain diseases but also information to help you participate in your own family's care. It is important to state, however, that you should always follow your doctors' advice rather than what you read in this book if there is a disagreement. Every individual's medical condition is different, and your doctors will know about your particular situation. We have to discuss the general case, and often at a very basic level. Furthermore, with the pace of brain research today, it is possible that new treatments and medications will become available to you.

To help you keep up with those advances, *The Dana Guide to Brain Health* provides you with two more important resources. Toward the back of the book is a listing of the many organizations devoted to people who have brain disorders and

to their families. These groups can often provide more detailed information on diseases, referrals to doctors, moral support, and tips on dealing with chronic or fatal conditions.

The CD-ROM included with this book extends your reach even farther, providing updated additional Web sites selected by our expert contributors to help you use the Internet and all its vast resources effectively. Use the CD-ROM to search for articles, books, treatment facilities, Web pages on specific disorders, and even Web pages about the brain for children.

This book and its CD-ROM will guide you to a deeper understanding of our most complex organ, the brain. To keep on top of new developments in brain science, turn to The Dana Foundation Web site, www.dana.org, for news releases, coverage of current studies, and information about public events. There you will also find a wealth of free publications such as fact sheets, newsletters, and periodicals that cover the latest findings in all areas of The Dana Foundation's interests: brain science, immunology, and arts education. Sign up for e-mail alerts to know when there is a new publication or a Dana event near you. Our discovery of the brain is an ongoing journey, and www.dana.org will keep you onboard.

The Dana Guide to Brain Health is the product of many people's work: not simply ours and that of the many fine contributors, but also that of all the scientists whose studies of the brain have led us to this point. We hope that you will enjoy learning from this book as much as we have enjoyed preparing it for you.

Floyd E. Bloom, M.D.
M. Flint Beal, M.D.
David J. Kupfer, M.D.

HOW TO READ THIS BOOK

Because the brain is connected to so many parts of life, *The Dana Guide to Brain Health* is a hefty volume. You may be wondering just how you can find what you want inside it. Here are some guidelines for getting the most out of this book.

If right now you are interested in a specific brain condition (such as depression, amnesia, cerebral palsy, migraine, or myasthenia gravis), use the index or table of contents to turn to that section.

After you satisfy any immediate interest or curiosity, we recommend that you read Part I, Understanding Your Brain. These chapters explain in brief how to think about the brain, how we have come to know what we do, the best steps for taking care of your brain, and finally the connection between brain health and body

health. Together with our colorful "brain primer" (located after page xxxii), Part I will give you the concepts and the "lingo" to get the most out of what follows. At that point, you have your choice of several pathways through *The Dana Guide to Brain Health.*

Part II, Your Brain Through Life, traces the brain's development. Chapters 5 and 6 provide an overview of the birth and growth of the brain in the prenatal period and childhood. They help explain why so many brain disorders arise in childhood. Those years are crucial to the growth of healthy brains, though the young brain can also be surprisingly resilient. These two chapters will be especially interesting to parents and people who are soon to be parents. Part II then goes on to discuss brain development in adolescence and adulthood. Scientists once thought mature brains reached a static point, not growing and perhaps declining. More recent research has shown that our brains continue to develop in middle age and beyond.

Part III, The Healthy Brain, describes all the remarkable operations your brain monitors and regulates throughout your body, usually without you even being aware of them. Each of the three chapters in this section is divided into several sections, one for each set of brain functions. They explore how we sense the world around us; how our brains regulate our breathing, blood flow, temperature, and even blood sugar; how our brains move our bodies through the spaces in which we live and work; how we recognize pain and why; how humans can learn, remember, imagine, and create; and even how scientists are theorizing about the mysterious state we call consciousness. This part of the book is where we delve most deeply into how the healthy brain performs.

In contrast, Part IV describes what can go wrong. Conditions of the Brain and Nervous System explores dozens of diseases and illnesses you might encounter. We have organized these problems into eight groups:

■ conditions that appear or arise in childhood

■ disorders of the senses and the brain's internal operations

■ problems with emotions and control of behaviors, generally called psychiatric disorders

■ infectious diseases and problems that arise when people's immune systems inappropriately turn on their brains or nerves

■ disorders of the nerves and muscles that control our movements

■ pains, either chronic or episodic

■ injuries to the nervous system, whether arising within the body or from physical wounds or poisons

■ troubles with thinking and remembering

Within each chapter of related disorders, we have organized the problems generally from the most to the least common.

When you see a designation in boldface, such as **B10** or **C67,** you will find more information by turning to the corresponding section in Part III or IV. These cross-references may lead you directly to what immediately concerns you. For instance, you may worry about whether a sudden headache means you are having a stroke. That would indeed be an *emergency.* The sections on ischemic and hemorrhagic strokes (**C59, C60**) can prepare you to recognize these problems in yourself or others so you can obtain immediate care. Fortunately, the section on headache (**C54**) will reveal that there are less dire explanations for that symptom. That could relieve your worries, help you identify the more likely problems, and lead you to the proper medical care.

In the book's end matter, you will find a glossary immediately after Part IV. Although technical terms in the book are explained when they are first used, the glossary is a quick way to track down the meaning of a term that was defined earlier. Finally, if you are educating yourself in detail about the brain or a particular disorder or treatment, you should be able to gather a great deal of additional information through the extensive resources listed in the appendices and through even more Web sites suggested by our expert contributors included in the CD-ROM that complements this book.

CONTRIBUTORS

(IN ALPHABETICAL ORDER)

Marilyn S. Albert, Ph.D.
Director
Division of Cognitive Neuroscience
The Johns Hopkins Medical Institutions
Baltimore, Maryland

Nancy C. Andreasen, M.D., Ph.D.
Andrew H. Woods Chair of Psychiatry
Director
Mental Health Clinical Research Center
University of Iowa Carver College of Medicine
Iowa City, Iowa

Arthur K. Asbury, M.D.
Van Meter Professor of Neurology, Emeritus
Hospital of the University of Pennsylvania
University of Pennsylvania School of Medicine
Philadelphia, Pennsylvania

Richard Balon, M.D.
Professor of Psychiatry
Wayne State University
Detroit, Michigan

Eduardo E. Benarroch, M.D.
Professor of Neurology
Mayo Clinic College of Medicine
Rochester, Minnesota

Peter McLaren Black, M.D., Ph.D.
Franc D. Ingraham Professor of Neurosurgery
Harvard Medical School
Neurosurgeon-in-Chief, Brigham
    and Women's Hospital
Chair, Department of Neurosurgery
Children's Hospital
Boston, Massachusetts

Patrick J. Bosque, M.D.
Assistant Professor of Neurology
University of Colorado
Denver, Colorado

John C. M. Brust, M.D.
Professor of Clinical Neurology
Director, Harlem Hospital Neurology Service
New York, New York

Thomas N. Byrne, M.D.
Clinical Professor of Neurology and
    Health Sciences and Technology
Harvard Medical School
Massachusetts General Hospital
Senior Lecturer, Department of Brain
    and Cognitive Sciences, MIT
New Haven, Connecticut

David Caplan, M.D., Ph.D.
Professor of Neurology
Neuropsychology Lab
Massachusetts General Hospital
Boston, Massachusetts

Louis R. Caplan, M.D.
Chief, Cerebrovascular Disease
Beth Israel Deaconess Medical Center
Professor
Department of Neurology
Harvard University Medical School
Boston, Massachusetts

Gregory Youngnam Chang, M.D.
Chief of Neurology
Los Angeles County and University of
    Southern California Medical Center
Associate Professor of Neurology
Keck School of Medicine
University of Southern California
Los Angeles, California

Abe M. Chutorian, M.D.
Professor of Neurology and Pediatrics
Attending Neurologist, Hospital
    for Special Surgery
Weill Medical College of Cornell University
New York, New York

Jonathan D. Cohen, M.D., Ph.D.
Director, Center for the Study of
    Brain, Mind and Behavior
Professor of Psychology
Princeton University
Princeton, New Jersey

H. Branch Coslett, M.D.
Professor of Neurology
Section Chief, Cognitive Neurology
University of Pennsylvania School of Medicine
Philadelphia, Pennsylvania

Jeffrey L. Cummings, M.D.
Director, UCLA Alzheimer's Disease Center
Augustus S. Rose Professor of Neurology
Professor of Psychiatry and
    Biobehavioral Sciences
University of California at Los
    Angeles School of Medicine
Los Angeles, California

Antonio R. Damasio, M.D., Ph.D.
Director
The Brain and Creativity Institute
University of Southern California
Los Angeles, California

Lisa M. DeAngelis, M.D.
Chairman, Department of Neurology
Memorial Sloan-Kettering Cancer Center
Professor of Neurology
Weill Medical College of Cornell University
New York, New York

Mahlon R. DeLong, M.D.
Professor and Director of Neuroscience
Department of Neurology
Emory University School of Medicine
Atlanta, Georgia

Richard L. Doty, Ph.D.
Director, Smell and Taste Center
Professor, Department of Otorhinolaryngology
University of Pennsylvania Medical School
Philadelphia, Pennsylvania

Daniel B. Drachman, M.D.
Professor of Neurology and Neuroscience
Johns Hopkins School of Medicine
Baltimore, Maryland

David A. Drachman, M.D.
Professor and Chairman Emeritus
Department of Neurology
University of Massachusetts Medical Center
Worcester, Massachusetts

Stanley Fahn, M.D.
Movement Disorders Division Chief
H. Houston Merritt Professor of Neurology
Columbia University Medical Center
    Department of Neurology
New York, New York

Martha Farah, Ph.D.
Professor of Psychology
Director, Center for Cognitive Neuroscience
University of Pennsylvania
Philadelphia, Pennsylvania

Jan Fawcett, M.D.
Professor of Psychiatry
University of New Mexico School of Medicine
Albuquerque, New Mexico

Carl Feinstein, M.D.
Professor, Department of Psychiatry
Stanford University School of Medicine
Stanford, California

Howard L. Fields, M.D., Ph.D.
Professor of Neurology and Physiology
Ernest Gallo Clinic and Research Center
Vice Chairman, Department of Neurology
Director, Wheeler Center for the
    Neurobiology of Addiction
University of California, San Francisco
Emeryville, California

Kathleen M. Foley, M.D.
Senior Attending Neurologist
Department of Neurology
Pain and Palliative Care Service
Memorial Sloan-Kettering Cancer Center
New York, New York

Ellen Frank, Ph.D.
Professor of Psychiatry and Psychology
Western Psychiatric Institute and Clinic
University of Pittsburgh Medical Center
Pittsburgh, Pennsylvania

J. M. Friedman, M.D., Ph.D.
Professor of Medical Genetics
University of British Columbia
Vancouver, Canada

Albert M. Galaburda, M.D.
Chief, Division of Behavioral Neurology
Beth Israel Deaconess Medical Center
Emily Fisher Landau Professor of
    Neurology and Neuroscience
Harvard Medical School
Boston, Massachusetts

Patricio C. Gargollo, M.D.
Surgical Resident
Massachusetts General Hospital

Boston, Massachusetts

Claude P. Genain, M.D.
Assistant Professor, Department of Neurology
University of California at San Francisco
San Francisco, California

Apostolos P. Georgopoulos, M.D., Ph.D
McKnight Presidential Chair in
    Cognitive Neuroscience
Director, Brain Sciences Center
Minneapolis VA Medical Center
University of Minnesota
Minneapolis, Minnesota

Donald H. Gilden, M.D.
Professor and Chairman,
    Department of Neurology
University of Colorado Health Sciences Center
Denver, Colorado

Elkhonon Goldberg, Ph.D.
Clinical Professor of Neurology
New York University School of Medicine
New York, New York

Gary W. Goldstein, M.D.
President and Chief Executive Officer
Department of Neurology
Kennedy Krieger Institute
Baltimore, Maryland

Jack M. Gorman, M.D.
Lieber Professor and Vice-Chair for
    Research, Department of Psychiatry
Columbia University
New York, New York

Susan A. Greenfield, D.Phil.
Director, Royal Institution of Great Britain
Professor of Pharmacology
Oxford University

Oxford, England

Katherine A. Halmi, M.D.
Professor of Psychiatry
Weill Medical College of Cornell University
White Plains, New York

John J. Halperin, M.D.
Professor and Chair, Department of Neurology
North Shore University Hospital
Manhasset, New York

Barry Jay Hartman, M.D.
Clinical Professor of Medicine
Division of International Medicine
    and Infectious Disease
Weill Cornell Medical Center
New York, New York

Stephen L. Hauser, M.D.
Robert A. Fishman Distinguished
    Professor and Chair
Department of Neurology
University of California, San Francisco
San Francisco, California

Kenneth M. Heilman, M.D.
James E. Rook, Jr. Distinguished Professor
Department of Neurology
Program Director and Chief
North Florida/South Georgia Veterans
    Affairs Medical Center
University of Florida College of Medicine
Gainesville, Florida

J. Allan Hobson, M.D.
Director
Laboratory of Neurophysiology
Massachusetts Mental Health Center
Boston, Massachusetts

Alexander H. Hoon, Jr., M.D., M.P.H.

Associate Professor of Pediatrics
Johns Hopkins University School of Medicine
Director, Phelps Center for Cerebral Palsy
  and Neurodevelopmental Medicine
Kennedy Krieger Institute
Baltimore, Maryland

Earl Hunt, Ph.D.
Professor, Department of Psychology
University of Washington
Seattle, Washington

Jerome H. Jaffe, M.D.
Clinical Professor, Department of Psychiatry
Division of Alcohol and Drug Abuse
University of Maryland School of Medicine
Baltimore, Maryland

Joseph Jankovic, M.D.
Professor of Neurology
Director, Parkinson's Disease Center
  and Movement Disorders Clinic
Department of Neurology
Baylor College of Medicine
Houston, Texas

Peter J. Jannetta, M.D.
Vice Chairman, Department of Neurosurgery
Allegheny General Hospital
Professor of Neurosurgery
MCP Hahnemann University
Pittsburgh, Pennsylvania

Peter S. Jensen, M.D.
Ruane Professor of Child Psychiatry
Director, Center for the Advancement
  of Children's Mental Health
Department of Child Psychiatry
Columbia University
New York, New York

Richard T. Johnson, M.D.

Distinguished Service Professor of Neurology,
  Microbiology and Neuroscience
The Johns Hopkins University
  School of Medicine
Adjunct Professor
Department of Molecular Microbiology
  and Immunology
Bloomberg School of Public Health
The Johns Hopkins University
Baltimore, Maryland

Michael V. Johnston, M.D.
Professor of Neurology and Pediatrics
Johns Hopkins University School of Medicine
Chief Medical Officer, Kennedy Krieger Institute
Baltimore, Maryland

Jerome Kagan, Ph.D.
Professor of Psychology, Emeritus
Department of Psychology
Harvard University
Cambridge, Massachusetts

Walter Kaye, M.D.
Professor of Psychiatry
University of Pittsburgh
Western Psychiatric Institute and Clinic
Pittsburgh, Pennsylvania

James R. Keane, M.D.
Professor of Neurology
Los Angeles County and University of
  Southern California Medical Center
Los Angeles, California

Dennis K. Kinney, Ph.D.
Director, Genetics Laboratory
McLean Hospital
Associate Professor of Psychiatry
Harvard Medical School
Belmont, Massachusetts

William C. Koller, M.D., Ph.D.
Assistant Professor
Department of Neurology
University of North Carolina School of Medicine
Chaple Hill, North Carolina

Edwin H. Kolodny, M.D.
Bernard A. and Charlotte Marden Professor
  and Chairman, Department of Neurology
New York University School of Medicine
Director, the Eunice Kennedy Shriver Center
New York, New York

James W. Lance, M.D., F.R.C.P., F.R.A.C.P.
Emeritus Professor of Neurology
Consultant Neurologist
Prince of Wales Hospital
Sydney, Australia

Anthony E. Lang, M.D., F.R.C.P.C.
Jack Clark Chair in Parkinson's Disease Research
Division of Neurology
Department of Medicine
University of Toronto
Director, Movement Disorders Clinic
Toronto Western Hospital
Ontario, Canada

Henrietta L. Leonard, M.D.
Professor of Psychiatry and Human behavor
Director of Training, Brown University
  Child Psychiatry and Triple
  Board Residency Programs
Division of Child Psychiatry
Providence, Rhode Island

Adam C. Lipson, M.D.
Resident Physician, Department
  of Neurological Surgery
University of Washington Medical Center
Seattle, Washington

Michael D. Lockshin, M.D.
Professor of Medicine and
  Obstetrics and Gynecology
Weill Medical College of Cornell University
Attending Physician, Hospital for Special Surgery
Director, Barbara Volcker Center for
  Women and Rheumatic Disease
Co-Director, Mary Kirkland Center for Lupus
  Research Hospital for Special Surgery
New York, New York

Richard Mayeux, M.D., M.Sc.
Gertrude H. Sergievsky Professor of
  Neurology, Psychiatry, and Epidemiology
Director, Sergievsky Center
Co-Director, The Taub Institute
Columbia University
New York, New York

Jerry R. Mendell, M.D.
Helen C. Kurtz Professor
Chairman of Neurology
Ohio State University
Columbus, Ohio

Emmanuel Mignot, M.D., Ph.D.
Professor
Stanford University School of Medicine
Stanford, California

Alireza Minagar, M.D.
Assistant Professor of Neurology
Louisiana State University
  Health Sciences Center
Department of Neurology
Shreveport, Louisiana

J. P. Mohr, M.D., M.S.
Sciarra Professor of Clinical Neurology
Columbia University
New York, New York

Michael A. Moskowitz, M.D.
Director, Stroke and Neurovascular Regulation
Massachusetts General Hospital
Professor of Neurology
Harvard-MIT Division of Health
   Science and Technology
Harvard Medical School
Charlestown, Massachusetts

Joseph B. Nadol, Jr., M.D.
Walter August Lecompte Professor and Chair
Department of Otology and Laryngology
Harvard Medical School
Chief of Otolaryngology and
   Director of Otology Services
Massachusetts Eye and Ear Infirmary
Boston, Massachusetts

Benjamin H. Natelson, M.D.
Professor of Neurosciences
University of Medicine and
   Dentistry of New Jersey
New Jersey Medical School
Newark, New Jersey

Thomas C. Neylan, M.D.
Medical Director, Post-Traumatic
   Stress Disorder Program
Veterans Affairs Medical Center
Assistant Professor, In Residence,
   Department of Psychiatry
University of California at San Francisco
San Francisco, California

Charles P. O'Brien, M.D., Ph.D.
Kenneth E. Appel Professor
Vice Chair, Department of Psychiatry
University of Pennsylvania
Philadelphia, Pennsylvania

Timothy A. Pedley, M.D.

Henry and Lucy Moses Professor and
   Chairman, Department of Neurology
Columbia University
New York, New York

Fred Plum, M.D.
University Professor
Weill Medical College of Cornell University
New York, New York

Jerome B. Posner, M.D.
George C. Cotzias Chair in Neuro-Oncology
Department of Neurology
Evelyn Frew American Cancer Society
   Clinical Research Professor
Memorial Sloan-Kettering Cancer Center
New York, New York

Richard W. Price, M.D.
Chief, Neurology Service
San Francisco General Hospital
Professor and Vice Chair
University of California at San Francisco
San Francisco, California

Steven R. Pritzker, Ph.D.
Adjunct Professor of Psychology
Saybrook Graduate School
San Francisco, California

Stanley B. Prusiner, M.D.
Director and Professor, Institute for
   Neurodegenerative Diseases
Department of Neurology and Biochemistry
University of California at San Francisco
San Francisco, California

Rivka A. Rachel, M.D., Ph.D.
Research Fellow
National Cancer Institute, Frederick
Frederick, Maryland

Ruth Louise Richards, M.D., Ph.D.
Professor of Psychology
Saybrook Graduate School
San Francisco, California
Associate Clinical Professor of Psychiatry
University of California, San Francisco
Research Affiliate, McClean Hospital
Belmont, Massachusetts
Lecturer, Department of Psychiatry
Harvard Medical School
Boston, Massachusetts

Janet Sweeney Rico, M.S.N., M.B.A., R.N., C.S.
Assistant Professor
Simmons College Graduate
    School for Health Studies
Boston, Massachusetts

Allan H. Ropper, M.D.
Chief, Division of Neurology
St. Elizabeth's Medical Center
Chairman of Neurology
Tufts University School of Medicine
Boston, Massachusetts

Roger N. Rosenberg, M.D.
Professor of Neurology
Zale Distinguished Chair in Neurology
Department of Neurology
University of Texas Southwestern Medical Center
Dallas, Texas

Leslie Gonzalez Rothi, Ph.D.
Program Director, Brain Rehabilitaion
    Research Center
North Florida/South Georgia
    Veteran Health System
Professor of Neurology
University of Florida
Gainesville, Florida

Lewis P. Rowland, M.D.
Professor of Neurology
Neurological Institute
Columbia-Presbyterian Medical Center
New York, New York

Clifford B. Saper, M.D., Ph.D.
Professor and Chairman
Department of Neurology
Beth Israel Deaconess Medical Center
Harvard Medical School
Boston, Massachusetts

Herbert H. Schaumburg, M.D.
Edwin S. Lowe Professor and Chairman,
    Department of Neurology
Albert Einstein College of Medicine
Bronx, New York

Nicholas Schiff, M.D.
Assistant Professor of Neurology
    and Neuroscience
Director of Laboratory of Cognitive
    Neuromodulation
Weill Medical College of Cornell University
Assistant Attending Neurologist
New York Presbyterian Hospital
New York, New York

Bruce K. Shapiro, M.D.
Associate Professor of Pediatrics
Johns Hopkins University School of Medicine
Vice President, Training
Kennedy Krieger Institute
Baltimore, Maryland

Gordon M. Shepherd, M.D., D.Phil.
Professor of Neuroscience and Neurobiology
Department of Neurobiology
Yale Medical School
New Haven, Connecticut

Ira Shoulson, M.D.
Louis C. Lasagna Professor of
   Experimental Therapeutics
Professor of Neurology
University of Rochester
Rochester, New York

Larry J. Siever, M.D.
Professor of Psychiatry
Director, Mood and Personality
   Disorder Research Program
Mount Sinai School of Medicine
Bronx, New York

Larry R. Squire, Ph.D.
Distinguished Professor of Psychiatry,
   Psychology, and Neurosciences
University of California, San Diego
Research Career Scientist
Veterans Affairs Medical Center
San Diego, California

Christian Stapf, M.D.
Research Scientist
Columbia University
Stroke Center, The Neurological Institute
New York, New York

Murray B. Stein, M.D.
Professor of Psychiatry, In Residence
University of California at San Diego
La Jolla, California

Jacek Szudek, Ph.D.
Dalhousie University
Halifax, Nova Scotia

Michael E. Thase, M.D.
Professor of Psychiatry
University of Pittsburgh School of Medicine
Pittsburgh, Pennsylvania

B. Todd Troost, M.D.
Chair, Department of Neurology
Wake Forest University School of Medicine
Winston-Salem, North Carolina

Michael Vickroy, Ph.D.
Investigator
Neurobehavioral Research Laboratory
VA New Jersey Health Care System
East Orange, New Jersey

Peter C. Whybrow, M.D.
Director, Semel Institute for Neuroscience
   and Human Behavior
Physician-in-Chief, Resnick
   Neuropsychiatric Hospital
Judson Braun Distinguished Professor
   and Executive Chair
Department of Psychiatry and
   Biobehavioral Sciences
UCLA School of Medicine
Los Angeles, California

Rachel Yehuda, Ph.D.
Director, Post-Traumatic Stress
   Disorder Program
Bronx Veterans Administration Medical Center
Professor of Psychiatry
Mount Sinai School of Medicine
Bronx, New York

Wise Young, M.D., Ph.D.
Professor and Founding Director
W.M. Keck Center for Collaborative
   Neuroscience Chair
Department of Cell Biology and Neuroscience
Rutgers, The State University of New Jersey
Piscataway, New Jersey

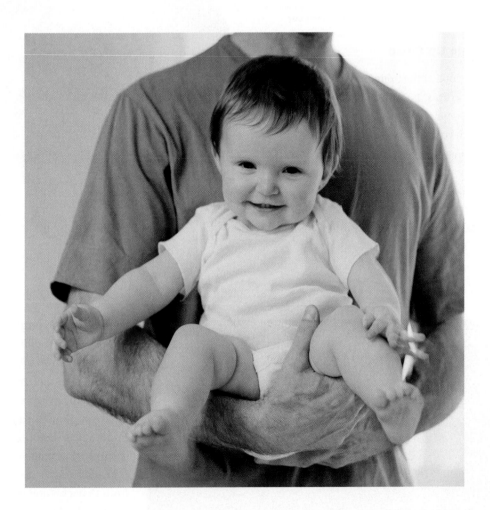

The Brain as Life

As we grow from infancy to adulthood, so do our brains—changing and maturing through a combination of genes, biology, and experience. Our brains let us think, feel, plan, and remember; they govern how we eat, breathe, and move. We depend on our brains when we interact with other people, from subtle responses to language and ethical beliefs. In many ways, we are our brains.
PHOTO © LAURA DOSS/CORBIS

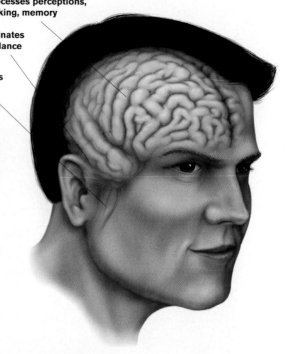

Cortex: processes perceptions, thinking, memory

Cerebellum: coordinates movement and balance

Spinal cord: communicates with the body

The Brain Up Close

When we look at the brain, most of what we see is the **cortex**. Its surface is wrinkled because so many brain cells are squeezed into that layer of tissue (see chapter 1). Also visible, below the cortex, is the **cerebellum**. All vertebrate animals' brains have a cortex and cerebellum, but the size and complexity of our cortex set humans apart. Extending from the bottom of the brain is the **spinal cord**. ILLUSTRATION © ROBERT FINKBEINER

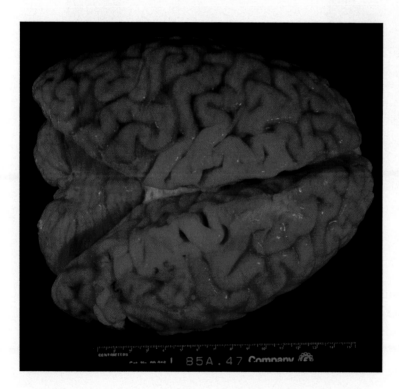

Seen whole and intact in this photo, the brain has a pinkish hue from the many tiny blood vessels that provide it with oxygen and nutrients. Considering their importance, our brains are surprisingly small—this one is just over six inches from front to back—and they weigh only about three pounds. PHOTO © CLARK OVERTON/PHOTOTAKE/PICTUREQUEST

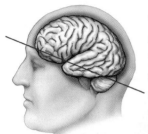

This slice through the cortex *(left)* reveals that the brain contains spaces, called **ventricles**, and that, although the two sides of the brain appear symmetrical, they are not exact mirror images. The ventricles and spaces surrounding the brain and spinal cord are full of **cerebrospinal fluid (CSF)**, which cushions these vital organs against life's bumps. In the middle right image, the butterfly-shaped form visible between the cortex and cerebellum is called the **pons.** It contains some of the brain cells involved in behavior such as sleep and facial expression. Just visible in the pons, looking like a pair of dark eyebrows, is the **substantia nigra**, which makes dopamine, a brain chemical important in both movement and our feelings of pleasure. Near each tip of the "butterfly's wings," you can see part of the curved structure called the **hippocampus**, which is essential to the formation of memories.

Looking up at the brain from underneath shows the many nerves running into it *(lower right)*. The thickest and busiest is the **spinal cord**, which connects to the brain stem. In addition, there are twelve pairs of **cranial nerves**, each with a different set of functions: **1.** smelling (olfactory nerves); **2.** seeing (optic nerves); **3.** moving the eyes, constricting the pupils; **4.** moving the eyes downward; **5.** chewing, sensation in the face (trigeminal nerves); **6.** moving the eyes outward; **7.** moving the face, tasting, salivating, crying; **8.** hearing, balancing; **9.** tasting, salivating, swallowing; **10.** tasting, swallowing, speaking; **11.** moving the head and shoulders; and **12.** moving the tongue.

ILLUSTRATIONS © ROBERT FINKBEINER

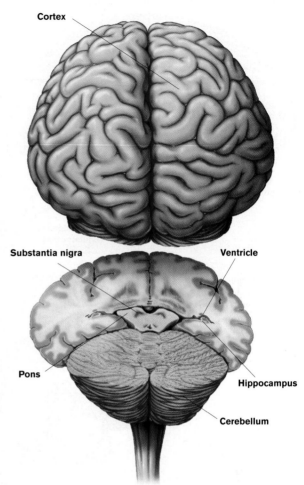

Cortex

Substantia nigra

Ventricle

Pons

Hippocampus

Cerebellum

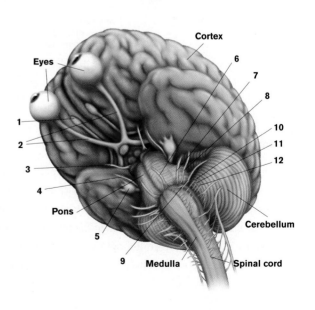

Cortex

Eyes

6

7

8

1

2

10

3

11

4

12

Pons

Cerebellum

5

9

Medulla

Spinal cord

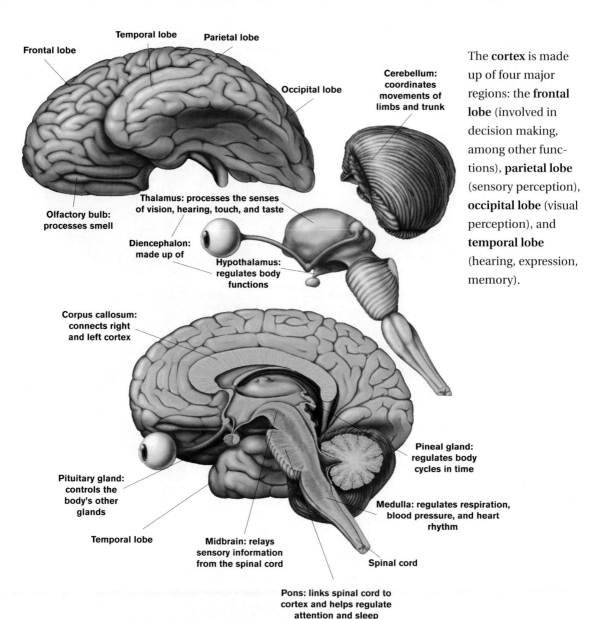

Frontal lobe

Temporal lobe

Parietal lobe

Occipital lobe

Cerebellum: coordinates movements of limbs and trunk

Thalamus: processes the senses of vision, hearing, touch, and taste

Olfactory bulb: processes smell

Diencephalon: made up of

Hypothalamus: regulates body functions

Corpus callosum: connects right and left cortex

Pineal gland: regulates body cycles in time

Pituitary gland: controls the body's other glands

Temporal lobe

Midbrain: relays sensory information from the spinal cord

Medulla: regulates respiration, blood pressure, and heart rhythm

Spinal cord

Pons: links spinal cord to cortex and helps regulate attention and sleep

The **cortex** is made up of four major regions: the **frontal lobe** (involved in decision making, among other functions), **parietal lobe** (sensory perception), **occipital lobe** (visual perception), and **temporal lobe** (hearing, expression, memory).

Important Structures in the Brain

Opening up the brain reveals many more parts, protected deep inside the cortex and cerebellum. Almost all of these parts come in pairs, though we usually speak of each pair as a single object. With some exceptions, regions on the left side of the brain gather information from and govern the right side of the body, and the other way around. Here is where much of the brain's work goes on.

Our brains are linked to nerves running throughout our bodies. The brain and spinal cord make up the **central nervous system**. All other nerves form the **peripheral nervous system**.

ILLUSTRATIONS © ROBERT FINKBEINER

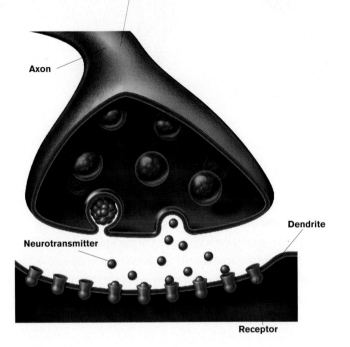

Brain Cells at Work

The nervous system cells that receive and pass on information are called **neurons**. In addition to containing the **nucleus** common to all cells, each neuron has a long fiber called an **axon**. Most neurons' axons are sheathed in layers called **myelin**, which helps speed signals along. Axons can grow several inches long. They link to other neurons at specialized sites called **dendrites**, as in the lower right foreground. A neuron can receive signals from one other neuron or several, and, based on its structure and the strength of that signal, can pass on signals to one or several cells. Some neuronal circuits are in continuous activity, such as those that drive breathing in and out.

A link between neurons is called a **synapse**. It is not a direct connection, with one neuron touching another. Instead, there is a small space between the cells. The axon of the first cell, or sending neuron, transmits a chemical message to the receiving neuron by secreting a **neurotransmitter** from the axon's terminal (this is called the "presynaptic," or sending, side). The receiving neuron (postsynaptic side) gets the message through receptors on its surface, mainly on its **dendrites** but often on the surface of the cell body.

ILLUSTRATIONS © ROBERT FINKBEINER

Dendrite

Nucleus

Axon

Myelin

Axon

Neurotransmitter

Dendrite

Receptor

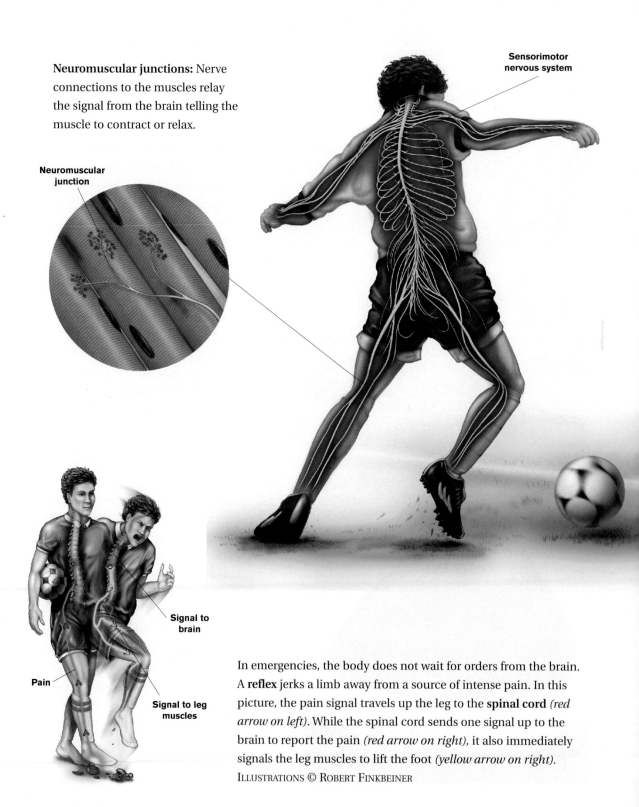

Neuromuscular junctions: Nerve connections to the muscles relay the signal from the brain telling the muscle to contract or relax.

Neuromuscular junction

Sensorimotor nervous system

Signal to brain

Pain

Signal to leg muscles

In emergencies, the body does not wait for orders from the brain. A **reflex** jerks a limb away from a source of intense pain. In this picture, the pain signal travels up the leg to the **spinal cord** *(red arrow on left)*. While the spinal cord sends one signal up to the brain to report the pain *(red arrow on right)*, it also immediately signals the leg muscles to lift the foot *(yellow arrow on right)*.

ILLUSTRATIONS © ROBERT FINKBEINER

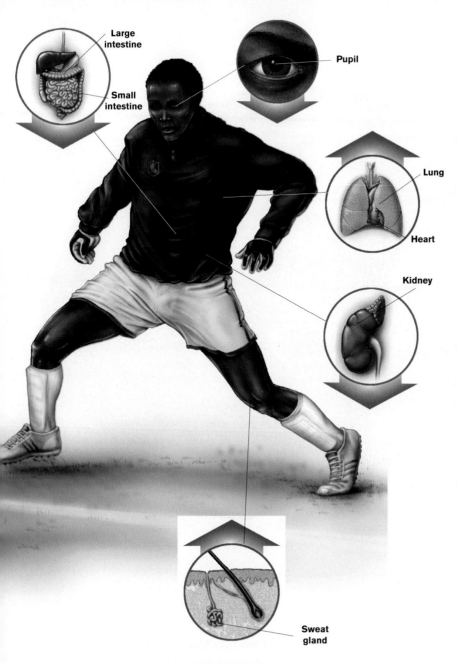

Large intestine

Small intestine

Pupil

Lung

Heart

Kidney

Sweat gland

Included in the peripheral nervous system are the nerves known as the **autonomic nervous system**. Because this system works automatically, we rarely think about its actions, but these nerves direct our body responses from moment to moment, turning up some responses and turning down others. As the soccer player on the left enters play, his autonomic nerves produce these (and more) responses in his body: **pupils** constrict to focus vision; **heart and lungs** send more oxygen to muscles; **sweat glands** activate to cool the body; **intestines** stop digesting, freeing blood for muscles; **kidneys** slow to conserve fluid.

The Peripheral Nervous System

In the soccer player above, we see the **sensorimotor nervous system**. These nerves generally follow the lines of our bones, then branch into smaller fibers. Each **motor nerve** ends at a **neuromuscular junction** in the muscle cell that it signals to contract or relax. The **sensory nerves** connect to (or **innervate**) all parts of the body, monitoring touch, pain, temperature, and other sensations. ILLUSTRATIONS © ROBERT FINKBEINER

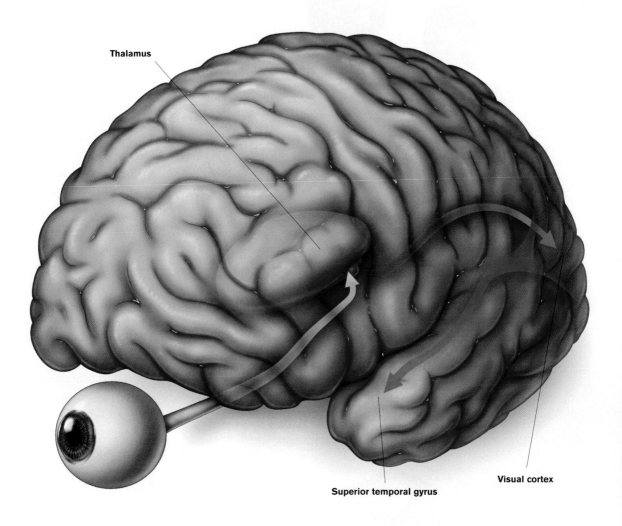

Thalamus

Superior temporal gyrus

Visual cortex

A regular series of synapses forms a **pathway** in the brain. The pathway used for recognizing a familiar face starts with each **eye** sending information to the **thalamus** on the brain's opposite side *(yellow arrow)*. Identifying the information as visual, the thalamus relays signals to the **visual cortex** *(green arrow)*. Different parts of that region process motion, lines, color, and other qualities. The visual cortex then signals the **superior temporal gyrus**, which handles the emotional memories involved in recognizing a friend or foe *(blue arrow)*. All this signaling can take place in far less than a second, or can drag on as we struggle to recall where we have seen a face before. ILLUSTRATION © ROBERT FINKBEINER

Blood Flowing to the Head

Positron-emission tomography (PET) is a way to trace blood flow in the brain and, thus, determine which regions are active in a given period. The process starts with injecting a briefly radioactive tracer into a volunteer's bloodstream. The PET scanning machine then captures "snapshots" of where the tracer is in the brain before and during a stimulus or task. A computer produces a map of the brain with color-coded areas showing which regions received the most new blood.

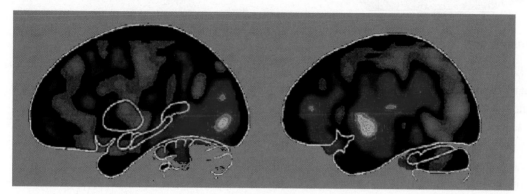

Imaging language: These PET scans show some of the different ways in which our brains work to perceive words. (In both images, the active brain areas are shown as bright yellow spots.) In the image on the left, the person was asked to read words. This led to activation in the back of the brain, where the visual cortex is found. On the right, the person listened to words, which activated the auditory cortex, located at about the middle of the brain. In both cases, the language system was being activated, but the form of presentation of the words was different.

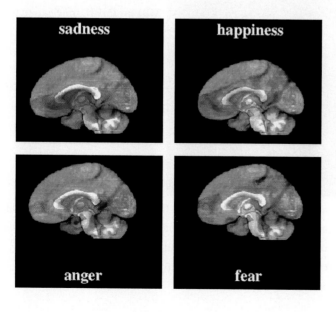

Emotions: These PET scans hint at why the brain's "limbic" region is sometimes called the emotional brain. *Limbic* refers to the inner edge of the brain, where, as the scans show, particular brain areas are especially activated by tasks evoking the volunteers' emotions. IMAGES COURTESY OF DR. ANTONIO DAMASIO, UNIVERSITY OF IOWA COLLEGE OF MEDICINE

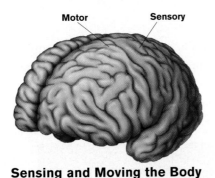

Motor   Sensory

Sensing and Moving the Body

Within the cortex, interconnected neurons that share a function are usually arranged in columns. The strip of columns that process the body's physical sensations is the **sensory cortex**. The columns that govern voluntary movements form the nearby **motor cortex**. ILLUSTRATION © ROBERT FINKBEINER

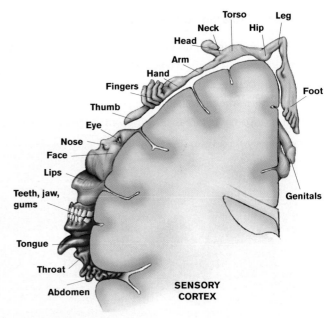

Torso Leg
Neck Hip
Head
Arm
Hand
Fingers
Thumb
Eye
Nose
Face
Lips
Teeth, jaw, gums
Tongue
Throat
Abdomen

Foot

Genitals

SENSORY CORTEX

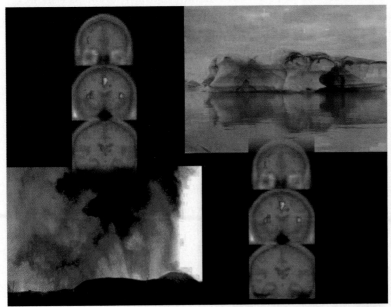

Magnetic resonance imaging (**MRI**) machines sense structures inside the body through a combination of radio waves and a magnetic field. Properly programmed, as **functional MRI** (or **fMRI**), they can map blood flow in the brain over short periods, showing which areas are most active. These fMRI images show a person's brain during arm movement and sensing heat and cold.

Sensing pain: We can perceive both hot and cold sensations as painful. In these images, a person's brain is responding to the pain of painfully hot and painfully cold stimuli applied to the hand. The responses (appearing as bright-colored patches) involve many brain areas, particularly in the limbic region (the "emotional brain"), which appears to be responsible for the sense of unpleasantness associated with both painful stimuli. IMAGES COURTESY OF DR. IRENE TRACY, CENTRE FOR FUNCTIONAL MAGNETIC RESONANCE IMAGING OF THE BRAIN, OXFORD UNIVERSITY

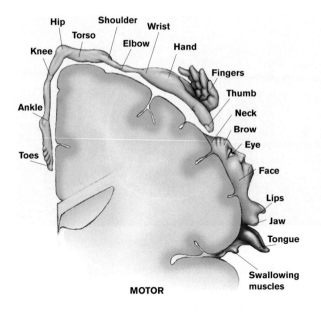

Hip
Shoulder
Torso
Wrist
Knee
Elbow
Hand
Fingers
Thumb
Ankle
Neck
Brow
Eye
Toes
Face
Lips
Jaw
Tongue
Swallowing muscles

MOTOR

Different segments of the sensory and motor cortices are devoted to each part of the body. More sensory brain cells are devoted to our well-innervated lips and fingers than to our back and legs. Similarly, the body parts we move most adeptly, such as the tongue and fingers, occupy a relatively large chunk of the motor cortex. These drawings show the relative size of each body part according to the proportion of the sensory or motor cortex devoted to it.
ILLUSTRATION © ROBERT FINKBEINER

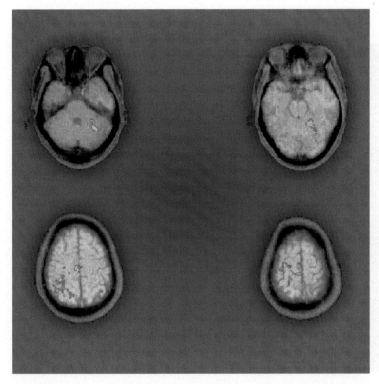

Arm movement: These images show the brain as a person reaches for an object. The movement involves integrated activity (appearing as bright yellow patches) by the brain's perceptual, motor planning, and execution centers. The upper left image shows the areas active in motor planning and execution, while the upper right image shows the brain's spatial perception activity. The lower images show activation of the cerebellum, or hindbrain, during this task. IMAGES COURTESY OF DR. R. CHRIS MIALL, DEPARTMENT OF PHYSIOLOGY, OXFORD UNIVERSITY

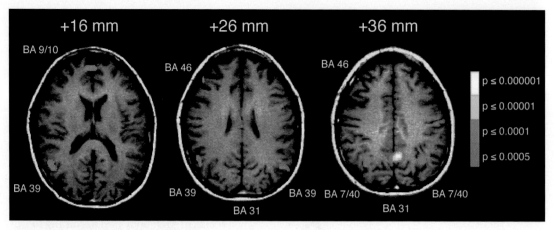

+16 mm   +26 mm   +36 mm

BA 9/10

BA 46   BA 46

p ≤ 0.000001

p ≤ 0.00001

p ≤ 0.0001

p ≤ 0.0005

BA 39   BA 39   BA 39 BA 7/40   BA 7/40

BA 31   BA 31

Exploring Timeless Questions

Moral reasoning: In these fMRI scans, researchers explored how the brain deals with moral reasoning. The researchers described different moral dilemmas to volunteers during brain scanning. They found that the brain responses varied according to how much the dilemmas engaged emotional processing. For some dilemmas, the reasoning process "turned on" brain areas involved with emotional processing, while other dilemmas activated regions associated with working memory and logical problem solving. These differences aligned well with how the volunteers said they would behave in the dilemmas, supporting the idea that moral reasoning can include emotional evaluation. IMAGES COURTESY OF DR. JOSHUA GREENE, PRINCETON UNIVERSITY

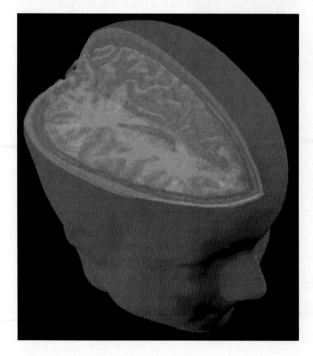

The brain's active areas during moral reasoning. IMAGE COURTESY OF DR. JONATHAN COHEN, PRINCETON UNIVERSITY AND UNIVERSITY OF PITTSBURGH

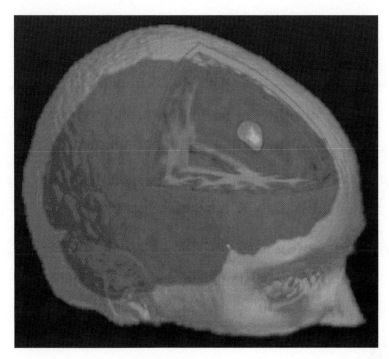

Decision making: This three-dimensional rendering using MRI shows that, when we are faced with two conflicting conditions and need to select an appropriate response, an area of the brain called the anterior cingulate gets busy. IMAGE COURTESY OF DR. JONATHAN COHEN, PRINCETON UNIVERSITY AND UNIVERSITY OF PITTSBURGH

Green
Blue
Red
Yellow

To challenge your anterior cingulate or a friend's, try the famous Stroop Test *(left):* Say out loud the color in which each word is printed, not the color the word names. The brief uncertainty you feel is the conflict provoked by your immediate instinct to read the word rather than say the color of the ink.

The Electric Brain

The flow of charged chemicals through neurons creates weak electrical currents, which provide other ways to measure brain activity.

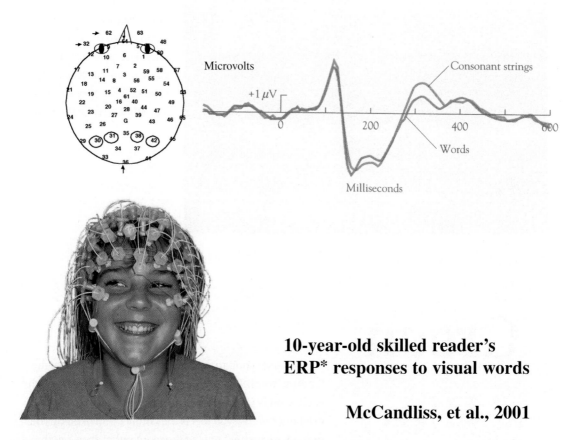

10-year-old skilled reader's ERP* responses to visual words

McCandliss, et al., 2001

This young girl is wearing a cap full of electrical sensors that produce an **electroencephalogram (EEG)**, or tracing of the brain's electrical activity. These electrical readings are accurate to within thousandths of a second and are valuable to researchers trying to understand how different regions of the cortex signal (or malfunction). The numbered circle is a schematic representing the girl's skull; it identifies the sensors from which the readings are taken. IMAGES COURTESY OF BRUCE MCCANDLISS, PH.D., WEILL MEDICAL COLLEGE, CORNELL UNIVERSITY

---

* event-related potentials (the brain's activity in response to a stimulus)

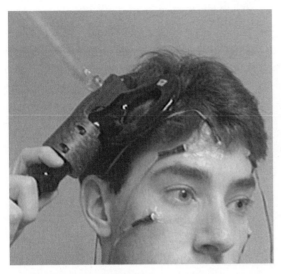

Combining Technologies

Combining two technologies can produce maps of brain activity that one technique alone is unable to do. Two technologies that researchers combine are **MRI scans** and **transcranial magnetic stimulation (TMS)**. TMS focuses magnetic fields on specific brain areas, halting electrical activity there for a few thousandths of a second—so quickly that volunteers often notice no effect. In these images, researchers investigating the visual cortex used TMS to produce brief blind spots in a volunteer's right and left visual fields. They projected the pattern of results onto an MRI of the person's brain to create an accurate map. Green dots represent areas where TMS had no effect; red dots indicate where it disrupted vision in the right visual field; and blue dots show disruption in the left visual field. Photo above courtesy MIT AI Lab; Images below used by permission, *The Journal of Clinical Neurophysiology* 15(4), pp. 344–50, 1998

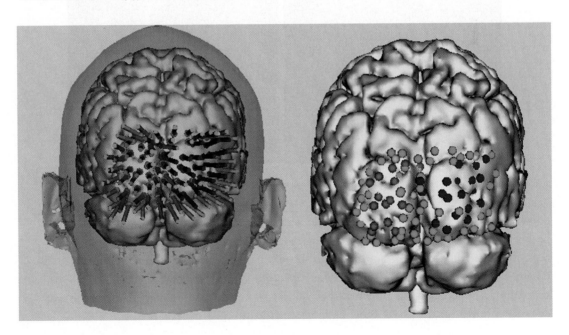

Brain Repair:
A Hint of Things to Come?

As complex as our nervous system is, we can now make some rudimentary repairs to it.

The **cochlear implant** is the most advanced replacement for nerves in common use. It turns sound vibrations into weak electrical signals and sends those signals to the brain through the **auditory nerve**, bypassing the eardrum. The brain's channels for processing information from the ears must be able to adapt to the device's signals; implants are still as yet less sensitive than good natural hearing. ILLUSTRATION © ROBERT FINKBEINER

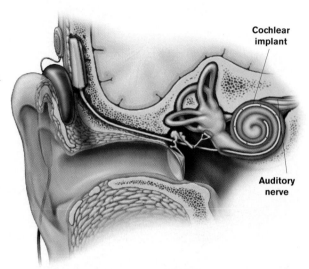

Cochlear implant

Auditory nerve

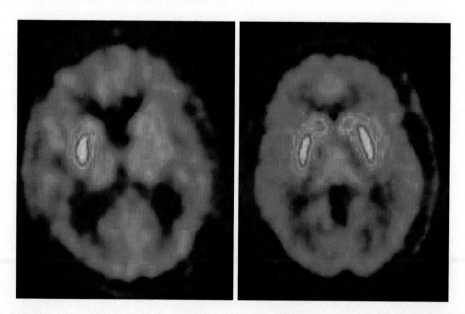

Another technique for repairing the brain, still experimental, involves **implanting cells**. The brain of a person with Parkinson's disease (**C41**), left, shows very low levels of the neurotransmitter **dopamine**. On the right is the same brain after neurologists implanted cells from the dopamine-producing **substantia nigra**. The procedure has been tried experimentally in several groups of patients around the world. For some patients, the new cells produced too much dopamine, so this potential treatment is still being refined. Researchers also hope to use other specialized cells, or **stem cells** that might develop into those specialized cells, to repair the damage caused by other disorders. IMAGES COURTESY OF DR. PAOLA PICCINI, HAMMERSMITH HOSPITAL, LONDON

PART I

Understanding Your Brain

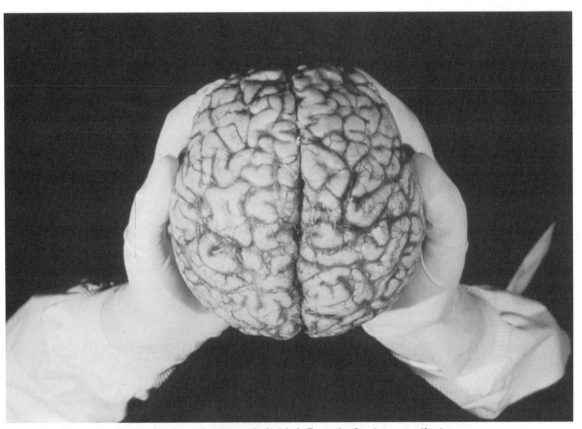

The human brain weighs about three pounds (1.5 kg). From the front, we see the two hemispheres of the cortex, with dark blood vessels covering their outer surface. PHOTO © GEOFF TOMPKINSON/SCIENCE PHOTO LIBRARY

CHAPTER 1

How to Think About the Brain

Since a human brain weighs on average some three pounds, it is easy to hold one in your hands. This simple fact somehow makes it even harder to imagine how such a small mass of tissue can be the source of all that we think of as human. Yet that is what the brain is, and how that can possibly be is one of the most fundamental questions in brain science. What *is* the link between the anatomy of a brain and the workings of a human mind? The big challenge is that there are no obvious moving parts within the brain—it does not operate mechanically as our hearts and lungs do. If we simply look at the brain, our only remote clue about how it works is that it seems to be made up of different parts, easily discernible to the naked eye (see illustrations on page 4). In addition to the cerebral hemispheres (resembling a pair of large walnuts pressed together), the smaller structure that sits behind them (the cerebellum) is visible, as is the stalk that connects to the spinal cord (the brain stem). But there are many more regions than these three.

One easy way to think about the brain would be to view each of these different regions as having a clear function. Every part would be a sort of independent minibrain, controlling one aspect of our mental and behavioral repertoire: movement, emotion, ethics, balance, mathematical thinking, and so on. Simple and attractive though this idea is, it quickly runs into problems. After all, such a

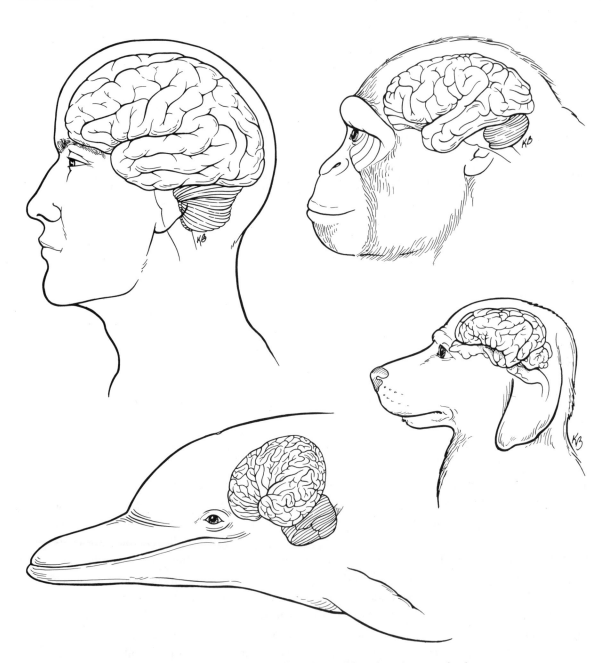

Every mammal's brain—human, chimpanzee, dolphin, and dog—has the same basic structure: a wrinkled cortex atop a creased cerebellum, with a brain stem leading to the spinal cord. More intelligent animals have more cortical surface, however. The human cortex is much larger in proportion to the overall brain than any other animal's. ILLUSTRATIONS © KATHRYN BORN

scenario would merely be miniaturizing the problem, not solving it; we would still have to figure out how each of those minibrains operates. And, as neuroscientists have learned through extensive observations and experiments, the brain just doesn't work that neatly.

Let's start with a straightforward way of trying to match up the brain's physical structures with specific functions. We know that within the animal kingdom, each species has a very different range of abilities and behavior patterns. If the brains of different animals diverge in form, that would give us significant clues about what structures are important for what kinds of functions. For instance, no animal has a language function anywhere near as sophisticated as ours. If there is a particular structure for language, it should be especially well developed in human brains, and small or nonexistent in the brains of other species.

However, the brains of very different creatures, such as a reptile, a bird, and a mammal, differ mainly in size. In all cases we can make out the same big features: the hemispheres, the brain stem, and the cerebellum. So whatever makes one species so different from another—and above all makes the human species so different even from other primates—is not some new, clearly conspicuous structure in their brains that no other animal has.

If, however, we look at various animals' brains for a difference not in *quality* but in *quantity*, then one clue about the physical basis of mental differences becomes apparent. The biggest discrepancy appears in the surface of the outer layer of the hemispheres. This layer is called the cortex, after the Latin for "bark," because it wraps around the brain the way its namesake wraps around a tree. In a rat or rabbit, for example, the surface of the cortex is completely smooth. In a cat it has clear

convolutions. By the time we look at monkeys and apes, and eventually humans, the cortex takes on an ever more wrinkled appearance. Why?

Imagine trying to hold a sheet of paper in one fist. The more you crumple the paper, the more the sheet will fit inside your fingers. In a way, this is what has happened to the cortex within the skull. As species have become more sophisticated, the surface of their cortices has increased faster than the limited confines of their heads. The only way to develop more "working surface" in the cortex was to fold and wrinkle it. We can see this same evolutionary trend in the development of an individual human. The brain of the six-month-old fetus has a completely smooth cortex. But in the final three months of pregnancy, the baby's neurons proliferate at an astonishing 250,000 a minute. The cortex expands enormously so that by birth it has become as walnutlike as we know it. (For more on the brain's prenatal development, see chapter 5.)

Mapping the Regions—
The Top-Down Approach

We can call this method of thinking about the brain—looking at its physical regions and their traits—the top-down approach. The surface area of the cortex and the degree to which it is wrinkled seem to hold a clue about how a species' brain relates to its mental abilities. Small wonder, then, that the cortex has fascinated many brain researchers. But how might it accommodate the uniqueness of our human traits?

The top-down approach has given us some valuable insights into how the cortex is organized and how it plays a part in brain function. We know, for example, that despite the way its surface looks the same everywhere, different parts of the cortex participate in different processes. Certain areas, along with many deep brain structures below the cortex, seem to relate directly to the processing of each of the senses: vision, hearing, smell, and so on. As an example, let's take one thin strip of cortex that straddles the brain a little like a hair band. This region is called the somatosensory (that is, body-sensing) cortex. (See pp. 138–39 for more about it.) The cells in this strip collect signals from other brain structures, which in turn are activated by impulses buzzed up the spinal cord that report on touch, pain, or temperature felt in certain parts of the body. Clearly, this strip of cortex must contain some sort of representation of the body. How else would you know that a pain was in your toe as opposed to your hand?

So far, so good. The most logical way of thinking about your body being "mapped" in the brain would be in direct relation to size. A large part of the body like the back would have a large allocation of brain territory, and a small area like the fingertips or the tongue would be represented by a correspondingly meager area of cortex. But here is a simple experiment you can do at home to prove that this "obvious" scenario is wrong. All you need are a pair of sharp pencils, or unbent paper clips, and a willing friend.

Ask the friend to close his or her eyes and turn away. Hold the pencils so their points are close together—three-eighths inch or so. Gently touch both pencil points to your friend's skin in different parts of the body, and ask if you are applying one or both points. (You can also try touching just one point at a time to see if your friend feels a clear difference between one and two points.) When you touch both pencils to your friend's back, he or she will almost always report feeling a single point. Now position the points much closer, only one-sixteenth inch apart, and apply

them to your friend's fingertip or (with permission) tongue. Surprisingly, this time your friend will be able to feel two distinct points. Even though the fingertips and tongue represent only small fractions of our bodies, they are extremely sensitive to physical detail. Despite their small size, the fingers and the tongue have the lion's share of territory in the relevant strip of brain. That's because our brains are organized according to the functional needs of our bodies rather than simple physical size. Our fingers and tongue have to be more sensitive to touch than our back—so they have more brain territory allocated to them.

Thus we can start to see that the structures of our brains are in tune with our daily lives. But testing such primitive processes as touch doesn't help with the question of how our cortex works differently from those of other species. So let's go back to what is arguably the monopoly of us humans, language. Surely if we understood how our brains process language, we would have a route into understanding the physical basis of what makes us so special.

Paul Broca was a physician working in Paris during the mid-nineteenth century. He has earned his place in neurological history thanks to one of his patients, a Monsieur Leborgne. Everyone knew this unfortunate man by his nickname, "Tan," because that was all he could say. Leborgne had a severe speech problem, an aphasia (**C70**), which meant he could not articulate words. When Tan died, Broca examined his brain and discovered a clear hole in the side of its left hemisphere. Tan's aphasia was obviously related to the damage in this region, henceforth known as Broca's area. But does this mean that Broca had discovered the mind's center for speech? Far from it.

Within a decade, a German physician, Carl

Wernicke, identified a second site, also on the left-hand side of the brain but clearly well behind Broca's area, where damage gave rise to a different type of speech problem. Wernicke's aphasia is also referred to as jargon aphasia because although a person with this problem can articulate words perfectly well, all that comes out of his or her mouth is a string of gibberish.

By the end of the twentieth century, scientists had come to realize that there are still more brain regions involved in speech. Imaging techniques have made it possible for us to see the brain at work in conscious humans without causing any pain or harm. Positron-emission tomography (PET) and functional magnetic resonance imaging (fMRI) exploit the facts that the brain is very greedy for oxygen or glucose and that the hardest-working brain regions are hungriest of all. (For more on these technologies, see chapter 2.) Studies have now revealed that, during such seemingly simple behaviors as using language, many brain regions are working together, rather like the instruments in an orchestra. Each region will be making a specialized contribution, but the whole is somehow more than the sum of its parts. What we don't know yet is how all the different brain regions involved in any one task, be it language or vision or memory, somehow come together.

But what might we learn about the particular contribution of one brain region? Let's look at an area toward the front of our brains, the prefrontal cortex. This area is twice the size it should be for a primate of our body weight. Could this contain the secret of our awesome mental abilities?

Again, as long ago as the mid-nineteenth century people realized that there was something special about the prefrontal cortex. This was demonstrated in 1848 in a most dramatic way by Phineas Gage, a railway worker in Vermont. One day, Gage was working to clear the path for a new railroad when the gunpowder he was using exploded prematurely. As a consequence, the bar with which he had been tamping down the explosive shot right through his prefrontal cortex. In effect, he had speared himself through the head. Surprisingly, Gage lost sight in one eye but otherwise appeared to be unaffected by this horrific accident. His movements and senses all were as before, and he actually went back to work. Only then did his workmates start to notice a difference. Gage was not badly affected in how he walked, pronounced words, ate, or did other normal human activities, but a far more subtle change had occurred. He had become very unpleasant and antisocial, cursing in inappropriate situations. So could the prefrontal cortex be the brain's center for character (or good character)?

In fact, in the decades since Phineas Gage had his accident, scientists have studied many other patients suffering damage to the prefrontal cortex. More recently, they have observed the region's activity in healthy people. The prefrontal cortex has now been implicated in a welter of seemingly disparate functions, ranging from "forward planning" to "working memory." In people suffering from clinical depression this area appears overactive, and in those with schizophrenia it can be underactive. There is clearly no single common, easily identifiable theme to these findings. So where does that leave us in our effort to localize functions within the brain, to match up different functions with different structures?

The emerging picture is certainly not a brain composed of autonomous minibrains. Rather, every function is divided among many brain regions, and every brain region participates in the

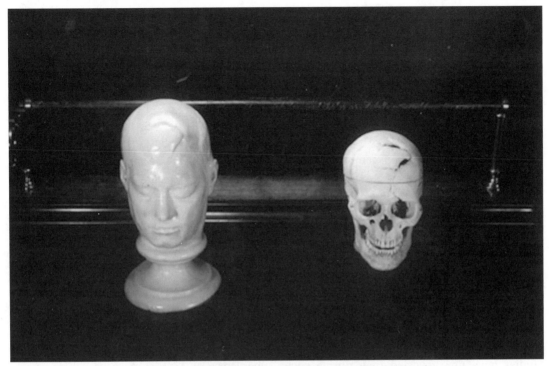

The most famous brain injury patient, Phineas Gage, underwent a complete change of personality after an explosion drove an iron bar through his prefrontal cortex. Photo © The Warren Anatomical Museum, Francis A. Countway Library of Medicine, Harvard Medical School

many functions that make up the human behavioral repertoire. We can say that certain regions of the brain are more active than others when it comes to certain functions, but we can't say those functions are confined to particular areas. And we are still a long way from knowing how to assemble the different structures of the brain to make up a human mind.

Studying the Cells—
The Bottom-Up Approach

We can also think about the brain in the opposite way, or "bottom up." This alternative approach involves starting with the brain's most basic components and then figuring out how they connect with each other.

The most basic working unit of the brain is a special type of cell, the neuron. You have approximately 100 billion neurons—as many trees as there are in the Amazon rain forest. But neurons are not the only cells in the brain: they are actually outnumbered ten to one by another type, glial cells. These cells maintain a healthy and nurturing microenvironment within our heads for the neurons to operate at their best.

So what do neurons actually do? Since the 1920s, neurologists have known that neurons generate minute electrical signals. Each neuron alive in your brain at this moment is producing a tiny voltage, a potential difference between the charge

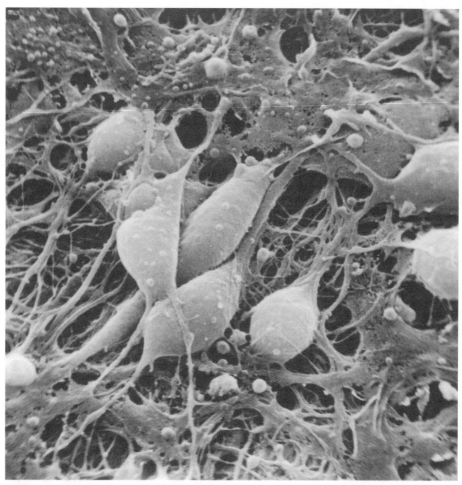

This image is a scanning electron micrograph (SEM) of nerve cells in the human cerebral cortex. These cells make up the outer, heavily folded gray matter of the brain. IMAGE © CRNI/SCIENCE PHOTO LIBRARY

inside the cell and the charge outside. Under certain conditions, such as when a signal comes in from a neighboring cell, tiny channels open in the wall of the neuron so that there is a sudden, brief interchange of ions (atoms with an electrical charge, in particular sodium and potassium). This ion interchange causes a temporary shift in the neuron's charge—an electrical blip called an action potential. Action potentials last for only about one thousandth of a second. Yet a neuron will typically fire off a hundred or so every second. This traffic in charges represents the "moving parts" of the brain, the actions that make it work. Ultimately all that we are—all our memories, hopes, and feelings—can be boiled down to the banal transfer of a few ions across the membrane wall of our brain cells.

Using the right sensors, we can read those electrical signals through the bone of the skull; the result is the valuable diagnostic tool called the

DO WE USE ONLY 10 PERCENT OF OUR BRAINS?

There is a common myth that we use only 10 percent of our brains. We're not sure exactly where this idea came from, but one possibility is that in experiments recording brain tissue's electrical activity, some scientists assume that at any one time roughly 10 percent of neurons will be spontaneously active—firing off action potentials. But it is important to remember that the lab is hardly a natural environment. The brains under investigation either belong to anesthetized animals or are thin slices of tissue kept alive in a dish. Imaging technologies look at regions of the brain over time, so the pictures they create are too general to allow us to count how many neurons are firing at any one time. Even apart from these qualifications, we must consider that neurons that are temporarily silent may well be fulfilling some important role by *not* being active. Single neurons, just like larger brain regions, do not operate in isolation. Once again, and on a much tinier scale, the whole is more than the sum of its parts.

electroencephalogram (EEG; for more information, see chapter 2). Over the last few decades, furthermore, technology has enabled neurophysiologists to record the activity of a single neuron. Therefore, we have a fairly good idea of what makes those little building blocks of our brains work.

What happens once a neuron has generated an action potential? This tiny blip, some eighty thousandths of a volt in amplitude, buzzes away at speeds up to 250 miles per hour along the biological equivalent of a wire: an axon. But unlike any household electrical circuit, the brain isn't wired so that all neurons form one single continuous network. Instead, in most cases, there is a gap between the axon of one neuron and the next neuron. This gap is called a synapse. It is as impossible for the action potential to cross a synapse as it is for a car to screech down a road and then float across a river. This might seem to be a cumbersome weakness in our wiring, but it is actually a powerful advantage.

The brain has an alternative way to send a signal across the fluid-filled gap. When the electrical impulse invades the end of the axon, it triggers the release of a chemical that can spread across the synapse and activate the target neuron. This chemical, because it transmits a signal, is known as a transmitter (or a "neurotransmitter," if we want to make absolutely clear that it is at work in the brain). Once the transmitter hits the target cell, it enters into a kind of molecular handshake with a custom-made protein, a receptor, on the outside of that cell. This molecular handshake then causes the opening of the tiny channels into that neuron so that ions can cross over, once again generating the electrical signal. The brain therefore is not like a computer or any other electrical device, because it operates by means of a cascade of alternating electrical *and chemical* events.

Furthermore, there are many different transmitters in the brain, each with several different subtypes of receptors. So unlike a standard electronic circuit within a computer, which can only be on or off, the brain has a powerful spectrum of functions. Different chemicals will trigger different states within the brain. To appreciate just how important chemical signaling is to brain function, and hence to our mental abilities, let's take a look at drugs.

All drugs that modify moods and feelings, whether prescribed or proscribed, do so by changing the availability or the efficacy of different transmitters within the brain. For example, some 30 years ago scientists discovered that the drug morphine worked by imitating a naturally occurring neurotransmitter called enkephalin (literally, "in the head"). But that does not mean that it is natural or safe to take the most abused derivative of morphine, heroin. Enkephalin is released in minute amounts as and when it's needed in the brain; then, even more important, it is disposed of very rapidly. Not so with heroin. First, it is not released in a small quantity exactly where it is needed; a heroin user effectively marinates his or her whole brain, setting the drug free to act wherever there are appropriate receptors. Second, when heroin does encounter a receptor and enters into a molecular handshake, the drug can't be removed as readily as its natural counterpart. Because heroin is a different chemical, it will remain stubbornly in place. The result is like a handshake with an excessively strong grip. And just as the hand being gripped quickly starts to turn numb, the brain's special receptors become less sensitive. The heroin user needs increasing amounts of the drug to obtain the same effect, one sign of an addiction (**C29**).

The powerful effects of drugs on the brain surely demonstrate the importance of transmitters and, above all, of the connections over which they operate. Even the awesome number of neurons in our brains is dwarfed by the number of connections between them. There can be as many as 10,000 inputs to any one neuron. One estimate has it that counting each connection in your cortex alone, one a second around the clock, would take you 32 million years!

Making Connections— The Dynamic Approach

Looking at the connections our brain cells forge is a sort of middle approach, halfway between studying large brain regions and examining single cells. It is this aspect of the brain that will most likely allow us to discover what it is about these squishy organs that makes humans such an intelligent species, and makes each one of us unique.

As you'll see in more detail in Part II of this book, we are born with pretty much all the neurons we will ever have. (In fact, many brain cells die off during childhood.) But the marvelous feature of being human is that many of the *connections* among those neurons are laid down after we are born. This forging of connections in the most basic and broadest sense underpins what we refer to as learning. We have highly adaptable brains that reflect and benefit from our experiences. In contrast, simpler organisms like bugs operate at the dictates of their genes, following preprogrammed instincts.

We call the adaptability of our human brains plasticity. Our brains reflect each new experience. As a consequence, we become individuals. Everyone undergoes different experiences, and everyone's brain develops differently. Of course genes play an important part in constructing the molecular machinery at work on each side of your synapses. But there are about 1 billion more connections in your brain than genes in your chromosomes; it is impossible for each connection to be programmed by a gene. Instead, the connections are shaped by your experiences.

The basis of this adaptability is the growth of connections between cells, strengthened and promoted by the activation of the relevant neurons. An axon coming from one neuron makes contact with the next neuron along the circuit by means of what are called dendrites on the receiving neuron. The more dendrites a neuron has, the more connections it will be able to make and the greater the circuitry underpinning a particular process or function. Just as a muscle grows with appropriate exercise, so selective circuits in the brain branch out and expand as they are worked. We can see this change even at the level of a single neuron. In one study with adult rats, half were housed in humane but isolated cages while the other half were housed collectively and exposed to interactive objects, such as ladders. The neurons from the group in the temporarily "enriched" environment showed more dendrites emanating from a single cell than those in the nonenriched group.

The more sophisticated a species, the longer it takes for an individual to grow to adulthood. We humans are the most sophisticated animals of all, so we take many years to develop. Our brains need that much time to collect and store the experiences that shape our minds. Childhood is usually a time of exploration, of making the mental connections that go along with the growing connections among our brain cells. That is why an individual's circumstances in youth help mold that person's personality, skills, and other qualities. (For more on brain development in childhood and adolescence, see chapters 6 and 7.)

But learning doesn't have to stop in childhood. The plasticity of our brains means that they can usually adapt to further challenges. A recent study showed that London taxi drivers, who have to memorize all the street names and routes of that huge city, have a larger part of the brain relating to memory than do other adults of a similar age. Another striking example of our brain's ability to learn entails not a lifetime at a profession but

merely five days spent practicing a piano exercise—this study showed that over such a short time the brain territory allocated to the fingers became enhanced. Even more amazing, mere *mental* practice has a similar effect on the brain.

But is the brain's power to learn limited as we get older? We have already briefly explored the physical basis of "blowing the mind" with drugs. Sadly, old age can bring the horror of "losing one's mind" because of degenerative diseases like Alzheimer's (**C67**). In this disorder, still not fully understood, the connections that a person's brain has so painstakingly accumulated throughout life gradually become dismantled: increasingly, everything around the person comes to "mean" less. Imaging techniques have now revealed that certain brain regions in Alzheimer's patients shrink far faster than in healthy individuals of a similar age. This finding has an encouraging implication: the symptoms of senile dementia that come with this disease are not a natural consequence of aging but are due to some special factor or factors that are as yet a matter of conjecture.

In fact, healthy older brains retain their plasticity. We can see this in the often remarkable recoveries of people who have had strokes (**C59, C60**). Parts of their brains suffered severe damage, having been deprived of blood and oxygen for significant periods. Nevertheless, many of these people are able to offset the damage and regain functions they initially lost. Their brains create new neural pathways, or start to use old ones, to bypass the damaged areas. Once again, the brain responds to experience by creating new connections and new functionality. (For more about the brains of older adults, see chapter 8.) In the near future the brain sciences will be shedding more light on these mechanisms of plasticity, as well as giving us insight into the specific losses that characterize Alzheimer's disease and other disorders.

Because of plasticity, as we go through life, our brains become increasingly personalized. Everything we encounter will be interpreted in the light of all that we have seen before. It is this personalization of the brain that gives rise to the mind. Viewed in this way, the mind is not some airy, whimsical alternative to the physical brain, but the aspect of it that makes each of us unique.

The Director of the Royal Institution of Great Britain, Dr. Susan Greenfield, has a memory that captures nicely the mystique of the physical human brain and its relationship to mind. Here is how she tells it:

"Once upon a time, over 25 years ago, I was undertaking a dissection of the human brain as part of a college class. Each pair of us students had our own plastic bucket, containing in preservative liquid the organ that had once defined a unique person. I stared down at this odd object in my fingers, resembling two compacted giant walnuts with a smaller walnut on the back. A macabre thought struck me: What if I weren't wearing protective gloves and got a piece of this brain stuff stuck under my fingernail? Would that be a thought or a memory, a habit or a feeling? Exactly what part of the individual would be nestling on top of my finger?"

Evocative, fundamental questions remain to tantalize. We are at an exciting time, when we no longer need to think about the brain as a collection of static anatomical regions, nor as a mere mass of generic cells and chemicals. We can now peek into the brain and see it shaping and reshaping every moment of our lives. It is truly the most dynamic and the most personal part of our bodies.

CHAPTER 2

How We Know: Learning the Secrets of the Brain

The human brain, the three pounds of soft tissue inside your cranium, is a marvel of complexity. Nobel laureate James Watson, codiscoverer of DNA's structure, has called the brain "the most complex thing we have yet discovered in our universe." In round numbers, the organ contains some 100 billion nerve cells, each of which branches out to hundreds of thousands of others, forming trillions of connections, all told. The cells' communication and activity produce electrical currents and the ebb and flow of chemicals, with millions of operations occurring simultaneously. How do we trace all these tiny elements to create a composite picture of the brain and nervous system?

For thousands of years scientists, philosophers, and other scholars tried to understand the workings of their own brains, to little avail. But in the twentieth century, with progress in techniques and technology, brain research began to gather momentum, and as the century closed, a much-repeated theme among neuroscientists was that more had been learned about the brain in the previous 25 years than in all of human history. A key advance, made a century ago, paved the way: the discovery of dyes that would make the cells in brain tissue visible under a microscope, a feat that won a joint Nobel Prize for two fierce scientific rivals, Santiago Ramón y Cajal of Spain and Camillo Golgi of Italy. Subsequent decades brought better ways to see and perform experiments on those cells and their chemical and electrical activity, especially with the inventions of the electron microscope and, in the 1950s, new devices that could record the firing of single brain cells in living, behaving animals, starting with cats and rabbits and later with monkeys and rodents. Such investigative tools were remarkably productive in the hands of skilled scientists. Those researchers' pioneering demonstrations of the brain's dynamic activity spelled out fundamental principles, such as that some brain circuitry will simply not operate if deprived of stimulation from the external world, that neurons communicate using both electrical action and chemical messengers (the neurotransmitters), and that the vast network of cells in the brain includes precise "pathways" participating in various functions. These "first principles" established a frontier to which new cadres of neuroscientists would flock in the 1980s and 1990s to make the brain yield more and more secrets of its advanced functions. Now scientists can draw on a host of new tools to probe the human brain in exquisite detail. This technology includes not only the repertoire of genetics and molecular biology but also a valuable array of brain imaging or scanning devices handed to neuroscientists by the similarly exuberant field of physics, permitting researchers to study the living human brain's machinery in action.

With these powerful tools, knowledge of the brain has spread from the laboratory to the clinic, and from there to the world at large, where, in places as different as the classroom and the courtroom, everyone is learning about the brain's structure and function, gaining insight on such basic tasks as learning, memory, thinking, and feeling. We are also discovering what can go wrong: how injury, disease, and developmental miscues can make these vital functions break down. As neuro-

science progresses, we all—scientist and layman alike—are peering with ever better vision inside the once unseeable "black box" of the human brain and understanding some of the mysteries that have intrigued us for so long.

A note about the more recent findings described in this chapter: after one research group publishes any scientific study, other laboratories must examine, replicate, and refine the findings before the scientific world as a whole accepts its value. That is how progress takes place in medicine, or in any science. Most of the examples you will read about here fall into the category of promising results still under scrutiny as the new century opens. Many have a bright future as definite statements about how our brains work, but all are illustrations of the creative ferment in which teams of scientists all over the world are engaged, wedding their fascination and curiosity to new technology and new ideas to explore the brain.

Brain Exploration: Past and Present

While visiting London in 1873, Mark Twain entered the office of Lorenzo N. Fowler, a "practical phrenologist." During the examination, Fowler informed Twain of a cavity in his brain in a place where, according to phrenologists, humor normally resided.

This dubious assessment of Twain, one of the world's great humorists, highlights the fallibility of phrenology—a long discredited attempt to judge human character and intellect by the size and shape of bumps on the head. First promoted in the early 1800s by the Austrian physician Franz Joseph Gall, phrenology associated specific bumps on the skull with brain regions responsible for mirth, dexterity, wit, amativeness, and

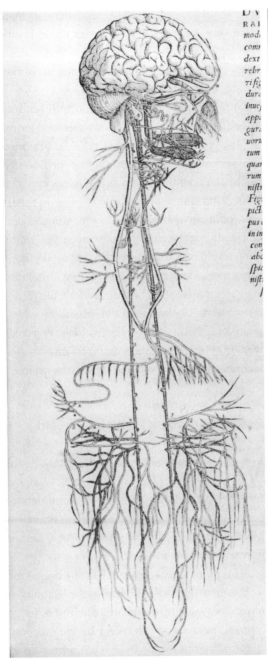

Andreas Vesalius, a Flemish anatomist at the University of Padua, showed this brain and spinal cord in his sixteenth-century book, based on his dissection of human cadavers. IMAGE COURTESY OF THE NATIONAL LIBRARY OF MEDICINE A027048

other qualities. The theory attracted followers in Europe and the United States for many decades, but the medical community ultimately rejected it as pseudoscience. Researchers concluded long ago that the organization of the brain's soft tissue has absolutely no bearing on the shape of the skull. Nevertheless, phrenology had stumbled onto a significant aspect of how we understand the brain today: different parts of the brain are indeed involved in executing different tasks, though with an intricacy and subtlety that Gall's fanciful theory had no hope of explaining.

More authentic scientific approaches have provided a more direct, and less conjectural, means of exploring brain structure and function. The most venerable and still valuable technique, and certainly the most straightforward way to inspect the human brain, is to slice it open after its owner has died. The Greek physician Galen, for example, dissected the brains of humans and other animals in the second century A.D. He concluded that the brain's vital parts are its fluid-filled cavities rather than its soft tissue—an erroneous notion that prevailed for nearly 1,500 years. Centuries before Galen, around 300 B.C., investigators in Egypt also probed human anatomy through dissection. Herophilus, a physician with a keen interest in the brain and nerves as well as other organs, distinguished nerve networks from the tendons and blood vessels throughout the body. He also noted that nerves come in two varieties, sensory and motor. His successor, the anatomist Erasistratus, differentiated the cerebrum, the brain's main component, from the cerebellum, the smaller section behind it. Shortly after that, Egyptian religious authorities decided that the human body should remain intact after death, bringing a sudden end to such dissections. Yet the basic approach, called postmortem exam or autopsy, was revived in re-

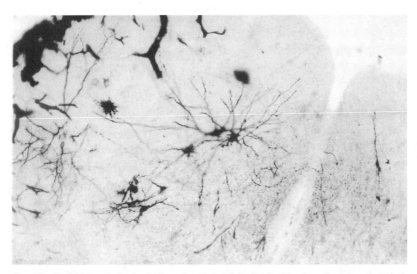

Camillo Golgi invented a technique for staining individual brain cells, revealing their axons (which scientists call "processes"), as shown by the microphotograph of rabbit spinal cord neurons taken from one of Golgi's original slide preparations. IMAGE COURTESY OF MARINA BENTIVOGLIO, M.D., UNIVERSITY OF VERONA

cent centuries, providing a fertile avenue for scientific and medical progress.

Relying on microscopic examination of brain cells and nerves from dead humans and animals, scientists began to trace the circuitry of the nervous system. A pioneer in this area, Camillo Golgi of Italy specialized in histology—the study of how tissue is organized at various levels, from single cells to an entire organism. In 1873, Golgi introduced a staining technique that selectively darkened neurons with silver nitrate. This made the cells and their fibrous extensions—axons, which transmit nerve signals, and dendrites, which receive signals—easy to see under the microscope. About 15 years later, the histologist and neuroanatomist Santiago Ramón y Cajal of Spain improved on Golgi's stain, using gold to reveal the structure of the nervous system in even finer detail. Ramón y Cajal focused in particular on how neurons communicated through a "synapse," a tiny gap between one cell and the next. Golgi dis-

agreed with this finding, maintaining that nerve cells formed a physically interconnected net. (Ramón y Cajal eventually proved to be right.) Despite their differences, the two scientists shared the 1906 Nobel Prize in medicine for their contributions in making the nervous system visible.

Scientists have also gained hints about the brain by studying human behavior. This strategy was especially fruitful when doctors came across patients who behaved oddly and whose brains— it was learned after their death—were impaired in specific, obvious ways. The approach came to be called lesion studies because it focused on the location of lesions, or damaged areas, in these people's brains. Of course, researchers also need to look at healthy brains, which serve as controls, so that they can spot the deviations caused by disease, injury, or congenital defects. In the 1860s, for example, the French neurologist Paul Broca conducted postmortem exams of stroke victims, linking damage to a region in the left frontal lobe (now

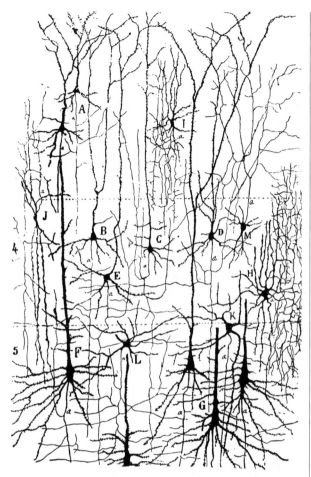

Santiago Ramón y Cajal improved on the Golgi staining technique. More important, he realized that neurons do not quite touch each other, but communicate chemically across a small gap (called a synapse). This is his drawing of cerebral cortex neurons from his 1911 textbook of the nervous system. IMAGE COURTESY OF MARINA BENTIVOGLIO, M.D., UNIVERSITY OF VERONA

called Broca's area) with the inability to speak. A decade later the German neurologist Carl Wernicke discovered that damage to a part of the left temporal lobe (Wernicke's area) affects the ability to understand language. In 1906, the German physician Alois Alzheimer described an autopsy of a 51-year-old woman who had suffered from memory problems. Her brain was riddled with two kinds of microscopic protein clumps, "plaques" and "tangles"—the first reported case of Alzheimer's disease (**C67**).

Lesion studies, now sometimes called clinical pathologic correlations, remain an important research avenue. For example, many physicians have used the method in postmortem studies of brain tissue to try to find the roots of schizophrenia (**C25**), a complex disorder that affects many functions of the brain. Teams at the University of California at Los Angeles examined the brains of people who had had schizophrenia and reported misplaced neurons in the hippocampus—a seahorse-shaped structure involved in learning and the formation of long-term memories. Other analyses of schizophrenics' brains, performed at the University of California at Irvine, found out-of-place neurons in various parts of the cerebral cortex. Researchers at the Brain Tissue Research Center of McLean Hospital in Massachusetts have found that the brains of schizophrenics have more excitatory neurons and fewer inhibitory neurons than normal individuals—a finding consistent with evidence that people with the disorder are often overwhelmed by sensory stimulation.

Similar studies of people who succumbed to Huntington's disease (**C47**) have shown a marked deterioration in the brain's caudate nucleus—an area involved in controlling movements, among other responsibilities. Investigators are exploring strategies for curbing brain cell death in that region by blocking the action of a protein responsible for the devastation.

Electric Avenues

For decades, neuroscientists have measured electrical currents in the brain and seen how this activity goes haywire in conditions like epilepsy (C13). Efforts to understand the physiology of animals and humans through electrical stimulation of the brain and other body parts have a long tradition. In 1791, the Italian scientist Luigi Galvani (from whose name we have the term *galvanic*) made disembodied frogs' legs jerk spasmodically when he ran a current through them. His colleague Alessandro Volta (for whom the volt is named) extended this research over the next several years, finding he could induce motions in an unconscious frog by stimulating nerves rather than muscles. Reports like these established that our nervous systems depend on bioelectrical currents.

In 1879 the German researchers Eduard Hitzig and Gustav Fritsch brought this line of research to the brain. Hitzig and Fritsch demonstrated that electrically stimulating certain areas of a dog's cerebral cortex produced movements in the animal's limbs—a pioneering approach to localizing function in the brain. Continuing this work, the American neurosurgeon Wilder Penfield began a series of operations in the 1930s to locate the source of seizures in human patients. To identify sites with abnormal electrical activity, Penfield placed small exposed wires called electrodes throughout the cerebral cortex of hundreds of patients. He used the electrodes to stimulate particular areas and observed the effects. Penfield found that simulating adjacent parts of the cortex, for example, affected adjacent parts of the arm. Specific sections of the cortex, he concluded, correspond to specific parts of the body surface.

Brain surgery is unusual among major operations in that patients can be awakened to respond to their surgeon's questions and actions, after their scalp, skull, and meninges (the covering around the brain) have been cut open under local anesthesia. In one such operation, Penfield stimulated a particular part of a teenage girl's brain, and she suddenly recalled a terrifying incident from her youth when a man holding a sack appeared and asked, "How would you like to get into this bag with the snakes?" In this way, Penfield showed that vivid childhood memories could be retrieved by stimulating parts of the temporal lobes. A similar procedure caused a young woman to laugh whenever one area of her left cerebral cortex was stimulated. Her doctors asked why, and she replied that she suddenly found them very funny.

Although electrical stimulation techniques yield interesting results and avenues for further exploration, they can be used only on patients already undergoing brain surgery. So their greatest value remains medical: assisting neurosurgeons in identifying important areas to protect in surgeries for illnesses such as epilepsy and brain cancer. This would be a significant research limitation except that many other approaches, all noninvasive, have become available.

Lessons from the Animal World

To probe more deeply into the human brain, scientists have always studied animal anatomy and behavior. One of the most famous experiments involving animals began when the Russian scientist Ivan Pavlov noticed that his laboratory dogs salivated at the sight of the white-coated attendants who brought them their food. The dogs barked before they saw the food itself. By ringing a bell or flashing a light before mealtimes, Pavlov was able to condition the animals to salivate in response to those stimuli as well. They even came to salivate and wag their tails when they received electric shocks, so long as those shocks were consistently followed by food. Pavlov thus showed how events could condition the brain to produce a specific physical behavior.

Other animal studies involve making small brain lesions, implanting electrodes to monitor activity, or disrupting peripheral, sensory, or motor nerves to see how these nerves can repair themselves. Many people find it hard to read about this, and thus it is important to take a moment here to point out that cruelty has never been an intended consequence of research using animals, except in extremely rare instances by unprincipled scientists who were readily stopped by their peers. Taking good care of animals to keep their health and environment as humane and near normal as possible has been the rule. This means cages are kept clean, the animals are well nourished, procedures that cause pain are done with anesthesia, and if pain itself is the object of study, the least amount necessary to make the needed observations—such as a hot pepper ointment on a paw—is used. Why? Not only because gratuitous suffering in animals offends most scientists, who are decent people, but also because findings cannot be trusted if unnecessary pain and its biological responses have crept in. That said, studies of fruit flies, yeast, snails, worms, mice, rats, birds, and certain fish are the mainstay of neuroscience, providing useful models for understanding the human brain and nervous system and disorders, particularly at the genetic and cellular level. Monkeys, dogs, cats, and other animals are studied mainly at the stage when the research question must be pursued in a nervous system closer to that of humans. Most responsible investigators consider animal subjects indispensable for basic research; almost every scientific and medical advance described in this book passed through an animal testing stage. The al-

ternative, to experiment on or prescribe treatments and medications for humans without first confirming safety and efficacy in animals, is unthinkable.

Scientists took a big step forward in the 1950s and 1960s by learning how to record the electrical activity of individual neurons in live laboratory animals, at first with cats and rabbits, then later with monkeys and rodents. In this technique, researchers anesthetize the animal and insert extremely fine electrodes directly into the targeted brain cell. When a neuron is active, it discharges an electrical impulse. Once the electrodes are surgically implanted, the scientists can record the animals' brain activity repeatedly, during wakefulness and sleep, without causing them harm. The technique offers a way to gauge the response of cells to various stimuli, confirming ideas about nerve cell function in particular brain regions. Such exquisitely fine observations of living brain activity would not have been possible without electrode recording.

In 1957, National Institutes of Health neuroscientists Eric Kandel and Alden Spencer obtained the first recordings of cell activity in a mammal's hippocampus. Kandel's goal was to understand the cellular basis of memory, and he soon switched to studying how that worked in a simpler brain: the sea snail *Aplysia californica*, which has the largest nerve cells of any animal. Studying this creature at Columbia University over several decades, Kandel showed that when the snail (like Pavlov's dogs) learned a response to a repeated stimulus, the synapses between its nerve cells strengthened as well. Scientists now believe that this process, called long-term potentiation, is vital to the formation of memories in humans as well as in snails. Kandel won a Nobel Prize for this work in 2000.

Around the same time that Kandel and Spencer started probing the hippocampus with microelectrodes, David Hubel and Torsten Wiesel began using such miniature electrodes to probe animal brains, one cell at a time. In 1958, while studying the primary visual cortex of cats at Johns Hopkins University, Hubel and Wiesel made an astonishing discovery: neurons in one part of the visual cortex responded only to vertical lines moving across the cat's field of vision. Nearby brain cells responded just to horizontal lines, and still others responded to diagonal lines. This showed just how specialized brain cells can be. Hubel and Wiesel also learned that the cells that responded to the same kind of stimuli—such as shapes of a specific orientation—were stacked in vertical columns extending from the top of the visual cortex to the bottom. In later studies, the two discovered that a newborn cat must be able to see in order to develop vision—that is, to "wire up" the visual cortex. They closed a kitten's eye using surgical sutures and removed them when the kitten was about eight weeks old. The kitten was left without vision through that eye for life. This finding led to today's understanding of the "critical" period for vision in infants, when an impairment, such as a cataract, with which some babies are born, must be corrected for sight to develop normally (see chapter 6). Hubel and Wiesel collaborated for two decades, earning a Nobel Prize for their labors in 1981.

In the early 1960s, the American physiologist Vernon Mountcastle uncovered more details about the vertical organization of the cortex. By applying movable electrodes to the brains of anesthetized animals, Mountcastle showed that the neurons that respond to stimulation of the body's surface are also arranged one on top of another. Each column within this part of the brain seems to have a particular function in sensing the outside world. Another pioneer of neurophysiology, Edward Evarts, had developed the systems for these motor recordings, and Mountcastle later advanced them to allow recording in animals that were awake.

In the 1980s and 1990s, the University of Minnesota neuroscientist Apostolos Georgopoulos found additional evidence of brain cell specialization in experiments with monkeys. Georgopoulos and his colleagues showed that neurons in the motor cortex—the part of the brain that directs simple movements—can be active even when an animal remains still. By monitoring the firing of individual cells in the motor cortex, Georgopoulos could accurately predict the direction in which a monkey would extend its arm *before* the movement took place.

Scientists at Johns Hopkins University have studied the physiological basis of attention by recording brain cell activity in monkeys. The investigators placed microelectrodes in a part of the cortex located in the parietal area of the monkeys' brains. The animals performed visual tasks for seven to eight minutes, picking out targets on a computer screen, and then performed tactile tasks in which they manipulated a touch pad and keyboard for a similar period. When the monkeys switched between these two different kinds of tasks, each shift in attention was accompanied by sharp "spikes" of neurons firing together in the cortical region under study. The researchers suggest that a "chorus" of neural activity, with multiple nerve cells firing in unison, may help the brain focus attention on one item amid the flood of incoming sensory information.

Surgery on laboratory animals has also yielded revealing results in a burgeoning area of brain research: "plasticity," the brain's ability to change. In

BEYOND THE LABORATORY WALLS

Not all brain research depends on discoveries in the laboratory or clinic. Sometimes scientists are fortunate enough to find useful information that people have collected themselves. For instance, the order of nuns called the School Sisters of Notre Dame has been helping researchers at the University of Kentucky study aging and the brain, specifically Alzheimer's disease (C67). These women have agreed to be observed and interviewed, to undergo blood tests and other examinations, and to let their brains be studied after their death. What makes their cooperation more useful than a random group's is that the order also has detailed information dating back decades on each member's health, socioeconomic background, and education.

One part of this "Nun Study" looked at the handwritten autobiographies the nuns wrote in their youth, describing their lives before they joined the order. Researchers measured how grammatically complex the young women's sentences were, and how many ideas each presented. They found that these factors did not depend on how much education the women had when they wrote. But the complexity of their writing did correlate with how well the nuns performed on cognitive functioning tests decades later, and even with whether their brains showed evidence of Alzheimer's disease after death.

Other Nun Study researchers have examined the women's nutrition, a task made easier because nuns at a particular convent were all exposed to basically the same diet, environment, and health care. The scientists tested each group's blood for a variety of nutritional markers and, after the women died, examined their brains. One study found that a low level of folic acid in the blood was associated with atrophy of the cerebral cortex.

In another example of using evidence from outside the laboratory, a number of researchers have studied families' home videotapes of babies who developed schizophrenia (C25) as young adults. They looked for unusual behaviors that might identify infants at risk for developing this disorder. Different teams have reported a number of such signs, ranging from inability to make eye contact with others to an awkward manner of rolling over. At present, these signs are so subtle that researchers must be very well trained to spot them on the videotapes, and so far the studies have involved small numbers of infants. Nevertheless, this approach may contribute to a better understanding of the development of schizophrenia.

experiments at the Massachusetts Institute of Technology published in 2000, scientists "rewired" the brains of newborn ferrets so that signals from the eyes traveled to the auditory cortex—the part of the brain devoted to hearing—instead of to the visual cortex. The scientists rerouted nerves in the ferrets' brains in the same way that a mechanic might switch around wires in a car's engine. They tested the ferrets after the animals had matured into adults, finding physical changes in the auditory region that made it more closely match the visual center. The studies demonstrated the brain's remarkable ability to adapt—a capacity that might be exploited in the future to treat people's brain disorders during early stages of development.

New Tools for Illuminating the Brain

Spurred by rapid advances in computers over the past several decades, new technologies for brain imaging have helped change the way we look at the brain and suggested new ways to think about it. Although the imaging tools we use today still cannot tell us everything we would like to know about how the brain works, they provide important clues on where to look for answers in the near future.

The oldest technology for "looking" at what is going on in the living brain is electroencephalography (EEG), which measures the electrical activity of neurons inside the brain by means of electrodes attached to the patient's scalp. A major application of EEG, employed clinically for more than 50 years, has been to monitor brain activity during sleep and chart the different sleep phases, including the rapid eye movement (REM) and non-REM (slow-wave) stages. (For more on sleep, see **B3.**) Another common use of EEG is the clinical investigation of brain wave activity in epilepsy, in an effort to locate and understand the misfiring neurons. And researchers studying infant behavior have found EEG particularly useful because it easily picks up signals from within a baby's thin skull and involves simply placing a cap covered with sensors on the baby's head. Using EEG and these little caps, investigators studying how babies acquire language have made dramatic observations of changes that occur in infant brain waves in response to sounds in the language of their parents, compared with sounds in foreign languages (see chapter 6). But EEG cannot map the entire brain in detail because it lacks the resolution to monitor activity deep within the organ. Nevertheless, it remains a valuable research device for scientists studying important areas lying close to the surface.

X-ray computed tomography (CT), developed in the early 1970s, offered the first opportunity to produce X-ray images of the body's soft tissue, including the brain. (Traditional X rays can see only the skull, not the brain.) During brain scans, which may take just a few minutes, patients lie on a table that slowly moves through a doughnut-shaped scanner. X-ray beams pass through the brain at various angles and are collected as they emerge, changed by their interactions with brain tissue of varying density. A computer takes the information obtained from numerous X-ray transits to draw a three-dimensional picture of the brain. Clinicians commonly use these pictures to identify brain abnormalities.

Then physics joined computer science to produce positron-emission tomography (PET), invented soon after CT scans. PET was the first technology that could peer beyond anatomy to infer changes in brain activity as mental acts were performed. In typical PET studies, patients are injected with water in which the oxygen molecule bears a radioactive "label" that emits a low level of radiation for about 15 or 20 minutes. Researchers then track brain activity by monitoring blood as it flows through the brain, delivering the labeled oxygen to brain cells. The highest level of radioactivity indicates the site of the greatest blood flow and therefore the most cellular activity at any given fraction of a second.

Early PET used a chemically modified form of glucose, the fuel of brain cells, but because the cells trap this nutrient, it was not easy to tell when activity stopped—in other words, it was difficult to distinguish whether the cell was still using fuel or just sitting there. As a result, researchers had to keep their study questions very simple, so that

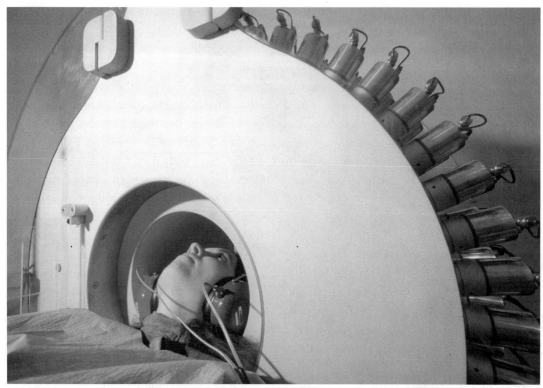

In positron-emission tomography (PET), the doughnut-shaped scanner detects low-level emissions from radioactive tracers injected in a subject to monitor blood flow increases in the brain's most active areas. The scan data are fed into a computer that produces images of the brain activity. PHOTO © DAN MCCOY/RAINBOW/PICTUREQUEST

some neurons would do a lot more work than usual and would therefore stand out from all the other neurons that already normally used a lot of glucose. Some favored early experiments were to move one hand or wriggle a few fingers to image that part of the motor cortex that represents the hand, and to flash lights in one eye to image the primary visual cortex. In contrast, oxygen molecules and their radioactive labels wash away when the cell is through with them. Also, the oxygen isotope (oxygen 15) that's used to emit positrons decays many times faster than the modified glucose. This meant scientists could observe many more patterns and much finer mental

activity, such as seeing, reading, speaking, and rhyming words.

In the late 1980s and early 1990s at UCLA, Michael Phelps (who with Michael Ter-pegossian had invented PET while both were at Washington University in St. Louis, Missouri) and John Mazziotta used the device to study the process of learning. Among their findings was that the extent of brain area devoted to a task shrinks and energy consumption diminishes as people learn to perform the task better. Moreover, responsibility for the action shifts over time from the cortex, a "high level" brain region, to more primitive brain structures, where the task is carried out with much less

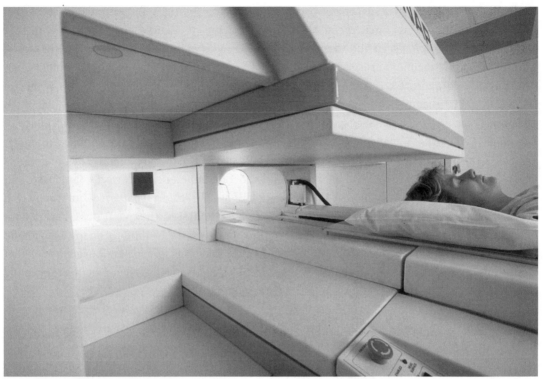

Magnetic resonance imaging (MRI) machines use radio waves and magnets to produce different kinds of images. A regular MRI shows structures of the brain in fine anatomical detail. Functional MRI (fMRI) is able to produce images of brain activity. Photo © Dan McCoy/Rainbow/PictureQuest

deliberation. In sum, tasks we do often truly do become easier and more routine.

In an intriguing 1996 experiment, Harvard researchers used PET to watch the brain making a mistake. Experimenters read a list of words to adult subjects. Ten minutes later, the subjects looked at another list and tried to identify the words they had just heard. The brain scans revealed a difference between those who remembered correctly and those who remembered incorrectly. Both sets of scans showed heightened activity in an area near the left hippocampus, a region important for memory formation. But scans associated with the correct memories also showed activity in the left temporal parietal area, where word recognition occurs, providing the researchers with a way to distinguish between accurate memory and errors—if only in this controlled situation.

The next advance, magnetic resonance imaging (MRI), is similar to CT technology, except that it probes the body with a combination of radio waves and a powerful magnetic field rather than X rays. Like CT, MRI yields anatomical, not functional, images of the brain and other interior zones of the body that have many useful medical applications. Neuroscientists usually use it to identify structural differences in the brain associated with psychiatric and neurodegenerative conditions. For example, researchers at Massachusetts General Hospital used MRI to spot early warning signs of Alzheimer's disease (**C67**), long before symptoms appeared. The entorhinal cortex, a tiny brain structure connected to the hippocampus, was 37 percent smaller (presumably due to nerve cell death) in patients who later developed Alzheimer's, as compared with subjects who remained disease-free.

As the inventors of PET technology had confirmed, blood flow increases in active parts of the brain. But the oxygen-carrying red blood cells also alter those areas' magnetic fields—and MRI machines are set up to measure magnetic fields. Therefore, in the early 1990s, scientists at Massachusetts General Hospital, the University of Minnesota, Washington University in Saint Louis, the University of Pittsburgh, and Carnegie Mellon developed ways to use a series of MRI scans to monitor blood flow and oxygen consumption. Scientists now compare MRI images of the brain at rest and in the midst of an activity such as listening to music, looking for the areas of increasing and decreasing activity. This technology, which came of age in the 1990s, is called functional MRI (fMRI).

Functional MRI made brain scanning a hugely popular research technique, not only because of its fine resolution but also because fMRI does not require the injection of radioactive tracers, which makes it safer for study volunteers, including children. Thus, researchers are using these scans in an effort to understand a wide variety of activities in a healthy brain, such as reading, speaking, looking at pictures, hearing a joke, experiencing pain, or recalling a disturbing memory. They are able to do this because, with fMRI, people's brains can be imaged while they participate in traditional cognitive psychology ex-

periments. In 1998, for instance, scientists at Massachusetts General Hospital in Boston used fMRI to capture what they suggested was "the birth of a memory." During the experiments, volunteers looked at a series of words while researchers monitored brain activity. Much of the neural firing occurred in the left parahippocampal cortex, a structure in the temporal lobe that is linked to the hippocampus. However, people who remembered those words later also displayed a characteristic pattern of brain activity in their left frontal and temporal lobes. That pattern did not appear in the fMRIs of people who forgot. For the first time, researchers looked inside other peoples' heads and predicted whether they would remember what they were seeing.

Functional MRI has also provided the first direct means of monitoring neural activity in a developing fetus, an impressive technological feat. Researchers at the University of Nottingham in England reported detecting changes in the fetal brain—namely, the activation of the temporal lobe—in response to the mother's voice.

But the utility of these techniques is not limited to providing insights only into normal brains. Both PET and fMRI have enabled researchers to find new aspects of brain activity to examine in the study of brain disorders, including addiction (**C29**), autism (**C5**), depression (**C20**), dyslexia (**C1**), epilepsy (**C13**), and schizophrenia (**C25**).

Of course the creative minds of imaging inventors are not leaving things there. Most recently, computer programmers have improved fMRIs by exploiting the technology's reliance on advanced mathematical computations to assemble a series of readings into a single picture of a brain. By applying more sophisticated mathematical tools, programmers can improve the resolution of these images, almost as if they were focusing a microscope lens. For example, researchers at the National Hospital for Neurology and Neurosurgery in London used computer software to compare MRI scans of people who experienced cluster headaches with those who did not. The computer analyzed tiny portions of the brain, one cubic millimeter (about six hundredths of a cubic inch) at a time. Before this study, conventional wisdom held that the brains of people who suffered from cluster headaches were structurally normal. But the London researchers reported a very slight increase in gray matter in the hypothalamus on the side where the headaches occurred. A cubic millimeter holds a few hundred neurons, so while it still has a long way to go, the technology is heading in the right direction.

Combining Technologies

Another tool, transcranial magnetic stimulation (TMS), relies on a pair of electromagnets to focus magnetic fields on specific brain areas, briefly inactivating them. The basic idea is to figure out what a brain structure does by seeing what happens when it is immobilized for a few thousandths of a second—a time so short that experimental volunteers often do not realize anything is amiss. Applying TMS to the area called V5 (the fifth relay level of the visual system after information has reached the visual cortex), for example, interferes with the perception of motion, supporting theories that V5 is the brain's motion detection center. When a magnetic pulse is directed to a region on the left side of the head, people momentarily lose the ability to talk, showing the importance of the area for speech. Scientists are combining imaging techniques, such as PET or fMRI, with TMS to see how different parts of the

cerebral cortex are connected. Other researchers are investigating how to use TMS to treat such conditions as depression (**C20**).

Magnetoencephalography (MEG), a technique for measuring neurally generated magnetic fields, can also complement fMRI. Although fMRI has good spatial resolution—it can accurately determine where in the brain something is happening—it is not nearly as good at pinpointing *when* events happen. Many brain processes occur within about a millisecond. MEG can clarify the picture by detecting rapid shifts in brain activity and describing what is happening millisecond by millisecond. As is the case with PET, MEG's resolution is enhanced when it is combined with MRI.

Scientists have also begun to combine tools from molecular biology with imaging techniques—a trend that should become even more prevalent in the future. PET scans, for instance, have become more versatile because scientists have learned how to create radioactive tracers that bind to specific molecules in the brain, including neurotransmitter receptors. Using PET scans to watch where these tracers end up can reveal, for example, a deficiency in receptors in a particular part of the brain. Researchers can now assess the course of Parkinson's disease (**C41**) by using tracers with imaging to reveal the extent to which dopamine-producing neurons have died—a hallmark of the disease. The technique thus allows for the evaluation of new therapies to see how well they stave off that damage. Similarly, targeting specific dopamine receptors with PET may identify people at risk for Huntington's disease (**C47**) before symptoms are evident.

It is important to note that these exciting tools for examining the brain have definite limits: while the scans reveal pathways and sequences of brain

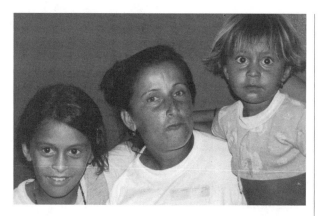

The people of Lake Maracaibo, Venezuela, have a high incidence of Huntington's disease (C47). Starting in the 1970s, they cooperated with scientists to help identify the cause of this fatal neurological disorder, providing medical histories and blood samples. Photo courtesy of Julie Porter/Hereditary Disease Foundation

activity, as well as many of the brain structures that participate, they do not resolve all the molecular questions about, for example, what genes and neurotransmitters are in use and what they contribute to the brain activity. For that, scientists must return to their petri dishes, jars of fruit flies, and cages of mice and rats and perform their traditional labors. These technologies have not replaced earlier methods but augmented them.

At the Level of Our Genes

Probably the greatest advance in medical research in the last half-century has been the discovery of the role of genes. Neuroscience has benefited from this knowledge as much as any other branch of medicine. Since the 1950s, we have known that each brain cell, like almost every other cell in our bodies, contains 23 pairs of chromosomes and that each chromosome is a long, twisted strand of deoxyribonucleic acid (DNA). In

2000 we learned the currently estimated number of segments—30,000 to 40,000—of that DNA that contain the blueprints for proteins that we need to live. These segments are what we call genes. Genes do much more than determine the traits that we are born with; they operate throughout our lives, turning on and off at particular times to initiate functions or when triggered by experiences or other cues.

The field of genetics is aiding brain exploration in many ways. In 1996 scientists at the Massachusetts Institute of Technology used a gene-splicing technique to create a breed of "knockout" mice that were missing the gene that makes a particular receptor for the neurotransmitter glutamate in the hippocampus. Lacking the receptor, the mice had difficulty figuring out how to navigate through a maze—a finding that supports theories tying molecular processes in the hippocampus to spatial learning.

In recent years, scientists have identified genes associated with a variety of neural conditions. The gene responsible for Huntington's disease (**C47**), for instance, was discovered in 1993 after an exhaustive search lasting more than 15 years. The first breakthrough came in 1983, with the discovery of a genetic marker for the disease: a DNA variation found only in people who had Huntington's. That marker provided a hint about the general location of the defective gene. Ten years later the gene itself was identified, owing to a telltale pattern—a "triplet" of DNA bases repeated an abnormally high number of times. Further research showed that the more repetitions that appeared in an affected person's genes, the earlier he or she showed the signs of Huntington's.

These discoveries about the Huntington's gene have inspired scientists to link genes with

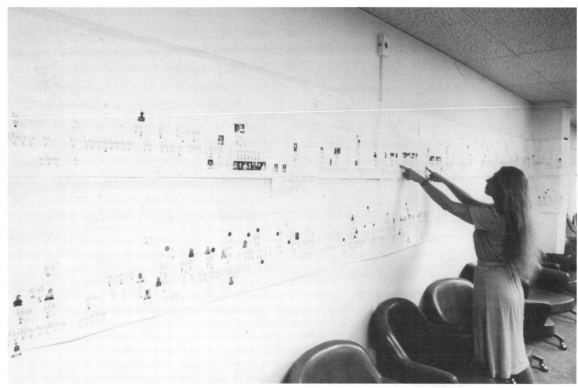

Dr. Nancy Wexler assembled a family tree of people near Lake Maracaibo who developed Huntington's disease, showing that they were all related to one woman and that the disease thus had a genetic basis. Further study revealed that a faulty gene on chromosome 4 is the source of this disorder, which allows doctors to identify people at risk. PHOTO © STEVE UZZELL

similar patterns of increasing repetitions to other diseases, thus suggesting how those diseases are passed down in some families with earlier and earlier onset as the number of repetitions grows. When Huntington's disease is inherited, the age at which the disease begins to be recognized gets younger and younger: a father shows it at 35; sons may show it in their 20s—a phenomenon called anticipation. Researchers also hope that by experimenting with the Huntington's gene in the laboratory, they will learn the basic mechanisms of the disease and be able to develop new therapies. So far there is increasing evidence that the dysfunctional Huntington's gene causes

problems with other genes, leading to the disorder's neuronal breakdown. Years after the discovery of the original gene, however, no effective treatment has been developed, and the research continues.

Frontiers of Neuroscience

When we deal with a system as complicated as the human brain, we can ask simple questions but cannot expect many simple answers. Nor can we hope to comprehend such sophisticated mental processes as attention, awareness, and consciousness just by seeing which parts of the brain "light up" during scans as a person performs all manner of tasks. Through imaging studies, animal experiments, and research in genetics and biology, we are clarifying some elements of brain function, bit by bit. The challenge ahead lies in putting these pieces together to form a cohesive picture. Through that effort, we hope to understand how the brain coordinates myriad processes and assimilates vast amounts of information to function as an integrated whole.

Do not expect a grand synthesis anytime soon, as progress toward this goal can be difficult to gauge. Indeed, sometimes it may seem as if we're going backward. Further explorations of the brain will uncover more, rather than less, complexity, bringing to light things we cannot yet fathom.

Given the immensity of the challenge, it may take a century or more to truly understand how the brain works.

This is no cause for despair, since—as scientific disciplines go—neuroscience is still in its relative infancy. Indeed, there is good reason for optimism, given that the brain is not the inscrutable black box it once was. The field has made great strides since Franz Gall tried to divine the brain's inner properties from the contours of the skull. With new tools at our disposal, and other powerful instruments continually being developed, it is now possible to study the brain in a much more systematic fashion. As a result, scientists are making steady progress, uncovering some of the brain's tightly held secrets, while leaving many other mysteries for future explorers.

CHAPTER 3

Basic Brain Care: Protecting Your Mental Capital

Each of us has just one brain, so probably the smartest single thing you can do in life is to treat your brain with care. What exactly does that mean? Although the development and organization of the brain are amazingly complex, taking care of it is really quite simple. The basics include sleeping well, eating well, staying fit, drinking in moderation, and taking routine precautions like fastening seat belts and wearing bicycle helmets. Obviously, some brain-related problems—such as a head injury (**C61**), stroke (**C59, C60**), a bout of depression (**C20**), or anxiety (**C21**)—require the attention of a neurologist, psychiatrist, or other specialist. But there is still a lot you can do on your own to get the most out of your brain and, in so doing, the most out of life.

To illustrate the value of basic brain care and to show how researchers are continuing to probe and refine these principles, we describe several recent studies in this chapter. As we said earlier, however, neuroscience is a never-ending process of refining ideas. Some of the research we cite may still need to be replicated and analyzed. It is important to state, therefore, that these studies are far from the only ones that support this chapter's basic advice. They are merely the latest investigations into the best way to take care of our brains.

The Slumbering Brain

Your parents probably told you about the benefits of a good night's sleep—especially on nights when they wanted one themselves. But what does sleep actually do for us? Surprisingly, science cannot yet answer this question in full. We cannot say exactly why we sleep nor what happens during the different stages of sleep. One thing we know for sure is that sleep keeps us alive. If rats are deprived of sleep for a couple of weeks, their appetite drops off, their body temperature becomes unstable, and they die. Researchers are convinced that humans, too, cannot survive a prolonged stretch of sleep deprivation. Fortunately, this theory has never been put to an empirical test.

Rest must be at least a partial answer to the question of why we sleep, but again, scientific knowledge is spotty on this issue. It is true that some parts of the brain are relatively tranquil at night, but other parts keep busy, performing critical jobs while the rest of the body goes on break. A number of recent studies suggest that at night our brains process information received during the day. In particular, the brain "consolidates" learning and memory during sleep, especially during the rapid eye movement (REM), or dream; phases. (For more about sleep stages, see section **B3**.)

Many researchers are now investigating sleep with the help of the latest technologies. In a study in 2000 at the University of California at San Diego, functional magnetic resonance imaging (fMRI) brain scans showed that sleep-deprived

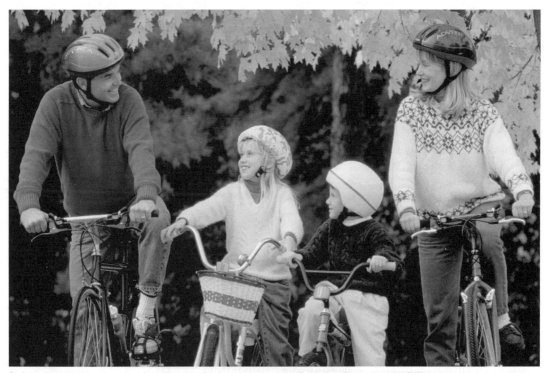

Safety first is the top rule of brain care. Brain injury is one of the leading causes of disability in the world. PHOTO © DAVID STOVER/STOCK SOUTH/PICTUREQUEST

subjects performing verbal tasks had to work harder—and recruit different parts of the brain to help out—than well-rested subjects performing the same tasks. In another brain imaging study that same year, this one using positron-emission tomography (PET) scans, researchers at the University of Liège in Belgium found that people learning a task at a computer displayed the same pattern of neuronal firing in the brain as they did that night during REM sleep. The team concluded that some sort of mental training goes on in the REM sleep phase to solidify the memories we acquire during the day.

A third study in 2000, at the Harvard Medical School, illustrated the drawbacks of cutting sleep short. Undergraduate volunteers learned to pick out visual targets on a computer screen and were tested on that skill later in the day. They showed no gain in proficiency. The students took the same test the following day. Those who had had more than six hours of sleep found the targets more quickly than before, but those who had slept less showed no improvement. As one of the researchers described it, this was "one of those 'your mother was right' studies." With any kind of learning, it is a good idea to sleep on it. Meanwhile, more studies are under way to explore the relationship between sleep and memory.

Food for Thought

For living, breathing, and thinking humans, just staying in place takes energy. Each of us needs energy, for example, to power our heart so that it can pump blood carrying oxygen and nutrients to the brain (among other spots in the body) to sustain the brain cells that keep our vital systems running. An active, learning human requires even more energy than a stationary one. Like any high-performance machine, the brain

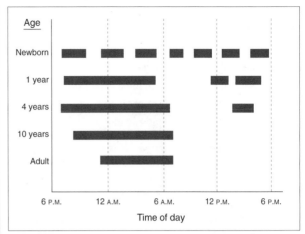

Our sleep patterns and needs change strikingly between infancy and adulthood, reflecting how intricately sleep is tied to the brain's health and development. Research is finding growing evidence of the vital importance of sleep for the brain at every age. Brain functions that depend on sufficient sleep include consolidation of memory, overall cognitive functioning, and body regulation, such as maintenance of body temperature and weight. CHART © LEIGH CORIALE

needs fuel, the higher quality the better. A good diet is essential for developing and maintaining a healthy nervous system—another thing your parents might have told you, although they probably put it in more general terms.

We all need protein to survive, but it is especially important for people undergoing rapid growth. For humans, the brain grows the most during the last several months in the womb and the first two years of life. (For more on this growth, see chapters 5 and 6.) In addition to protein, dietary fat is also critical for the formation of nerve and brain tissue during the first few years. Accordingly, parents and other caregivers should feed infants whole rather than skim milk, despite our national obsession with fat consumption. Undernourished babies can end up with lighter brains, with smaller brain cells that are fewer in

PROTECTING THE FORTRESS

Accidental injury—from car and motorcycle crashes, sports accidents, and falls—is one of the most common causes of brain trauma and death in the United States. Every year, about 2 million Americans suffer blows to their heads that can impair their thinking and physical functioning. An additional 15,000 Americans injure their spinal cords each year, leaving them partially or totally paralyzed. Yet there are many simple things we can do to minimize the odds of serious harm.

- Drive safely and wear seat belts to keep from getting thrown out of the vehicle or tossed around inside the vehicle.

- Dive into water only in safe areas, with no obstructions, where the water is at least ten feet (3 m) deep.

- Wear a helmet when motorcycling, bicycling, rollerblading, skateboarding, horseback riding, or playing such sports as hockey, football, and baseball. A 1996 study of 3,390 injured bicyclists in Seattle, published in the *Journal of the American Medical Association,* found that bike helmets reduced the risk of head and brain injury by 65 to 70 percent. Make sure that children get into the habit of wearing helmets, too, because the protection offered by helmets might be even better for them: a 1996 study in the journal *Pediatrics* concluded that if every child cyclist wore a helmet, bike-related injuries in the United States would decline by 83 percent and accidental deaths by 75 percent.

- Anyone who loses consciousness as a result of a blow to the head should be examined by a physician. However, people should also take seriously minor concussions, where there is no loss of consciousness. You should see a doctor after hitting your head if you experience lethargy, drowsiness, persistent nausea, visual disturbances, or abrupt changes in temperament.

- If a person sustains potentially serious neck or spine injuries from a fall, collision, or other cause, you should not move him or her, because you might damage the spinal cord. Instead, summon trained medical technicians to take the injured person to the hospital.

- Doctors have recently become concerned about "second impact syndrome"—a second head injury that closely follows a first. Even if the initial blow was relatively minor, the second trauma can lead to serious brain damage and even death. Athletes who have hit their heads should check with a doctor before returning to their sport, or consult guidelines devised by the American Academy of Neurology to minimize the risk of second impact syndrome.

number, with less extensive dendrite branching than average, and with less insulation of nerve fibers by the fatty coating called myelin—conditions that may be irreversible.

If taken by women of childbearing age before and during early pregnancy, the B vitamin folic acid can prevent birth defects of the brain and spine. Other B vitamins are required for the synthesis of neurotransmitters. Minerals such as iodine, iron, manganese, and zinc are also vital for the proper functioning of the nervous system, but they must be taken in the proper quantities: too

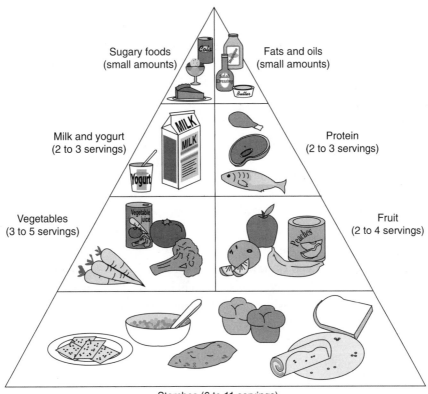

Sugary foods
(small amounts)

Fats and oils
(small amounts)

Milk and yogurt
(2 to 3 servings)

Protein
(2 to 3 servings)

Vegetables
(3 to 5 servings)

Fruit
(2 to 4 servings)

Starches (6 to 11 servings)

Good brain care is about the basics: eating healthfully, getting adequate sleep, and protecting your brain against traumatic injury. Since your body does not manufacture its own vitamins, eating the right balance of foods for good nutrition is necessary to keep your brain and nervous system in peak condition. SOURCE: CENTERS FOR DISEASE CONTROL; CHART © LEIGH CORIALE

much can be as bad as, or even worse than, too little.

Timing is significant in nutrition. Scientists have not worked out a precise feeding schedule that optimizes brain performance, but studies have demonstrated the importance of a good breakfast. Elementary school children, for example, improved their academic performance and had fewer behavioral problems after participating in a national school breakfast program, according to research at Massachusetts General Hospital and Harvard Medical School.

By now, it is common knowledge that a high-cholesterol diet, rich in saturated fats, can contribute to the clogging of arteries. That condition may in turn lead to a stroke that kills brain cells, impairing speech and other brain functions (**C59, C60**). A healthy diet helps keep your cholesterol level down, but eating for health does not mean you have to cut fat from your diet altogether. Cholesterol, for example, comes in two varieties: low-density lipoproteins and high-density lipoproteins. The first clog the arteries with fatty buildup, while the second clear arteries of such deposits. In addition, one type of fat commonly found in fish (omega-3 fatty acids) is needed to keep the nervous system running smoothly. Because fish is such a rich source of these essential fatty acids, it is sometimes called brain food or, as described in one article, "Prozac of the sea."

Although fats are a necessary part of sound nutrition, most Americans consume too much and would benefit from eating lower-fat foods. A recent study at Case Western Reserve University suggests that people with a genetic predisposition for Alzheimer's disease, having a susceptibility gene called ApoE-4, should consider a low-fat diet loaded with fruits and vegetables. The study found that people with the ApoE-4 gene had eight times the risk of getting the disease if they ate a high-fat, as opposed to low-fat, diet. Though more research is necessary on this question, the prescribed diet already makes sense for most people on nutritional grounds.

As a general rule, good nutrition for the body is good nutrition for the brain. Be wary of diets and products advertised as "brain food," which can throw off your nutritional balance. If you use common sense when it comes to diet, normally your brain will do just fine.

Special Diet for Epilepsy

Some doctors now recommend a special high-fat diet, in which most of the calories one gets each day come from things like butter and cream, for certain patients suffering from severe epilepsy (C13). The idea behind this "ketogenic" diet is that some of the fats are digested and converted into "ketones" that enter the brain and act as a sedative, damping down electrical disturbances. Although the diet offers potential benefits for those who have frequent seizures, it can also have harmful side effects. People should not try this diet without strict medical supervision.

Metaphysical Fitness

Working out does more than keep your muscles toned and your body trim; it can also keep your mind sharp. Although the mechanisms responsible for the benefits are not entirely clear, many studies are exploring how physical exercise helps the brain. The following is a sample of some promising experiments in this field.

One of the most straightforward benefits of exercise is that it promotes blood flow through the brain, supplying nerve cells with more oxygen and nutrients. Psychologists at the University of Illinois tested the benefits of exercise on three groups of laboratory rats. Two groups of rats were put on different exercise regimens, while the third remained sedentary. Autopsies revealed that the rats that exercised developed more capillaries around their neurons, which were capable of supplying their brains with more oxygen and nutrients.

A 1995 study at the University of California at Irvine concluded that the mental gains from exercise stem from more than just increased blood flow. Rats that exercised on treadmills had enhanced levels of brain-derived neurotrophic factor (BDNF), a "growth factor" or protein that sustains the function and survival of many types of neurons. The effect became more pronounced as the animals logged more miles; the animals that ran the farthest produced the most protein. The biggest increases in BDNF appeared in parts of the brain associated with memory and higher mental processing, including the hippocampus.

Many people consider exercise on a treadmill a mindless activity, but a 1999 study at the Salk Institute suggests otherwise. This project found that mice that exercised regularly on treadmills performed significantly better when tested in a maze than mice denied access to the treadmills.

Postmortem exams indicated that the mice who ran also had twice as many hippocampal cells as those who did not. Furthermore, when physical exercise is combined with mental exercise, there may be different, even more direct benefits to the brain. As part of the University of Illinois study mentioned above, researchers sent a fourth group of rats through a daily obstacle course that demanded balance and manual dexterity. This group formed relatively few new blood vessels around their neurons but a significant number of new synapses connecting them.

Although findings from animal experiments cannot be directly translated to humans, some of the foregoing results appear to be born out in human studies as well. In a University of Illinois study, researchers divided 100 sedentary adults, 60 to 75 years old, into two groups. One group walked vigorously three times a week; the other engaged in gentle stretch-and-tone exercises. Six months later, the walking group had quicker mental reaction times, performing "task switching" tests on a computer up to 25 percent faster than the stretch-and-tone crowd.

Regular aerobic exercise can also help you sleep better, especially if you do it three or more hours before bedtime, according to a 1997 study from the Stanford University School of Medicine. In addition, exercise can reduce stress, which takes its own toll on the brain.

Keeping Stress in Check

It's hard to deny that we live in a stressful society. Many of us are busy from the instant we wake up to the moment we fall asleep, taking care of children, commuting to and from work, putting in a solid eight to twelve hours at the office, keeping up with our reading and e-mail and phone correspondence, and then having to confront 100-odd cable TV channels. The human response to stress—an increase in heart rate, blood pressure, breathing, metabolism, and blood flow to muscles—has evolved over millions of years and is responsible, in no small measure, for the survival of our species. It also contributes to peak performance under pressure—an asset to athletes, firefighters, and countless others. But the inappropriate activation of the stress response, in a world where people rarely face life-or-death situations, can eventually damage both the heart and the brain.

Researchers have examined how stress affects people in various ways. As one example, in a five-year study published in 1998, psychologists gave memory tests to people in their 70s and asked them to find their way through different mazes. The subjects who did the worst on the tests had the highest levels of cortisol, a stress hormone in the glucocorticoid family. Over the years these same people had lost the most brain cells from the hippocampus, a brain structure critical for memory.

Some studies imply that there is a link between a shrinking hippocampus and chronic exposure to glucocorticoids like cortisol. We see this most clearly in an extreme condition called Cushing's syndrome, in which the adrenal glands release large quantities of glucocorticoids. This condition is accompanied by memory problems known as Cushingoid dementia. MRI brain scans performed at the University of Michigan showed that the hippocampus shrinks in Cushing's patients. People who secreted the most glucocorticoids suffered the most serious memory problems and the worst hippocampal atrophy.

However, other studies question whether the glucocorticoids alone are responsible for the de-

CELL PHONES AND YOUR BRAIN

More than 80 million Americans now use cellular phones, and that number is rising fast. With that growing use has come increasing popular concern that the radio waves emitted by these phones may cause brain cancer. Worries of this sort have continued for years despite the fact that no one has been able to produce firm evidence of a health hazard or show that the type of radio waves that cellular phones emit can penetrate beneath the skull.

Epidemiologists—scientists who study the prevalence and common factors of diseases in large groups—have examined health records of cellular phone users and people who have had brain diseases, and have found no unusual overlap between them. A report published in 2000 in the *Journal of the American Medical Association,* for instance, showed that people who spend more time talking on their cell phones do not have more cancers than people who use their phones less often. A study appearing the next year in the *New England Journal of Medicine* reached similar conclusions. In both cases, the researchers acknowledged that long-term studies are needed, given that people have not been using cell phones for very long. However, no cause for worry has emerged so far.

More studies will surely follow. Science cannot claim absolute certainty about these findings or any other. It is worth keeping in mind, however, that at the moment, the only documented health hazard posed by cell phones comes from using them while driving. A 1997 *New England Journal of Medicine* study found that the odds of having a crash increase fourfold when people drive while on the phone. So you don't need to give up your cell phone, but you ought to seriously consider turning it off when you drive.

generation of hippocampal neurons. A 1999 study performed at the University of Washington exposed aging rats to elevated glucocorticoid concentrations for 12 months without increasing their exposure to stress. The average size of the hippocampus in these rats, as well as the number and density of neurons in that region, remained the same as in an unexposed control group. Hippocampal damage, the researchers concluded, must arise from other effects of stress, perhaps in conjunction with elevated glucocorticoid levels but not due only to them. These results hint that the organic effects of stress on the brain are complex and unlikely to yield to a simple remedy.

Unfortunately, stress is not the only thing we have to worry about. Research at Washington University School of Medicine in St. Louis shows that chronic depression can also harm the hippocampus. In a 1999 study, investigators scanned the brains of 48 women, ranging from age 23 to 86. In women who had a history of depression, the size of the hippocampus was 9 percent to 13 percent smaller. The hippocampal volumes were smaller in women who had been depressed more often, but age was not a factor. Glucocorticoids may be involved here, too, as depressed patients produce abnormally high quantities of this stress hormone.

Fortunately, there are techniques for managing stress. Physical conditioning can help by lowering your blood pressure and resting heart rate. Exercise—such as aerobic workouts and competitive sports—can also provide an outlet for relieving some of the stress and frustration that build up in a day. Some people achieve deep relaxation through contemplative activities like yoga and meditation, while others may prefer listening to Mozart or wild dancing. People who handle stress well generally have strong social ties with others. Whenever possible, they avoid putting themselves in situations in which they feel helpless, buffeted by forces beyond their control. However, when things don't go their way, they try to take it in stride. (For more on the "mind-body connection," see chapter 4.)

Stimulation Throughout Life

Proper development of the brain requires stimulation through the different senses—touch, sight, sound, smell, and taste. The maturation of the nervous system, including the building and strengthening of connections among neurons, is shaped by stimulation of this sort and fine-tuned by years of experience. The importance of talking to children, exposing them to music and art, and keeping them involved in playful, creative activities as well as emotionally engaged, is clear. Despite all the marketing related to the "Mozart effect" and other forms of stimulation for young children, there is little hard evidence for the notion of achieving additional benefits—some kind of "mental bonus"—through superenriched environments and enhanced stimulation. In fact, overstimulating children can be counterproductive by causing stress.

Many researchers are now skeptical of the idea of a "critical window" of opportunity during the first three years of life. The brain is, without question, extremely malleable in the early years, but recent studies show that it does not become un-

bendable, or "hardwired," at the end of childhood or even in adolescence. Indeed, the phenomenon of "neural plasticity"—the brain's ability to generate new cells, forge new connections, and strengthen old ones—persists into adulthood. And we get the most from our brains by keeping them exercised, a strategy sometimes called "use it or lose it."

A 1995 Harvard Medical School study of 1,192 people aged 70 to 79 found that intellectual vigor and physical fitness can both keep people mentally sharp and keep more brain cells alive. The researchers speculate that by having more brain cells "in reserve," people may be able to stave off memory loss and dementia—conditions once considered almost inevitable by-products of old age. A steady dose of novel challenges and stimulating tasks, it appears, may be the ticket to cerebral fitness for both young and old.

Similar results have been found from studying the world's oldest people, centenarians. In 1992 researchers at the Harvard Medical School launched the New England Centenarian Study (NECS) to systematically analyze all people 100 years old and over in an eight-town area around Boston to learn how they reached such advanced ages while avoiding the common age-related diseases. Several findings have emerged from this pioneering work.

Part of the reason many centenarians maintain a high cognitive level is that they keep their minds active in a variety of ways: they may continue to work, read challenging books, play bridge, or do crossword puzzles. Learning a foreign language promotes the growth of dendrites, forging new connections between neurons. Complex activities like music, painting, and dance, which involve different parts of the brain, can provide a "whole-brain workout," the NECS authors conclude. By expanding neuronal networks, these people may build up a "functional reserve" that helps them compensate for changes associated with aging.

Healthy centenarians also keep physically active, as much as possible, and do not smoke. They avoid alcohol and drug abuse—practices that can lead to memory problems, dementia, and other forms of mental impairment. Not surprisingly, most have found ways to keep stress under control, either because of their innate dispositions or because of deliberate choices. One centenarian in the NECS study, after realizing that "worrying didn't do any good," decided to become a "fun guy" who wouldn't worry about anything.

It is unrealistic to assume we can all become stress-resistant personalities by an act of will. Some people seem to be born with temperaments that make them more prone to anxiety than others (**B9**). Nor can we all expect to live to 100. But by pursuing a healthy lifestyle as best we can, we can lead richer and fuller lives, while preserving the mental capacity to enjoy them.

The Brain-Body Loop

If someone you love is gravely ill, you say you are "sick at heart." You may have a boss who makes your stomach churn. At sixteen, you blush when someone you secretly adore sits next to you in the library. Occasionally, you may be so worried you can't sleep, feel your head pounding at the end of a frustrating day, or find your heart racing when you spot a police car with its light flashing in your rearview mirror. These feelings show the brain's power to control your body.

That power flows in the opposite direction, too: eating, sex, exercise, illness, injury, and other physical experiences also affect what you think and feel. As simple an event as the enjoyment of a good meal will likely boost your sense of overall well-being and tranquillity. Jogging, swimming, or even a brisk walk around the block can make you feel energized and upbeat. Having a cold, the flu, or an aching back may make you cranky, perhaps even blue. Even minor everyday physical insults such as a paper cut or a stubbed toe may briefly upset your mood, while small positive physical encounters—a dental assistant's hand on your arm when you're getting a tooth drilled—can lessen pain and anxiety.

Most of us are familiar with the idea that our mental states and emotions influence a host of bodily functions and that the opposite is also true, but the ebb and flow of our feelings are just the beginning of the story. As scientists take advantage of

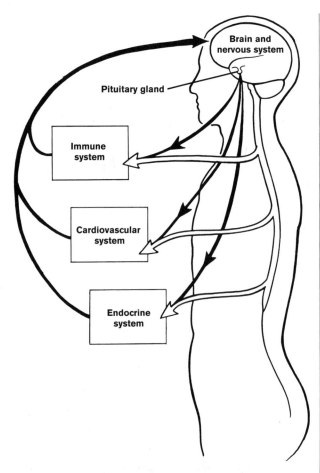

The brain-body loop. The main communications systems of the body—immune, cardiovascular, and endocrine—are influenced by the brain through direct nervous system activity and circulating hormones. In turn, they feed back signals to the brain—completing the loop. ILLUSTRATION © KATHRYN BORN

ever more refined information about how cells work—the physics and chemistry of both the brain and the body, and how our genes function—the picture of brain and body interactions is beginning to gain detail and become vastly more interesting. Already medical and scientific research to understand how brain and body communicate has provided fascinating clues to the different systems

that link brain and body in constant dialogue and feedback. Whole disciplines in brain research are developing around the many ways in which the brain acts as the body's central command post (see chapter 9, "The Body Manager").

The brain is connected to every part of the human body, and to the outside world, by a communications network dominated by two major components, nerves and messenger chemicals, primarily neurotransmitters and hormones. Nerves form circuits that extend from the brain to the spinal cord and then to both the interior and the farthest reaches of the body. Hormones produced by the body's glands and internal organs speed messages along these nerve pathways. The brain is able to interpret these hormonal messages with the help of special receptors and then send out messages of its own. These busy communications circuits—and we have quite a few of them, often performing simultaneously—make up, in effect, an intricate "brain-body loop."

The brain-body loop orchestrates the most familiar routines of our lives: the daily rhythms by which we sleep, wake, and go about our activities, our eating behavior, sex life, and the very act of navigating our environment from minute to minute. The interaction of brain and body managed by this system is also proving to be an important influence on the state of our overall health and mental vitality, often in ways we modify.

Circadian Rhythms

The sun rises, and night gives way to day. Light fades, and night returns. The brain uses these daily signals to set the body's own internal clocks. Researchers estimate that people have more than 100 daily cycles, known as circadian rhythms, *cir-*

cadian meaning "about a day." Some of our rhythms, such as the menstrual cycle, are much longer than a day, and others, such as the several cycles that make up a night's sleep, are shorter (or "ultradian"). The best known circadian rhythm is the sleep-wake cycle, but others include the daily rise and fall of body temperature, hormone levels, and urine production. An internal biological clock, or "pacemaker in the brain," generates and regulates the rhythm of cellular activity. Messages then travel from the pacemaker to the appropriate part of the body. Various genes function as off-and-on switches to keep the clock ticking. External signals—sunlight is by far the most potent—provide time cues to synchronize bodily functions.

The pacemaker is housed in two small clusters of cells in the hypothalamus known as the suprachiasmatic nucleus (SCN). The SCN takes its name from its location, which is "supra," or above, the optic chiasm, a major junction for nerves that transmit information from the eyes to the brain.

The sleep-wake cycle illustrates how the SCN regulates circadian rhythms. Studies of humans living in time-isolation laboratories—research apartments with no windows, clocks, or other time cues—show that people naturally sleep about one-third of the time and remain awake about two-thirds of the time, living on days that are slightly longer than 24 hours. Their schedule thus drifts slowly around a real-time clock. In the outside world, sunlight anchors the sleep-wake cycle to Earth's 24-hour rotation, programming us to stay awake in the day and to sleep at night. Sunlight enters the eyes, where it is converted to electrical impulses in the retinas, the nerve cells in the back of the eye. Light signals then travel to the SCN.

Once we are awake, the clock begins ticking on

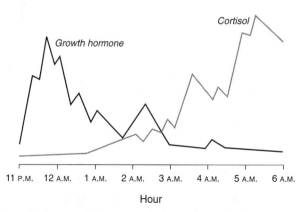

The brain regulates many body cycles. The chart shows secretion patterns of growth hormone and cortisol during sleep. Growth hormone levels, responsive to biological rhythms, drop during the night. Levels of cortisol, one of the stress hormones, increase as the night goes on, to help the body gear up for the stress of waking and the activities of the coming day. Graph © Leigh Coriale

the ultradian rhythms that cause fluctuations in our attentiveness throughout the day. The output pathway probably extends from cells in the SCN to other parts of the hypothalamus, the pituitary gland, and the pineal gland, as well as to portions of the brain stem involved in sleep regulation. A number of different hormones act on nerve cells in this circuit, to either induce sleepiness or facilitate wakefulness. For instance, cells in the SCN contain receptors for melatonin, a sleep-inducing chemical produced by the pineal gland that increases in quantity at night and falls after dawn. Other neurotransmitters involved in the sleep-wake cycle include acetylcholine, noradrenaline, serotonin, and histamine; these act in the brain, in the cortex and thalamus, where attention and consciousness are maintained. It is still not clear exactly how all these neural circuits induce sleep or stimulate wakefulness, but there appears to be a seesaw mechanism:

in the *pons* (meaning "bridge"), which connects the medulla, atop the spinal cord, and the midbrain, the activity levels of certain neurons rise and fall, and cells in the thalamus and cortex speed up or slow down in response.

When the body's daily rhythms fall out of sync with those of the outside world, the result can be physical fatigue and mental sluggishness. A common example of this is jet lag, which occurs after travel across multiple time zones, when our biological clocks take a few days to adapt to the new local time. People who work at night or rotate shifts face similar difficulties.

Eating Behavior

Until almost the end of the twentieth century, those of us carrying around extra pounds could say only, "I'm naturally big" or "It runs in the family." The only role in weight control that we ascribed to the brain was a moral one, responsibility for willpower. Brain research beginning in the 1970s, however, began to show that body weight is not that simple. In the early part of that decade scientists began to identify the chemicals the brain uses to direct us to eat and to learn how messages of hunger and fullness sent from the body are processed in the brain. It now seems likely that controls in the brain set a person's body weight, and if they work properly, we will be healthy, though quite possibly at a point slightly above or below what is fashionable. Metabolism is more clearly a task of the brain, and genes that may contribute to weight problems are active in the brain, too.

The most basic brain-body circuit governing eating behavior consists of the brain's control through the autonomic nervous system together with blood-borne hormones that carry messages from the body back to the brain. When you taste food, nerves from both your taste and smell receptors activate processing structures in the brain that signal the hypothalamus. The hypothalamus then relays that information to autonomic neurons that control the gastrointestinal tract, to begin the process of secretions that allow food in the stomach to be digested and moved on. As food reaches the stomach, a number of digestive hormones, known collectively as satiety factors, are released. As the stomach fills, levels of these hormones rise, signaling the brain and prompting a decision to stop eating.

Several recent discoveries suggest that other neural pathways may be involved as well. In the past few years, scientists have identified hormones in other parts of the body besides the stomach that also appear to signal the hypothalamus and thereby influence eating behavior. These include leptin, a protein contained in fat cells, and dopamine, a neurotransmitter in the brain involved in the regulation of some hypothalamic eating and drinking circuits. As researchers have studied the traffic in these hormones and neurotransmitters, they have come to believe that body weight is maintained within a narrowly defined "setpoint" as the brain increases or decreases appetite and metabolism to keep the body's fat stores stable. Enthusiastic publicity for some of these findings has raised high hopes for new weight-loss drugs that may precisely target the brain systems for eating behavior. But many questions remain about how this complicated brain-body system actually works. Research advances in this area will also likely benefit people with disorders such as compulsive eating and anorexia, which may be related to flaws in one of the brain-body loops that govern eating behavior.

Sexual Response

We are animals at heart when it comes to sex. What may seem like magic—that first tingle of attraction, the pleasurable muscle contractions of orgasm—actually shares the same chemical and electrical genesis as any other biological event. In fact, animal research has provided some intriguing clues about this particular brain-body connection. In rats, for instance, scientists have found that the hormone estrogen increases the electrical activity of cells in the medial hypothalamus of the female brain. Progesterone enhances the effects of estrogen by increasing sensitivity to touch. An excited female rat, responding to both a male's touch and her own hormonal flood, will crouch and raise her rump. This posture, which facilitates intercourse and fertilization, results when hormones begin racing along several neural circuits that extend from the medial hypothalamus to the midbrain, and then down to the spinal cord, where motoneurons activate muscle spasms and stretching. At the same time, the medial hypothalamus is sending other signals, which affect heart rate and breathing.

Still, as anyone knows, it's not all hormones and mechanics. In people, cultural values, personality, and social cues also affect sexual behavior, although scientists do not yet know the biochemical pathways that underlie this influence. But, clearly, the cerebral cortex also plays a role in physical sexual arousal and behavior.

Navigating Our Environment

We see a car coming toward us in the street and step out of the way. We smell some chocolate-chip cookies baking and walk into the kitchen to get some. Every day we use our senses to detect changes in our environment—some good, some not—and then act on them. Our ability to navigate our environment in this way depends on our brain's ability to detect and interpret signals and then send its own commands to parts of the body that can respond. To figure out how the brain's command and control systems work, scientists must break things down into almost absurdly small components. For example, a study of how the brain may cause movement may consist of scanning the brain while a volunteer lies perfectly motionless except for tapping a finger. But this kind of careful investigation does pay off, and in recent years scientists have learned more about how our brain guides our body in ordinary ways.

In addition to the five major senses (sight, hearing, touch, taste, and smell), the brain also works with the body to maintain a sense of balance (equilibrium), monitor body and limb positions (proprioception), and keep track of movement (kinesthesis). Additional sensing systems continually track body temperature, blood chemistry, and hormone levels. With all this sensing going on, it's a wonder our brains don't collapse from sensory overload. Fortunately, the brain is as skilled at sorting sensory information as it is at detecting it in the first place. Each piece of sensory information is channeled into a specific neural pathway in the brain and then relayed upward through a series of hierarchical circuits. For instance, after you taste something sweet, the information is relayed first to the medulla, in the brain stem, then to the thalamus, and finally to the somatosensory cortex, at which point you decide whether you want to eat more of this substance.

As efficient as the brain is at sensory processing, these complex systems sometimes break

REWIRING THE BRAIN

Until recently, scientists believed that the death of brain cells after a stroke meant permanent loss of function. An intriguing study of stroke survivors by a team at the University of Alabama, however, suggested the brain may be able to rewire its circuitry to improve the chances of accomplishing former tasks again.

In this study the researchers first mapped the activity of the area of the brain's cerebral cortex that controls an important hand muscle. They then examined this area in 13 stroke survivors, finding it smaller on the side of the brain damaged by a stroke than the comparable area on the brain's nondamaged side. Next, they restrained each person's "better" arm, the one less affected by the stroke, keeping the subjects from using this arm in most of their waking hours for two or three weeks.

Forced to use their damaged arm more, the patients gradually acquired more power to move it. They regained their ability to hold silverware, brush their teeth, and carry objects. Moreover, the critical area of their brains also increased in size, starting as soon as the first day after treatment began.

The rehabilitation technique, the researchers reported, recruited additional areas of the brain to participate in the production of movement following a stroke. The study authors proposed that the use of this or other rehabilitation techniques or even medications may prompt certain areas of the brain to take on functions disrupted by a stroke or other injury, a process termed cortical reorganization.

Other studies are attempting to confirm or clarify the significance of this "forced-use protocol," since actively trying to induce cortical reorganization would be a sea change in strategies for poststroke recovery.

down. In an unusual disorder, an agnosia (**C72**) called hemisomatopagnosia, damage to the brain from stroke or trauma can leave a patient adamantly denying the very existence of an arm or a hand or even one whole side of the body. And many scientists believe flaws in sensory processing may contribute to some of the symptoms of more common disorders, such as autism, schizophrenia, and dyslexia.

Learning from the Body

The remarkable phenomenon that researchers call plasticity is the brain's power to build new connections among neurons and, under certain conditions, reroute whole pathways. Plasticity underlies all growth and development in the brain, from infancy to the end of life, and is the basis of learning, a process we tend to consider abstract and intellectual. But the brain is a learning machine, and now researchers are discovering ways that it also learns purely from the body's experiences.

If you are trying to master a new skill or improve one you already have, brain plasticity offers you a distinctly novel way to think about your progress. In the mid-1990s, researchers in Germany conducted brain imaging studies on professional violinists, whose instrument requires intricate finger movements by one hand. The scans showed that in the violinists' brains the area of the motor cortex that commands finger movement had become larger than the same area in the brains of nonplaying study participants. And in further examining their data, the researchers found that the younger the violinists were when they started playing, the bigger the corresponding area in the motor cortex was. The scientists believe the musicians' brains responded to the greater and more complex finger use needed for professional-level skill by producing many times more connections in that area. Thus, if you decide to learn a physical skill, from piano playing to roller-skating, you can talk yourself through the hard times by reminding yourself that you're making some site in your brain sizzle.

Also mining the brain-body connection are researchers who suspect that this interaction can bring advances in the treatment of physical disabilities. Two fields in which interest is particularly strong are those of stroke treatment and spinal cord injury. In both fields, recent experiments—none yet widely replicated and involving a very small number of patients—have sought evidence for the proposition that messages from the body can stimulate recovery in the brain and spinal cord. These experiments involve long, intensive, and sometimes grueling sessions of coaxing the paralyzed limbs back into use. The theory is that enough stimulation from the moving muscles can induce rewiring in the damaged brain or cord well enough to improve, if not restore, mobility and reduce the patients' disabilities.

For the most part, brain-body systems are self-directing, but we do have a degree of control over them. Thus, most obviously, we can consciously decide whether or not we will do anything about a powerful sexual attraction. We can take steps to reset our Miami- or New York–based body clock if we travel to Los Angeles or London, and we can keep practicing piano or guitar until we play without a hitch. It is unclear whether we can adjust comfortably to a lower body weight than our setpoint if we have an urgent reason, such as damaged knees from playing sports in school. In such circumstances, we can probably get used to reduced food intake, but most studies show that keeping weight down is not a simple set-and-forget operation like our circadian clock's ability to adapt when we visit a different time zone.

Two other areas of brain-body interaction have come under increasing study in recent years and, as a result, present excellent opportunities for patients and physicians to use the brain-body connection to assist in maintaining health and improving healing in illness. These are the stress response and the emotions, two systems that appear to share some neural circuitry and that can do both good and harm.

The Stress Response and Disease

In the early twentieth century, the pioneering physiologist Walter Cannon fed dogs their food mixed with barium and then, using a fluoroscope, watched the progress of that material through the dogs' intestines. He discovered that whenever a dog perceived a threat, the barium would stop moving. In effect, the dog's gastrointestinal tract shut down. Eventually, Cannon linked this effect to the secretion of a hormone he called sympathin from the adrenal medulla, a gland in the abdomen closely controlled by the autonomic nerves. He theorized that by halting the digestive system, this hormonal signal freed up more of the dog's energy to either combat whatever had

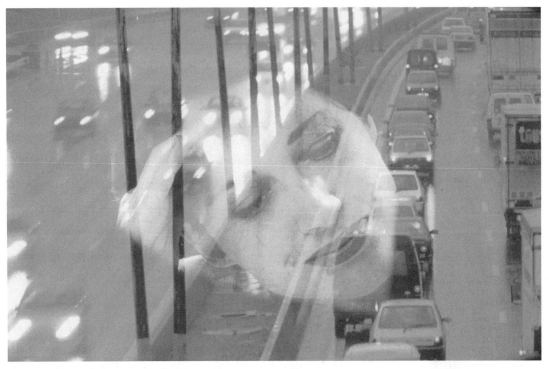

© IFA/eStock Photography/PictureQuest

aroused it or to run away. Cannon termed that response to stress "fight or flight," and it has become a basic part of how we think about our own brain-body connection.

We all encounter stresses—good and bad—every day. We face deadlines, hit traffic jams, quarrel with spouses, worry about children. We fall in love, hear praise for a job well done, score the winning run. Without such peaks and valleys, our lives would be flat and dull. Any experience may frighten some of us but delight others: consider how you feel about riding a roller coaster or giving a speech. "Strange to say," Barbara Kingsolver writes in *The Poisonwood Bible*, "if you do not stamp yourself with the words 'exhilarated' or 'terrified,' those two things feel exactly the same in a body."

If you hear footsteps behind you while walking in the dark, you will likely respond much as your ancient ancestors did when they heard a vicious beast crashing through the forest. Your brain alerts your adrenal glands to dispatch stress hormones throughout your body to prepare you to wrestle or run. These hormones, epinephrine (adrenaline) and norepinephrine (noradrenaline), make your heart beat faster, your blood pressure soar, your muscles tense, and the pupils of your eyes open wider. You become more energized and more focused. Blood drains from your stomach and intestines as digestion is put on hold. It goes to the limbs to fortify your muscles. Your awareness of pain falls, distracting you from a sprained ankle or other injuries you might suffer as you act. Like Cannon's dogs, you are ready for fight or flight.

If those frightening footsteps turn out to come from a passing jogger, you will probably calm

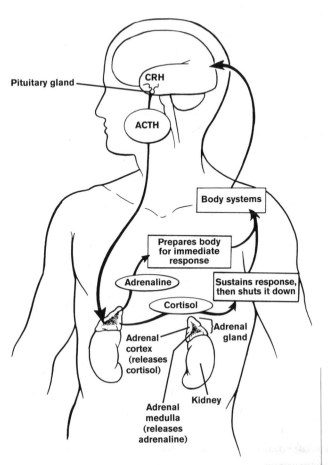

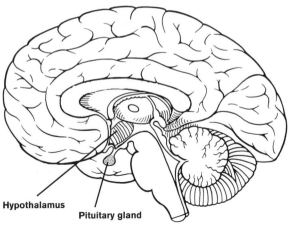

The major communication center for brain-body interaction, the hypothalamus works with the pituitary gland to regulate your body's hormones. When you have a "stress response," these two structures throw the adrenal glands into high gear for "fight or flight." ILLUSTRATION © KATHRYN BORN

When the brain perceives a stress stimulus, it immediately releases adrenaline from the adrenal glands, and corticotrophin-releasing hormone (CRH) from nerve cells in the hypothalamus. CRH travels to the pituitary gland, where it triggers the release of adrenocorticotrophic hormone (ACTH), which then stimulates the production of cortisol in the adrenal glands. Cortisol sustains energy, but it also curbs the surge of adrenaline and turns off CRH. ILLUSTRATION © KATHRYN BORN

While this genetically programmed response may help you face an attacker, the stresses we encounter in our daily lives do not often demand intense physical action. Nevertheless, our bodies may still respond that way. According to the National Institute for Occupational Safety and Health, one in four employees views his or her job as the number one stressor in life. Running from or fighting off a saber-toothed tiger may have kept your distant ancestor alive, but facing a snarling boss requires different behavior. Your body's evolutionary responses can give you the energy to work longer, but they can also make it harder to think or speak clearly in a tense meeting. Either way, you can feel chewed up inside.

Individuals respond to stress in different ways, however. Some people seem to remain unruffled—eating and sleeping normally, remaining physically healthy. Small hassles leave others feeling constantly "stressed out"; Bruce Springsteen

down fast. You *need* to calm down to avoid overtaxing several of your body systems. The next night, you may feel your heart thump as you approach the same spot. That is your brain working, warning you of possible danger.

describes this state in "For You" when he remembers a woman beset by crises: "Your life was one long emergency." Our reactions to different types of stresses help define our individual psychologies. Even infants display wide variation in how they respond to novelty and stress, a demonstration of our innate basic temperaments (**B9**).

Stress and Some Common Illnesses

To study stress, researchers assess an individual's responses to a wide variety of challenges and compare them with those of other people in similar circumstances. Emotional stress tests include being asked to do mathematical computations, give a speech, watch scary movies, or perform certain exercises. Researchers may measure levels of epinephrine, norepinephrine, and other biological markers of stress in blood and urine, or assess volunteers' blood pressure around the clock. They may also use techniques such as functional magnetic resonance imaging (fMRI) to study areas of the brain that become active as people engage in different mental tasks.

In one study of life stress, 276 healthy volunteers completed questionnaires about their life stressors, personality traits, social networks, and health practices. The researchers then gave these men and women nasal drops containing a low dose of a common cold virus. Over the next five days, the research team monitored the volunteers to see whether they developed infections and congestion, runny nose, sneezing, and other symptoms of illness. Blood tests showed 84 percent of the participants had been infected by the virus, but only 40 percent of them developed cold symptoms. What accounted for the difference? The people who reported job stress or problems with family or friends in the previous year that had lasted for a month or more were two to three times more likely to get sick than those without such troubles.

Chronic stress, as well as anger and hostility, may increase the concentration of acid in the stomach, possibly triggering peptic ulcers, stress ulcers, or ulcerative colitis. While a chronic infection of the stomach lining by the bacterium *Helicobacter pylori* is the prime culprit in nearly all peptic ulcers, many people with this infection do not develop ulcers. Stress may be what makes some individuals more susceptible than others. Air traffic controllers at busy major city airports, who clearly have high-stress jobs, report peptic ulcers more frequently than both controllers working in less-populated areas with lower flight traffic and air industry workers with less stressful jobs.

These findings, in a sampling of diverse diseases, remind us how the brain affects the body at many levels. And the body's general well-being affects the brain. Everyone knows it's no fun being sick, and trying to keep up with tasks at home or work while you're sick can cause stress. Thus, people can enter a cycle in which stress makes them vulnerable to illness, illness causes them stress, and so on. This is the brain-body feedback loop at its most troublesome.

Fortunately, stress management has long been a popular area of concentration in many fields, and good techniques and strategies are easy to find. They are available in every conceivable setting, from business seminars and health clubs to the offices of psychologists and family doctors. If you feel that your stress response is "on" more than it should be, a careful canvass of the stress management approaches that seem appropriate to you should lead you to one that will be helpful. Oftentimes, in the reinforcing company of people with the same goal, you can lower your stress response simply by reforming stress-related bad habits: smoking, too much drinking, careless eating, and staying up too late too many nights.

Chronic, inescapable stress, such as that incurred by taking care of a terminally ill family member or facing a long-term financial crisis, may have serious health consequences. If you or someone you care about is ensnared in a deeply stressful state of affairs that may not be resolved for months or years, confiding in a trusted medical or mental health professional is important. Plans for a respite schedule, guidance to support groups, and many other valuable coping strategies can be the beginning of lightening the load. It is extremely hard for anyone in a chronic stress situation to go it alone.

Mood and Health

When brain scientists refer to "mood" and "emotions," they are being much more precise than most of us are when we say we "got up on the wrong side of the bed" or are "happy as a clam." To the scientist, mood—more often called affect—and emotions are the mental states related to specific chemicals and pathways in the brain. And because these brain circuits undeniably communicate with the body, researchers are beginning to look for potentially important connections between mood and health. And in this respect, the likelihood that mood, emotions, and stress all share some pathways seems to offer an especially valuable relationship for study.

Depression and the Heart

Most people know that the stress of sudden shock or fright can trigger heart attacks. News reports of an earthquake, hurricane, or other natural disaster often include the number of people brought to hospitals after suffering heart attacks.

For example, immediately after the Northridge, California, earthquake in 1994, the local incidence of sudden death from heart attacks jumped sixfold.

But emotional stress can be comparable in effect to moderate physical stress for people with heart conditions, according to one study. Researchers asked 132 people with heart disease to wear a device that monitored their heart activity for 48 hours. The volunteers also kept diaries in which they noted their activities and emotional states roughly every 20 minutes. Fifty-eight people had episodes in which the blood supply to their hearts fell too low, a condition known as ischemia. Feelings of tension, frustration, and sadness produced changes comparable to moderate or light physical activity. By contrast, participants experienced fewer episodes of ischemia when they reported feeling happy or in control.

In any year, about 7 percent of Americans, 17 million people of all ages, experience mood disorders such as depression (**C20**). Depression is an independent risk factor for heart disease, many controlled studies show. These include an ongoing study of nearly 1,200 male medical students who enrolled at the Johns Hopkins University School of Medicine between 1948 and 1964. About 12 percent of these students eventually developed depression. These men were more than twice as likely to have heart attacks as peers who were not depressed, even decades after first being diagnosed with the mood disorder.

After suffering a heart attack, people with depression also tend to be sicker than people whose moods remain stable. A group of researchers analyzed data from 8,000 people enrolled in the first National Health and Nutrition Examination Survey (NHANES I). Participants were healthy when they entered the study between 1982 and 1984 and completed a standard test for depression. The researchers assessed their health again in 1992 or after they had had a heart attack. Depressed people proved nearly twice as likely to have suffered a heart attack as those who had no depression. Other studies have found that depression also hastens death from heart disease.

But associations, even when they are as clear as these, are not hands-down proof that mood affects health and vice versa. Certainly the studies offer intriguing clues that this might be so, but the nature of this particular brain-body interaction remains sketchy at best. Still, the observed link between depression and heart disease is the strongest evidence so far. Researchers have found that about 65 percent of patients will suffer depression immediately following a heart attack. One in four of them will develop severe and recurrent clinical depression. At the same time, other studies have suggested that depressed people are more likely to develop heart disease. In one large population study, 18 percent of depressed people had coronary artery disease, compared with only 5 percent of those who were not depressed. Other intriguing clues come from reports that regular aerobic exercise—which improves cardiovascular health—can also improve mood. In fact, one recent study found that moderate exercise might be as effective as medication in treating depression.

But which comes first, depression or heart disease? The fact that the two appear together so often suggests the existence of a distinct brain-body circuit. Scientists do not yet know what such a circuit might consist of, but they have identified several chemical messengers that may be involved. It has been reported that specific neurotransmitters—serotonin and the catecholamines epinephrine (adrenaline) and norepinephrine (noradrenaline)—are found in reduced levels in the cerebral spinal fluid of people with depression or anxiety. These same substances, acting as hormones in the body, also have a role in cardiac function by increasing heart rate, raising blood pressure, and strengthening the contractions of the heart. Catecholamines also increase the "stickiness" of blood platelets, which help to form clots, and decrease anticlotting compounds in the bloodstream. The brain's mood-regulating systems and the heart clearly share some chemicals. Whether this constitutes a bona fide brain-body link remains to be seen.

Depression and Stroke

The same NHANES data also showed that people with depression are nearly twice as likely to suffer strokes as their nondepressed counterparts. On the other side of the brain-body loop, almost everyone who suffers a stroke experiences some feelings of depression, either soon after the event or some months later. About half suffer what doctors call clinical depression, mood changes serious enough to require medication or other treatment. Most of these people did not experience depression before suffering a stroke, suggesting that the mood disorder arises from both biological factors provoked by their brain injury and their response to being impaired.

Anger

In one large study, researchers followed nearly 13,000 healthy participants for six years. These people completed a self-test by responding to statements such as "I am a hotheaded person" and "When I get angry, I say nasty things," ranking their experience with anger on a scale from "almost never" to "almost always." Those who identified themselves as highly prone to rage proved nearly three times more likely to have a heart attack in the following years than people with even tempers. A high propensity for anger, the researchers found, put people at higher risk of heart attacks regardless of whether they also smoked, were obese, or had high blood pressure.

Given findings about anger as a trigger for heart attacks, researchers wondered about its impact on strokes (C59, C60), so one group analyzed findings from an eight-year study of some 2,100 middle-aged men in eastern Finland. The men had completed a questionnaire similar to the one used in the heart study to describe their usual ways of dealing with anger. Men prone to outbursts proved almost twice as likely to have a stroke as those who were more easygoing.

Researchers offer several hunches about how and why stress and anger boost the risk of heart disease and stroke. We know these states raise blood pressure and that sustained high blood pressure weakens the heart and blood vessel walls. In addition, long exposure to stress-related hormones such as epinephrine, norepinephrine, and dopamine may damage the arteries and heart muscle and disrupt the electrical rhythms that keep the heart beating regularly. These hormones may also promote platelet "stickiness," leading to clots that block arteries that feed the heart muscles. In addition, they prompt fat to accumulate in the abdomen and in the arteries, where it may block the passage of blood or break off in globs that circulate until they plug smaller blood vessels.

You should be careful to remember, however, that indications such as these still leave plenty of room for debate: If people who have experienced clinical depression are more vulnerable to certain diseases, is that because of hormonal or immune system changes in their bodies, or because their depression has made them less likely to take care of their bodies? People under chronic stress are more apt to smoke, overeat, and skip regular exercise than people with less emotionally charged lives. So is the stress itself the cause of their increased health problems, or are their unhealthy behaviors at fault? Some studies have tried to isolate one factor from another by identifying people who smoke, overeat, and so on. The evidence may lean toward an independent health effect for stress and emotions, but the case is still far from open-and-shut.

With that warning in mind, however, if you are of an activist inclination when it comes to your health, the very nature of the brain-body loop suggests all sorts of ways to encourage that interaction to keep working for you. Strategies that favor biochemical harmony in these systems range from cognitive to nutritional to medicinal.

We can choose many different ways to respond to the stressors in our daily lives. Many people find relief in exercise, hobbies, volunteer activities, and their families. Others respond by eating too fast or too much, missing sleep, skipping exercise, and drinking or smoking or using other drugs. People in the first group usually report better health and overall quality of life. People in the second group more often report such symptoms as tension headaches (C54) and other muscle aches; nausea, diarrhea, or other digestive problems; rapid heartbeat; and shortness of breath. When stress persists, normal bodily care and repair activities get short shrift. This condition can make us more vulnerable to colds, flu, herpes, and other infections, and to more serious illnesses, including obesity, heart disease, and cancer.

The Search for a "Mind-Body Medicine"

When you think of "mind-body medicine," you might think of meditation, relaxation

TROUBLE IN THE LOOP

Certain disorders markedly interfere with brain-body connections. Sometimes they originate in the body and bring trouble to the brain, and sometimes it's the other way around. When this process begins, the trouble it produces can feed on itself in the very definition of a vicious cycle.

Because of the tight feedback between brain and body, what affects one part of ourselves usually affects the other, even if only mildly. A disorder affecting the brain may also toggle switches along the brain's circuits to the body, and a disorder of the body changes the messages the brain receives.

Diabetes provides a good example of how a disorder can create trouble in a feedback loop. Type 2 diabetes, the form that affects about 90 percent of diabetics, is tied to excess weight. Approximately 20 percent of people known to have diabetes also have depression, about double the rate in the population as a whole. Depression can cue some people to overeat; it certainly makes it more difficult for people to take care of themselves. Thus, depressed people with diabetes are less likely to stick with a recommended diet than diabetics who are not depressed.

Unfortunately, diet is very important in managing diabetes. After people learn they have diabetes, they must adapt: watch what they eat, lose excess weight, and often carefully monitor their blood glucose levels. Glucose is the basic fuel for brain cells, and stability in supply is important to everything from good mental function to consciousness itself. (That is why if insulin overdose is not corrected quickly, the lowering of blood sugar can lead to coma.) On top of that, the stringent diet requirements imposed by diabetes may seem almost punishing and can cause some individuals to suffer anxiety, stress, and a feeling of not being in control. Thus, at the bodily end of the loop, a single physical ailment can affect both our fundamental brain activity and our emotional states.

In the worst case, the physical and mental troubles associated with a disease can turn the brain-body loop into a spiral. Diabetics who feel too stressed or depressed to control their glucose levels are at greater risk for high blood pressure. That condition in turn increases their risk of heart attacks and strokes, causing more worry in the short term and perhaps serious disability in the long term.

Fortunately, we have ways to break such vicious cycles before they spiral out of control. When people with diabetes receive treatment for their depression, both their moods and their control of the diabetes improve. Exercise not only helps keep weight down and cardiovascular fitness up but helps relieve stress. In other words, the brain-body loop can spiral the other way, too, leading us to a healthier, happier life.

techniques, guided imagery, and other approaches that are said to harness the body's natural healing power. These are often lumped together with thousands of other unconventional treatments. In 1998 the National Institutes of Health set up an office of Complementary and Alternative Medicine to evaluate such approaches. So far there have been few studies as large and rigorous as have been done for most standard treatments.

Consider the connection between stroke and depression that we described earlier. One research team studied 50 people admitted to the hospital after suffering strokes and followed them for the next two years. People who reported having a difficult relationship with their "closest other" before their stroke and a limited social life proved most likely to be depressed both right after their stroke and many months later. To lessen the chance of entering a depression, the researchers concluded, survivors need social support and contact most in the first few weeks after a stroke. One to two years after a stroke, another study showed, depression alone limits how well people have recovered physically regardless of their social functioning. The study also found that people who suffer depression after a stroke are three times more likely to die earlier than stroke survivors who are not depressed.

Futhermore, for many stroke patients, relief of their depression actually restores lost mental function. Researchers randomly assigned 21 people who had had strokes to take an antidepressant and gave 26 other stroke survivors a placebo. Those taking the antidepressant showed significantly greater improvement in both mood and mental function over the next 6 to 12 weeks. Nearly three fourths of people with strokes who took an antidepressant drug in this study improved their orientation, memory, language, and hand-eye coordination.

Similarly, most people who have cancer suffer distress and a depressed mood after hearing their diagnosis. One in four becomes clinically depressed. Improving their mood lowers pain, curbs anxiety, and improves the quality of their lives. It improves various markers of immune system functioning, and, some studies suggest, may even increase longevity.

One of the underpinnings of belief in the mind's healing power is the "placebo effect," a concept with decades-long standing in medical research. This doctrine holds that if we expect our health to improve, it often does. With that assumption, the best medical studies are designed to cancel out the placebo effect.

The term *placebo* is Latin for "I shall please." It found its way into medical dictionaries in the early nineteenth century, when treatments often involved much more art than science. Doctors began to believe that their patients' expectations affected how they responded to treatment. For instance, at that time people often sought medicines that made them vomit or defecate quickly so they would know the drugs were effective. (Today we generally view such reactions as side effects, and drug manufacturers strive to minimize them.) Every patient wanted to receive *some* medication, so physicians often prescribed harmless substances that would please the people who took them—hence the name placebo. But these prescriptions seemed to benefit some patients' health, and not just in their own perceptions. So with this in mind, as research grew more sophisticated and bent on accuracy, scientists began making sure they measured all sorts of apparent placebo effects.

Scientists account for placebo effects by trying to make sure that all volunteers for treatment studies believe that the medication or procedure they receive has the same chance of being effective as that which every other subject gets. Researchers typically assign subjects randomly to receive an active or inactive treatment. They instruct all subjects the same way, not telling them whether they will get the study treatment or the placebo. To avoid subtly influencing the results, the people who dispense the treatments are often also kept in the dark as to which treatment is active; such a study is termed double-blind. The randomized, double-blind, placebo-comparison study has long been the gold standard for research on how well treatments work: To be deemed effective by the U.S. Food and Drug Administration, a new drug or procedure must significantly outperform placebos. That is why when you hear or read news of a finding about a drug, the results are explained in comparison with "a sugar pill" or a "sham treatment." This is good research trying to screen out the placebo effect.

However, the venerable placebo-controlled research concept took a blow in 2001 when the *New England Journal of Medicine* published a careful study suggesting that the placebo effect may be overblown, if not nonexistent. The study analyzed a large number of clinical trials and looked at the differences between placebo and no treatment. The conclusion the study offered was that perhaps the effect researchers were reporting was actually a disease or problem retreating according to its normal ebb and flow. The report looked for instances in which studies had adjusted for this possibility and they found none. Some news reports raised fears that this revelation might mean that drugs tested against placebos are not as good as thought, but while that may be possible in some cases, a drug that works better than waiting out a disease is probably an effective drug. However, the placebo report did underscore the need for caution in turning mind-body clues too hastily into mind-body medicine. The leap from placebo to assumptions about the power of the mind has always been a long one, and the study questioning the placebo's reality suggests it may be a false one.

Some forms of brain-body interaction have become entwined in the idea of the placebo effect. For example, most doctors believe the placebo effect is part of every doctor-patient interaction, but many base this assumption not on a positive but a negative effect. Specifically, some

research has estimated that one in four individuals experiences higher blood pressure during a visit to the doctor, a condition called white coat hypertension. Many people with this reaction relax after a few minutes, and their blood pressure falls to its usual level. For this reason, physicians who see an initial high reading usually take further readings before the visit is over. Some people don't settle down until after they leave, however, and are mistakenly diagnosed as having chronic high blood pressure. Thus, it bears considering whether too easily crediting the placebo effect interferes with more constructive medical thinking—for example, wondering if a patient is prone to stress that should be discussed and perhaps treated.

Expect more to come on the question of placebos, because the challenge to them calls for an answer, and surprisingly few studies have ever focused directly on how placebos work or if they do. While the new doubt raised by the report is being explored in follow-up studies, placebos will remain an important standard in clinical trials of new drugs. Some experts think that the use of a placebo may lower a patient's stress and anxiety over symptoms, thus easing stress-related changes in hormones, blood pressure, and other body systems and perhaps letting the immune system resume its normal functioning. Studies show that people who believe a placebo will ease pain secrete the natural pain-killing substances called endorphins that block pain signals to the brain. Still, for many conditions, from the common cold to well-set broken bones, healing occurs naturally with time.

While many mainstream researchers distrust studies that claim the power of the mind acting by itself to heal, even people on the distant opposite sides of the mind-body question do respect well-designed research that takes both body and mind carefully into account. Mind-body medicine is an attractive goal, as the tantalizing brain-body links suggest. Such research with modern methods is still in its infancy, so an open mind is important. The hope is that the National Institutes of Health's Office of Complementary and Alternative Medicine will produce much more, and much better, science in this area.

Challenges Ahead

Physicians still have a hard time defining, assessing, and treating such subjective or "invisible" symptoms as fatigue and pain. Anyone can see a rash, a broken bone, or the reading on a thermometer. But how do we measure a person's pain from one day to the next except through what he or she reports? As the pathways in body and brain for such symptoms become better understood, the opportunities to devise tests to detect their chemical markers and to intervene in their operations are increasing, and the outlook, particularly for the treatment of pain, is very promising.

Another challenge is that in most countries, including the United States, some medical-practice trends march in the opposite direction from the highly individualized treatments to which the mapping of brain-body connections would lead. The average doctor visit has shrunk to only a few minutes, while health insurers seek to standardize care and minimize costs by treating all patients with particular diagnoses as similarly as possible—even though individuals can respond to the same condition and treatment in very different ways. Many health insurance plans also reimburse people for care of so-called mental illnesses at lower rates than they provide for illnesses classified as medical. This practice works as a disincentive to seeking combined brain and body treatment. The more that is learned about the brain-body loop, the harder it becomes to make such distinctions.

Although a viable mind-body medicine is very much a work in progress, already hard science on brain-body interaction, sparse as it is, has given mainstream medicine more ability to recognize and respond to both emotional and physical dimensions in the diseases doctors treat. A back-to-the-future component has even popped up, as a few doctors around the country adopt the old-fashioned practice of making house calls. While the difficult work of defining and explaining the brain-body loop goes on, such a desire to focus not just on a particular disease but on our total experience of an illness—what neurologist Oliver Sacks calls a patient's "predicament"—can only improve our confidence in medicine and add optimism to the quality of our health.

PART II

Your Brain Through Life

CHAPTER 5

Prenatal Development

The first signs of pregnancy are subtle. A woman's menstrual period does not arrive on time. Her breasts may feel sore to the touch, and she may need to urinate more often. Perhaps she feels more tired than usual. She may suffer from nausea when she smells certain foods, or might crave others. But all these signs can have other explanations besides pregnancy. To confirm their suspicions, many people buy a home pregnancy testing kit, available in any pharmacy. Such tests work as soon as the first missed period, but they are more reliable if you wait another two weeks. By that time, the develop-ing fetus is about a month old. And the basic com-ponents of its brain have already formed.

Many people do not realize just how early a child's brain begins to develop—and how long it continues to mature after birth. The process starts between the second and third week of fetal devel-opment, and it continues well into early adult-hood. No other organ in the human body takes so long to develop as the brain does or goes through as many changes. This unique growth process ex-plains the brain's complexity and amazing activi-ties, as well as its vulnerability to injury.

MILESTONES IN DEVELOPMENT

Scientists have studied prenatal brain growth in two main ways. By examining fetuses that did not survive until birth, they learned about the anatomical changes that take place at different stages of human development. Researchers have also conducted experiments in animals, particularly in monkeys (whose brains most resemble those of people), to learn more about normal development and what can disrupt it. Today it is also possible to use imaging technology, while a child is still a fetus in the womb, to examine the developing brain.

With these methods, we have a good picture of how a fetus normally develops. It takes about 38 weeks for a single fertilized egg to grow into a baby. Pinpointing the exact date of conception is often difficult, however, so pregnancy is most often said to last for 40 weeks from the date of the woman's last period. The timeline below shows how your baby's brain develops during the various months of pregnancy.

MONTH 1

BRAIN: A preliminary structure known as the neural tube forms. Part of this eventually becomes the spinal cord, and the other part the brain.

OTHER MILESTONES: All major organs are forming by the third week of development, and the heart begins to beat.

MONTH 2

BRAIN: The major structures of the brain begin to form, including the cerebral cortex. As the brain grows, the embryo's head begins to look more human.

OTHER MILESTONES: All major organs have now developed. The eyes, ears, nose, and mouth begin to take shape.

MONTH 3

BRAIN: The brain continues to grow new cells and make connections between those already in place. The fetus develops physical reflexes.

OTHER MILESTONES: The eyes are in place, and eyelids are beginning to form. The fetus cannot control its movements, but it can react to stimuli by moving its arms and kicking.

MONTH 4

BRAIN: Parts of the brain begin to receive signals from the developing ears and eyes. The fetus can detect bright lights and hear sounds like its mother's voice, although it will not yet know how to interpret them. As facial muscles develop along with the brain, the fetus can squint and frown.

OTHER MILESTONES: The lungs begin to function, although the fetus still receives its oxygen through the placenta. Taste buds form on the tongue. Eyebrows and eyelashes grow.

MONTH 5

BRAIN: As the brain makes more and more connections, the fetus begins to control its movements, turning and stretching, perhaps even somersaulting. The fetus also begins to react to sounds outside the mother, such as music.

OTHER MILESTONES: The sex organs become visible on an ultrasound. The beginning of an immune system emerges.

MONTH 6

BRAIN: The cerebral cortex is now the largest part of the brain and has started to separate into lobes. As this part of the brain develops, a primitive type of memory and conscious behavior emerge. You may notice the fetus reacts more to some noises and music than others. Some experts believe the fetus will remember music and voices "heard" at this stage and unconsciously react with comfort to them after birth.

OTHER MILESTONES: The facial features are so developed that the fetus looks almost like a newborn. All muscles are in place, and the bones begin to harden.

MONTH 7

BRAIN: The once-smooth fetal brain has begun to form the grooves and indentations typical of a more mature brain. An electroencephalogram (EEG) can detect fetal brain waves. Myelin begins to form a protective sheath around nerves from the brain, like insulation keeping wires from crossing; this sheath enhances communication among nerve cells.

OTHER MILESTONES: The fetus gains weight as it builds up fat stores that will later help to maintain temperature. Eyelids open, the fetus begins to "see" inside the womb. It may swallow or suck its thumb.

MONTH 8

BRAIN: The auditory cortex, the visual cortex, and Broca's area have begun to function. The fetus is thus developing a primitive ability to interpret sights and sounds and distinguish language.

OTHER MILESTONES: All organs except the lungs have now matured. As the eyes develop further, the fetus can begin to focus. The fetus has grown so large that it can no longer easily move about.

MONTH 9

BRAIN: The brain continues to grow, and by this time most of the neurons your child will ever have are in place. Just before birth, the brain is one fourth the size and weight of an adult brain.

OTHER MILESTONES: The fetus gets into position for birth, usually with its head facing downward toward the mother's cervix. The lungs mature. The immune system continues to develop.

Nature and Nurture

You have probably heard the phrase nature versus nurture. It tends to pop up whenever we gain some new insight into human development. Has some aspect of personality or intelligence come about as a result of genes, part of our inborn nature? Or because of the influence of parents, teachers, or other aspects of the environment that nurtured us?

When it comes to the brain, the answer is really both. Some neuroscientists have compared the building of a human brain to the weaving of cloth: some threads are supplied by genes, others by the environment. In the resulting fabric, the different strands are so tightly woven that they are virtually indistinguishable. Other theorists have compared the brain to a seedling, which is full of potential but needs the right mixture of nutrients, sun, and rain in order to grow into a tree. So the debate in brain development is not one of nature versus nurture, but of how these factors interact and which is more important in the development of particular traits, behaviors, and disorders. The consensus on these questions tends to change as we learn new information.

The brain is malleable because it develops

WHY FOLIC ACID COUNTS

Chances are, you have heard about folic acid. This B vitamin, once overlooked, has burst into public awareness in the past ten years or so. And if you are concerned with your child's developing nervous system, it bears special attention.

In 1989 researchers reported that folic acid deficiency could result in devastating brain and spinal cord abnormalities. These include spina bifida, in which the spinal cord develops outside the vertebrae (C9), and anencephaly, where most of the brain fails to develop. Each year, about one baby out of a thousand suffers some type of neurological damage caused by folic acid deficiency. Fortunately, studies have reported that folic acid supplements can decrease the risk of neurological birth defects by as much as 70 percent.

Why is folic acid so important? It is essential for forming new cells because it promotes enzymes that help build genetic material. Folic acid is thus most important when cells are multiplying rapidly—as in early fetal development. Although a mother-to-be needs adequate folic acid throughout her pregnancy, the vitamin is essential in the first few weeks, when the embryo's neural groove closes to form the neural tube and the brain begins to develop. Since a woman may not even realize she is pregnant during this time, most experts recommend that all women of childbearing age make sure they get enough folic acid.

You can obtain folic acid naturally by eating fortified cereals and green leafy vegetables. Or you can take a supplement. An expectant mother should aim for at least .4 mg (400 mcg) of folic acid a day during the first trimester and, ideally, throughout pregnancy. Some experts recommend as much as 1 mg per day. Check with your physician to determine the best strategy for you.

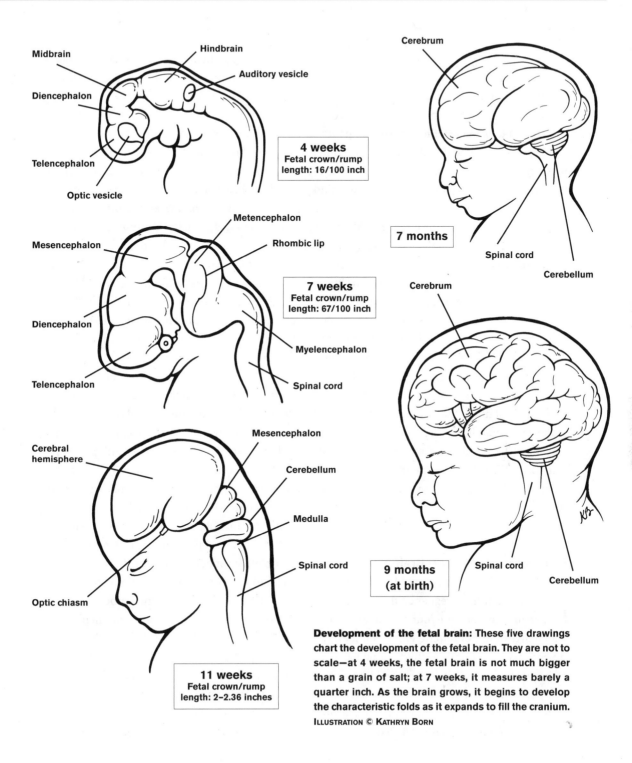

4 weeks
Fetal crown/rump
length: 16/100 inch

Midbrain
Hindbrain
Auditory vesicle
Diencephalon
Telencephalon
Optic vesicle

7 weeks
Fetal crown/rump
length: 67/100 inch

Metencephalon
Rhombic lip
Mesencephalon
Diencephalon
Telencephalon
Myelencephalon
Spinal cord

11 weeks
Fetal crown/rump
length: 2–2.36 inches

Mesencephalon
Cerebellum
Medulla
Spinal cord
Cerebral
hemisphere
Optic chiasm

7 months

Cerebrum
Spinal cord
Cerebellum

**9 months
(at birth)**

Cerebrum
Spinal cord
Cerebellum

Development of the fetal brain: These five drawings
chart the development of the fetal brain. They are not to
scale—at 4 weeks, the fetal brain is not much bigger
than a grain of salt; at 7 weeks, it measures barely a
quarter inch. As the brain grows, it begins to develop
the characteristic folds as it expands to fill the cranium.
ILLUSTRATION © KATHRYN BORN

partly as a result of the preprogrammed instructions encoded in genes, and partly as a result of exposure to the outside environment. Genes govern the type of brain cell produced, its location and function, and what type of neurotransmitters it will respond to. But whether a particular neuron will develop further and realize its full potential, or go unused and wither away, depends on external stimulation—everything from sight to sound to stress.

In the beginning your developing child follows a standard and predictable course of development. And what you or your mate continue to experience may feel like a straightforward, linear process: the baby becomes steadily larger in the womb, the ultrasound reveals more and more features, the mother feels more vigorous activity. But while a baby's nine-month gestation includes many clearly defined stages, at the cellular level these processes tend to overlap. Some are repeated several times. This development is guided by the genes built into every cell of the embryo. It is by following those genes' complex instructions that your child's brain is able to develop from a group of primordial cells into one of the most powerful organs in the universe.

Building Blocks of the Brain

In the first month of pregnancy, the changes you notice in your body (or your mate's) are subtle; the changes the developing embryo undergoes are enormous. At birth the child's brain will consist of 100 billion neurons, organized into groups that perform such particular functions as interpreting sounds, storing memories, and learning new skills. Yet this complex organ, like every other part of the human body, must grow from a single fertilized egg. The brain develops at a phenomenal rate in the nine months from conception to delivery. At the height of this process, a quarter of a million new brain cells are born every minute.

In the first week, the fertilized egg goes through a series of divisions, giving birth to a hundred or so progenitor cells, all exactly alike. The cells are clustered in a small ball known as a blastocyst.

During the second week, the original generation of cells has given birth to others, which begin to differentiate, or take on unique characteristics that distinguish them from their cousins and forebears. As the cells differentiate, the developing embryo evolves from a small round cluster of cells into an elongated disk that consists of three layers of tissue. The upper layer of the disk, or ectoderm, will eventually give rise to the outer covering of a person (skin, fingernails, and hair) and—with help from the middle layer, or mesoderm—to the brain and central nervous system. The bottom layer, or endoderm, gives rise to internal organs, such as the lungs and stomach.

Brain development begins with a process known as induction, which takes place in the third week of embryonic growth. Cells multiply rapidly along the lines of the ectoderm so that a structure called the neural plate forms. This process is not completely understood, but it seems to be sparked by contact between the ectoderm and mesoderm. Chemical factors produced in the mesoderm create a reaction in the neighboring ectoderm, pushing some cells along the developmental pathway that leads to skin and hair, and others on a different developmental pathway that leads to brain and spinal cord.

By the fourth week, part of the neural plate has folded in on itself to form a neural tube. At this point, primitive brain cells called neuroepithelial cells begin to divide rapidly, or proliferate. At first the wall of the neural tube is composed of only a single layer of such cells. Yet this initial layer grows, forming additional layers. Cells proliferate at a furious pace, in part because the neuroepithelial cells begin to divide into three new cells rather than two.

Three bulges emerge from the top of the neural tube, eventually giving rise to the forebrain, midbrain, and hindbrain. The rest of the neural

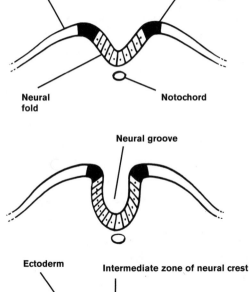

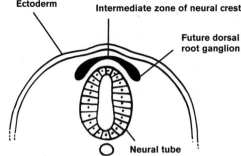

At about the third or fourth week after conception, the neural tube begins to form and to show bulges that will become parts of the brain and spinal cord.
ILLUSTRATION © KATHRYN BORN

plate becomes the neural crest, which will become the spinal cord. As cells proliferate in the three primitive brain structures, the brain begins to grow and fluid-filled spaces known as ventricles form in the middle. Even at this early stage, primitive brain cells are organized into distinct groupings known as neuromeres, visible as tiny grooves on the ventricles. Although the neuromeres disappear in another two weeks, they are precursors of the large-scale differences between parts of the brain that we can easily see.

Thus, as the embryo enters its second month of development (before the mother may even realize she is pregnant), the brain and the central nervous system have already begun to take shape. That's one reason it is so important to take care of your health, even at this early stage.

Growing by Leaps and Bounds

By the second month of pregnancy, you may know that you are pregnant, or that your mate is. A mother may feel morning sickness, but aside from that the external signs of a pregnancy are still subtle. But probably you have begun to wonder what this child might be like when it is born. Will it be a boy or a girl? Will it have its mother's eyes, or its father's? Will this child grow up to be an athlete? Or an astronaut? A gifted musician?

While you daydream and speculate, your developing child is busy building a brain that will one day allow him or her to do the same. During this second month of fetal development, the brain grows by leaps and bounds. Construction begins on all its major components. What happens in this month will lay the foundation for your child's ability to see, hear, speak, and one day imagine his or her own child.

During the second and third months of fetal development, the growing brain begins to take shape. The hindbrain gives rise to the medulla oblongata and the pons (part of the brain stem), which are involved in many functions essential to life, such as breathing and heartbeat. The cerebellum, the part of the brain involved in maintaining balance and coordinating movement, emerges partly from the hindbrain and partly from the midbrain.

But it is the forebrain that undergoes the most complicated changes. The forebrain divides into two distinct structures: the diencephalon and telencephalon. The diencephalon develops into the thalamus and hypothalamus, which will affect everything from emotions to sensory perception. The telencephalon gives rise to several parts. First come the hippocampus, which eventually will be involved in short-term memory, and other structures involved in the olfactory pathways, which will enable your child to smell. Next, the telencephalon produces the basal ganglia, which will eventually contain structures that control movement, sensory information, and some types of learning. The amygdala will eventually help the brain attach emotional significance to signals it relays elsewhere.

The last structure to evolve out of the telencephalon is the cerebral cortex, one of the most complex parts of the brain and the site of what are considered "higher functions": learning, language, and abstract thought. The cerebral cortex begins to develop in the eighth week of embryonic growth but will continue to form during much of the prenatal period. The connections between neurons in the cerebral cortex continue to mature into early

adulthood, and some experts say they never stop maturing.

This tremendous growth is possible because the neurons are still proliferating. Although cells have been dividing since the moment of conception, this activity builds to a fevered pace about day 40 (or in the sixth week) of embryonic development. This process, known as neurogenesis, continues until day 125 (around the seventeenth week). Even then, it does not completely stop but only slows down.

In these early months of prenatal development, cells not only proliferate—they begin to take on particular identities. This process starts when some of the cells in the ventricular zone stop dividing and begin to do a microscopic dance. Precursor cells divide on the innermost surface of the neural tube, which borders the ventricles, then move to the outermost surface to synthesize DNA, the blueprint of life. Then the precursor cells return to the ventricular surface to divide again. The cells repeat these steps a set number of times, depending on their types.

With all this back and forth, patterns of similar cells develop into columns, or what the neuroscientist Pasko Rakic has suggested is a protomap for the fully developed brain. According to this model, columns of cells form on the surface of the ventricles with genetic instructions on how many particular cells the brain needs, where they will eventually be located, and what they will do. The result is both a prototype of the brain and a map of it—hence the term protomap. Some neuroscientists have challenged this theory as too simplistic, but it offers a helpful way to picture how the parts of the brain develop.

The primordial cells in the neural tube eventually become either neurons or long, thin glial cells. The neurons are the brain cells that do the actual work of thinking and controlling movement. The glial cells have been compared to scaffolding that helps guide the building of the brain, especially the cerebellum. These glial cells sprout from the ventricular zone, extending upward to the outer surface of the developing brain. Neurons begin to migrate in different directions, depending on their preprogrammed roles.

Guiding all this movement are genes, which we can compare to blueprints. Each contains instructions for creating a protein, which in turn might induce cells to divide or perform particular functions. Early embryonic cells divide and give rise to progenitor cells, which then give birth over several generations of divisions to more specialized cells. No one gene contains a master plan. Rather, one set of genes controls the initial phase of development, other genes then kick in and take it to the next level, and so on.

The First Glimpse and Flutters

During the first months of pregnancy, you probably do not notice much external change. If you are the mother, perhaps your waist has begun to thicken a bit as your uterus grows. You may have trouble wearing some tighter-fitting clothing but are probably not yet in maternity clothes. As the middle period of pregnancy arrives, however, you are likely to become more aware of the life growing within.

Your earliest glimpse may come from an ultrasound, often performed for the first time in the third month of pregnancy. (A second ultrasound may be performed later in pregnancy as well.) Though its image is blurry, the fetus is starting to look human. An expert can usually point out the

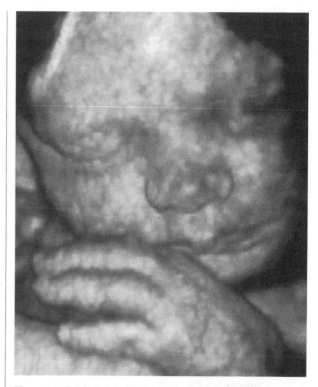

The use of 3-D fetal ultrasound imaging has helped doctors detect development problems such as harelips and spina bifida early in the pregnancy. This scan of the face and hand was produced using a transducer, which emits high-frequency sound waves that are reflected off internal structures. IMAGE © BERNARD BENOIT/ SCIENCE PHOTO LIBRARY

large head, fingers and toes, even tiny eyes and ears. As the ultrasound technician prods your abdomen with the probe, the fetus might dart away. Its movements are jerky and uncoordinated, and you probably will not be able to feel them. At the end of the third month, the fetus is still very small—about 3.5 inches (9 cm) from head to rump, and weighing only 1.7 ounces (48 g).

An expectant mother's experience changes at the end of the fourth month, or more likely the beginning of the fifth. Many women then feel the

HOW TO FEED DEVELOPMENT

When it comes to nutrition and the pregnant woman, "experts" abound and the advice is often contradictory. Eat for two. Eat for your baby. Eat for yourself. Give in to your cravings for pickles and ice cream. Don't give in to your cravings. Give up coffee and switch to herbal tea. Don't drink herbal tea.

What's a woman to do? First of all, relax. The best advice nutritionists give pregnant women is remarkably similar to the advice they give all of us: eat a balanced diet low in fat, heavier in carbohydrates, and rich in fruits and vegetables. Of course, there are a few cautions for pregnant women based on the needs of the developing fetus. The best thing you can do is talk with your obstetrician about your particular nutritional requirements. Many physicians recommend that pregnant women take a multivitamin or a special "prenatal" vitamin each day to supplement their diets.

Here are a few guidelines for eating well during pregnancy:

- Add 300 to 800 calories per day to your diet to provide the extra energy your body needs. The amount your physician recommends will depend on your weight and activity level. A woman who weighs 125 pounds (56 kg), for instance, might normally consume 2,000 calories a day before pregnancy but should increase that by about 300 calories a day while pregnant.

- Fresh food is best when it comes to nutrients; frozen foods are next best.

- Protein is essential throughout pregnancy. Your baby's vital organs all develop during the first trimester, but the brain continues to grow in spurts throughout pregnancy (and even after birth). All this growth requires energy, so your need for protein increases by one third when you are pregnant. Aim for six to seven ounces (200 g) of protein-containing foods per day. The best sources are cheese,

first slight movement, or a fluttering in the abdomen. Known as quickening, this is the first physical sign a mother has that the fetus has begun to move. This is often the most exciting time for parents, the point at which they start to become acquainted with their child and anticipate its birth. The fetal movements, which will grow to somersaults, jabs, kicks, and the like in the sixth and seventh months, can seem deliberate. And in a way, they are. Your child is helping to develop its own brain, with each turn and move accelerating processes that have been under way for some time.

Moving, Thinking, Being: The Cerebral Cortex

The middle part of pregnancy is a significant time in fetal development, when the brain evolves from a primitive structure into a much more complex form. Cells continue to proliferate and differentiate during this phase, but they do much more besides. They have begun to travel (migration), form communities (aggregation), and make connections that facilitate the communication necessary to brain function (synaptic formation). All of this lays the foundation for what

eggs, fish, meat, milk, and poultry (all animal sources, which also provide amino acids that you and your developing baby need). But the FDA recommends that pregnant women not eat shark, swordfish, king mackerel, or tilefish, as they may contain enough mercury to harm your baby's brain.

- Make sure you get enough vitamin D and calcium in your diet (either through dairy products or supplements), since these build your baby's bones and teeth. Aim for four glasses of milk, or 1,200 to 1,300 mg of calcium and 400 IU of vitamin D per day.

- Drink plenty of fluids. While you are pregnant, the volume of blood circulating in your body (and to your fetus) increases by almost 50 percent. Since water is a component of blood (as well as every other part of our bodies), getting enough to drink is important. Aim for at least eight glasses of water or fruit juice per day.

- Make sure you get enough iron in your diet. This helps build red blood cells, which supply oxygen to your body and the developing fetus. Since iron supplements may cause stomach irritation (and thus worsen morning sickness), some women prefer to postpone taking them until the second trimester. That's fine, since maintaining sufficient blood iron levels is most important in the latter part of a pregnancy. Aim for 48 to 78 mg of iron per day, from a supplement or through foods like dried beans, liver, and meat.

- Many herbal teas are fine, but avoid herbal supplements. To be on the safe side, drink only those herbal teas that contain ingredients naturally found in your diet. These include apple, orange, and mint tea. Some experts advise staying away from ingredients such as chamomile and hibiscus, whose effects during pregnancy are not known.

makes us human: movement, learning, conscious thought, and memory.

Although all of brain development involves some combination of cell growth, migration, aggregation, and synaptic formation, this process is most dramatic in the cerebral cortex. This is the largest part of the human brain and the site of the so-called higher functions. The cerebral cortex builds itself from the inside out, with the neurons of the deeper layers being made before those of the outer layers. But all the neurons are born deep inside the brain, in the ventricles, so some must travel to the outermost reaches of the organ. At about the eighth week of embryonic development, primitive brain cells begin to migrate outward from the innermost part of the brain and start to build the first layer of the cerebral cortex. Succeeding groups of cells follow, slowly building all six layers of the cortex, a process that continues for most of gestation.

Meanwhile, neurons continue to proliferate, creating new cells. The peak growth occurs in the fourth and fifth months of pregnancy, when the cortex (also known as the brain's gray matter) grows much more rapidly than the supporting structures underneath (known as white matter). By the time the cortical growth spurt ends, in the

WHAT TO AVOID (OR REDUCE)

Fetal development, and especially brain development, is full of peril and promise. With millions of cells multiplying each day, and the brain building itself inside out, much can go wrong. Fortunately, the brain has its own built-in repair systems. But if you ingest certain drugs and substances during pregnancy, not only do you increase the risk that a developmental mistake will happen, but you also may prevent the fetal repair systems from working properly. Listed below are some substances to avoid while pregnant.

ALCOHOL: It is best to avoid alcohol altogether while pregnant, and to give up drinking if you are trying to conceive. Alcohol can interfere with brain development. It sometimes causes fetal alcohol syndrome, which involves central nervous system abnormalities, mental retardation, and stunted growth. Because alcohol in the mother's bloodstream passes into the placenta so easily, the developing fetus receives almost as much from a drink as its mother does. Some experts, in fact, estimate that 2.5 percent of all birth defects are caused by alcohol. If you had a few drinks before discovering you were pregnant, it is likely that any damage to the fetus will be overcome as long as you stop drinking. But speak with your physician if you have any concerns.

DIETARY SUPPLEMENTS: Herbal and dietary supplements, often sold in health food stores and increasingly showing up in grocery stores as well, are not regulated by the U.S. Food and Drug Administration. For the most part, physicians have not studied their use in pregnant women. Most experts therefore recommend avoiding such supplements altogether during pregnancy.

ILLEGAL DRUGS: Substances such as cocaine, heroin, and marijuana can have a devastating effect on fetal development and should be avoided completely during pregnancy. These drugs wreak havoc with brain development and can result in premature delivery, behavioral problems, and learning disorders.

MEDICATIONS: If at all possible, it is best to avoid both over-the-counter and prescription medications during pregnancy, and especially during the first trimester, when your baby's vital organs are developing. Even some medications you might consider harmless, such as some cough medicines, contain alcohol. If you have a medical condition requiring medication, talk the issue over with your physician. He or she might be able to recommend a strategy that will balance your needs with those of your developing child.

SMOKING: Smoking any form of tobacco can badly affect the fetus's physical development and perhaps brain development. Smoking has been linked to low weight at birth and a greater risk of miscarriage. Some studies (although the evidence is less conclusive here) have reported that a mother's smoking may contribute to learning difficulties and behavioral problems later on in her child's life. Certainly the safest strategy is not to smoke; if you cannot give up the habit, at least cut back as much as possible.

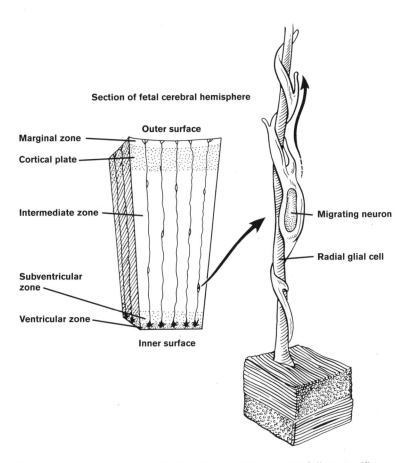

Section of fetal cerebral hemisphere

Outer surface

Marginal zone

Cortical plate

Intermediate zone

Subventricular zone

Ventricular zone

Inner surface

Migrating neuron

Radial glial cell

Neuron climbing a glial cell: During development, neurons follow specific cues and migrate along glial cells (the support cells that act as the "road" on which the neurons travel) to their designated locations in the brain, spinal cord, and nervous system. Scientists say this journey, for some neurons, is like walking from New York to California. ILLUSTRATION © KATHRYN BORN

sixth or seventh month of development, 70 percent of the brain's neurons are located in the cerebral cortex. At the same time, the fetal skull has begun to harden as cartilage turns to bone throughout the body. Both the rapid growth and the hardening skull help explain why the cortex acquires its characteristic folds, but that wrinkling is far from random. The fully developed cortex has peaks and valleys that are generally the same from one person to the next, pointing to some underlying genetic blueprint. Even so, there are many small differences between individual brains, even the brains of identical twins, who share the same genes. The exact contours of the cortex are thus a product of both nature and nurture.

As cells migrate, they travel along particular pathways to reach their preprogrammed destination. Exactly how the cells know where to go is not entirely clear. Rakic's theory suggests that the protomap contains instructions that point the cells in the right direction and then, as the cells head out, other signals guide them along the way. Most cells use other neurons' offshoots, known as axons, and chemical signals to guide their journey. Others climb along glial cells, which are so elongated they resemble strings or small plants; when these glia are no longer needed, they either degenerate or become permanent supporting cells in the white matter of the brain.

Sometimes, in spite of all the signals and directions, migrating cells lose their way through the layers of other cells. About 3 percent arrive at the wrong place. If too many neurons lose their way, part of the cerebral cortex may never develop. Some neuroscientists believe that errors in cortical cell migration contribute to certain types of mental retardation (**C3**), epilepsy (**C13**), developmental delays, and perhaps even schizophrenia (**C25**). In extreme cases, the cortex will be smooth rather than wrinkled, a condition known as lissencephaly. A dramatic example of problems with cell migration appeared in the aftermath of the nuclear blasts over Hiroshima and Nagasaki. Many people who were exposed to the radiation between the tenth and seventeenth weeks of their fetal development grew up with impaired higher brain functions; they could not hold jobs and were institutionalized. Autopsies revealed not only that these victims' cerebral cortices were thinner than normal (indicating that not all cells had migrated successfully), but also that errant cortical neurons were scattered throughout the supporting white matter.

Cells Settle In and Start to Talk

Much as people do when they move to a new place, cells that have recently arrived at their proper destination seek out similar cells and begin to form their own versions of communities. The technical term for this is *aggregation.* The cells recognize each other by their distinct biochemical properties and receptors. Cell adhesion molecules, sometimes called sticky molecules, help the cells bind.

Once settled, a neuron sprouts an axon for sending signals to other brain cells, and numerous dendrites for receiving signals from others. In forming connections, neurons do not simply reach out randomly to the closest cells. They seem to be programmed to seek out specific targets. In some parts of the brain, such as the cerebral cortex, the cells even align themselves in the same way, axons pointing down and dendrites pointing up.

The axons that send signals and the dendrites that receive them communicate for this purpose at specialized contact zones, where the sending axon physically connects to the dendrite. These specialized contact zones are called *synapses;* they were named from the Greek word that means "to grasp." Although there is a thin gap between the axon and the dendrite at such connections, the chemical signals (neurotransmitters) from the axon can diffuse rapidly across it to deliver the signal to the dendrite. As the signal spreads from the cell body of the sending neuron, a wave of activity flows down the axon, caused by the movement of sodium ions from outside the cell into the axon. As the wave of activity reaches the nerve terminal at the synaptic contact point, calcium ions also enter the axon and trigger the release of the neurotransmitter. The neurotransmitters bond with receptors on the target cell, prompting a new electrical signal to surge through that neuron. In this fashion, brain cells can send many different messages to each other with varying degrees of urgency.

Although most neurons connect to a limited number of other brain cells, some send signals to as many as 10,000. This web of communication helps explain the brain's vast computing power. Scientists are still trying to explain how so many connections are made, and so precisely, in the developing brain. In some cases, the distance an axon travels before reaching its target is astounding, as much as a thousand times the diameter of the cell itself. At other times, axons must twist and turn along their route. Some grow as long as a few inches. Although more remains to be discovered, several mechanisms have been identified that help explain how synapses form.

For starters, time determines, to a great degree, when a neuron will first sprout an axon and begin making connections. We believe that neurons form the bulk of their connections during a particular period in their development, soon after they arrive at their destinations and sprout axons. At that time, they can make connections only with cells already in place. If other cells arrive later, the neuron will no longer be able to forge a link. Neurons that arrive early seem to connect to their neighbors. Later, when the communities grow in number, cells need additional help to find the right targets for their connections.

Although the sprouting of an axon is directed by every cell's genetic instructions, the path of further growth is aided by various chemicals and molecules in the surrounding tissue. The tip of the axon, known as the growth cone, sprouts tiny filaments (filopodia) that continuously extend and retract, almost as if they are testing the environment and feeling their way ahead. Meanwhile, target cells produce various chemicals, called chemotrophic factors, that both encourage an axon to grow and attract it in the desired direc-

tion. (Cells that are not appropriate targets produce chemicals that repel the axon.) These factors spread through the tissue, and axons with receptors that can bind with them grow in that direction. Meanwhile, filopodia that do not encounter the appropriate chemicals retract, so that the growth does not go off in the wrong direction.

In this way, the axons find their targets by taking the cell equivalent of baby steps, rather than one long leap into the unknown. They grow toward higher concentrations of chemicals that they find attractive, avoiding cells that produce chemicals that are repugnant.

Chemotrophic factors are usually present in small, well-defined areas. When the journey is long, still other molecules function almost as beacons, or what the neuroscientist Per Brodal has called signposts, along the way, helping guide growing axons on their journey so that they reach their proper targets. Other axons come up behind, following their lead.

Like-minded axons, which share the same sorts of targets, also ease the process by squeezing out sticky substances called neuronal cell adhesion molecules, or N-CAMs. These N-CAMs help keep individual axons from getting lost. Such axons may actually huddle together, forming collective groups known as fascicles. Like any clique, these groupings are exclusive; axons that do not express the same N-CAM, or express none at all, are discouraged from coming near.

External stimuli also help cells in the developing brain make connections and strengthen them. When the fetus kicks or sucks its thumb, the neurons that control movement are exercised and form more connections between more axons and dendrites. Typically, for instance, a fetus be-

PRENATAL TESTS AND THE BRAIN

ULTRASOUND is a standard test performed on almost all pregnant women in this country because it reveals a great deal, is not invasive, and has minimal risk of complications. As its name implies, ultrasound uses high-frequency sound waves to produce a picture of the developing fetus. It is generally performed twice during a woman's pregnancy: first between the eleventh and thirteenth weeks, and then again between the eighteenth and twentieth weeks.

The images generated by an ultrasound reader may appear blurry to you at first, but a trained technician can help identify the head, arms, and legs of a developing fetus. This test helps a physician check how many babies a woman might have, the sex of each fetus, and overall growth and development. For parents, ultrasound provides the first glimpse of the fetus and a chance to listen to its heartbeat. Although most ultrasound scans reveal nothing out of the ordinary, these tests can detect abnormalities such as spina bifida (where the spinal cord has not closed properly; **C9**) and anencephaly (where most of the brain fails to develop). Further tests, such as those described below, are needed to confirm these diagnoses.

The **NUCHAL TRANSLUCENCY SCAN**, a form of ultrasound, examines the fetus to see if it has excess fluid between its skin and the underlying tissue along its back. Such excess fluid could be a sign that the fetus has Down's syndrome (**C3**) or certain inherited heart abnormalities. The diagnosis is confirmed by amniocentesis. The test is usually done between the eleventh and fourteenth weeks of pregnancy.

The **ALPHA-FETOPROTEIN (AFP)** test is usually performed between the sixteenth and eighteenth weeks of pregnancy. High AFP levels in the mother's blood may be a sign that the fetus has hydrocephalus (**C8**) or spina bifida (**C9**). Low levels of this blood chemical may signal Down's syndrome (**C3**). But the screening is inexact and must be confirmed with another test.

SERUM SCREENING measures blood levels of AFP, estriol, and human chorionic gonadotropin. It provides a

---

gins moving its arms and legs around the tenth week of development. At first these movements are uncoordinated and random. But gradually the fetus becomes more purposeful in its movements (as any pregnant woman knows). The child's increasing ability to coordinate movements, which continues to grow after birth, is due to the gradual development and strengthening of the appropriate transmitters, receptors, and connections between all the cells involved. Practice helps make perfect.

Preparing for Birth

During the last stage of pregnancy, parents and fetus both are preparing for birth. You may take childbirth classes, decorate the nursery, and be guests of honor at a shower. The developing fetus, meanwhile, has grown so large that it has difficulty moving within the uterus. Its brain is maturing rapidly. By month seven, electroencephalography (EEG) can detect fetal brain waves. The fetus can see and hear, although these senses

rough estimate of how likely it is that a mother might give birth to a baby with Down's syndrome (C3). The test, generally done at the sixteenth week of pregnancy, requires further confirmation by amniocentesis.

AMNIOCENTESIS is usually performed only after a screening test has identified a possible chromosomal abnormality in the developing fetus, or if a woman is older than 35 and therefore more at risk for conceiving a baby with Down's syndrome (C3). Amniocentesis can detect abnormalities with greater accuracy than other tests. It also carries a small risk of causing miscarriage, which is why the test is performed only when its results might affect a couple's decision about whether to continue the pregnancy.

An amniocentesis begins with taking an ultrasound image of the fetus to determine its location. A physician then inserts a thin needle through a woman's abdomen into her uterus to extract a small sample of the amniotic fluid surrounding the fetus. This fluid contains fetal cells that can be cultured and tested to detect any abnormalities.

Amniocentesis cannot be performed before the sixteenth week of pregnancy, and results usually take two to three weeks, so waiting for the test or the results can be anxious periods for parents.

CHORIONIC VILLUS SAMPLING (CVS) also detects chromosomal abnormalities, but in a way that eventually allows cells to be tested for specific genes as well. In this procedure, a physician takes a tissue sample from the placenta and analyzes it. (To reach the uterus, the doctor may insert a needle into the abdomen or insert a catheter into the vagina and through the cervix.) This test can be done earlier than amniocentesis (generally between the tenth and twelfth weeks of pregnancy). The results are also faster: physicians can offer an initial diagnosis within a day or two, and confirmation within seven days. If a woman decides to have an abortion after learning the results of the test, it can thus be done earlier, which is safer for her. As with amniocentesis, there is a small chance this test might result in miscarriage, so it is performed only on women with a family history of certain disorders, or those who are 35 and older.

are only in the earliest stages of development and will become much more refined outside the womb. During this last phase of development, the earlier processes of cell proliferation and migration continue to some degree, and synapses continue to form all over the brain. But two new processes begin in earnest: a pruning of unnecessary cells and connections, known as apoptosis, or programmed cell death, and the protection, known as myelination, of vulnerable neurons and connections.

Until this point, everything about brain growth has been about *more:* more cells, more axons and dendrites, more synaptic connections. And the result is more than the brain needs. The brain overproduces cells and synapses. Apoptosis provides balance. This large-scale elimination of neurons affects some parts of the brain more than others. Relatively few neurons in the spinal column die, as compared with five in ten motor neurons (which control muscle movement), and nine in ten cells in the cerebral cortex.

Structures That Differ in Male and Female Brains

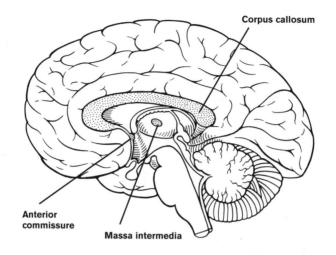

Corpus callosum

Anterior commissure

Massa intermedia

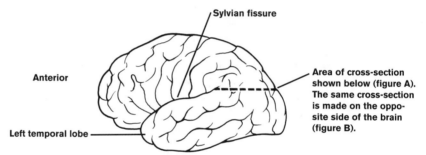

Sylvian fissure

Anterior

Left temporal lobe

Area of cross-section shown below (figure A). The same cross-section is made on the opposite side of the brain (figure B).

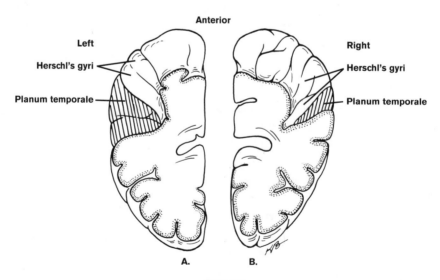

Anterior

Left

Herschl's gyri

Planum temporale

Right

Herschl's gyri

Planum temporale

A.

B.

Posterior

ILLUSTRATION © KATHRYN BORN

BOY BRAIN OR GIRL BRAIN?

Is it a boy or a girl? This is probably one of the first questions expectant parents are asked, or may ask themselves. But when it comes to the brain, it may not matter all that much. Certainly there are both anatomical and hormonal differences between male and female bodies, and these differences begin quite early in development. Some researchers say that there are also differences in the way the sexes think and behave, but not everyone agrees on this. Other scientists point out that most differences in ability emerge after adolescence, suggesting that either hormones or the different socialization of boys and girls may play a role. And they cite recent studies that show that men and women differ only in narrowly defined skills, such as the visual-spatial task of determining how a flat paper with perforations will look when it is folded. With broader challenges, of the sort that come up in daily life, the differences disappear. For instance, men and women usually differ on a test of verbal fluency: coming up with as many words as possible in a given category. They score the same, however, on tests of vocabulary and reading comprehension. The natural differences between male and female brains are so subtle, it seems, that people usually compensate for them.

At the anatomical level, the brains of men and women look remarkably alike. Neuroanatomists have so far identified only four structures that differ in any way:

- The CORPUS CALLOSUM, a bridge between the left and right hemispheres, is larger in women than in men, according to some studies but not others.

- The ANTERIOR COMMISSURE, another structure that connects the two hemispheres, is larger in women than in men.

- The MASSA INTERMEDIA, which connects the left and right sections of the thalamus, may be larger in women than in men.

- The PLANUM TEMPORALE, the name for the uppermost level of the temporal lobe, is usually larger on the left hemisphere, where it overlaps the part of the brain involved in language. In some women, it may be larger on the right side.

So what does all this mean? It's not clear. There is some evidence that the brains of men and women are organized slightly differently. Typically, the right hemisphere of men's brains is involved in visual and spatial activities, while the left side is involved in language. But studies of people who have suffered brain damage have revealed that while that left-right split holds true for men, it does not seem to matter for women. This has led researchers to speculate that brain skills are distributed differently between the sexes. It is also uncertain what effect hormones exert on the brain. Most of the information we have about this comes from studies of people born with mutations in their sex chromosomes. These mutations include one responsible for a rare condition called idiopathic hypogonadotropic hypogonadism, in which boys do not produce testosterone when they reach puberty. Men with this condition do poorly on visual-spatial tests, suggesting that testosterone may help the part of the brain involved in spatial tasks to mature.

The bottom line is that boys and girls are born with brains that are equal in most ways. And with the right encouragement and challenges, they grow up with a full range of abilities, regardless of their sex.

How all this happens is still a matter of investigation and conjecture. We know that when a cell undergoes apoptosis, its DNA begins to fragment and it eventually dies. What is not as clear is what triggers apoptosis. One theory is that cells need growth factors in order to survive, much as people need nutritious meals on a regular basis. Once a neuron makes the right connections with other brain cells, it receives the growth factors it needs. Cells unable to make appropriate connections "starve" and die. Another theory is that neurons are preprogrammed to self-destruct but that exposure to growth factor inactivates the genes that contain these instructions.

In the final months of pregnancy, the brain also begins to protect itself. Around the eighth month of prenatal development, myelination begins; it will continue well into childhood. Myelin is a protective membrane produced by oligodendrocytes, which are types of glial cells. The membrane extends from the oligodendrocyte's body and wraps itself many times around an adjacent axon, forming layers. Myelin has sometimes been compared to the rubber that coats electrical wires, but it is actually even more useful. Myelin not only protects the brain cells; it helps them communicate by facilitating, and speeding, the transmission of their signals. Since electrical signals can

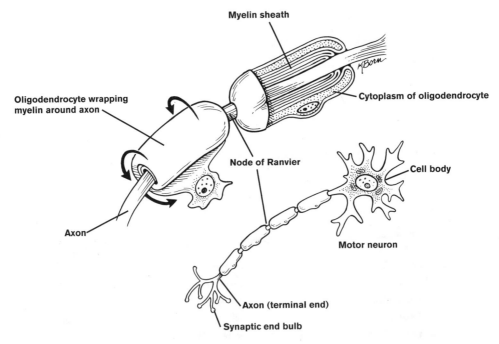

Myelin—the white fatty insulation around axons—helps move the electrical impulses more efficiently. Myelin sheaths are formed by a type of glial (supporting) cell known as an oligodendrocyte. As the brain and nervous system develop in the embryo, the oligodendrocyte wraps around and around the axon in layers resembling an onion. Lengths of oligodendrocytes wrap around the entire length of the axon in a pattern much like links of sausage. Illustration © Kathryn Born

enter and exit the axon only where it is exposed, the myelin covering ensures that those signals will pass quickly to the target brain cell. In multiple sclerosis (C33), Guillain-Barré syndrome (C49), and other conditions, the myelin covering is damaged; the axon is thus exposed to signals from neurons it normally does not communicate with, and the result is something like an electrical short circuit, causing loss of motor control and other problems.

Myelination occurs at different times in different parts of the brain. Generally, motor and sensory brain cells are protected first, before birth. The last area to be myelinated is the cerebral cortex, and that happens long after birth, in childhood. The process of myelination coincides with the development of more advanced and coordinated skills. Your child will become better able to control arm and leg movements, and will thus be better able to crawl and walk. Over the same period your child's cerebral cortex becomes myelinated, he or she will start to form words, string them into sentences, and finally form abstract thoughts, one of the highest brain functions of all.

Breathing Lessons—and Bedtime Stories

By the eighth and ninth months of pregnancy, you are probably practicing your breathing in preparation for the birth. (You may be eager to get this over with at last!) As the baby's due date approaches, many parents wonder if they should begin to talk to the developing fetus, or even begin to teach it in some way, such as exposing it to music. Certainly some intriguing research shows babies pick up on prenatal experiences. Newborns suck harder when they hear their own mothers' voices than when they hear another woman's, for instance. In one set of experiments, researchers asked women to read a Dr. Seuss book aloud twice a day in their eighth and ninth months of pregnancy. Subsequently, the newborn babies sucked more energetically when their mothers read that book to them than when they read another.

Other researchers have gone so far as to assert that a program of stimulation before birth can produce a brighter, more active baby afterward. But most neurologists are not so sure. They worry that well-intended parents may overstimulate their offspring in the womb. A large part of the meaning that babies pick up from their parents' talk and play is emotional, based on the tone of the interactions; if parents are stimulating babies in an anxious way, or doing so without happiness because they feel obliged to, the effect may be counterproductive.

The consensus advice is fairly straightforward:

- Remember that the major developments your fetus undergoes in the womb are physical rather than mental. The best advice for mothers is to eat well and avoid such toxic substances as alcohol and drugs.

- As long as you do it in moderation, talking with your fetus and exposing it to music and stories can't hurt. This is best done in the eighth and ninth months, when your fetus has developed the brain capacity to hear and perhaps even remember sounds.

- A fetus needs periods of rest, just as we all do. As active as the fetus may seem at times, it also needs to drowse quietly. Overstimulation can disrupt these rhythms and may even be stressful.

■ Be wary of any "fetal development" program that is sold commercially, especially if it carries a hefty price tag. When the marketing pitch comes across more clearly than the medical research, it is wise to be skeptical. When in doubt, check with your obstetrician or pediatrician.

If nothing else, remember that your child's brain continues to develop well into young adulthood. You will have plenty of time to interact with, and challenge, your child after he or she is born. And then you will also have the satisfaction of seeing your child react, learn, and grow.

CHAPTER 6

Brain Development in Childhood

In the first moments after birth, as you and your spouse cradle this new child and stare down with wonder (and some exhaustion), you are probably not thinking about brain development. If you are thinking about your baby's head at all, it may be only to provide it with enough support, or to be careful to avoid touching the "soft spots" where the bones of the skull have not yet joined.

But your obstetrician is thinking about your child's brain, and the tests he or she performs soon after the birth are designed in part to measure brain function. The standard Apgar evaluation provides preliminary information about your baby's overall health and development. The doctor looks at skin color, breathing, pulse, reflexes, and muscle tone. This examination takes only a few minutes and is done mainly to identify newborns that might need special assistance in the nursery.

A few days later, your child will undergo a more thorough examination, known as the Neonatal Behavioral Assessment Scale (NBAS). This test takes 20 to 30 minutes and evaluates your baby's physical health, reflexes, and overall well-being as he or she adjusts to life outside the womb. While your baby sleeps, your pediatrician will use a light, a rattle, and other stimuli to see whether the infant can tune out these external distractions. This provides insight into the functioning of your baby's central nervous system. The pediatrician will also evaluate your baby's reflexes. Stroke a newborn's cheek, and he or she will turn toward the finger (hoping to find a breast). Slip the tip of your finger into a newborn's mouth, and the baby will suck. Support the newborn's body across the palm of your hand so that his or her feet touch something solid, and the baby will take one step and then another, displaying the "walking reflex"—a foreshadowing of his or her first steps. These abilities, though rough and immature, show just how much brain development has already taken place before birth.

Your Baby's Brain: A Work in Progress

Most parents know they must cradle a baby's head carefully. A newborn's neck muscles are not yet able to support the weight of its head—and just look at the size of that head! It is by far the largest part of an infant's body. At birth, your baby's brain is already one fourth the weight of an adult's, even though his or her whole body weighs less than a tenth of an adult's. This is the marvelous result of the prenatal development described in chapter 5, when billions of neurons form, axons grow, and synapses start to connect the neurons.

All of those cells and links are sometimes referred to as the brain's "hard wiring." But that phrase implies that your baby's brain at birth is equivalent to a circuit board in a radio, ready to be plugged in and played. It might be wiser to compare a newborn's brain to early roots in a spring garden. The environment, the human version of sun and rain, will play an important part in how your child's brain actually grows and the unique talents and personality traits he or she develops.

You don't have to be a neuroscientist to notice the amazing development that takes place after birth. The same child who was so helpless as a newborn will be babbling at six months, and walking and talking with abandon as a toddler. These developmental milestones are matched by growth of the brain as an organ. In the first year, your baby's brain triples in weight. By the end of the second, your toddler's brain weighs three quarters that of an adult's. The brain's activity increases with its weight. The metabolism of a baby's brain, as measured by how much blood sugar it uses, builds steadily from birth until the age of 3. At that point, your child's brain is more than twice as active as yours, and it will remain so until he or she reaches puberty.

All that internal energy and growth is matched by the toddler's external activities: exploring the world, reaching out for objects, gurgling and practicing sounds (the building blocks of language). And elements of your baby's personality will begin to emerge sooner than you think. Some toddlers are shy, others bold. Some are rambunctious, others quiet. Some are easily soothed, others hard to calm down. (For more on these variables of temperament, see **B9**.)

So what's going on? Although new cells are born in the rest of your baby's body every day, the brain adds comparatively few cells after birth. Instead, the existing neurons grow larger and more powerful, sprouting axons and dendrites and connecting with neighbors. Some researchers have compared this blooming to the growth of a tree: branches emanate from the trunk of a cell's body and reach out all around. These connecting branches account for the brain's growth. And the synaptic connections enhance the brain's computing power, its ability to accept sensory input from the outside world and make sense of it. Perhaps not surprisingly, synaptic growth is most significant during your baby's first few years of life—when he or she is taking in all sorts of new input and acquiring new skills. By the time your child turns 3, each neuron has formed as many as 10,000 connections, making a total of about a quadrillion (1,000,000,000,000,000) throughout the brain. (That's double the number of connections in your own brain.) Synapse formation slows after the toddler years, but continues throughout childhood and into adolescence, finally reaching adult levels when your child is anywhere from 15 to 18 years old.

Meanwhile, the process of myelination, which also began before birth, continues throughout childhood. As discussed in chapter 5, myelin not only protects the growing nerves, it helps them communicate better. The brain undertakes this task in stages. Those neural networks involved in early life skills (such as sucking and swallowing) are myelinated during pregnancy. The prefrontal cortex, the part of the brain involved in higher forms of learning, may not be completely myelinated until your child is 10.

But the first few years of life are not only about growth. This is also a time of selection. As your baby begins to see better, to explore his or her environment, and to interact with adults, the neurons in his or her brain transmit signals to each other. The neural networks that are used grow stronger; those that are not wither away, just as unused brain cells started dying in the last weeks before birth. This process is known as pruning. It is similar to the way a tree is pruned of excess or dead branches but is much more extensive. The death and removal of excess brain cells and connections truly sculpts a person's brain. Growth and pruning continue throughout our lives, but the relative balance of the processes changes. Until your baby is 3, growth far outpaces

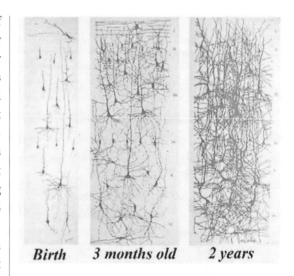

Birth   3 months old   2 years

Neuronal branching: dendrites and synapses. According to the "critical period" theory, while in the womb the brain overproduces synapses to ensure that it will be able to capture important experiences in relatively narrow time frames. After birth, as the child begins having experiences, certain networks of synapses will activate and become stronger, creating more complex connections between other neurons. By age 3, each neuron will form as many as 10,000 connections; those not used will eventually be pruned. Different parts of the brain will go through critical periods at different times, depending on the skills needed. IMAGES FROM THE POST-NATAL DEVELOPMENT OF THE HUMAN CEREBRAL CORTEX, VOLS. I–VII, BY J. L. CONEL, UNIVERSITY OF HARVARD PRESS, CAMBRIDGE, 1939, BY PERMISSION

pruning. From then until the age of 10, the formation of new connections is balanced by the elimination of unused ones. When your child reaches puberty, the balance finally shifts and the pruning of connections exceeds the formation of new ones.

Plasticity and Critical Periods

This whole process of synaptic formation and subsequent pruning helps explain the plastic-

EARLY DELIVERIES, LATER PROBLEMS?

Babies born prematurely face development risks ranging from mild learning impairments to more severe problems, like blindness, cerebral palsy, deafness, and even mental retardation. Fortunately, as our technology to care for these infants has improved, so have many aspects of their development.

About one in ten babies born in this country is premature. However, the newborns most at risk for future problems are those weighing less than 3 pounds, 4 ounces (1.5 kg). Only about one infant out of a hundred is in this group. The proportion of such preemies has increased since the 1980s, mostly because of the increased use of fertility treatments.

One of the major difficulties facing premature babies is that their central nervous systems are still developing. The carefully timed construction of their bodies lacks its finishing touches. Vision, for instance, is not yet mature. Although patches can protect a preemie's eyes from the bright lights of the intensive care unit, doctors can do little to speed the development of the blood vessels that nourish the retinas. These vessels begin growing from the optic nerve at about the fourth month of prenatal development and, in full-term babies, reach the retina at about the time of birth. In preemies, the blood vessels have not yet connected. Sometimes they can go astray, so that the retina is not nourished and becomes detached. This can result in retinopathy, which, untreated, can lead to blindness. Fortunately, the condition can be treated with laser surgery.

A newborn's sense of hearing is also developing as his or her auditory cortex forms synapses. Preemies are often in intensive care units full of artificial beeps and loud noises. They do not primarily hear a mother's voice, as other newborns hear both in the womb and after birth. That may be why preemies sometimes experience a delay in recognizing patterns of speech.

Other researchers have found that preemies may suffer brain hemorrhages, probably because their developing nervous systems cannot properly regulate blood flow yet. This can damage the brain, resulting in cerebral palsy (C4) or learning disabilities later on.

If you have a child who has been born prematurely, your best course is to talk at length with your pediatrician and hospital workers to find out what special services your child might need to develop his or her full potential. Be aware that many of the studies of development in preemies are based on children born in the 1960s and 1970s. Since then, technology has improved. Given the right medical and educational supports, most premature babies born today will grow up to live normal and productive lives.

ity that is central to understanding the brain. Once your baby is born, his or her brain develops partly because of genetic instructions (nature) and partly because of exposure to the outside world (nurture). Experiences help determine which synapses grow stronger and which are pruned. Sometimes certain experiences are even necessary to "turn on" genes and unlock their natural coding. This interplay seems to be lifelong. Even the brain of an adult can continue to rewire itself and make connections after exposure to new situations. The result of all this is that the brain is custom-designed to function in its owner's environment. In this way, the brain differs from the heart, lungs, and other organs, which follow a more standard and predictable developmental process.

We do not entirely understand why activating neural networks ensures their survival. It may be similar to the case of a muscle, which becomes stronger the more it is used. External stimuli send electrical impulses racing from one part of the brain to another. The more that a particular brain network is activated, the stronger the signal becomes. At some point, the signal becomes so strong that it triggers a resiliency in the network, so that these connections cannot be pruned away.

And timing may be everything. Neuroscientists believe there are "critical periods" for development, when a particular network of neurons and their connections are best made and strengthened. According to this theory, the brain overproduces synapses to ensure that it will be able to capture important experiences in relatively narrow time frames. Once the experience occurs, certain networks of synapses have been activated and become stronger. Those not used are pruned. Different parts of the brain go through critical periods at different times, depending on the skills needed.

One dramatic example is how your child learns to see. Look your newborn in the eyes, and he or she might look puzzled, as if coming out of a deep sleep. Both eyes and brain have to develop more before your baby will be able to see in the way that adults do. At first, babies can focus only on objects 8 to 15 inches (20–40 cm) away, and may go cross-eyed when trying to follow motion. By the time your baby is six months old, he or she is able to track all sorts of movements and focus on objects several feet away. As his or her first birthday approaches, your baby can see even small toys located across a room. Not until the second birthday, however, does a child's vision reach mature levels.

All of this is the result of the interplay between genes and environment. Genes contain instructions for how to organize cells initially in the visual cortex, but these "ocular dominance columns" become functional and sophisticated only when a child begins to use his or her eyes to take in the outside world. Researchers who kept a kitten's eye shut for several months after birth found that the cat was *never* able to see from that eye. Anatomically, the eye was fine, but the nerve pathway into the cortex had not developed because no sensory input was available. There have been similar findings about humans, though not because of deliberate experiments. At one time, the standard treatment for amblyopia (a form of crossed eyes) in newborns was to cover one eye with a patch until the muscles that controlled it had developed enough to be operated on; often, the eye was covered for so long that its nerve pathway never developed and it became useless.

Researchers believe that the same "use it or lose it" principle applies to other aspects of brain development—everything from hearing and moving to thinking and feeling. But just how the environment interacts with the underlying network of brain cells and connections is not well understood. Researchers have studied the phenomenon of critical periods most in the visual cortex. The issues get murkier when it comes to other types of learning.

For that reason, many neurologists and educators prefer to talk about "prime times" for learning and development. According to this theory, we can learn most skills any time in life, but they come most easily during particular periods. In some cases, these prime times can extend for years. So if your child is developing normally,

EXPECTED VISUAL PERFORMANCES

BIRTH TO 6 WEEKS OF AGE:

- Stares at surroundings when awake
- Momentarily holds gaze on bright light or bright object
- Blinks at camera flash
- Eyes and head move together
- One eye may seem turned in at times

8 WEEKS TO 24 WEEKS:

- Eyes begin to move more widely with less head movement
- Eyes begin to follow moving objects or people (8–12 weeks)
- Watches parents' face when being talked to (10–12 weeks)
- Begins to watch own hands (12–16 weeks)
- Eyes move in active inspection of surroundings (18–20 weeks)
- While sitting, looks at hands, food, bottle (18–24 weeks)
- Now looking for, and watching, more distant objects (20–28 weeks)

30 WEEKS TO 48 WEEKS:

- May turn eyes inward while inspecting hands or toy (28–32 weeks)
- Eyes more mobile and move with little head movement (30–36 weeks)
- Watches activities around him or her for longer periods of time (30–36 weeks)
- Looks for toys he or she drops (32–38 weeks)
- Visually inspects toys he or she can hold (38–40 weeks)
- Creeps after favorite toy when seen (40–44 weeks)
- Sweeps eyes around room to see what's happening (44–48 weeks)
- Visually responds to smiles and voice of others (40–48 weeks)
- More and more visual inspection of objects and persons (46–52 weeks)

12 MONTHS TO 18 MONTHS:

- Now using both hands and visually steering hand activity (12–14 months)
- Visually interested in simple pictures (14–16 months)
- Often holds objects very close to eyes to inspect (14–18 months)

- Points to objects or people using words "look" and "see" (14–18 months)
- Looks for and identifies pictures in books (16–18 months)

24 MONTHS TO 36 MONTHS:

- Occasionally visually inspects without needing to touch (20–24 months)
- Smiles, facial brightening when views favorite objects and people (20–24 months)
- Likes to watch movement of wheels, egg beater, etc. (24–28 months)
- Watches own hand while scribbling (26–30 months)
- Visually explores and steers own walking and climbing (30–36 months)
- Watches and imitates other children (30–36 months)
- Can now begin to keep coloring on the paper (34–38 months)
- "Reads" pictures in books (34–38 months)

40 MONTHS TO 48 MONTHS:

- Brings head and eyes close to page of book while inspecting (40–44 months)
- Draws and names circle and cross on paper (40–44 months)
- Can close eyes on request, and may be able to wink one eye (46–50 months)

4 YEARS TO 5 YEARS:

- Uses eyes and hands together well and with increasing skill
- Moves and rolls eyes in an expressive way
- Draws and names pictures
- Colors within lines
- Cuts and pastes quite well on simple pictures
- Copies simple forms and some letters
- Can place small objects in small openings
- Visually alert and observant of surroundings
- Tells about places, objects, or people seen elsewhere
- Shows increasing visual interest in new objects and places

REMEMBER: All the age ranges given above are approximate. Lags of a week or so are not unusual, but any definite developmental delay or nonperformance should be given every necessary attention. The performances listed above are important. All are preparatory to school readiness and are visual skills that are essential to lifetime activities.

Excerpted from: A Reference Guide for Preschool Children's Vision Development © Optometric Extension Program, 1995

there will be plenty of opportunity for growth; should a problem develop, there is usually time to fix it. An example of this is language development.

From First Words to First Book

At six months, babies may gurgle and babble. At nine months, they have progressed to "dada" or "mama." By the time they are a year old, they may voice those sounds when they see their parents, connecting sounds and meanings to make actual words. Language is a skill woven from many threads: hearing sounds, mimicking them, speaking words, learning their meanings, stringing them together into sentences (**B14**). Some aspects of language seem to be innate to us as humans, but most we have to learn. Mastering one set of skills leads to the next. And when language does not develop normally, the fault may lie in a problem with any one of the basic skills involved.

Long before a baby learns to speak, he or she is literally learning to listen, at least in a very basic way: distinguishing the various sounds of speech that add up to words and sentences. Between the ages of six months and a year, your baby is primed to be multilingual. Infants can distinguish the basic sounds used in every language, such as the consonants used in Thai but not in English. But consistent exposure to only one language, especially from hearing their parents and other family members, makes infants' brains focus on the sounds that are meaningful in that language. By his or her first birthday, a baby who hears only English can no longer distinguish among those Thai consonants, because their subtle differences have no meaning in English. And a baby who hears only Chinese does not notice a difference

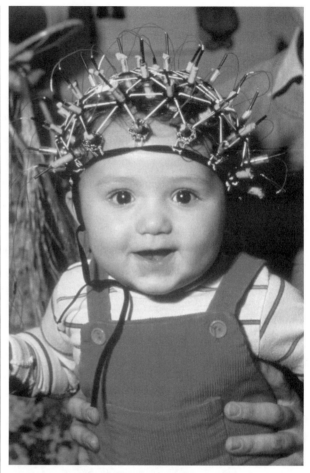

Electroencephalography (EEG) allows researchers to study how babies use their emerging brainpower. This young subject is participating in a study of how quickly infants can detect changes in speech sounds, and which brain areas may be involved. PHOTO © JACK LIEU, JACKLIEUPHOTO@HOTMAIL.COM

between the syllables "ra" and "re," which are not used in Chinese.

The next step, from distinguishing sounds to actually speaking, takes place gradually. According to one leading theory of language (but not the only one), when your baby hears you say something, signals received in his or her auditory cortex are then relayed to Wernicke's area, the part of

MILESTONES OF CHILDHOOD

The brain continues to develop and mature throughout childhood, and even longer for some higher functions. A child's first 6 years see the maturing of the auditory cortex (hearing), the visual cortex (seeing), the angular gyrus (understanding language), and Broca's area (speaking). The prefrontal cortex, site of learning and thinking, matures until age 15 and perhaps beyond.

How do parents experience these changes? Here are some general developmental timetables. It is important to remember, however, that individual children follow their own schedules. They develop at different rates, often regress before making a leap forward, and sometimes appear to be at different levels of development in different areas.

4 TO 6 WEEKS: First smile (usually during a feeding)

6 TO 9 MONTHS: Baby sits up on own and babbles

9 MONTHS TO 1 YEAR: Baby crawls and stands; recognizes own name when spoken; says a few words

8 TO 14 MONTHS: First steps and many words

18 MONTHS ON: Toddler builds up more words, sentences, meanings

3 YEARS: Average age when toilet training begins, as a child begins to understand the concept, to imitate adults, and to respond to simple instructions

4 YEARS: Memory matures just as preschool often begins

5 YEARS: Language and learning skills build, and abstract thinking begins to develop; the first day of kindergarten approaches

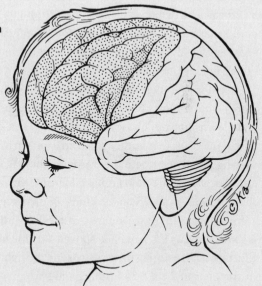

Frontal lobes

Age 3–6
Areas of rapid myelination

Possible effect:
Alertness, attention span

From age 3 to age 6, the brain's frontal lobes undergo rapid myelination, in which the neurons' axons are sheathed in signal-speeding insulation. The improved neuronal communication is thought to help the child's developing alertness and attention span. ILLUSTRATION © KATHRYN BORN

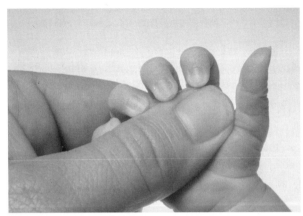

© Mark Miller/Photo Network/PictureQuest

the brain that recognizes words. As your child starts to talk, he or she activates several areas of the brain in rapid succession. The basic components of the word form in Wenicke's area, which then sends signals to an adjacent structure known as Broca's area, which calculates the lip, tongue, and throat movements necessary for utterance and then signals the motor cortex to alert the required muscles.

Reading is a more advanced language skill, with a more complex neural pathway. When your child learns to read, his or her eyes send signals first to the visual cortex, then to an area known as the angular gyrus, where the words on the page are associated with sounds your child heard when the word was spoken. Those sounds, in turn, are communicated to Wernicke's area, where the word is understood as if it had been spoken. Writing is a further skill, requiring the brain to send the right instructions to the child's writing hand (or typing fingers).

In most children, this progression from hearing to speaking to reading and finally to writing goes without a hitch. And when something goes wrong, the brain is amazingly plastic. Some infants have had to undergo surgery to remove the

left hemisphere of their brain because of spreading tumors. This hemisphere typically controls language, yet these children usually develop normal speaking and reading skills. The brain merely rewires this ability into the right hemisphere.

The First Three Years: Myth or Mandate?

Given all this emphasis on critical periods and prime times for learning, parents can feel awfully pressured. If you are not already concerned about what you should or should not be doing for your child, pick up a book or magazine on parenting; you will become a worrywart in no time. Today the popular media seems to emphasize your baby's first three years, as if everything that follows depends on what happens during this initial period. Should you turn off the Top 40 radio station and play Mozart instead? Take away the teddy bear and invest in flash cards? Or throw up your hands and feel like a failure because your child is already older than 3?

The first thing to do is relax. Most insight into brain development during the first three years has come from research into extreme deprivation and adversity. For instance, we know how important individual attention and contact are for infants from what happened to orphans housed in institutions without such nurturing care. Though their physical needs were provided for, these children never received sustained attention from particular caregivers. As a result, they suffered from high rates of mortality and other problems. We saw heartrending examples in the Romanian orphanages that did not have enough staff to care for the many infants they housed. After spending their first few years in these settings, some of these orphans were adopted by well-meaning American parents. But in spite of loving homes and supportive care, many continued to suffer developmental delays and behavioral problems.

Many researchers argue, however, that studies of deprivation and adversity of this sort cannot be worked backward into a model of healthy brain development. And they point out that even severely deprived children can be remarkably resilient. Some Romanian orphans, for instance, are doing well.

Furthermore, most experts agree on one point about early child development. In the first three years, the most important things parents can do is to establish a strong, nurturing relationship with their baby. This primary attachment creates the groundwork for self-confidence, the ability to learn new things, and the capacity for getting along with other people. Building a healthy relationship means picking your baby up, cuddling, responding to his or her cries. It means playing games, singing nursery rhymes, and reading aloud at bedtime. These seemingly innocuous activities, which many parents do without prompting, provide sensory input (sights, sounds, touch) that stimulate the young neurons and connections in your baby's brain. This is an important form of learning.

Sadly, if adults ignore a baby, or do not respond to his or her needs, that child will later have trouble forming attachments or empathizing with others. And the care has to be consistent. If it is not, the child may become anxious and clingy later on, almost as if he or she has decided the world is an unstable place.

Physically, all of this has to do with hormone levels in the child's brain, which in turn affect his or her ability to regulate emotions. Although hormones are governed in part by genes, a child's ex-

perience of interactions with his or her family helps fine-tune them. Specifically, attachment with a parent or primary caretaker helps modulate the levels of cortisol, the so-called stress hormone. When people experience stress, their cortisol levels rise to increase their heart and breathing rates (the "fight or flight" response). In the brain, high cortisol levels induce other chemical changes that can actually destroy neurons and unravel synaptic connections.

Researchers have found that babies who form a strong bond with a nurturing caregiver by their first birthday do not experience elevated cortisol levels in response to relatively low levels of stress. And when their cortisol levels do rise, these children are able to shut the response down faster and more efficiently than other children. On the other hand, children who experienced trauma or abuse, or who did not form a secure attachment, suffer from chronic high cortisol levels. Those babies raised in Romanian orphanages had elevated cortisol levels, researchers found. Such children are often slower to learn, walk, and interact with others than children whose cortisol levels remain normal.

What researchers cannot answer yet, and perhaps will never be able to say for sure, is exactly how much supportive care is necessary to rear an emotionally well-balanced child. Every parent occasionally loses his or her temper with a toddler (or teenager), or doesn't feel up to playing at the end of a long day at work. And probably that is fine; it is long-term care rather than isolated instances that seems to matter. And much remains unknown. The *mechanics* of brain building in childhood are not understood as well as the right ingredients. It is as if parents receive a recipe that states only approximate measurements, temperatures, and cooking times. Following those directions can usually produce a good dish, sometimes an exquisite one, and sometimes one that needs a little help.

Encouragement and Enrichment

Your child's brain matures in stages, as you can see in the gradual building of skills. Take walking, for instance. Few moments are as exciting as a baby's first steps. You may view this moment as a whole new stage in your child's development (and of course it is), but it is also the end of a long developmental journey deep within his or her brain.

Newborns' movements have a jerky, spastic quality to them. But by the second or third month, your baby will be grasping objects and may seem more in control of other movements. As the months pass, infants can lift their heads and look around when placed on their stomachs. They will kick and rock and finally learn to sit up. They will learn to crawl, then to "cruise" by holding on to furniture and taking steps. Some babies prefer to scoot along the floor instead of crawling, and some stand up later than others (especially those in large, busy families). Almost all children pass through these stages as part of our natural human urge to reach further and move under our own power. And finally the big day arrives: your child takes those first wobbly but unsupported steps.

Your baby's brain has been building toward this moment for a while. Those months of learning to sit up and crawl have helped build synaptic connections. Circuits have linked the visual cortex and motor cortex, helping your baby assess space and move within it. Muscle strength and control have improved, as has balance. The basal ganglia and the cerebellum are also involved, relaying messages back and forth. Toddlers use their legs to walk, but they also rely on their brains.

Higher-level skills also appear to develop in stages. Memory first emerges as a very simple function involving only the hippocampus, the part of the brain that receives and organizes new information. Infants as young as two months can recognize when they see something new, as shown by how long they stare at it. A child's ability to consciously recall information at will does not begin to develop until his or her first birthday, however, and this system must mature during the next few years. One reason that people typically cannot remember much that happened to them before the age of 3 or 4 is that the parts of the brain necessary for recalling such memories are not "wired" then. The synaptic connections that link the hippocampus to the cerebral cortex have not yet been made. These connections become circuits as your child enters preschool. Meanwhile, other parts of the brain, notably the prefrontal cortex, are also developing. This enables a growing child both to understand why it is important to remember certain things and to develop tricks and strategies for recalling those things.

We also see how children's minds develop in stages by looking at what they *cannot* do at different ages. Following the discoveries of psychologist Jean Piaget in the mid–twentieth century, development experts have recognized many ways in which children do not think like adults. For instance, preschoolers consistently believe that a tall glass can hold more than a shorter one, even if the shorter glass is significantly wider, and that there are more books and toys if they are spread all over the floor than if they are stacked away. Not until about school age do children realize that different people can have different knowledge of the world. And researchers are still debating when

THE DAY-CARE DILEMMA

Few decisions create as much anxiety for working parents as the decision about whether to enroll their child in day care, at what age, and in what setting. The experts are also divided, although there is some consensus on some core issues.

Most child development specialists agree that by the time a child reaches his or her first birthday, day care is not a problem. By then, most babies can handle playmates and new situations. The issue is whether day care at an earlier stage interferes with the formation of a primary attachment to a caregiver. Some experts say it cannot help but do so, while others say children are resilient enough to adapt. But obviously, not all parents have a choice about whether to work during a child's first year, and not all can make stable, long-term arrangements with a grandparent, other relative, neighbor, or friend, or bring in a daily sitter.

When it comes to day-care facilities, therefore, these are some of the most important variables to examine:

- **Quality of services.** Individual states license day-care centers, and the regulations vary. These rules are primarily concerned with safety, which is indeed important. But you should also assess a facility's general atmosphere. How does it provide opportunities for your child to play and learn? Are the children about your child's age? Do you feel as if you could relax there if you were tired?

- **Number of children in the group, and number of adults looking after them.** Do babies receive individual attention and care? Are adults with the children at all times? The National Association for the Education of Young Children recommends that day-care centers have only 6 to 8 children in an infant group, 6 to 12 in a group of 1-year-olds, 8 to 14 in a group of 2-year-olds, and no more than 20 children aged 3 to 5 together. For a group of any age, these standards recommend that at least two adult caregivers be present.

- **Continuity and quality of staff.** High employee turnover does not allow children to enjoy consistent caregiving. And most employees should have experience and/or accreditation in caring for children. They should understand that day care is not simply a way to keep young children out of trouble, but a chance for them to learn and grow.

children can clearly sort out the real world from what they vividly imagine. Experience plays a role in moving children to the next level of cognitive development, but it seems that the brain has to be ready for that step as well. Parents and teachers can hurry a young child along only so much.

In movement, memory, and other functions, therefore, you will see your child develop preliminary skills, refine them, and then build on them to achieve more advanced skills. Inside your child's brain at this time, neurons are firing signals, selected synaptic connections are growing stronger, and myelin is coating the nerves to make them more efficient. What educators see is potential: the more your child uses his or her brain, the more it grows. How can you facilitate this process? You can enrich your child's environment and encourage him or her to explore it (even if that results in a few mistakes).

FIVE STEPS TOWARD ENRICHMENT

How do you help your child grow mentally as well as physically throughout childhood? As we said before, the first step is loving children so that they feel secure and confident. After that, parents can encourage their children to explore the experiences offered by the physical world around them and the possibilities of the mental worlds inside their heads. Here are just five suggestions for making that happen:

1. Read aloud to your child, from infancy until he or she is old enough to read alone (and then take time to listen). As you read, talk about the stories you are sharing. Encourage your child to think about what's coming next, or about the issues and choices the books portray.

2. Encourage imagination and exploration. Don't force your child to play with a particular toy when he or she might prefer to make believe with the help of the cardboard box that contained it. The educational value of a toy is determined by what a child does with it, not by its expense or the research behind it.

3. Even before your child enters school, play number games to encourage openness to math lessons later on.

4. Don't ban passive TV watching, but try to minimize it. Discuss the programs, the work that goes on to create them, and the choice to watch TV. Provide alternatives like books and games as well.

5. Get outdoors and exercise. This is the best way for you to encourage your child to do the same. The brain benefits from improved blood flow and oxygen; the spirit benefits as well.

Researchers have seen the importance of enrichment clearly in rats' brains. Rats who live in an "enriched" environment (full of toys and other rats) are better able to navigate mazes than rats raised in more austere environments. Furthermore, autopsies show that the enriched rats develop more synapses in the parts of their brains that control memory and vision. Intriguing research on people shows a similar pattern: learning particular skills changes the brain. One often-cited study of violinists found that the part of their somatosensory cortex devoted to controlling left-hand movement is larger than the area that governs their right hands. This is significant because violinists use the fingers of the left hand on the fingerboard which requires more motor control than their right hand needs to hold the bow.

Furthermore, the change was largest in musicians who had begun taking lessons before the age of 10, suggesting that parts of the young brain literally grow with experience.

Bold or Bashful?

One toddler cowers and cries at the sight of a birthday clown; another rushes up and hugs the entertainer's leg. What has created such a difference? Like cognitive skills, your child's temperament is partly inborn and partly modified or enhanced based on interactions with parents, siblings, peers, and teachers.

Jerome Kagan's work on shyness suggests that temperament is influenced by the amygdala, a small, almond-shaped area in the brain that functions almost like a relay station. The amygdala receives all sorts of sensory input about sights, sounds, tastes, and so on. It communicates that news to other parts of the brain involved in thought, emotional reactions, and behavior. The amygdala is also the part of the brain involved in the fight or flight response. When a child becomes frightened, the amygdala alerts the hypothalamus, which in turn triggers the release of cortisol. The hypothalamus also activates the sympathetic nervous system, causing a rise in heart rate, breathing rate, and temperature.

Kagan theorizes that some infants are born with amygdalas that are highly reactive, triggering a stress reaction in response to even a moderate stimulus. These infants will tend to be shy. Others, born with amygdalas that are not as reactive, will be less inhibited. He began testing babies before they were even born. Three weeks before a mother's expected due date, Kagan measured the heart rate of the fetus. Then he asked the mothers to return with their babies at four months old, when his team exposed the babies to new experiences, such as a bright mobile or an unfamiliar voice, and monitored their heart rates. The researchers watched for the babies to smile and gurgle to signify comfort, or to flex their limbs and arch their backs to signify distress. The children were studied again at fourteen months, twenty-one months, and $4\frac{1}{2}$ years old.

Kagan and his colleagues found that children who tended to react with fear to new situations when they were four months old were more likely to by shy when they got older. The babies who were less fearful tended to develop into outgoing children. Interestingly, whether an infant would show a fearful reaction could be predicted, with a high degree of accuracy, by its heart rate in the womb. Infants who were low reactive tended to have fetal heart rates lower than 140 beats per minute; those who were highly reactive tended to have heart rates over that level.

So is biology destiny? Not necessarily. Kagan's work also showed that only one in ten of the children who were highly reactive at four months turned out to be extremely shy by the time they were $4\frac{1}{2}$. Although the inborn tendency remained, most children were able to modify or overcome it with the encouragement of their parents and the accumulation of positive experiences. Few became as outgoing as the low-reactive infants, though. For most people, it seems, an inborn temperament remains a tendency for life.

Further evidence for the impact of environment appears in the way boys and girls start to behave differently by the age of 2. By that point, most of the shy children are girls, while most of the outgoing children are boys. Yet at four months, there were no differences between the sexes. Kagan theorizes that parents try harder to encourage their sons to overcome initial timidity, guidance then reinforced by a culture that expects boys to be bold. Other studies have shown that when adults play with an infant they have not met before, they consistently pick different toys depending on whether they believe the baby is a girl or a boy. It seems clear that we often place different expectations on boys and girls well before they turn 2, so it should not be surprising if different behaviors and even different thought processes result.

What Neurological Impairments Reveal

Many parents worry about what can go wrong in brain development. Fortunately, most children grow up in the normal range. And when something does go seriously wrong, it is usually beyond a parent's or child's control. In fact, one of the biggest contributions of brain imaging studies has been to show that the most difficult mental disorders are connected to abnormal chemistry in the brain, not to anything that parents or children have done.

Take autism, for example. Children with this developmental disorder withdraw from the world and are not able to communicate well or build relationships with other people. The underlying problem seems to be that autistic children do not know how to gauge and interpret other people's expressions. Yet at the same time, people with autism may be extremely skilled and talented in other ways.

As late as the 1960s, psychiatrists thought autism resulted from cold, unemotional parents. Although that theory has been soundly rejected, the cause of the disorder remains unknown. Evidence now points to several possible culprits: abnormal genes, some sort of virus, or environmental poisons. Whatever the cause, an autistic brain functions differently from a healthy one. Imaging studies show that when someone with autism looks at another person's face, the inferior temporal gyrus lights up; this part of the brain usually reacts only to inanimate objects, like blocks and trees. Cells in an autistic person's limbic circuits, the brain circuits that control emotions, are not as well developed as they are in healthy people. Other research has revealed that subtle differences in brain chemistry may be present at birth.

Behavioral interventions to treat autism have shown promise, so both physicians and families are eager to find ways to diagnose the condition as early as possible. Children who develop the dis-order can appear perfectly normal until they are toddlers, but then parents perceive their behavior changing: the child may resist being held, stop talking, and avoid making eye contact. Some subtle signs may even show up before a child's first birthday: researchers who have analyzed home videos of autistic children in their first year have detected subtle abnormalities in their eye contact, gestures, and responsiveness to their names. For now, the American Academy of Neurology recommends consulting a pediatrician if your child has not babbled, pointed, or gestured at something by twelve months; has not spoken a single word by sixteen months or a two-word phrase by twenty-four months; or has shown any loss of verbal or social skills. These signs could mean anything from a hearing problem to a developmental disorder like autism. There are several types of screening tests to help you determine the possible problem and the best way to help your child develop. (For more on autism, see section **C5**.)

Like autism, attention deficit/hyperactivity disorder (ADHD) was once thought to be a behavioral problem, not a biological one. Children with this disorder, fidgety and less apt to pay attention, were once regarded as willfully acting out. But researchers at McLean Hospital in Massachusetts have used functional MRI to find evidence of differences between the brains of healthy children and at least some of those with ADHD—specifically, reduced blood flow to the putamen, a part of the brain involved in movement and some components of attention. While these findings have yet to be confirmed and explored, most researchers now believe there is at least some biological basis for ADHD. It is still not clear why the condition develops in the first place, or what the best treatments for it are. (For more on ADHD, see section **C2**.)

Sometimes we know the source of a brain impairment but see its effects only years later. Studies of children who suffered damage to the prefrontal cortex before they were sixteen months old, because of either surgery or an accident, show that they can grow up with a normal ability to learn but may lack certain social skills and moral reasoning. This implies that even social behavior, which most of us treat as entirely a product of the right sort of nurturing, may in fact be partly due to "nature," or biological in origin.

But parents or other caretakers can still be to blame. Neglect and abuse can have devastating effects on children's brains. Using brain imaging techniques and other tests, McLean Hospital researchers recently identified four distinct types of brain abnormalities in adults who were abused or neglected as children. These include electrical disturbances in the limbic region (sometimes referred to as the emotional brain); arrested development of the left hemisphere; reduced size of the corpus callosum, which links the hemispheres; and increased activity in the cerebellar vermis, which is involved in emotion, attention, and regulation of the limbic structures. The researchers theorize that people with such irregularities have been "hard-wired" to survive in a hostile world and suggest (though the evidence is less clear) that such damage may lead to the development of anxiety disorders (C21), ADHD (C2), and depression (C20) in adulthood.

Other studies of physically and sexually abused children show that about a third of them go on to develop post-traumatic stress disorder (C28). Symptoms of this disorder include disruptions in sleep, inability to concentrate, and recurring nightmares and are thought to be related to underlying changes in the brain. What is not clear is whether the damage is caused by particular traumatic episodes of abuse or by long-running deprivation or stress in the child's home.

Helping Children Explore the World

The first day of school is a big step in your child's life—and in yours. Even if your child was in day care, the transition to school is a significant, life-changing milestone. As your child progresses from preschool to kindergarten to grade school, you will notice his or her individual talents emerge and bloom. Your child's crayon drawings may reveal the skills of a budding artist. Or an early facility with numbers may hint at a future career as an engineer or mathematician. At the same time, your child is developing in other important ways: making friends, playing team sports, and joining clubs and other after-school activities. This can be a bittersweet time for parents, as they proudly watch their babies become increasingly independent individuals. It can also be stressful; many parents worry about whether they should be doing more to help their children grow and mature.

Neuroscientists point to several signs that a child's brain is especially primed for learning in the years between toddlerhood and puberty. Axons and dendrites are plentiful, creating a synaptic net that can capture many new experiences. Brain metabolism, as measured by blood sugar consumption, remains high. So does a healthy child's energy. And while it is possible to learn new skills at any age, many researchers believe some are easiest to learn between the ages of 6 and 12. One dramatic example is language: children sometimes seem like sponges soaking up new words, both in the family's primary language and in others they regularly hear. Not surprisingly,

DEALING WITH DEPRESSION

The "baby blues" is a pretty phrase for a common and sometimes severe condition: postpartum depression. There is strong evidence that, when it comes to the brain, the "baby blues" affects both mother and child. As many as 8 in 10 mothers experience mood swings and crying jags after the birth of a baby. This behavior is typically caused by the fluctuation in hormones that occurs right after birth, and for most it disappears in a week or so. But 1 in 10 women suffers from clinical depression by her baby's first birthday, and another 1 in 15 suffers prolonged bouts of the blues.

In terms of brain development, a mother's depression seems to have the most consequences when her baby is between the ages of six and eighteen months. That is when the neural connections that will later support the child's learning and behavior are being built and strengthened by his or her interactions with a supportive caregiver. But a mother's depression can cause effects in her child no matter what age. This may be because depressed mothers are less able to respond to a child's crying, or even to interact. Depressed mothers may show more negative emotions than positive ones, or try to control their children's behavior rather than encouraging them to find their own way. The result, some researchers have reported, is that such babies are later withdrawn and detached themselves. They have higher heart rates and cortisol levels. And they may not be able to pay attention to things as long as other children do.

Geraldine Dawson and colleagues used electroencephalography (EEG) technology to track how children used their frontal cortex, the part of the brain involved in regulating emotion. They found that about four in ten children of depressed mothers showed reduced activity in the frontal cortex. The left frontal cortex is the birthplace of expressed emotions, such as happiness and anger. In 90 percent of the children born to mothers who did not suffer from depression, its activity was high. By contrast, in 75 percent of babies born to depressed mothers, that part of the brain showed low levels of activity; presumably they were less able to express joy and displeasure.

Some research even suggests that if a mother is depressed while pregnant, her baby will be less active and less likely to respond to social cues than other babies. Fortunately, there is also good news. If a mother's depression is treated, she will be better able to respond to her baby, and the child's brain activity and hormone levels will remain normal. So it is wise to seek treatment for depression (C20).

studies show it is easier for people to learn second languages before the age of 10 than after.

For most other skills, however, the guidelines are less clear-cut, and we must always recall that learning continues throughout life. Harvard educator Kurt Fischer believes that learning does not progress in a strict linear sequence (which he likens to rungs on a ladder), but instead flourishes as a result of growth cycles in which a child ac-quires preliminary skills and then uses them to build new capacities. Fischer has identified several growth cycles, involving everything from basic reflexes to abstract thinking, between birth and the age of 30. As a parent, it is also important for you to remember that each child is unique and will develop at his or her own pace.

So how can parents best help their children meet the challenges of the school years? Perhaps their most useful role is to continue to provide a warm, loving, supportive, and consistent environment. At times, your children need help with homework or special tutoring, but they *always* need to know you love them. Don't worry if you're a klutz at sports and can't train your child into becoming the next Tiger Woods or Venus Williams. That's a coach's job. As parents, your job is to show your pride when your child plays hard and plays well. Another important part of the school years is learning to work with others; though children build these relationships mostly on their own, they start from their foundation of emotional support at home. There are many ways you can provide your school-age child with an enriched environment, but in order to explore any new activity, he or she needs to feel secure.

Challenge your child with new opportunities, but don't overdo it. Many well-intentioned parents overstimulate their children and miss subtle and not-so-subtle signs that the kids just aren't interested or have had too much. Exposing children to Mozart may make them more receptive to classical music. But it does not guarantee that they will grow into musical prodigies or even like such music later on. Sometimes it is more healthy to let a child discover his or her own interests. Educators and psychologists agree that when children enjoy an activity, they become more attentive and more motivated to improve. Although all parents want their children to become well-rounded, it is also important to give your child the time and freedom to pursue activities on his or her own. This builds self-confidence, discipline, and motivation, which are all important as your child approaches the teen years. And a child needs opportunities to explore, directed by his or her own brain.

Pay attention to your growing child's physical health as well, because that affects his or her brain. Establishing healthy eating habits in childhood is one of the best ways for people to avoid becoming overweight, which could lead to diabetes, hypertension, and eventually an increased risk of stroke (**C59, C60**). Immunizations and regular checkups at the pediatrician can head off some neurological problems. Requiring your child to wear a helmet while bicycling, skateboarding, or doing similar activities, and to wear a seat belt while riding in a car, can greatly reduce his or her chance of suffering a serious head injury (**C61**). School-age children have the mobility and the energy to explore their worlds, but they don't always have the experience to know what is unsafe.

Finally, if you can, relax and enjoy childhood while it lasts. Puberty and the turbulent teen years follow soon enough.

CHAPTER 7

The Adolescent Brain

The years between childhood and adulthood are a stage of life that brings out strong feelings in just about everyone. For the young person ready to dash full speed ahead into adolescence, as well as for the adult getting ready to see adolescence from the other side as a parent, the prospect stirs up a mixture of impatience, anxiety, excitement, and just plain curiosity. The next several years will include many "firsts": receiving a driver's license (or sitting in the passenger seat while your baby daughter drives); landing a real job (or seeing your self-effacing son brandish his first paycheck); suddenly being (or welcoming) the newest participant in dinner-table discussions of world politics; experiencing (or reliving) the ter-

rors and the bliss of a first love. Perhaps no amount of reading can prepare adolescents and their families for the explosive growth ahead, but some understanding of the brain in adolescence can offer a helpful perspective.

Research into adolescent brain development now makes use of such techniques as brain imaging and very precise hormonal probes, plus new methods to make observations and analyze information in ways that are sensitive to the context in which the information is collected. Sophisticated, long-term investigation promises a wealth of findings yet to come, but today's scientific understanding already provides the outlines of the picture.

Sorting Out Adolescence from Puberty

What can a 20-year-old brain do that a 14-year-old brain cannot, and what takes place in between those ages to make the difference? Although the answer to this basic question is still incomplete, one point that has been firmly established in recent years is that, despite our inclination to think of adolescence and puberty as a single stage of development, each has its own timetable and its own distinct effects on mind and body.

The series of biological changes called puberty is concerned with ushering in our reproductive ability and begins well before the teenage years, often as early as age 8 or 10. This is when the adrenal glands (best known for producing the heart-racing, artery-tightening hormone adrenaline) reach maturity and sharply increase their production of the hormone dehydroepiandrosterone (DHEA), which is geared toward sexual development. Meanwhile, the hypothalamus, a small but powerful structure that regulates heart rate, appetite, and other vital systems, sends a chemical message in the form of gonadotropin-releasing hormone to the pituitary gland, just below it. The pituitary gland then sends the hormones known as gonadotropins to the gonads (the ovaries or testes). Interestingly, the same chemical message produces parallel results in the two sexes: in the female, egg cells begin to develop into fertilizable eggs and the ovaries begin to produce estrogen, while in the male, the testes begin to produce both sperm and testosterone. The rising levels of estrogen or testosterone bring about some of the more noticeable changes in an adolescent's body: breast

CHANGES IN SLEEP

The physiological changes of puberty produce powerful effects on the brain. One of the most striking examples appears in patterns of sleep. The bedtime established in childhood no longer seems late enough; most adolescents begin to move it along by a good hour or more, even if this makes it more difficult to wake up at the usual time in the morning. For a long time, experts thought this shift was due entirely to peer pressure or to the typical adolescent's expanding social life, but most now agree that some biological factor plays a role here as well. The identity of this factor is still in question; so far, the best evidence points to a time shift in the body's daily production of melatonin, a hormone associated with the onset of sleepiness.

Keeping later hours on weekends may not pose a serious problem, but during the week a teenager pays a heavy price. If school hours require rising as early as ever, the upshot is that the teenager will be sleep-deprived by at least an hour a day, five days in a row, which can add up to a sleep deficit that drags along from one week to the next. The result, apart from the teenager's feeling tired and perhaps emotionally on edge, is an eroded ability to learn and to remember. A great deal of research now suggests that sleep plays an important role in the brain's consolidation of long-term memory; thus, a chronic sleep deficit during these later formative years may take a toll that goes beyond mere weariness. In addition, studies suggest that sleep deprivation raises the risk of drug or alcohol use, perhaps by hobbling reasoning and judgment.

disorganized and inconsistent is actually undergoing important physical changes within the skull, all taking place in precise coordination throughout billions of brain cells. Biological changes in the brain (which we will discuss in more detail below) lay the groundwork for new modes of thinking and behaving, at the same time the young person is striving in school and outside of it to master more abstract concepts, more nuanced explanations, and a greater perspective on life in general.

Behind the Scenes in the Adolescent Brain

A large part of adolescent development takes place in the frontal lobes, which house an incredible number of faculties that we use many times each day. Here are the brain sites that enable us to make sense of the floods of information constantly being gathered by our five senses; to know when we are experiencing an emotion, and even to think about it while we feel it; to understand and keep track of the passage of time; and to hold a thought or object briefly in the forefront of our mind while we proceed with another thought (an ability known as working memory). According to a recent animal study of frontal lobe development, several different "transporter" molecules, which help the neurons to take in neurotransmitter molecules and break them down for reuse, either increase in density during adolescence or reach a plateau, which in turn alters some signaling pathways and stabilizes others. Partly from refinements in the signal circuits of the frontal lobes and partly through accumulated experience, adolescence gradually brings greater independence along with new capacities to plan,

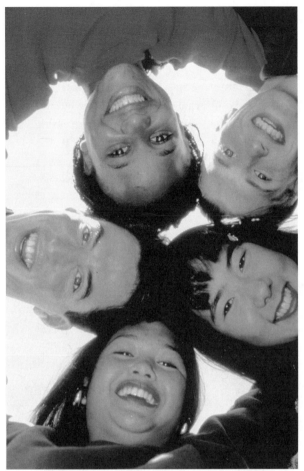

Adolescence is a time of tremendous changes in the brain, as hormones are secreted and neurons are either strengthened or pruned, depending on use or inactivity.
PHOTO © SW PRODUCTION/INDEX STOCK IMAGERY/PICTUREQUEST

development, pubic hair, and a fuller figure in females; more muscular development, voice change, pubic hair, and, finally, facial hair in males.

In contrast to puberty, the process of adolescence is aimed toward mental and emotional adulthood, and it is all but invisible because it takes place entirely within the brain. Inside that confined space, a great transformation is under way. An adolescent who may outwardly appear

to consider the possible consequences of an action, and to take responsibility for the conduct of one's life.

Not surprisingly for a major executive center, the frontal lobes must reorganize to meet new demands, and they do so at more than one level in the years leading up to adulthood. One of the most significant changes (which actually continues well into adulthood) is a major increase in the myelination, or insulation, of the nerve fibers going both into and out of the frontal lobes. Greater insulation here means faster signaling, and perhaps more highly branched signaling pathways, between frontal lobe neurons and those in any distant region of the brain. This is a development that we can understand on an everyday level. Clearly, the more information the executive center can gather in various modes—visual signals, the emphatic tone of someone's voice, the emotions of the moment—the more nuanced and appropriate the brain's responses can be.

At a day-to-day level, adolescents encounter increasing demands on their attention. For starters, entering middle school or high school means a lot more to keep track of. Instead of being with one teacher in one classroom all day, students move among a half-dozen different classrooms, with a homeroom somewhere else and a locker at yet another place. And, typically today, it quickly becomes necessary to juggle various homework assignments and projects and to balance them against sports or after-school activities, paid or volunteer work, and an ever more complicated social life. Is it any wonder that researchers, psychologists, and sociologists alike are becoming concerned about the long-term effects of these very crowded schedules on the young, developing brain? Some experts warn that our society may be overencouraging the development of quick responses and mental multitasking in young people, at the expense of equally valuable life skills: planning, thinking things through, and predicting the consequences of actions.

Whether such trade-offs are taking place on a large scale, and how they may affect the brain and behavior throughout adulthood, will become clear only with studies that can follow young people for a decade or more. Meanwhile, today's adolescents have their hands full trying to manage conflicting demands on their time, energy, and attention. Which would be a better use of time—attending an extra soccer practice in order to start in next week's game or finishing a history project now to avoid having to work on it over the weekend? Is being in charge of your family's recycling as worthwhile as volunteering two hours a week at a local soup kitchen? Young adolescents may resent or shy away from making such decisions, aware only of the appeal of each option. This behavior, although frustrating to others, is not really surprising, since their prefrontal cortex (the furthest-front portion of the brain) is not yet mature enough to offer much help either in setting priorities or in weighing the likelihood that it may not be possible to do everything at once.

Fortunately, a brain development that begins in the midteens, just in time to help with such difficulties, is the maturing of the anterior cingulate gyrus, a ridge in the middle of the frontal lobes that controls our ability to maintain attention, or to shift attention from one object to another. A young person may gradually notice an ability to focus thoughts more sharply than before or keep his or her mind on topics for longer periods. Others will also be struck with this development as they hear the adolescent delve into more complex ways of thinking. In making plans, for example, adolescence means getting better at allowing for the un-

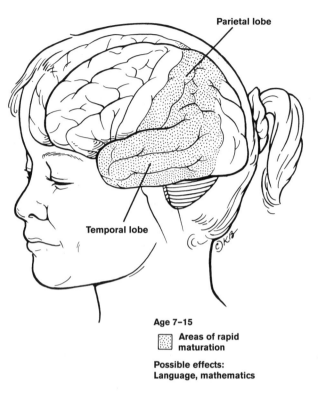

Parietal lobe

Temporal lobe

Age 7–15

▦ Areas of rapid maturation

Possible effects:
Language, mathematics

As a child enters adolescence, the brain undergoes a new surge of maturation. ILLUSTRATION © KATHRYN BORN

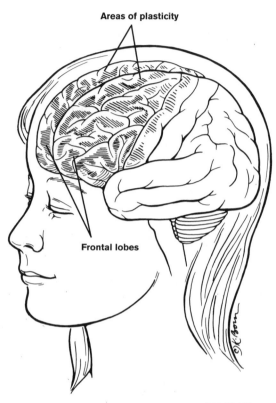

Areas of plasticity

Frontal lobes

Age 16–20

Areas of greatest change ▨

In the frontal lobes, continuing changes take place to lay the groundwork for new modes of thinking and behaving and a new way of looking at life in general. ILLUSTRATION © KATHRYN BORN

expected ("But if I'm not going to be there by 12, I'll call you"), and in conflicts, particularly where a friend is involved, it means considering a situation from more than one perspective ("I know he's angry, but he shouldn't take it out on his girlfriend").

Two brain structures involved in feeling and thinking—the amygdala, which plays an important role in the processing of emotions, and the hippocampus, crucial for the formation of memories—increase in volume up to age 18, adding many new synapses to enhance cell-to-cell communication. Intriguingly, the amygdala grows proportionately larger in males, which may explain why young men often seem to gain an extra measure of irritability and aggressiveness in early

adolescence (although young women can certainly show these traits as well). In contrast, the hippocampus increases proportionately more in females, perhaps laying the groundwork for their special adeptness at remembering complex social relationships, an ability that may have helped to promote the survival of our human ancestors.

Meanwhile, the corpus callosum, the thick bundle of nerve fibers best known for transporting signals between the left and right hemispheres, also undergoes physical change, increasing in size up to about age 18. The nerve fibers take on more myelin, a fatty white matter that acts as insulation, so that the speed of signaling between the hemispheres and among many sites within each region increases many times. In the hemispheres themselves, a wave of growth adds more nerve fibers to the "association" cortex, where the brain translates the data from our five senses into mental perceptions, and to the regions concerned with language. Taken together, these changes both enable and support an adolescent's sense of experiencing life with greater intensity, while he or she reaches for new language with which to convey this sense.

Contrary to what we'd expect, some of our mental abilities develop in adolescence not by the adding of new synapses, but by means of the process scientists have labeled pruning—eliminating synapses that are weak or underused. A study of pubertal monkeys, aged about 15 to 20 months, observed a significant loss of one particular type of synapse in the prefrontal cortex. These synapses, which allow rapid communication with nearby cells but not with distant ones, are distributed in a pattern that looks like stripes, and the authors of the study suggest that the narrowing of these stripes is responsible for the notable improvement in short-term, or working, memory that usually takes place by the end of adolescence.

Pubertal hormones appear to play a role in synaptic pruning. The general effect is to refine and reinforce, rather than replace, the brain's signal pathways, through which the nerve cells exchange chemical and electrical messages. When this intricate process unfolds in normal fashion, the rewards are considerable. A young person will have gained a new capacity for abstract thinking, the ability not only to dream but also to plan, and the consolidation of a core identity, which in turn opens the way for deeper love relationships and for enduring satisfaction in work, friendships, and many other areas of life.

If young teenagers sometimes appear to be thrown off course by their hearts and their hormones, they have good reason. Because puberty is usually well under way, urging young people toward romantic and sexual relationships several years before the brain developments of adolescence begin to take root, people at this age lack the moderating influence of the frontal lobes that they will later come to rely on. With little impulse control, critical judgment, or a steady self-image, it is no wonder that young loves or young flings seem to blossom so suddenly and fade so quickly.

To add to the confusion, puberty, the biological stage of development, comes to some young people earlier than to their peers, creating an uncomfortable "maturity gap." Parents may see a youngster's physical and emotional changes outstripping mental development, which runs on a timeline more closely linked to age or experience. Young people going through puberty early may spend years moving about in the adolescent world with a sexually mature body and hormonally activated brain, but still lacking the mental skills to meet adult-level challenges such as defusing anger and hostility (in themselves or in others), foreseeing the consequences of their actions, or delaying immediate gratification for the sake of a long-term goal. To a lesser extent, a feeling of being out of phase—with body, brain, and social self all at odds with one another—is a feature of adolescence for almost everyone.

Having both one's physical and mental self in flux is what makes puberty and adolescence such a unique stage of life. These years have their perils, but they also bring great opportunities to explore, to widen horizons, and to start taking charge of one's own future.

The Real Role of Hormones

If a teenager is moody, goofy, or infatuated, people often attribute that behavior to hormones. It is important to keep in mind, though, that hormones circulate in our bloodstream not just during adolescence but throughout our lives, and they serve many purposes beyond those of sexuality and reproduction. For example, every evening a gradual rise in the hormone melatonin entices us to sleep; in the morning, peak levels of the hormone cortisol help get us up and moving. Our weight and energy levels, along with fat storage, are subject to fine-tuning by a hormone known as leptin.

In fact, a rise in leptin is one of the hallmarks of puberty for both sexes. But whereas in girls this rise is dramatic and sustained, bringing along with it an increase in body fat, in boys the increase in leptin is soon suppressed by the much greater production of testosterone—which in turn brings about the dramatic increase of muscle mass often seen in boys during puberty.

At the cerebral level, pubertal changes in hormones represent a set of new challenges to a brain system that has successfully maintained regular hormone levels for years. The hypothalamus and the pituitary gland, the brain sites that coordinate and oversee hormonal systems, need time to mature and to adjust to new cycles and baselines. With the many interactions and biochemical feedback loops that take shape at this time, the brain's hormone-regulating system is like a living-room thermostat that has been adjusted to exactly the right temperature and then must suddenly contend with the lighting of a hearty blaze in the fireplace.

Just as males and females differ in the nature of their hormonal shifts and in their age of onset, they are also affected by hormones in different ways. These variations are possible because hormones do their job not by circulating passively in the blood but by binding to specific receptor molecules in various tissues: muscle, skin, fat, larynx, and so on. This is why the same chemical message delivered to receptors in different tissues can produce any number of different but complementary effects, such as the increasing muscle mass and deepening voice of a teenage boy, the filling out of the figure of a teenage girl, and the growth of underarm and pubic hair in both sexes.

Major hormonal shifts can affect the mind as well as body, of course, and in adolescence some of the most familiar effects occur in the realm of mood—witness the stereotype of a teen who's always bouncing from despair to elation and back again. In a less exaggerated way, almost all adolescents find that their feelings seem to have gained a new intensity and that they change and reverse themselves more often than before. Most evidence from the research attributes this not only to surges in the sex hormones themselves, which can act as mood-altering neurotransmitters in the brain, but also to the strengthening of signal circuits within "emotional" brain sites such as the hippocampus and the amygdala. Within these circuits, the signal receptors themselves respond not to overall levels of hormones, but to *changes* in levels. During puberty this response becomes more pronounced, owing to an increase in the density of receptors.

Toward the end of puberty, at about the age of 15 or 16, this system comes under the moderating influence of the frontal lobes, as signaling pathways between the two regions take on new layers of myelin to insulate the nerve fibers. With a sharp rise in signaling from the brain's executive center, adolescents of both sexes begin to gain the ability to moderate the powerful effects of hormones on their emotions and behavior. This crucial development can take years or even a decade, but the outcome lasts for many decades more. Although we never become fully able to choose and direct our own feelings (and how strange life would be if we could do this!), reaching adulthood brings more expertise in directing one's own behavior—that is, what we choose to *do* with our feelings.

The complicated mental and emotional shifts involved in a transition from childhood to maturity usually have a strong impact not only on the adolescent but on those around her or him. While the young person may be most aware of changing feelings and physical states—a greater need for sleep, inability to concentrate, or overriding preoccupation with one idea or project at a time—others in the family are more likely to notice and to be affected by intense and changeable moods, perhaps irritability, and often some withdrawal from family life (with greater attention to social life).

Healthy Risks

In the context of adolescence, the term *risk* all too often has alarming association: unprotected sex, drug use, drinking and driving, and more. But risk isn't always bad; in fact, human development would be impossible without it. Even our first baby steps came with a strong possibility of bumps and falls, yet we all took that risk willingly. A hallmark of maturity is the ability not to avoid risks but to weigh them carefully and manage them well.

Risk taking is a normal part of adolescence, most researchers agree. According to one school of thought, novel or slightly dangerous experi-

ences stimulate the release of dopamine, bringing great pleasure through the circuits of the brain's "reward system." As the chief neurotransmitter in the reward system, dopamine is also responsible for feelings of motivation. But thrill seeking and the love of novelty do not carry equal weight in every teenager—several studies suggest that up to 60 percent of a person's tendency to act on impulse is inherited in the genes and may therefore exist to a similar degree in other members of a family.

Many of the risks we expect adolescents to take—creating romantic relationships, finding and keeping a responsible job, perhaps traveling far from home for schooling or to live on their own for the first time—obviously are positive, major steps toward independence. At the same time, from the adult perspective, other risks, involving physical recklessness (say, stunt driving) or flouting the law (for example, experimenting with drugs), may appear not only dangerous but foolish. It's often said that young people embrace this kind of risk because "they think they're immortal," or at least immune from the consequences of their actions. But what may really be at work here is a crucial gap between what young people rationally *know* and what knowledge they *use* in making decisions—a gap that fills in gradually as they learn more from the outcome of each decision.

Sports

For a great many adolescents, of course, the greatest and most widely assorted kinds of thrill seeking are found in sports. Particularly in the early teen years, one or two sports may become the overriding preoccupation and organizing principle of a young person's life—and for many good reasons. Team sports such as football and soccer, and even relatively solitary sports such as tennis and cross-country, offer the satisfaction of both physical challenge and mental skill building, all with a built-in social network and a demanding yet sympathetic mentor or two. Persistent effort is rewarded, thus building up motivation (via the dopamine-based reward system discussed above), which in turn promotes more effort, and so on, in a gratifying and healthy cycle. There is even evidence to suggest that participating in sports may help reduce other kinds of risk taking: for example, a study of female adolescents found that fewer than one fourth (21 percent) of those who took part in sports were sexually active, as compared with half (50 percent) of those with no athletic activities. However, very intense athletic involvement carries its own risks: another study showed the likelihood of eating disorders increasing along with the level of competition in a given sport.

Unhealthy Risks

Risk taking in itself is normal and even necessary for learning to live in the world, but it becomes a problem when carried out in excess, or when it persists in the face of clear warnings about significant, needless danger. Some experts in this area point out that adolescents are most prone to risky behavior in situations presenting new, unexpected challenges—not because of some weak or trouble-seeking character, but simply because they are inexperienced. A desire to experience something new doesn't necessarily guarantee that we will know how to handle it. We all understand the dangers of, say, reckless driving, but young people may be less adept at keeping those rather impersonal, statistical warnings in mind when they suddenly have to make a real live decision with friends and peers looking on.

This is one reason that practice with risk-carrying situations, especially talking them over beforehand with people an adolescent trusts, can be very helpful. Forethought and discussion also put decisions into better context, enabling a teenager to take into account the thoughts of people close to them but detached from the immediate situation. The National Longitudinal Study on Adolescent Health, which surveyed more than 12,000 high school students throughout the country, has noted that feelings of "connectedness" (feeling close to people at school, fairly treated by teachers, and loved and wanted at home) helped significantly to lower an individual's likelihood of emotional distress, early sexual activity, substance abuse, violence, and suicide.

Brain Trauma

Traumatic injury to the brain is a disorder of major significance to public health, according to the National Institutes of Health, and among teenagers a leading cause of death. Roughly twice as common in males as in females, brain trauma most commonly results from car, motorcycle, and other vehicular accidents; falls; acts of violence; and even sports injuries. Partly because adolescents are the most drawn to risk and partly because they have not yet developed the multi-processing skills needed to judge risks accurately, the age group from 15 to 24 suffers the highest incidence of brain trauma. Depending on which regions of the brain are injured, a victim may lose physical, emotional, or mental functioning, or perhaps only a very specific faculty such as short-term memory or the ability to recognize faces—but the impact on quality of life may be terrible nevertheless. While it isn't practical to ask anyone to avoid all activities that carry a risk of brain trauma, it is possible to cut down on risk with some simple protective measures, such as not using a handheld cell phone while driving, driving more slowly in bad weather, and wearing a helmet when bicycling to shield the all-important frontal lobes.

Substance Abuse

When it comes to unhealthy substances, it is common nowadays for teenagers to experiment with tobacco, drugs, and alcohol—that is, to try them a few times or on an occasional basis. This certainly does not mean that those who abstain aren't normal; rather, it suggests they may have a more advanced ability than their peers to weigh nonsimple risks, in which negative consequences are unlikely but could be very serious.

Rarely does mild experimentation bring lasting harm; the greater risk, of course, is that it may open the door to long-term use or even to addiction. In such cases, lifelong well-being is on the line—and there is simply no way to know whether the odds will be on the experimenter's side when exposed to this possibility. Fortunately for young people who do become ensnared, alcoholism and drug abuse are no longer considered simply failures of willpower. Extensive research has established that a behavior pattern of acting on impulse, carrying out aggressive urges, and being attracted to danger—including the dangers of substance abuse—has its roots in both biology and psychology (**C29, C30, C31**). An old naturenurture debate over whether these tendencies are caused by an individual's genes or childhood environment has given way to the more fruitful question of how a gene-based "predisposition" may be reinforced or inhibited by the individual's environment.

Everyone is familiar with the list of grim health effects that can emerge after years of smoking, ranging from a decrease in the amount of oxygen available to brain cells to an increased risk of lung, prostate, and cervical cancer. What many people may not know, however, is that using tobacco while still in one's teens makes the risk of tobacco dependence even more dangerous. Because the brain in adolescence is so prolific at producing new synaptic connections and so keen at pruning away unused synapses while strengthening those that undergo intense use, addictions that develop at this time in life are much harder to break than those acquired later.

Substances known as recreational drugs have acquired that name because they serve no medical purpose. But that doesn't mean they are harmless—on the contrary, they carry serious risks in both the short term and the long term (**C29**). To take just one class of these drugs as an example, amphetamines and methamphetamines distort the brain's reward pathway and interfere with everyday living. Users can very quickly become dependent on them for short-lived feelings of boundless energy and euphoria, although these are often followed by severe anxiety, paranoia, or depression. The most recent form of methamphetamine, dubbed Ecstasy, is also one of the most dangerous: regular use of Ecstasy can interfere with mental abilities and with memory for new information, impulse control, and sleep—quite apart from its association with seizures, irregular heartbeat, and liver damage. Some research even suggests that using Ecstasy repeatedly can cause brain damage, particularly to neurons that produce or use the neurotransmitter serotonin. Given the key role of serotonin in the regulation of mood, this damage may gradually bring on a full-fledged mental illness such as major depression.

The problems of alcohol have long been with us, of course, and the fact that drinking alcohol is legal (at age 21) offers a rationale for people who wish to turn a blind eye to its dangers (**C30**). Yet the evidence of danger is all too clear. Who by now has not heard the sobering statistics on the numerous accidents and acts of violence associated with alcohol, or seen billboards showing the bright faces of young people whose lives were cut short by drunken driving?

In addition, research suggests that adolescents, whose brains have not yet reached their full development, are more vulnerable than adults to alcohol's ill effects. If you have a family history of alcoholism, and therefore a greater risk of developing alcoholism yourself, you may show a high tolerance for alcohol; people will say you "hold your liquor well." The inconvenient truth is that even before you begin to feel drunk, you may have lost a crucial edge in your working memory, your reflexes, and even—most important of all—your judgment. But by far the greatest danger for adolescent drinkers is that they may pave the way for long-term alcohol abuse. And this danger can become real very quickly: whereas an adult who drinks heavily may take anywhere from 5 to 15 years to become fully dependent on alcohol, his or her adolescent drinking buddy may reach this point in less than 18 months.

Mental Disorders

Unsettling behavior or feelings may come and go throughout adolescence, giving this stage of life an extra degree of unpredictability. But adolescence is also a time of extra vulnerability to certain mood disorders, particularly eating disorders and depression. Each disorder has its own characteristic warning signs, as discussed in the following sections, but all the warning signs have one important feature in common: unlike normally shifting moods, which tend to dissipate after a day or two, these conditions persist. A person who shows any of the signs described for longer than two weeks at a time should consult with the family physician or with a mental health professional.

Excessive conflict between adolescents and parents can also raise concerns about mental health. If parent-adolescent fights seem to be much more frequent or fierce than those of other parents and kids, each may wonder whether these struggles are simply due to the clash of strong personalities or are signals of an underlying mental illness. Consulting with a professional who is unaffected by the conflict and is trained to recognize such illnesses can be reassuring on this question or can point the family toward appropriate help.

Worries about mental illness are not far-fetched; the surgeon general of the United States has estimated that each year nearly 20 percent (one in five) of Americans experience a mental illness. In many cases, these brain-based disorders first become apparent during the teenage years. That is why health care professionals, counselors, teachers, coaches, and adolescents themselves should always be on the alert for possible indications of the most common mental disorders of these years—depression (**C20**) and eating disorders (**C27**)—as well as several less common but very serious ones: bipolar disorder (formerly known as manic-depressive illness; **C24**), schizophrenia (**C25**), and suicidal tendencies (**C32**).

Depression. Under the misleading label of a "mood disorder," depression all too often fails to receive the medical attention it warrants. Clinical depression is not a case of temporarily low spirits or a bad mood but a persistent state of fatigue, interruptions in sleep, and inability to concentrate;

loss of appetite, motivation, and feelings of plea-sure; and a pervasive sense of worthlessness and guilt. Changes in the brain's supply or use of neu-rotransmitters (norepinephrine and, especially, serotonin) appear to form the biochemical basis for depression, but the triggers for these changes can vary with the individual. Depression is twice as common in women as in men, but this skewed ratio does not appear until early adolescence, sometime between ages 10 and 15. Most re-searchers agree that an inherited susceptibility to depression, sharp changes in hormone levels and hormonal cycles beginning in puberty, and stress-ful "life events" of the midteens, particularly in a fast-changing social arena, are all factors in the risk of depression, but the relative weight of each factor can only be assessed one case at a time. De-pression generally responds well to therapy, par-ticularly to a combination of psychotherapy and medication.

Eating Disorders. Anorexia nervosa and bu-limia threaten the health and sometimes even the lives of millions of American teenagers, most of them girls. Both these eating disorders come with a psychological symptom, an obsession with thin-ness. However, whereas anorexia produces a loss of appetite that quickly progresses from mild to drastic, bulimia often allows normal eating but regularly causes episodes of bingeing followed by self-induced vomiting. People with anorexia often suffer dangerous levels of weight loss, while those with bulimia tend to maintain their usual weight. Both conditions have long been treated as purely psychological disorders or excessive reactions to our society's insistence that only thin bodies can be attractive. Now, however, scientific research has turned up an abnormality in the brains of anorexic and bulimic patients: their levels of serotonin are unusually high. This is significant in two respects.

First, extra serotonin may produce excessive lev-els of electrical signaling between neurons and thereby bring about the perfectionism and anx-iousness that often seem to drive the quest for an ever thinner body. Second, in a perverse feedback loop, a lack of food may make these patients feel briefly better, because it temporarily blocks the body's ability to make serotonin.

Bipolar Disorder. This disease, marked by be-wildering high spirits or irritability and limitless energy that alternate with paralyzing depression, is often difficult to recognize at first as a cyclical disorder, since the timing and length of the cycles can be so irregular. If bipolar disorder develops during adolescence, it can be even harder to spot, given the camouflage of hyperemotionality and unrealistic ambitions that most people expect to see in this age group. The root causes of bipolar disorder are not yet known, although it is clear that genes play an important role in an individ-ual's vulnerability to this illness. In late adoles-cence, the stress of a major life change such as leaving the family home, starting college, or en-tering the workforce for good may be a trigger for the biochemical cascade that sets the stage for bipolar disorder.

Schizophrenia. Affecting one in a hundred people throughout the world, schizophrenia is far from the rarest but is probably the most misun-derstood of all mental illnesses. The layperson's image of someone with schizophrenia is usually of a dangerous lunatic, but the truth is that schizo-phrenic patients are rarely violent, and many ex-perience lucid, realistic intervals. Much of the time, a person with schizophrenia is struggling desperately to make sense of his unique knowl-edge and impressions; his efforts appear senseless to us only because the things he is trying to ex-plain logically—the voices, visions, and hidden messages—are not real but hallucinated, the inventions of an unwell brain.

Clinicians and researchers have long observed that schizophrenia often makes its first appearance in the late teens or early twenties, but the reason for this timing is unclear. One candidate for a trigger is the hormonal surges and changes of late puberty, but another possibility lies in a physical change in the brain itself: the burst of myelination that begins in late adolescence. If certain "vulnerability" genes have subtly weakened the nerve fibers to begin with, the sudden rise in speed and quantity of signaling that comes with myelination might overload the circuits altogether, causing a great deal of misfiring and miscommunication among neurons—just the right circumstances to produce the hallucinations and disordered thinking that are classic signs of schizophrenia.

Suicide. The risk of suicide runs all too high among adolescents and young adults. While the vast majority of young people obviously don't attempt to destroy themselves or even seriously contemplate it, the number of those who do is on the rise. From 1980 to 1996, the suicide rate among people aged 15 to 24 increased by 14 percent, and among those even younger—aged 10 to 14—the rate doubled. Among adolescents, those most gravely at risk are males aged 16 and older who are struggling with both a mood disorder and a disruptive behavioral disorder, as well as with substance abuse. Other risk factors for both males and females under 30 include personality problems (including serious difficulties with impulse control), and severe trouble with interpersonal relationships. But you don't need to know someone's medical history to help prevent a suicide. We should all be alert to the warning signs and ready to summon help if we see them.

Currently, researchers are working hard to define the biological factors that may contribute to the risk of suicide. If certain genes, for example, are found to increase an individual's risk of suicide—not to *cause* or *foretell* a suicide, but simply to make someone more vulnerable to the possibility—finding these genes and developing drugs to counteract their effect may lower the risk considerably. In the future, if it becomes possible to identify people at greater risk when they are still quite young, then professionals (counselors or social workers, psychologists or psychotherapists) could help these individuals build up the factors that have been found to protect against suicide, such as developing a feeling of connectedness within their family, looking out for their own emotional health, and discussing problems rather than ruminating on them alone. According to some researchers, increasing the protective factors may be even more important than trying to reduce the risk factors.

Kaleidoscope of Changes

Common sense tells us that periods of major development, like that of the brain in adolescence, must include a certain amount of disruption and inconsistency. For this reason, "normal" adolescence is easier to recognize by its successful outcome than by any of the ups and downs of a few days or a few weeks.

The many different societies of the world define adolescence in their own way: some as the beginning of adult life, others as a distinct age that bridges childhood and adulthood. But whether a society marks this stage of life with an arranged marriage, training as a warrior, or the awarding of a driver's license, the message is that the young person will now take on more weighty responsibilities along with greater independence. The shifting expectations of people surrounding a new adolescent will create some of the frustrating constraints, as well as many of the most exciting opportunities, that await him or her in the next several years.

All the restructuring and rewiring in the brain that has been discussed in this chapter has one essential purpose: to provide the physical basis for the remarkable mental growth that is the work of adolescence. Childhood's "windows" of optimal time for certain kinds of learning (foreign languages, superior athletic or musical skills) have been left behind, but the windows for other, more far-reaching kinds of learning now appear. By late adolescence the brain has achieved the ability to sustain attention but also to manage several demands at once; to experience all the physical impulses and drives of an adult but also to decide consciously when to act on them; to think more precisely but also more profoundly. And the best is yet to come. Capable as the brain has now become, it will continue to grow and develop for many years more.

CHAPTER 8

The Brain in Adult Life and Normal Aging

You might expect that, after spending 20 or so years in continuous self-construction, the adult brain would rest on its laurels for two or three decades. And so it could, if you were to let it, but the years from your early 20s through your 50s are called the prime of life for a good reason. Your fully formed brain is prepared to take in stride anything you care to challenge it with, short of toxins, traumas, and unhealthy stress.

If the hallmark of the child's brain is "wiring up," and the greatest feature of the adolescent brain is frontal lobe development, the most important trait the brain brings to adulthood and through the end of life can be summed up in one word, *plasticity. Plasticity* is the term neuroscientists have coined to describe the brain's biological adaptations in response to new experiences or change. Scientists say the word in tones of awe in the context of child development, hope in the context of brain damage, frustration when the subject is certain mental and nervous system disorders, and admiration in the context of normal adult life and aging. It is plasticity that underlies our transit of all life's major passages.

Plasticity allows us to learn, to form new habits, to adjust to new circumstances—whether as simple as remembering to make enough morning coffee for two after marriage, or as complicated as learning to use information technology when your employer decides to carve out a place in the "new economy." Consider how nearly limitless may be the number of new things an adult brain must contend with: the first full-time, permanent job, and then, in future years, career changes; marriage, the birth and rearing of children, shopping and obtaining a mortgage for, and getting used to, a new home, and then doing it all over again in future years; helping offspring with schoolwork that looks nothing like what you remember, using tools that didn't exist when you were a student; forming new circles of friends and colleagues from time to time and acquiring the social behavior common to those circles; taking adult classes in new topics, picking up a hobby, traveling to another country with your rusty high school foreign language skills; reordering your days or seizing on a new occupation for your retirement. Effortlessly (or sometimes not), you modify everyday routines to reflect the changing world around you and to seek out and involve yourself in new experiences. But everything would remain forever raw, difficult, and uncertain, day after day, if you could not count on your brain to swing into action through a steady stream of change and make it all familiar and easy.

Your brain allows you to become familiar with new circumstances through the process of "habituation," in which its response to a sensory stimulus (pictures, music, the feel of a new pair of shoes) gradually decreases in intensity as the stimulus continues. In general, the brain is primed to focus on what changes, rather than what remains in a steady state. This is why, for example, city dwellers can truthfully say they don't hear the 24-hour traffic roaring past their windows but may be awakened during a night in the country by a single

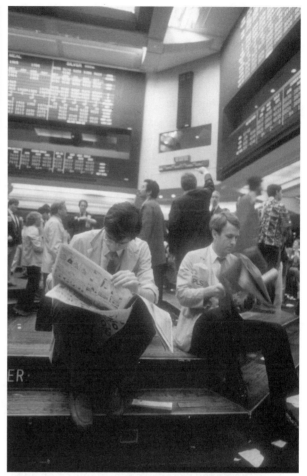

Habituation **is the term for your brain's ability to decrease its response to continuing stimuli. That is why these stockbrokers can read newspapers amid the noise and bustle of the exchange trading floor.** Photo © Steve Leonard/Black Star Publishing/PictureQuest

cicada. Being alert to new or unexpected sensations is not only essential for our survival, it's thrifty as well. By turning down the volume of signaling in response to things that happen steadily and consistently, the brain sets a fine example of energy conservation. At the same time, though, the brain invests considerable resources in paying attention to novelty and change, especially in the realm of sound. As if to underline once again the importance of this function, the brain carries it out by a circuit that redirects our attention to strange noises *involuntarily,* eliminating any hesitation or choice in the matter.

The brain also reallocates the precious resources of space and energy when a stimulus that once was novel becomes familiar; for example, recognizing the faces of people we have met recently is a job handled primarily in the frontal lobes, but once we've recognized them several times, the job is distributed along a larger neural circuit that even recruits some visual areas at the back of the brain for memory storage. And some well-practiced skills stake out additional territory in the brain, as has been seen in musicians: the cerebellum, which is thought to control a variety of sensory, motor, and cognitive functions, has a volume about 5 percent larger in musicians than in nonmusicians of the same age.

Perspectives on "Normality"

Given the reasonable constraints on opening the skulls of people who are alive and well, it is not a simple matter for scientists to find out how the normal brain carries out even the most ordinary tasks. (See chapter 2, "How We Know.") The more expertly and unobtrusively the brain performs a particular function, the more difficult it is for researchers to track down all its component tasks to the brain sites, synapses, or signals where these tasks originate. For instance, attention (**B10**), a faculty that seems to run on its own without any mental direction from us, is actually the output of a wide-ranging network that is partly built into the brain before birth and partly developed with de-

liberate effort by the individual. The ability to sustain attention is only one element of this feature, yet children attain it only after years of effort. The ability to shift attention from one object or task to another develops even more slowly, and the feat of *not* paying attention, of ignoring potential distractions, relies on a sophisticated filtering circuit that must be unique for each person and must even be able to change moment by moment as the person's circumstances require.

With memory (**B13**), too, it's easy for us to think of a great many capabilities as a seamless (although very extensive) whole, but the brain doesn't really work this way. The main aspects of memory will be described later in this chapter; suffice it to say here that remembering *who* Grandma is, how she *looks,* her *phone number, when* you're going to visit her again, *how* she makes that special noodle pudding, and how it *smells* when it comes out of the oven are all memories that draw some of their information from a wide variety of brain sites. This means researchers must focus their investigations very narrowly in order to be sure they're looking at exactly what they want to observe rather than at their research target obscured by other features. The result of narrowing the research focus can sometimes be a study that seems geared toward proving the obvious—for instance, that it hurts to dip your fingers into extremely hot water. But the goal of such a study is simply to clear the ground for the real inquiry: such as, does the anticipation of pain reduce or increase the actual pain when it occurs? Before investigators can produce, say, functional magnetic resonance imaging (MRI) scans that address this question, they must have images that establish a "baseline"—in this case, brain images of the volunteers' reactions during the first dip, before they knew the water would be painfully hot.

The normal brain at work can also be studied in terms of any of the innumerable functions it carries out each moment: directing the body's movements, for example, or selectively inhibiting them; producing language or interpreting someone else's utterances; retrieving a long-stored memory and actively bringing it into association with a new experience. While researchers continue their efforts to add detail to the composite picture of the normal brain, each finding must be evaluated carefully in terms of its own particular, and necessarily limited, perspective.

Generally, the combination of two or more perspectives gives clinicians and scientists a working consensus on what the normal brain looks like. At the same time, however, the consensus view must allow for considerable variation. Just to take one example, normal brains are not all the same size. The average male brain is larger than the average female brain, and this difference is generally thought to correspond to the larger muscle mass of the average male, which requires additional nerve cells and signal-transmitting fibers. Brain size can also vary greatly among individuals and is not an index of intelligence. It is not the volume of the brain but its large surface area—the famous wrinkles and folds of the cerebral cortex—that allow our neurons to build trillions of connections into the signaling pathways within which take place all the things that make each of us unique.

In time, neuroscience will discover all the circuitry, neurotransmitters, and hormones we use to achieve the astonishing performance of the adult brain, but two other interesting examples of what researchers are studying may give some sense of the elegant orchestration at work within this complex organ. One example is that of parenthood, a decades-long endeavor that includes in its early years exhaustion, frustration, logistical challenges, tedium, nagging fears, and occasional bewilderment—and later the stresses of piloting children through adolescence. If we were to depend only on objective, cognitive skills to be loving parents, we might choose easier ways to spend our prime years. But since survival of a species means rearing the next generation to maturity, some form of brain plasticity must help us give up our carefree ways in order to undertake this most important of all human ventures. Scientists exploring parenthood in the animal kingdom have seen intriguing clues about how that self-surrendering plasticity might be summoned, in the activity of a hormone, oxytocin, during mating and parenting. Oxytocin is produced in the hypothalamus, the brain site that maintains the body in a steady state by regulating such features as temperature, blood pressure, thirst, and hunger. Some researchers have been studying oxytocin and a closely related hormone, vasopressin, in a small, monogamous rodent known as the prairie vole, in hopes of finding "the neuroendocrine substrates for love." In the prairie vole, the brain's release of oxytocin at the time of mating appears to induce the female to develop a strong preference for the one male she is with; in the male it is vasopressin that seems to encourage this "partner preference." (Neither hormone produces this effect in another species, the montane vole, which is polygamous.) These hormones are also significant in the voles' new parenthood. With the birth of offspring, vasopressin floods the brains of both female and male prairie voles, along with extra oxytocin in females, and both sexes start behaving like parents: cleaning, feeding (exclusively the mother's job), and sheltering their young. With the release of oxytocin, even female montane voles show more caring behavior during this period than at any other time in their lives.

This transformation appears to be possible because the distribution of receptor sites in the brain for oxytocin actually changes within 24 hours of a vole's giving birth—plasticity at work for the survival of the species.

If it is perhaps too fanciful that hormones can ever explain how we develop parental love, it is beyond question that brain plasticity allows us to acquire expertise in a tremendous variety of areas beyond our basic survival skills. A case in point is music, which exists in all cultures, has been found in evidence going back millions of years, and yet cannot be said to be "hard-wired" into the brain like the regulation of breathing or eating or sleep. Listening to music may seem like a simple, low-key function, but it requires the participation of a number of sites throughout the brain, each performing its own specialized task. Research in this field suggests that the left hemisphere handles the perception of rhythm, while the right hemisphere focuses on pitch and the discrimination of single notes and melodies. Both the "language areas" in the left hemisphere and their right-hemisphere counterparts are active during music listening. Broca's area, which analyzes syntax when we hear someone speaking aloud, performs a similar function with music: it analyzes harmonic sequences. Wernicke's area, and particularly its right-hemisphere counterpart, appears to deal with temporal analysis (in music as well as in speech). And, in yet another example of plasticity at work, a study using electroencephalograms (EEGs) revealed a subtle difference in brain activity between people with musical training and those without. Notwithstanding the work of specific brain sites, in musically trained people the left hemisphere was dominant overall during music listening, whereas in nontrained music listeners the right hemisphere was dominant.

Taking Advantage of New Findings and New Thinking About the Adult Brain

Recent research on the brain has established two great principles. First, far from remaining static in adulthood, as we had long assumed, the human brain continues to grow and develop throughout our entire life span. This development takes place in two ways: by ongoing adjustments in signaling pathways and by the addition of new brain cells. Knowing this means that you should try, as you would with any fine, high-powered machine, to practice good maintenance to give it the best chance to provide peak performance. This means faithfully practicing basic brain care: plenty of rest, good nutrition, and good health habits. (See chapter 3, "Basic Brain Care.") But the brain offers a priceless opportunity that no man-made machine can provide: in many respects we can make a material difference in how it ages, and even induce it to perform better over time.

This is thanks to the second, equally powerful principle, that brain development in adulthood, as in childhood, is shaped largely by outside stimuli rather than by specifications within the brain cells themselves. Here is rich food for thought: beyond simply letting our brain carry us, we can consciously decide in what ways we would like our brains to grow. Just as we may choose to strengthen our muscles with challenging workouts, we can encourage brain growth by keeping engaged in many different mental activities.

Good "workouts" for the brain can be found in almost any area of life. Productive, satisfying work—whether in paid employment, volunteer programs, or a challenging hobby—provides exercise for the brain on a regular basis. Socializing with old and new friends and visiting with family in person or by long-distance communication;

analyzing new information (current events, for example, or the nitty-gritty of building a retirement portfolio) in the light of what is already known; and maintaining old skills or practicing a new one (sports, gardening, bird-watching, playing a musical instrument) all stimulate the brain in various ways.

When these activities include mild physical exertion as well, the brain receives a bonus; numerous studies now show that physical exercise at all ages makes a major contribution to the overall health of the brain. This link was suggested as long ago as the mid-1960s, when scientists compared the skull development of rats raised in an "enriched environment" (including running wheels and plenty of space for exercise) with that of rats raised in stark, "impoverished" conditions. More than 30 years later, another research team showed that not just the skull but whole populations of neurons benefited from an enriched environment. Researchers have established that even after its explosive growth during gestation and early development, the brain continues throughout life to give rise to new neurons, not only in rats and mice, but in humans as well. Strikingly, when normal adult mice are housed in an environment that is more complex than the standard laboratory setting, with more living space, greater social interaction, and more physical activity, the new neurons tend to survive at a higher rate, producing more brain growth. Of all the factors in this experiment, physical activity appears to be the most important: voluntary running, on a running wheel, led to the survival of as many new neurons as all the other enrichment conditions combined.

Exactly what takes place within and between brain cells to produce this effect is not yet clear, but studies in both animal and human subjects have produced evidence for several appealing possibilities. In Hannover, Germany, a small group of research volunteers displayed a higher velocity of blood flow in the middle cerebral artery after brief exercise of the arms or legs. The brain's metabolism, or use of energy—as measured, for example, by oxygen saturation—rose along with the velocity of blood flow. Of course, much of this additional energy goes into producing the brain signals that allow us to move our muscles; whether it provides the wherewithal for extra cognitive work as well is not yet clear. In middle-aged rats (fourteen months old), a daily one-hour swim improved the animals' memory, possibly by reducing the buildup of oxidatively damaged proteins in the brain. Conversely, when rats bred to run long distances are abruptly stopped from doing so, their brains show a sharp decrease in brain-derived neurotrophic factor (BDNF), a substance that is crucial for the nourishment of new brain cells. In a study that assigned previously sedentary men and women, aged 60 to 75, to one of two exercise groups for six months—one group performing aerobic exercise (walking) and the other anaerobic exercise (stretching and toning)—those carrying out the aerobic exercise showed significant improvement in "executive" (frontal cortex) skills, such as working memory, planning, and scheduling, as well as in the speed with which they could switch between executive tasks. The increased oxygen consumption that comes with aerobic fitness may be the physical basis for the improvements, but the question is still open.

Back in the laboratory, scientists are working to identify drug compounds that may support new cell growth in the brain at the molecular level; but this approach is expected to supplement, rather than substitute for, the important benefits of continually challenging the brain with new activities.

Disorders in the Adult Brain

As impressive as the adult brain is, it is not invulnerable. Almost any of the disorders to which the brain and nervous system are subject can occur in the prime of life, and some illnesses that strike in young adulthood or early middle age are a major challenge to the general picture of strength that the typical adult brain presents. The most incapacitating include schizophrenia (**C25**) and bipolar disorder (**C24**), which often emerge with the beginning of adulthood, multiple sclerosis (**C33**), which typically strikes in the forties, and Parkinson's disease (**C41**), which in many cases appears in late middle age.

Other, more common disorders typically appear in adulthood rather than in childhood or advanced ages. These particularly widespread problems—headache (**C54**), migraine (**C55**), back pain (**C56**), depression (**C20**), anxiety (**C21**), and alcoholism (**C30**)—can all become chronic or recurring and can be major impairments or even disabilities if they are not treated seriously as medical or psychiatric problems. Yet even in these disorders, the plasticity of the adult brain has a significant role—two roles, in fact. Sometimes it contributes to the problem, and sometimes, when treatment is undertaken, it can be recruited on behalf of recovery. The new "functional" imaging techniques that allow scientists and clinicians to observe the brain at work have now produced clear pictures of physical changes in the brain that take place as patients with major depression start to respond to treatment. Two studies published together, one using PET (positron-emission tomography) and the other SPECT (single-photon-emission computed tomography, in which the image is formed from many photos taken by a gamma camera that re-volves around the patient), showed changes in glucose metabolism and in blood flow (an indirect measure of brain activity) after 6 to 12 weeks of treatment. While it is reasonable to expect that in the course of recovering from an illness the brain would undergo some changes, it is still somehow startling to see them clearly. But the most intriguing observation from these studies is that the changes associated with psychotherapy and those associated with antidepressant drugs appear very similar. Does this mean the two forms of treatment are interchangeable, that one might as well take a pill as schedule a session? This is a question beyond the range of brain imaging. When it comes to exploring how physical changes in the brain may translate into changes in an individual patient's behavior or understanding, the research has so far just scratched the surface.

The possibility of enlisting plasticity in the treatment of disorders is one of the newest directions in neuroscience research. Hopes for its potential are implicit in most of the brain "repair" strategies being investigated for damage ranging from trauma to stroke to spinal cord injury. But, like the kindred mystery of stem cell development, the biology of plasticity is a story just beginning to be told. For example, can plasticity in the adult brain combat conditions present since childhood? In some circumstances, perhaps.

An informal report published in a major scientific journal late in 2001 reported an intriguing observation, concerning a mathematician who had been born with cataracts, opaque areas on the lens of the eye that prevent light from reaching the retina. He took eyedrops for 40 years to dilate his pupils around the cataracts, giving him limited vision. When he decided to have the cataracts removed, he invited two scientists with expertise in vision and perception to study his eyes before and after the operation. The scientists took baseline measurements before the surgery and conducted various tests for 56 days following the operation. During one test, as the researchers moved a light slowly across the pupil, the mathematician mentioned that the light seemed brighter at the far side of his eye. Startled by the comment, the researchers turned their attention to the patient's photoreceptors. These cells, located in the cones on the surface of the retina, usually point toward the center of pupils, where light is brightest. The researchers theorized that the mathematician's photoreceptors might be aligned to the side, where, because of lifelong squinting, his dilated pupils had been largest before the operation. To test their theory, they took a particular measurement, called SCE-I peak function, which indicates where a light shined into someone's pupil appears brightest. From this, they inferred the position of the mathematician's cones. In the first ten days after surgery, the patient's SCE-I peak function shifted to the center. In the left eye, peak function moved 1.6 mm, indicating a 4-degree shift in the cones. In the right, it moved 2.6 mm, indicating a 6.5-degree shift. Describing this unexpected adaptation by the retina, the researchers speculated that a simple feedback mechanism may control the orientation of photoreceptors in the human eye, allowing the receptors, like sunflowers in a field, to turn to the light.

Thinking About Memory

If plasticity is the name of the game in adulthood, the principal player and captain of the team is memory. In the healthy adult brain, memory is a lifelong resource that supports virtually all our cognitive abilities. Even in the most ordinary day, it is difficult to think of a single moment in which we are not using some combination of declarative memory, implicit memory, visual memory, emotional memory, and even auditory and olfactory memory, all at once. (See **B13**, "Learning and Memory.") We test new experiences against what we have stored away in these memory forms, and we use memory to guide everything from routine actions to major decision making.

Human memory is a reference library in constant use, and scientific research on memory at work bears out the vast flexibility and responsiveness that we count on in this everyday function. In one study, when 20 expert chess players underwent magnetic resonance imaging while they played chess against a computer, their brains showed the most activity in the areas of long-term memory storage. By contrast, inexperienced players showed the most brain activity in a region known for analyzing new information and forming long-term memories. The experts' brains were also seen to give off "focal gamma bursts" of signaling, a sign of memory-related activity, for several seconds after every move by the computer—a pattern explained by the theory that expert memory relies on large amounts of information available in "chunks," rather than numerous small items dispersed throughout the brain.

To appreciate the current scientific understanding of memory in terms of everyday experience, it helps to be familiar with several different but related aspects of this function. First, whatever we recall of our childhood, of a recent presidential election, or even of yesterday's lunch menu, is considered part of long-term memory. The small structure known as the hippocampus, deep in the middle of the brain, plays a major role in forming these memories, which are then stored diffusely throughout the brain. By contrast, a short-term memory, or working memory, such as a particular phone number that we are about to dial, is held in the hippocampus only as long as it is needed.

Second, memories can be divided another way as well. The human brain contains both declarative memory (information, descriptions, memories that can be stated verbally) and nondeclarative, or "implicit," memory (sensations, skills, procedures, and actions that can more easily be demonstrated than described, such as how to ride a bicycle).

Third, the feat of remembering actually consists of three steps. The memory must be formed, or encoded, with a unique pattern of nerve signals; it must be stored or maintained in its original state, whether for a few hours or a lifetime; and when needed, it must be actively retrieved.

Recognizing the three steps that are involved in remembering now adds an interesting new wrinkle to the discussion of memory problems: Do difficulties tend to arise during encoding, storage, retrieval, or some combination of the three? Recent work suggests that slight problems with memory in healthy older brains are mostly due to slower processing at the retrieval stage.

None of us will recall a story or commit a name to memory in exactly the same way at age 76 as we did at age 16, because the mental context in which we perform these functions may have changed entirely over half a dozen decades. But for the most part, what we have stored from life in our minds—the experiences and emotions, perceptions and information—remains there in safekeeping. It is the ease or speed with which we're able to *retrieve* something from memory that changes with the passing of time.

As early as age 20, before we have even begun to think about adapting to age-related changes in brain activity, signal transmission throughout the entire central nervous system begins to slow down very slightly, by just a few milliseconds each year, in a trend that will continue throughout adulthood. This is part of normal aging, and it takes decades to lead to a noticeable effect on everyday perceptions or movements. But the retrieval of a memory is likely to involve more signals and more intricate signal pathways, and then the numerous small slowdowns can amount to an unwelcome delay. Not all kinds of memories are equally affected, however: oft-repeated tasks that involve both physical and mental exertion, such as playing a musical instrument, are apparently less vulnerable to this age-related slowdown. Meanwhile, although our memory for the meaning and use of language is generally very well preserved, the slowdown may cause us to wonder why we can't remember the three or four grocery items we have just been asked to buy—when in fact the problem is not a mind full of holes but simply difficulty in processing rapid speech.

Almost everyone has a lapse of memory now and then, but often we worry more about these lapses as we grow older. Although many adults in midlife and later life fear they will eventually, and maybe inevitably, lose their memory completely, these fears are unfounded: years of study have established that the normal adult brain need not suffer a major loss of memory at *any* age. The notion of senility, or of an unavoidable loss of mental functions, dates back to a time when the diseases that attack such functions (Alzheimer's disease, **C67**, in particular) were impossible to diagnose in living patients; thus people with Alzheimer's disease were counted among the healthy, and their condition was considered a form of normal aging. Today the trained clinician can usually diagnose Alzheimer's disease at an early stage so that patients may benefit from treatment, and worried potential patients can learn about the difference between this serious disease and normal, benign age-related memory impairment.

It is true that the first stages of Alzheimer's disease can produce lapses similar to those of age-related memory impairment in a healthy person. The essential difference is that while the Alzheimer's patient will go on to develop more serious memory deficits, cognitive impairment, and finally dementia, memory impairment in the healthy individual will remain at the level of mere annoyance. While there is still no quick or foolproof way to distinguish between age-related memory impairment and early Alzheimer's disease, the doctor's general rule of thumb is this: if you take longer than before to learn a new piece of information, a new spatial structure, or a new skill, but then you remember it as well as anyone else, you do not have Alzheimer's.

The attention paid to mild memory slips common in the second half of life tends to overshadow the more important ability of the brain to compensate. In preparing to carry out a new task, for example, older adults may miss a point or two or may need to repeat the information about the chore once or twice. But having handled many smaller, larger, and equivalent tasks before, they are often able to fill in missing details for themselves—and to bring seasoned judgment to bear on the assignment as well. A similar power of compensation fills in if the normal older brain becomes less adept at carrying out a number of mental operations simultaneously: when it becomes more difficult to do many things at once, an older person may adapt by focusing on one thing at a time. For some individuals, this can also lead to greater awareness of the present moment and appreciation for what is important and what is not. "Depth of experience" becomes the watchword with increasing years.

Nevertheless, both clinical and research scientists are looking for ways to minimize the normal age-related memory snags and to supplement the brain's powers of compensation. The hormone estrogen, already well known for its crucial role in reproduction, has received considerable attention from brain researchers as well. Many studies have suggested estrogen may protect the brain to some degree from age-related memory decline, and may even bolster memory in the normal brain. The antioxidant vitamin E, which removes the highly reactive oxygen molecules that are believed to cause age-related damage in the brain, is also a center of interest, but the scientific jury is still out on its value in treatment or in memory enhancement. Another dietary supplement that has been proposed as a memory aid is ginkgo biloba, but the scientific study of this substance is still in progress.

The Brain at Midlife and Beyond

Like the body, the brain undergoes some predictable changes with age, but most of them are less intimidating when their basis in natural processes is understood. These natural biological processes include a small but significant decrease in the rate of cerebral blood flow from young adulthood to midlife, which may contribute in a minor way to the age-related slowing in signal transmission and a decrease in the amount of "white matter," the nonsignaling cells that sheathe and insulate the signal-transmitting fibers of the neurons around them. Oddly, the proportion of

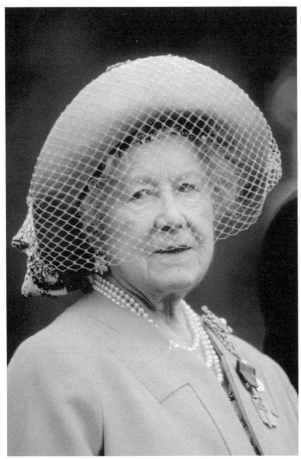

Living for more than a century, like the Queen Mother of Great Britain, who passed away in 2002 at the age of 101, has become far more common today. We have learned a great deal about the aging brain and how it can remain healthy, but some old myths about aging are surviving for a long time, too. Photo © Archive Photos/PictureQuest

"gray matter" (the neurons themselves) in the brain shows no significant difference for individuals under age 40 and those over age 69, hovering around 48 percent for both these groups, but it drops and then slowly rises again during the decades in between. The loss of the insulating white matter, meanwhile, probably accounts for most of the age-related slowdown. Also, sometime

in midlife the DNA of the brain's mitochondrial cells, which supply essential energy, start to show alterations that may interfere with the brain's ability to burn as much energy as it once did in sustained intense work or in meeting an impressive number of demands all at once.

A popular belief is that large numbers of brain cells die throughout the adult years. But to paraphrase that wise old author Mark Twain, the accounts of this death have been greatly exaggerated. Recent studies suggest that neuron death is restricted in normal aging, and physical evidence for great numbers of dead neurons in otherwise healthy brains has proven very hard to find. Since actual counts of neurons cannot be performed by even the most sophisticated imaging techniques but require a tangible slice of brain tissue, such a count can be performed only once on any individual, at the time of his or her autopsy. It isn't possible, therefore, to track one person's neuronal population at various ages. To measure the loss or survival of neurons, all that can be compared is the average count of one individual or group against another at autopsy. And when we take into account another finding, that the total number of neurons in the healthy brain can vary among healthy individuals by as much as 100 percent, any "average" extent of neuronal loss becomes even more fugitive. Instead, techniques such as magnetic resonance imaging are used to estimate change over time, and these show a consistent decrease in the *volume* of the brain after about age 40. It is likely that this "shrinkage" derives much more from the loss of white matter, as discussed above, than of neurons.

One specific area known to lose size with advancing age is the corpus callosum, the thick bundle of nerve fibers through which the brain's two hemispheres communicate with each other. This seems logical, since insulating white matter would account for a large amount of the corpus callosum's bulk. The gradual loss of white matter here takes a toll: as patterns of signaling shift very slightly and unpredictably, the two hemispheres lose a certain amount of electrical coherence—that is, the simultaneousness of their signaling. Just as in traffic, every driver lined up at a stoplight has a slightly different reaction time when the light turns green, and these slight differences add up to a long delay for the driver at the end of the line, so the small decrease in coherence between hemispheres can blunt the immediacy of the brain's responses.

Some adults in midlife or later also find themselves more easily distracted from a task or a line of thought than they used to be. Does the brain's intricate system for maintaining attention also change with age? The scientific answer to this question is both no and yes, depending on which aspect of attention we are discussing. The deliberate fixing of our attention on a specific object or task appears to be an ability that remains well into late adulthood. However, the ability to *shift* our attention efficiently begins to falter sometime after middle age, which may explain the annoying sense of distractability when a new demand or perception presents itself in the midst of an ongoing task. This age-related deficit must have a biological basis rather than a psychological one because it has been observed in studies of young and older adult monkeys as well as in people. It's not that our minds wander but that they may become less nimble than before at directing various circuits and brain functions toward a new target while keeping the previous target "on hold."

On the other hand, the ability *not* to pay attention, to ignore a large variety of environmental stimuli that our brains have judged unimpor-

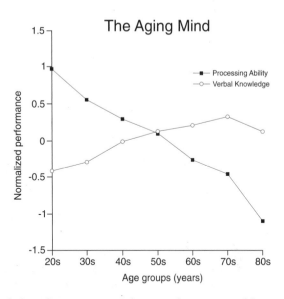

The Aging Mind

Aging slows our mental processing, measured by how quickly we process words and use various kinds of memory. But our actual verbal knowledge grows over our lifetime. GRAPH COURTESY OF DENISE C. PARK, PH.D., CENTER FOR APPLIED COGNITIVE RESEARCH ON AGING, UNIVERSITY OF MICHIGAN

tant—the ticking of a clock, the familiar view of a busy street, or a waving tree branch outside the window—is not permanently wired into the brain. It is a mental skill that we all had to learn in early development, and one that may lose a little of its strength in later adulthood. Losing some of the ability to filter out extra stimuli can add to the sense of being easily distracted. At the same time, the brain's creative powers of compensation allow older adults to draw on their experience and thereby anticipate and ward off potential distractors, or to reorient themselves quickly when they return to a previous task after an interruption.

Slowing reflexes, another common complaint, may be traced to the age-related decrease in the speed of signal transmission. We worry more about eyeblink-long lags in retrieving a

THE RHYTHM OF SLEEP

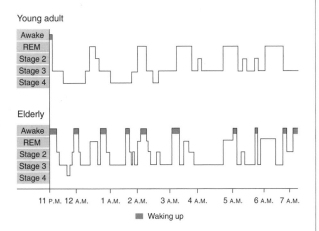

Sleep patterns change as we age. As these graphs show, a typical elderly person spends less time in deep sleep and more time actually awake than a young person. An older person also goes through more cycles of sleep stages during a night. ILLUSTRATION © BY LEIGH CORIALE

memory, as discussed in the previous section, than about a slight loss of speed in our movements; but the two effects arise from much the same cause, the slight pull of age on the speed of nerve signal propagation.

Another familiar age-related change occurs in sleep patterns. Sleep (**B3**) changes, not just because decades of rising early for school, work, child care, or all three, have left the brain ready to rebel, but because our inborn circadian rhythms seem to loosen their control somewhat with the passing of years. In general, we begin to need less sleep, but insomnia and other sleep disturbances (**C11**) also become more common after age 50 or so, starting at a prevalence of about 27 percent in the general population and gradually increasing to almost 40 percent after age 80. Problems such as difficulty falling asleep and repeated waking in the night have been reported in both sexes and across a number of cultures, so the condition evi-

dently arises from biological factors at least as much as from habits or lifestyle. In people who are subject to sleep disturbances, the direct trigger may be something as straightforward as snoring (your own or that of a fellow sleeper) or periodic leg or arm movements.

Finally, although it is not as freely discussed among adults as the occasional stiff knee or lapse of memory, a very serious but avoidable health threat to the brain in later years is depression (**C20**). Why this risk should increase with age is an unanswered question, but researchers are studying many possible contributing factors.

The brain's gradual loss of white matter, as discussed above, may cost most people only a small amount of speed in the transmission of nerve signals, but it may tip the balance of mood (of "affect," to use the proper professional term) in a system already under stress. One study has linked depression with illness elsewhere in the body, and not just because of sorrow about bodily illness, but because bodily illness may place an extra physiological burden on the brain. One particular kind of illness, heart disease, does seem to bring on a higher than usual risk of depression, but again, how this works in physiological terms is not yet known. Absent any other illness, clinicians and researchers of all stripes agree that lower levels of physical exercise bring a higher risk of depression, in older adults as in all age groups. The intensity of the exercise may also matter: mild activity brings the risk down, but not by as much as intense exertion.

Menopause has often been blamed as a trigger for depression, but this does not hold true for very many women. A study of more than 1,500 women in Melbourne, Australia, showed that menopausal status had no direct effect on well-being. Factors that did have an impact were general health, relations with other people, attitudes toward aging (and menopause), and lifestyle choices, such as smoking and physical exercise. Preliminary research on the male side of the picture reaffirms that hormonal shifts do play a role, if not a solo, in the risk of depression: in older males, those with depression were found to have the lowest levels of testosterone, and treating some of these men with testosterone relieved their depression.

Habits for Long-Term Health

In the maintenance of our well-being, long-term habits and lifestyles produce real results. The choices we make and the habits we keep, day in and day out, add up to about half of what determines how well we will be in our later years. Apart from luck in the genes we receive and the prudence to avoid fatal accidents, nothing counts more toward the well-being of our brain and body than what we ingest and how active we are.

The first important choice concerns cigarette smoking. Smoking damages the brain in ways that may take decades to appear. In a study of men aged 18 to 39 and 64 to 81, heavy smoking reduced the electrical coherence of several different "wave types" of signaling between the brain's two hemispheres. Even in the younger group, heavy smoking reduced the coherence of one type of wave. Long-term smokers were found to have significantly lower cerebral blood flow, independent of whether or not smoking had also contributed to hardening of the arteries in the brain. Smoking had a mixed effect on the consolidation of memories; low- and mid-intensity smokers (those smoking cigarettes yielding 0.8 to 1.3 mg of nicotine each) performed worse than nonsmokers on a memorization task after a half-hour delay but better than nonsmokers after a delay of one month. Long-term exposure to cigarette smoke and its by-products even makes itself felt in our ears: a study from a rural village in Kuala Lumpur revealed that long-term smoking nearly doubled the risk of some degree of hearing loss. In men aged 40 and older, the average rate of hearing impairment, about 30 percent, rose to 51 percent among smokers. Thus, for the senses and the mind as well as the body, not smoking is an obvious safeguard of well-being.

A related but less clear picture is that of alcohol use. While moderate drinking (one or two five-ounce glasses of wine per day is the usual example) has been found in a number of studies to reduce the risk of heart disease, excessive amounts of alcohol may increase the risk of brain hemorrhage. In any case, at any point along the spectrum, age is a factor in the effects of alcohol on the brain and body. Older adults have a declining ability to metabolize alcohol (to break it down into its component molecules) along with less water in the body to dilute it, allowing alcohol to act more rapidly and more intensely on the older brain. In later life, alcohol may also contribute to depression and to sleep disorders, which then take their own toll.

The health of our brain also bears the lasting effects of what we eat every day. It now appears that certain fruits and vegetables can do more than keep the body well—they may also help ward off the subtle but pervasive slowdown of nerve signaling that affects the brain in later years. In preliminary results from an animal model, spinach and an extract taken from strawberries were found to protect against the signaling slowdown; spinach was more effective overall, but in both cases the effect was substantial. The brain-friendly element in these foods may be vitamin E, an antioxidant—that is, a compound that shields cells from potentially destructive electrically charged molecules. Other studies of vitamin E, in humans as well as in animals, have found apparent protective effects. Although the formal medical jury is still out, enough evidence so far has led many doctors to admit they take vitamin E supplements for brain health, just in case.

It has often been said before, in this book as elsewhere, but still bears repeating: regular, habitual physical activity makes for a healthier brain. When undertaken as a conscious choice (even by rats voluntarily using a running wheel), exercise is proving in study after study to nourish brain cells, reduce the risk of many age-related brain illnesses, and generally buffer the effects of daily wear and tear on this extraordinarily busy organ.

The Myth of the Older Brain

In the last decade, the concept of "senility" has undergone a dramatic change: as the understanding of Alzheimer's disease and the ability to diagnose it have grown, the number of new cases of "senility" has shrunk to almost nothing. This is because once the evident cases of Alzheimer's disease and other specific disorders are weeded out, there is simply no general condition that can be called senility. Previous generations, unable to recognize the very gradual development of Alzheimer's in healthy-looking elderly people, had to assume that what they were observing was the typical course of old age.

Dementia (**C69**), too, has long had a distorted meaning as a fearful combination of insanity and feeblemindedness. But in medical discourse, *dementia* has nothing to do with insanity. Instead the term very specifically applies to a set of cognitive problems including memory impairment, loss of judgment, and inability to think in abstract terms, often accompanied by some changes in personality. Thus a person may be diagnosed with an ailment that may eventually bring about dementia, but no one need fear the sudden onset of dementia as a process in aging all by itself.

Neurodegenerative diseases, if they are going to occur at all, do tend to appear at a more advanced age. But although the diseases most people worry about developing in old age—Alzheimer's, Parkinson's, and Huntington's diseases and ALS (amyotrophic lateral sclerosis)—take a considerable toll, they are not typical risks of aging. By current estimates, Alzheimer's disease affects about 4 million Americans, or about 1 in 75, though it will become more common—affecting up to 1 in 20—as our population ages. Currently, Parkinson's disease has developed in about 1 million people, a rate of fewer than 1 in 250; about 50,000 people have Huntington's disease, 1 in 5,000; and ALS afflicts about 25,000 people, or fewer than 1 in 10,000.

For people diagnosed with these still incurable illnesses, and for everyone who cares about them, what matters is not the prevalence but where medicine and medical research stand in finding answers for them. The most encouraging news has been the demonstration that each of these illnesses almost certainly has a strong genetic basis. This offers the eventual prospect of decisive interventions, as genetic research develops into a more precise and systematic hunt for disease processes and points at which to interrupt those processes than has ever been possible. (It is important to remember that for most diseases a certain combination of genes does not mean an illness will definitely appear; it means only that a person may have more of a chance of developing it. Most of these diseases need other as yet unknown, biological events or triggers before they appear.) Chapters 16 and 19 discuss neurodegenerative diseases in greater detail.

Grateful Aging

Just as aging brings risks and predictable changes to the brain, it also opens new opportunities and consolidates the gains of a lifetime, a reason for gratitude. Our inclination to look to older adults for such desirable traits as patience, forbearance, and responsibility has a solid basis in reality. A study that followed more than 200 people over a 50-year period found that psychological health—not simple happiness but the qualities of being dependable, responsible, and productive, and of having good relationships with other people—increased steadily from age 30 onward. This happy flowering suggests still other ongoing processes in the brain, either deliberate or unconscious, have yet to be discovered, and many carefully designed studies and in-depth interviews have begun to search for such processes. Other research, begun in the late 1990s and early 2000s, may even help us understand how the accumulation of experience and the passage of time can work together in the mind to produce one of the most highly prized qualities of all—wisdom. In fact, seen in terms of lifelong development, the subtle attrition of neurons with age may represent not a sad loss but a progressive fine-tuning of cerebral networks.

Midlife and beyond is the optimal time of life to undertake challenges that require, above all, a larger perspective, as is assumed by the respected and esteemed role the elderly enjoy in many non-Western societies. In the Western context, this may translate to a spectrum of possibilities.

- More abstract or "philosophical" work in one's field or in a new profession altogether. The car salesperson who becomes a schoolteacher, the retired surgeon who creates a body of work as a painter, and other such second-career choices may be the natural and agreeable trajectory for the older brain.

- Volunteer work in the community or far from home (for example, in the Peace Corps). Keeping the brain's extensive library of experience and judgment in regular, vigorous use is a form of mental exercise that comes with obvious psychological benefits as well.

- Appreciating recreation and the company of family and friends. The gentler sides of life are too often dismissed because their value is hard to measure. But the older brain thrives on social contact and offers a constant resource to loved ones, whether by maintaining its fine-tuning in engagement with others, as in playing chess, where speed counts for nothing and years of experience add up to mastery, or finding thoughtfulness in solitary pursuits such as gardening, which rewards the ability to savor day-to-day efforts and rewards while also envisioning and planning for seasons far in the future.

PART III

The Healthy Brain

CHAPTER 9

The Body Manager

B1 The Major Senses: Sight, Hearing, Taste, Smell, and Touch   136

B2 Body Regulation   142

B3 Basic Drives: Eating, Sleeping, and Sex   150

B4 Movement, Balance, and Coordination   158

B5 Pain Perception   165

B6 Consciousness   171

All animals, from humans to oysters, need to regulate their bodies' internal workings, sense their surroundings, and move away from danger and toward food. These are among the most important tasks our brains handle for us, yet we rarely think about these functions. Right now your heart, lungs, and intestines are providing oxygen and nutrients for your body; your muscles are holding your head upright; and your eyes are open, correctly pointed, and focused to take in these words. All those normally unconscious tasks are regulated by your brain.

This chapter discusses various ways in which we sense the world around us and maintain our bodily health. Such functions rely largely on parts of the brain we share with all other vertebrate animals. In many animals these functions seem to operate on automatic, but for us humans they involve some conscious choice. For instance, we need to eat, but we choose when, how, and what we eat. We not only perceive the world, but we know we are perceiving it. That consciousness sets us apart from other animals, and hints at the greater power of our brains.

The Major Senses: Sight, Hearing, Taste, Smell, and Touch

The purpose of the major senses is to detect and discriminate among signals coming from our environment. These signals carry information necessary for us to support our vital functions, such as taste and smell in eating, as well as functions used in communicating with others and in our work, such as sight, touch, and hearing. In addition to the traditional five senses, other senses of which we are not aware are at work within our bodies, such as the sense of balance and the sense of muscle effort, called kinesthesia, and many senses involved in detecting chemical changes in the blood and other tissues.

All of these senses are present at birth in the human. Research on newborn babies has shown that when they are tested with different taste solutions before any exposure to feeding, they show the appropriate facial responses, such as smiling at a sweet taste and grimacing at a bitter taste. Since the higher brain centers, in the neocortex, of a newborn are not yet functional, these experiments have shown that our basic emotional expressions of pleasure and pain are hard-wired into our brain stem circuits from birth. Although sight and hearing appear to be rudimentary, careful testing has shown that babies of only a few months recognize their mothers by sight and sound.

Exploring the Senses

Sensory systems have been the subject of much modern research in neuroscience because they are accessible to testing and because one begins by knowing exactly what type of information is processed by them. In contrast, in many central brain systems, it is difficult to pin down what kind of information is being processed.

Each of the different senses has particular sense cells within its particular organs: for sight, photoreceptor cells within the retina at the back of the eye; for hearing, hair cells within the inner ear; for smell, olfactory sensory neurons within the olfactory epithelium at the top of the nasal cavity; for taste, taste cells within taste buds in the tongue and back of the mouth. For touch, there are many different types of receptors in the bare nerve endings in the skin that extend from nerve cells in spinal and brain stem ganglia: for pain, for tem-

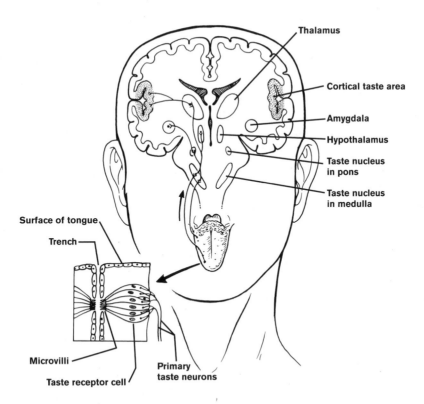

Our sense of taste is shown in this schematic drawing. It starts with specialized cells on the tongue that send information to the brain's taste nuclei in the medulla, atop the spinal cord. From these sites, signals go to the amygdala and the thalamus, which in turn alert the portion of the cortex that processes and stores that information. Notice that our taste buds are not the bumps on our tongue but actually line tiny trenches in the surface of the tongue. ILLUSTRATION © KATHRYN BORN

perature (heat and cold). In addition, there are specialized receptors in the skin and deep tissues for pressure and for light touch.

We move through the rough-and-tumble physical world with such ease that it is astonishing to realize the exquisite refinement of each of our sensory systems. Several aspects of sensory systems have been especially studied. One of the most important we are trying to understand is the mechanisms by which the signals from the external world are converted into nerve signals. That is, how can a passing molecule of diesel fuel, for ex-

ample, start the series of brain cell firings that result in our holding our nose? This process is called sensory transduction. One of the main principles emerging is that transduction begins with the sensory signal acting on a protein that sits in a sensitive part of the membrane of the sensory cell. For example, in the eye this protein is the photopigment rhodopsin, which is concentrated in membrane disks within the photoreceptor cells at the back of the retina. It is the first to receive that flash of light from a piece of paper as it flutters to the ground. In the nose, it is a receptor protein that is concentrated in fine hairs that extend from the ends of the sensory cells situated in a patch at the top of the nasal cavity. Research has shown that the sensory protein in the nose belongs to the same family of molecules as rhodopsin. Each protein is adapted to receive its particular sensory signal. They are called G protein-coupled receptors, because a molecule called a G protein (for guanosine triphosphate) must be coupled to them to continue to transmit a signal. When light or an odor activates these receptors, they in turn activate their G proteins.

Researchers have found that activation of a G protein then leads to the production of a small messenger molecule (cyclic adenosine monophosphate [cAMP] or cyclic guanosine monophosphate [cGMP]) that acts on a membrane protein to set up an electrical response in the membrane. Cyclic AMP and cyclic GMP are widespread throughout the body. They are called second messengers because they take the response to the first messenger (the initial signal from outside the cell), amplify it within the cell, and direct their response to an appropriate site within the cell. In the case of sensory cells, this is the electrical response, which in turn generates a discharge of impulses that encodes the strength of the sensory stimulation. Most sensory cells are set at near their physical limits for detecting very weak signals; for instance, the inner ear is set to detect a movement of the tympanic membrane (eardrum) of the width of a hydrogen atom, and the eye is set to detect single photons from starlight on a dark night.

The Senses' Specialties

It is important that sensory systems not only detect weak signals and determine the strength of a signal but also discriminate between different signals. In vision this includes the discrimination of fine details (called visual acuity) or different wavelengths of light (color discrimination); in smell it involves distinguishing between different smells; in taste it involves distinguishing among the basic tastes of sweet, salt, sour, and bitter; in touch it involves sensing the ways that different objects feel. Discrimination thus requires populations of sensory receptor cells that can respond to different aspects of the stimuli.

All sensory systems provide for such differently

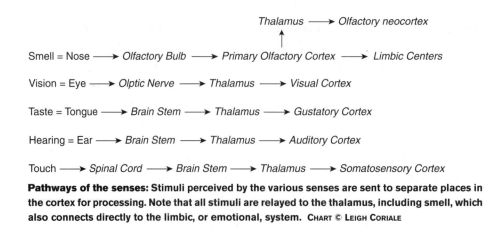

Pathways of the senses: Stimuli perceived by the various senses are sent to separate places in the cortex for processing. Note that all stimuli are relayed to the thalamus, including smell, which also connects directly to the limbic, or emotional, system. Chart © Leigh Coriale

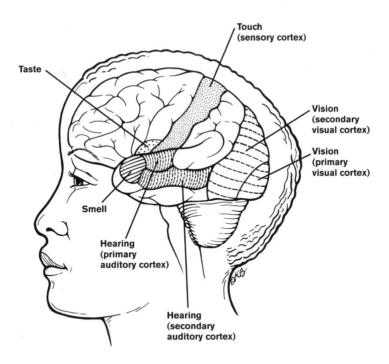

Each type of sensory information has its own area in the cerebral cortex for processing and storage. Vision and hearing take up the most space, smell and taste relatively little. ILLUSTRATION © KATHRYN BORN

sensitive receptor cells, which give rise to parallel pathways that carry the information to the higher centers where discrimination takes place. These pathways are gathered into nerve tracts that ascend through the lower parts of the brain to the highest centers. Thus, the optic nerves carry information in a highly ordered manner from the retina to a way station called the lateral geniculate body, in the thalamus, whence it is relayed to the primary visual receptive area of the neocortex. The auditory nerve carries the information from the array of hair cells in the inner ear to the cochlear nucleus in the brain stem, from where there are multiple relays through pathways that rise to the medical geniculate nucleus of the thalamus, from where the information is relayed to the primary auditory receptive area of the neocortex.

The sense of touch similarly has its pathway from the spinal cord and brain stem to its thalamic nucleus, for relay to the primary somatosensory receptive area of the neocortex. Smell information is carried in the olfactory nerves to the olfactory bulb, for processing and output to a first cortical station at the base of the brain, for output to the olfactory thalamic nucleus and further relay to the neocortical olfactory area. The taste nerves carry taste information from the tongue and oral cavity to brain stem nuclei for relay to the thalamus and on to the neocortical taste area.

Sensory discrimination generally involves conscious sensory perception. This usually takes place in higher sensory centers within the brain, at the level of the neocortex. The ways in which cortical neurons are able to sort out signals they receive allow the conscious individual to recognize differences in how strong a signal is, how one form of taste, visual, or sensory information varies from another taste, image, or touch. (These differentiations are known as discrimination.) Such physiological processes underlie the larger brain functions: perception, consciousness, memory, and other higher functions.

Differences

The basic functions of high sensitivity for the detection of weak signals, discrimination of increasing stimulus strength, and discrimination between different qualities of a stimulus are present in all humans. However, there can be significant differences. First of all, there are differences during early life. Although the basic sensitivity of the sensory cells appears to be laid down early, it takes time for the central pathways to mature, and the highest centers mature last. Thus the highest levels of sensory perception are generally not reached until the teens and twenties, having been refined by experience, training, and memory.

As we grow older, there are also differences. Hearing begins to fall off during the 40s and 50s, with loss of the highest frequencies first. There is evidence that this is directly due to damage to hair cells, particularly from excessive exposure to loud noise. Thus, while many middle-aged people may take great pride in the high fidelity of their stereo sets and speakers, most of that high performance is not actually available to them because of high-frequency hearing loss. Smell holds relatively constant until the 60s and then begins a slow decline, which also appears to be true of the sense of taste. Whether the loss is due to damage to the sensory cells or to changes in higher centers is not known.

There are also many kinds of individual differences among the normal population. Although there may be general agreement on the major types of smells and colors, there can be significant differences in making finer distinctions, as most of us know from personal experience. Some differences are related to gender. A well-known difference is the generally higher acuity of most women for smell, and the variation in this acuity for many women during the menstrual cycle.

Disorders

Some loss of function in the senses is just a sign of normal aging, as described earlier. In other instances, decline in function may be a symptom of a more serious problem. Hearing loss may be due to damage to the hair cells in the inner ear. Cochlear implants are effective in restoring serviceable hearing in young children. Loud noises and music, an allergic reaction to medications, immune system disorders, and tumors on the auditory nerve can also cause varying degrees of hearing loss (C16). Problems with vision, especially if they occur suddenly, may be the result of a stroke, or transient ischemic attack (TIA), which is caused by a blockage (usually cholesterol) of the retinal blood vessels (C15). Viral respiratory infections, tumors, or even a blow to the head that injures the olfactory bulb (C17) can cause loss of smell (anosmia) or taste (agensia).

The general rule is that because your senses are so dependable, an observation of loss of function in any of them should dictate a trip to the doctor. The doctor can determine whether the problem is a temporary malfunction due to another malady or refer you to the appropriate specialist for a more thorough examination.

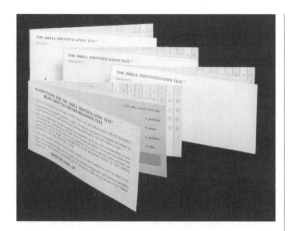

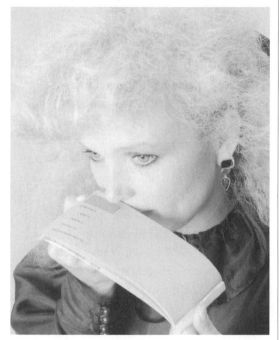

The science of smells benefited from the creation of smell identification tests, giving scientists a standard measure of people's olfactory powers. Researchers are now exploring whether losing the sense of smell is linked to other neurological disorders. PHOTOS COURTESY OF RICHARD L. DOTY, PH.D., SMELL AND TASTE CENTER, UNIVERSITY OF PENNSYLVANIA

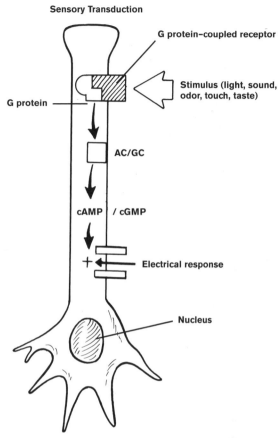

If you've ever wondered how a flickering light or a molecule of diesel smoke translates into a signal in your brain, this simplified schematic explains it. The sensory cell facing the outside world has a special receptor that scientists call a G protein–coupled receptor, which acts when a stimulus such as light or odor hits it. Its job is to stimulate a G protein inside the cell, which leads to the production of another molecule (cGMP) in the cell's membrane, launching the cell's signal into the sensory pathway to the brain. ILLUSTRATION © KATHRYN BORN

Body Regulation

Virtually every function of the body must work in coordination with others. For example, during competition an athlete needs more than a strong musculoskeletal system and keen senses—his or her cardiovascular system must increase blood pressure and heart rate to keep up with the physical exertion, the lungs must increase gas exchange, and the gastrointestinal system must provide adequate nutrients. Coordinating all of these systems is a crucial role of the brain. In particular, the brain stem, like a kind of autopilot, is responsible for reflexes that integrate bodily functions moment by moment. And the hypothalamus, processing signals from within the body and from the world around it, coordinates all these body systems with the way a person needs to behave.

Our brains collect information about the external world through the five senses: smell, taste, vision, touch, and hearing (**B1**). At the same time, our brains also need to monitor many things about our internal worlds. They do this in two basic ways. First, the brain collects information about the internal organs through what are called visceral sensory nerves. The most important of these is the vagus nerve. It tells the brain how full and acidic the stomach is, what the body's blood pressure is

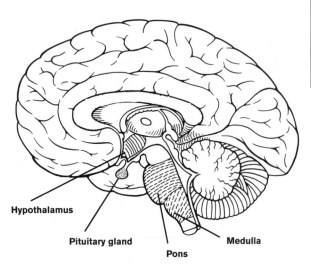

Hypothalamus

Pituitary gland

Pons

Medulla

The lower brain stem, made up of the pons and the medulla, is responsible for regulating such autonomic body functions as breathing, heartbeat, and gastrointestinal activity. The hypothalamus processes signals from both the body and the outside world and transmits the information to other brain regions. The pituitary gland releases a variety of hormones, triggering different responses throughout the body in response to such conditions as stress, fear, and hunger. ILLUSTRATION © KATHRYN BORN

and how fast the heart is pumping, and whether the body is under attack from microbial invaders.

The second main way in which the brain judges what is happening in a person's body is by monitoring the bloodstream. The brain shares the same blood as the rest of the body, after all. Its sensors detect the amount of oxygen and carbon dioxide in the blood, blood temperature, the presence of sugar and a variety of nutrients and minerals such as sodium, and levels of various chemical hormones, including the hormones made by white blood cells that signal infection or other inflammatory illnesses.

All of this information is necessary for the brain to detect disturbances in a person's internal bodily state, or to respond to such threats as infectious disease. At the same time, our brains must coordinate all of these functions with our daily sleep-wake cycles, as well as the seasons of the year. To do this, the brain uses an internal clock mechanism: this measures time and keeps track of cues, such as the length of the day, to synchronize its timekeeping with the outside world. The brain thus sets up circadian rhythms that affect periods of rest and activity throughout the body. The most important cue it uses is sunlight, which travels from the eye directly to the hypothalamus, which is sensitive to it. We have learned to use such bright light to resynchronize people's internal clocks if necessary (C11).

The hypothalamus is thus the master regulatory site in the brain. It is a tiny area: out of the brain's total three pounds (1,400 grams), it weighs only a bit more than an eighth of an ounce (4 grams). Yet the hypothalamus is necessary for a person to coordinate bodily function with behavior and the external world. It is the most protected part of the brain. It receives blood from all of the major blood vessels that supply the organ,

protecting it from damage if one of those vessels is blocked by an ischemic stroke (C59). It is also located in the deepest part of the brain, just behind the eyes in the middle of the head, so it is rarely injured by trauma (C61).

The hypothalamus regulates bodily functions by coordinating three main systems:

- the *autonomic system* of nerves that control all of the internal organs

- the *endocrine system*, which provides hormones that direct the body's organs

- *basic behaviors*, such as eating, drinking, sleeping, and reproductive behavior

In addition, the hypothalamus's activity influences the immune system.

The Autonomic Nervous System

The autonomic nervous system consists of three parts. The first is the sympathetic nervous system, which arises from the sympathetic ganglia, small collections of nerve cells lying alongside and in front of the spinal column. These ganglia are controlled by nerve cells in the spinal cord where it passes through the chest. The sympathetic nerves use norepinephrine as a neurotransmitter to chemically activate other tissues. One important component of the sympathetic nervous system is the adrenal gland, which releases epinephrine (also known as adrenaline). Sympathetic nerves prepare the body for "fight or flight": they increase a person's heart rate and blood pressure, cause sweating, make hair stand on end, and dilate the pupils. At the same time, they turn off systems, such as digestion, that are not immediately necessary in that situation.

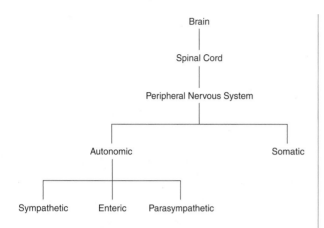

Brain
|
Spinal Cord
|
Peripheral Nervous System

Autonomic   Somatic

Sympathetic   Enteric   Parasympathetic

All the nerves outside the brain and spinal cord make up the peripheral nervous system. **That system consists of autonomic nerves regulating heartbeat, breathing, digestion, and other major body functions, and somatic nerves carrying messages about sensation and movement between the brain and the rest of the body.** CHART © LEIGH CORIALE

The second component of the autonomic nervous system is the parasympathetic system. The parasympathetic nerves for most parts of the body, such as the vagus nerve, originate in the brain. Those that control the bowel and bladder originate in the lowest part of the spinal cord. These nerves use acetylcholine as a neurotransmitter, and their primary purpose is to help us rest and digest. They cue the secretion of saliva, tears, and mucus (in the respiratory tract) and of acid and enzymes in the stomach and intestines. They slow the heart and increase the rate of digestion in the gut, thus reversing the actions of the sympathetic nervous system.

The third component of the autonomic nervous system, the enteric nervous system, is often underrated. This system consists of the nerve cells embedded in the walls of the intestines. That may

The Autonomic Nervous System		
Structure	Sympathetic Stimulation	Parasympathetic Stimulation
Iris (eye muscle)	Pupil dilation	Pupil constriction
Salivary glands	Saliva production reduced	Saliva production increased
Oral/Nasal mucosa	Mucus production reduced	Mucus production increased
Heart	Heart rate and force increased	Heart rate and force decreased
Lung	Bronchial muscle relaxed	Bronchial muscle contracted
Stomach	Peristalsis reduced	Gastric juice secreted; motility increased
Small intestine	Motility is reduced	Digestion increased
Large intestine	Motility is reduced	Secretions and motility increased
Liver	Increased conversion of glycogen to glucose	
Kidney	Decreased urine secretion	Increased urine secretion
Adrenal medulla	Norepinephrine and epinephrine secreted	
Bladder	Wall relaxed –sphincter closed	Wall contracted –sphincter relaxed

CHART © LEIGH CORIALE. USED WITH THE PERMISSION OF DR. ERIC H. CHUDLER,
DEPARTMENT OF ANESTHESIOLOGY, UNIVERSITY OF WASHINGTON

seem limited, but the enteric nervous system actually includes more cells than the other two branches of the autonomic nervous system combined. It controls the rate of peristalsis, or movement of food through the gut. This process is always going on, but it can be sped up or slowed down by the messages the enteric nerve cells receive through the parasympathetic or sympathetic channels.

All these autonomic reflexes are controlled by a person's brain stem. Nerve cells in the medulla, the lowest part of the brain stem, manage blood pressure and heart rate. They increase respiration when the blood needs more oxygen, and increase blood flow to meet tissue demands. Other nerve cells in the medulla monitor how full the gastrointestinal tract is, regulate digestion, and even cause vomiting when things go wrong.

At a slightly higher level of the brain stem are nerve cells that coordinate these autonomic reflexes with behavior. These cells are in an area called the pons, and they contain two significant structures: the parabrachial nucleus coordinates how we hold our breath, chew, and swallow and integrates control of blood pressure with pain and emotion; Barrington's nucleus controls bladder and bowel function, allowing us to rid our bodies of waste under socially acceptable conditions. However, the hypothalamus is necessary to tie all of these brain-stem reflexes together with ongoing behavior and emotion. For example, the hypothalamus increases blood pressure during an emotional experience.

The Endocrine System

The endocrine system controls how the brain and other tissues throughout the body produce and release hormones. The hypothalamus is the system's key site in the brain. It manages the pituitary gland just below it, and it regulates the glands elsewhere in the body through the autonomic nervous system.

The pituitary gland is made up of two lobes, anterior and posterior, with separate functions. The posterior pituitary lobe is really a part of the brain and contains the axons of special neurons of the hypothalamus. It secretes two main hormones: oxytocin, involved in controlling birth and milk production, and vasopressin, which controls blood pressure and the release of excess water through the kidneys. The oxytocin and vasopressin are made by nerve cells in the hypothalamus, in the supraoptic and paraventricular nuclei. These neurons send their axons down the pituitary stalk, allowing them to release their hormones in the posterior pituitary lobe.

The anterior pituitary lobe is a gland located just in front of the posterior pituitary and is connected to the brain only by a special set of capillaries from the hypothalamus. It produces five hormones:

- growth hormone, which stimulates growth and development throughout the body

- thyroid-stimulating hormone, which activates the thyroid gland in the throat

- adrenocorticotrophic hormone (ACTH), which signals the adrenal cortex to produce adrenal corticosteroids

- luteinizing hormone and follicle-stimulating hormone, which stimulate the production of reproductive steroid hormones

- prolactin, which prompts milk production

Neurons in the hypothalamus control the anterior pituitary lobe by secreting what are called releasing hormones. A portal vein carries these chemicals to the anterior pituitary lobe, which interprets them as signaling which hormones to release elsewhere in the body.

The rest of the endocrine system is made up of the gonads (ovaries and testes), the thyroid and parathyriod in the throat, the adrenal glands atop the kidneys, the islet cells in the pancreas, and the secretory cells lining the intestines (although there are many other organs that produce hormones, including the heart, which makes atrial natriuretic peptide, for example). These release a range of hormones, including estrogen, testosterone, and insulin. They direct everything from the body's metabolism rate to how much calcium it retains to whether breasts develop. The secretion of their many hormones is controlled, at least in part, by autonomic nerves. For example, the secretion of insulin is controlled by both sympathetic and parasympathetic nerves that extend into the tissue of the pancreas. (This extension of nerves into other tissues is what brain scientists mean by the word *innervation.*) The whole system thus connects back to the hypothalamus.

Basic Behaviors

The hypothalamus also plays a critical role in organizing basic behaviors necessary for us, or any large animals, to stay alive. It promotes specific behaviors that augment or, in some cases, go beyond what the hypothalamus can do through the other systems it directs. For example, virtually every animal needs to keep its temperature within a limited range around a setpoint. For humans, that setpoint is about 37°C (98.6°F). The hypothalamus regulates body temperature through the autonomic nervous system, which cues sweating,

shivering, goose bumps, and the movement of blood to or from the skin. But another way not to get too hot or too cold is to seek an environment that is the right temperature. Even primitive animals like reptiles, whose autonomic nervous systems cannot regulate their temperature as ours does, naturally seek an environment that produces an optimal body temperature. That behavior is driven by the hypothalamus.

Other fundamental aspects of behavior controlled by the hypothalamus include basic postures for feeding, sleeping, mating, or aggressive defense. The hypothalamus can also promote routine and repetitive behaviors, such as chewing, swallowing, shivering, or panting. These behaviors seem to be due to the hypothalamus's stimulation of neural networks in the brain stem, not in the higher brain; animals will perform them under the right conditions even if the rest of their forebrain has been removed. On the other hand, a person needs an intact forebrain to effectively coordinate these behaviors into long-term survival strategies. The hypothalamic neurons involved in producing these behaviors also have outputs to the cerebral cortex, which may promote the initiation of specific behaviors. For example, neurons in the lateral hypothalamus that contain melanin-concentrating hormone are activated during starvation. They send signals directly to the cerebral cortex, where they may be involved in activating behaviors that contribute to feeding.

The hypothalamus coordinates autonomic, endocrine, and behavioral responses to satisfy a person's basic life needs. Experiments by Walter Cannon and his colleagues at Harvard Medical School in the 1920s and 1930s showed that we need the hypothalamus to organize our patterns of behavior with coordinated autonomic and endocrine responses. Subsequent work has demon-

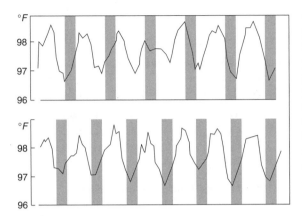

The brain times biological rhythms to a 24-hour day. The lower panel shows daily rhythms of body temperature during the day (white areas) and night (dark areas). When people were placed on a 28-hour schedule (upper panel, 19 hours of day and 9 hours of night), the same 24-hour rhythm of body temperature emerged, showing that the rhythm is an intrinsic, brain-directed pattern, not one that is imposed by the outside world. It is difficult for this internal clock to adjust by more than about 1 hour per day, which is why jet lag takes several days to wear off. Figure ADAPTED WITH PERMISSION FROM KLEITMAN, N., *SLEEP AND WAKEFULNESS*, © 1963, UNIVERSITY OF CHICAGO PRESS

strated that the hypothalamus operates the setpoints for a wide range of basic bodily functions: blood pressure, appetite, concentrations of glucose and salt in the blood, and others. It allows these functions to go only so far above or below the setpoint before it issues signals to restore the internal environment of the body to the healthful range. The hypothalamus is also critical for coordinating those functions with the external day-night and seasonal cycles. Furthermore, we rely on this part of the brain to provide effective responses to environmental challenges: an attack by a predator, invasion by a microorganism, hunger and thirst, and the presence of an appropriate mate. For more about how the brain works these basic drives, see **B3**.

Neuroimmunology

A new perspective on the hypothalamus is taking shape from evidence suggesting that its activities also affect the immune system, and researchers have begun carefully studying how this may influence a person's recovery from infections or some injuries. You might prefer to think of your immune system as a fully automatic response to viruses, bacteria, and other invaders, but the nervous system and immune system interact closely. Each constantly processes environmental cues and relays information to the other, using hormonal and other chemical messengers and the neuronal pathways.

These chemical messengers include interleukins—small proteins secreted by immune cells and other tissues. Interleukins in general act on the brain by causing cells along the blood vessels lining the brain to secrete prostaglandins. Prostaglandins cross the blood-brain barrier and cause manifestations of a systemic infection. You can block these with inhibitors of prostaglandin synthesis, such as aspirin. These proteins thus inform your brain when you are being affected by infection, inflammation, or any foreign substance.

A portion of the hypothalamus, the paraventricular nucleus, secretes a hormone called corticotrophin-releasing hormone. This hormone stimulates the pituitary gland, at the base of the brain, to secrete ACTH, which in turn stimulates the secretion of adrenal cortisol (a glucocorticoid). The pathway of this interaction is called the hypothalamic-pituitary-adrenal (HPA) axis. Cortisol at different concentrations has different effects. At natural concentrations—that is, concentrations not influenced by a drug treatment of some kind—cortisol suppresses immune responses. The HPA axis thus maintains a delicate balance and governs appropriate adjustments of the immune system during health.

When a person is exposed to stress, however, this balance breaks down, leading to increased susceptibility to infection or inflammation. During stress the brain releases large amounts of its stress hormones and induces the adrenal glands to produce more cortisol. High concentrations of cortisol suppress our immune responses and predispose the body to infection. Studies have shown that chronic psychological stress is associated with decreased immune responses, meaning more frequent and more severe infections. The following are some examples of these findings:

■ People exposed to greater perceived stress have an increased susceptibility to the viral-induced common cold.

■ Caregivers of people with Alzheimer's disease have a decreased immune response to influenza vaccination.

■ Medical students produce fewer antibodies after hepatitis B vaccinations during examination periods.

There are also nerves running to such immune system organs as the spleen, thymus, and lymph nodes as part of the sympathetic and peripheral nervous systems (that is, outside the central nervous system). Together these systems regulate local inflammatory responses. At the sites of inflammation, the peripheral nerves release neuropeptides. Immune cells express receptors for these neuropeptides, allowing the cells to respond by causing inflammation, which is then involved in protection against bacteria and viruses.

In sum, the brain and immune system interact across a wide network. These two systems constantly communicate to maintain a healthy balance of immune responses. Disruptions of this regulated balance may lead to disease.

Disorders of Bodily Regulation

A wide range of diseases can affect the ability of an individual's nervous system to govern his or her body's systems. Because these systems are crucial to life, when they cannot perform consistently a person can suffer a great deal of damage.

A person's autonomic nerves may degenerate in Parkinson's disease (**C41**) or in other disorders in which antibodies attack nerves, as in Guillain-Barré syndrome (**C49**) and other immune system diseases. The pathways in the brain that control the autonomic nerves may degenerate in certain neurological diseases, such as multiple-systems atrophy (**C42**). Either problem may result in a person's having difficulty maintaining blood pressure while standing, as well as a variety of digestive, bowel, and bladder problems.

Endocrine problems may result from a number of diseases that occur along the base of the brain, near where the pituitary stalk emerges from the hypothalamus. These include certain inflammatory diseases such as sarcoid, pituitary, and other rare tumors (**C64**).

When the posterior pituitary lobe stops producing vasopressin, a person must urinate excessively and thus must drink a great deal as well; this condition is known as diabetes insipidus. On the other hand, when the lobe releases too much vasopressin, the body is unable to eliminate water;

the resulting water intoxication may result in confusion or even seizures (**C13**).

If the anterior pituitary lobe cannot secrete luteinizing or follicle-stimulating hormone, the result may be atrophy of the gonads. A person may not be able to tolerate cold without enough thyroid-stimulating hormone, will remain short if growth hormone is not secreted adequately before adolescence, and will be unable to resist stressful stimuli if ACTH is cut off. Interestingly, of all the anterior pituitary hormones, only prolactin is normally held back by the hypothalamus; if that control is impaired, the body's levels of prolactin rise, which may result in unusual breast milk production and loss of menstrual cycles in women, or breast enlargement in men.

True hypothalamic injuries are very rare but very serious. Their effects depend on what part of the hypothalamus stops working correctly. If the medial hypothalamus is injured, a person may overeat badly and become obese. This problem can also cause atrophy of the gonads and loss of a woman's menstrual cycle. Individuals with these injuries may become exceedingly aggressive as well. People with a developmental disorder known as Prader-Willi syndrome have similar symptoms, but the focus of the problem in these patients' systems has not yet been identified.

Injuries to the lateral hypothalamus must occur on *both* sides of the brain to cause symptoms, and these are exceedingly rare. However, in rare cases such injuries may cause a person to stop eating and waste away (**C27**). They may also impair the sleep-wake cycles, resulting initially in sleepiness but ultimately in narcolepsy, in which a person falls asleep suddenly or remains awake but loses the ability to move (**C12**).

Occasionally, people with anterior hypothalamic injuries or developmental disorders have attacks in which their body temperature falls as low as 29°C (85°F), accompanied by coma. This rare regulatory disorder is called paroxysmal hypothermia, and its precise cause is not known.

Basic Drives: Eating, Sleeping, and Sex

We must eat to stay alive. We must have sex to reproduce, at least enough to carry on the species. We must sleep to remain healthy, though only recently have we begun to grasp how strong that connection is. The brain regulates each of these basic drives, controlling them automatically and unconsciously. At the same time, our conscious choices and unconscious psychological desires play important roles in how we express these needs. We generally decide when we will eat, what foods we eat, and how much. We choose when to go to bed, and when (or if) we set the alarm clock in the morning. Healthy sex is an inherently social act, requiring cooperation. Thus, while eating, sleeping, and sex are basic drives, our activities based on these drives are quite complex.

Given how vital and automatic these basic drives are, it is no surprise that the brain mechanisms serving them are located deep in the core of the brain. All three functions depend on nerve cells located in the hypothalamus, just above the pituitary gland. Through complex circuitry, other parts of the brain stem core orchestrate how these nerve cells are activated. The hypothalamus in turn connects to the limbic circuits, which organize the actions, emotions, and autonomic responses appropriate to satisfying each drive.

The drive to eat is a good example of how many factors are involved in these basic, life-sustaining activities. A complex interaction of pathways regulates hunger and feeding behaviors and involves the gastrointestinal tract, hormones in the blood, and pathways in the brain. In the brain, many different neurotransmitters play a role, with some stimulating and some inhibiting the drive to eat.

It seems that we are always primed to eat *except* when our brains sense certain appetite-suppressing neurochemicals, notably the hormone leptin. The stomach signals the brain when it is physically full, and the gut sends hormones with messages about what nutrients it has processed. The brain also seems to read the level of insulin in a person's cerebrospinal fluid, which reflects the amount of fat stores in his or her body. All of these signals reach a brain that is also conditioned to respond to certain psychological factors: whether the occasion is right for eating, whether the clock is showing a mealtime, whether a person wants "comfort foods," whether the available food has any appeal, and so on. Only after our brains balance all those factors do we sit down for a meal.

Most of us have experienced how difficult it is to diet in the long term. After a while, it gets harder and harder to reduce food intake, and often it seems like it gets harder to lose weight, even if we are not eating very much. While we do not understand why this is, it is interesting that many of the chemicals in the brain that we know inhibit or stimulate feeding also seem to be involved in the modulation of mood, and perhaps reward. It would be reasonable to guess that this link between feeding and mood may have developed as a way for Mother Nature to motivate animals to find food, whatever the dangers. Thus, in many people, chronic dieting may be associated with uncomfortable feelings, and feeding with some sense of satisfaction or reward.

Another important connection is that feeding and energy balance are linked to energy metabolism. That is, for many of us, the body seems to be able to make some adjustment in how vigorously it burns fuel. During periods of dieting (or starvation) the body may be able to slow down its metabolism, so that it becomes harder to lose weight. And this slowdown in metabolism makes it easier to gain weight back when people resume normal eating. It may be that genetic differences in the efficiency of their metabolisms cause a predisposition for some people to gain weight and for others to be lean.

The sex drive, in turn, is a good example of how much activity in the body the hypothalamus cues. Even though sexual behavior is regulated by the brain (parts such as the hypothalamus, the amygdala, and the nucleus accumbens), other parts of the body, such as the spinal cord and some endocrine glands, are also involved. The endocrine glands, namely testicles in men, ovaries in women, and adrenal glands in both sexes, secrete so-called sex hormones (also called sex steroids), such as testosterone, estrogen, and progesterone. The secretion of these hormones is partially influenced by the brain, but the hormones also provide information (feedback) to the brain and have an effect on some brain functions.

The regulation of sexual behavior is very complex and not fully understood. The sex drive motivates a wide range of planned behaviors, from making eye contact to (according to some theorists) buying red sports cars. An individual can be sexually aroused by a vast array of sensory experiences, and simply by his or her own imagination. Arousal and the sex act itself cause the autonomic nervous system to stimulate many parts of people's anatomy. Women and men experience its effects not simply in their genitals, but also in increased heart rate and breathing, sweating, erect nipples, muscle spasms in various parts of the body, and the pleasure of orgasm.

Modern science has broadened our understanding of human sexual functioning. Normal men and women experience a sequence of physiological responses to sexual stimulation. The sexual response cycle is usually divided into four phases: desire, excitement, orgasm, and resolution. Men experience one orgasm per cycle, women may experience more than one. Men and women may respond to different external erotic stimuli—men are more visual, women may respond more to romantic stories or tactile stimulation. The frequency and intensity of sexual intercourse vary from individual to individual. A person's satisfaction with his or her sexual life is important, and popular generalizations about specific frequency of sexual intercourse do not necessarily apply to everyone.

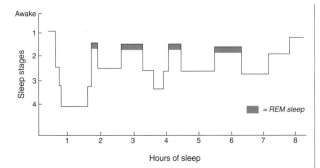

A typical night's sleep for an adult consists of four or five cycles, starting in deep sleep (stages 3 and 4) and rising to REM sleep (when we dream) before returning to deep sleep. Each cycle is one to two hours long. We dream the most just before we wake up. Graph © Leigh Coriale

Sexual behavior is diverse and determined by various factors. It is affected by relationships, life circumstances, stage of development, and culture. Some sexual behavior may be considered acceptable in one culture and not acceptable in another (extramarital sex, masturbation, oral sex). Sexual behavior develops throughout the life cycle. Early sexual experience may involve genital play in infants, which is considered part of normal development. Gender identity ("I am male/female") is established by the age of 2 or 3. Puberty is usually marked by a rapid development of secondary sexual characteristics and the ability to engage in sexual intercourse and reproduction. Sexuality usually peaks in early adulthood and gradually declines thereafter. However, contrary to popular beliefs, a satisfactory sexual functioning is possible even in advanced age (if the person is healthy and physically fit).

We know from daily experience how much thought can go into eating and mating, while sleep may appear to be a much simpler activity. In fact, it has complexities that we are only beginning to understand. There are really two states of sleep: rapid eye movement (REM) and non-REM (NREM). In REM sleep, a person's eyes move quickly back and forth behind his or her eyelids. The sleeper's muscles are still, but his or her brain is active: REM sleep is when most dreaming occurs, and the electroencephalograph (EEG) readings of a brain in that state can resemble those of an alert person. NREM sleep comes in stages, from light dozing to deep, sound slumber. A regular night's sleep for an adult includes several hours of both NREM and REM states, coming in cycles. And each of these states, studies have shown, serves a vital purpose for the brain.

Forming Concepts of the Basic Drives

The concept of a "drive" has undergone many changes over the last century. Sigmund Freud shaped the modern awareness of basic drives

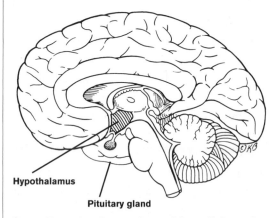

Hypothalamus

Pituitary gland

Our eating, sleeping, and sex drives all depend on the hypothalamus. Neurons in that structure serve as daily clocks, signaling periods of rest and activity for various body organs. The hypothalamus is connected to many areas of the body; it transmits information to other areas of the brain and signals through the pituitary gland's many hormones to other organs in the body, such as heart, lungs, and kidneys. Illustration © Kathryn Born

such as sexuality, aggression, and sleep, with a particular emphasis on dreaming. He championed the view that all of our mental life derives from deep instinctual forces of which we are unaware. Freud felt a keen need to anchor his psychoanalytic theory in brain science but, having little knowledge to build on, created it using only ingenuity, imagination, and clinical acumen. Since 1900, psychoanalysis has exerted a strong cultural and literary influence—without, however, advancing scientific status.

In the first half of the twentieth century experimental psychology focused strongly on the connections between human physiology and behavior. We learned a great deal about hunger, thirst, and sexual behavior, translating the concept of drives into the language of motivation and learning. Neuroscientists then began to focus on the brain circuits that underlie these motivated behaviors. Studying people with brain lesions and stimulating particular neural areas showed the importance of subcortical regions, especially the hypothalamus and the limbic system, but these techniques could not specify the precise regulatory mechanisms involved.

Since 1950, we have made considerable progress thanks to the ability to test the effect of particular chemicals on individual brain cells. Studying the flow of blood within the human brain through positron-emission tomography (PET) and magnetic resonance imaging (MRI) scans also helps us understand the importance of particular neural regions. Today we have a detailed picture of how, for example, chemically coded neurons govern the circadian rhythm of rest and activity, and the sleep-wake cycle. The next frontier to explore is the genetic basis of these systems. It is already clear that the activation of the brain cells that serve basic drives affects how

genes turn on or off and what proteins they produce.

Recent Discoveries About Basic Drives

For many years Western culture seemed to consider obesity to be a moral "weakness" that happened because people did not control their food intake. However, in the past decade, a number of strains of rodents were discovered that were very obese. This led to new discoveries of brain chemicals that played an important role in regulating feeding behavior. One finding that seemed to make an important change in the understanding of obesity was the discovery that some obese rodents had a disturbance of leptin, which resulted in their overeating and becoming obese. Leptin, a hormone secreted by fat cells, circulates in blood in proportion to body fat content. There are leptin receptors in the brain, and when leptin

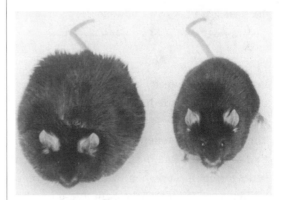

Healthy weight needs a good signal. The mouse on the left lacked the gene that creates the hormone leptin, a signal of fat levels, so its brain could not sense when it had stored enough fat. A similar mouse injected with leptin, on the right, lost its excess weight. The human gene for leptin is similar to, but not the same as, the mouse's. Our eating drive is also more complex, guided by emotions and social convention as well as biochemistry. PHOTO © AMGEN, INC.

SWITCHING ON AND OFF

The hypothalamus, which sits just above the pituitary (or master) gland, contains neurons that function more or less as clocks. They have a period length of about one day. The signals they put out trigger periods of rest and activity, and these signals in turn produce our states of waking and sleep. Via the sleep-wake windows, these neurons also affect our sexual and feeding control systems, each of which has its own rhythmic features, which we still understand only poorly.

A key feature of the hypothalamus is that it is intimately interconnected with organs throughout the body through the many hormonal outputs of the pituitary gland. It is also tightly linked with other control systems in the brain, especially the neurons in the midbrain, pons, and medulla that modulate other neurons. These neurons influence drive behavior as well as thinking because they control the chemical microclimate of the entire brain by projecting their chemical messages over wide areas.

To give but one example, REM sleep is characterized by the following changes:

■ activation of the thalamocortical system

■ activation of emotion and "drive" circuits in the amygdala

■ activation of sexual organs (erection and clitoral engorgement)

■ suppression of muscle tone

■ abandonment of central temperature control

And these are just a few of the drive-related functions that are altered.

is administered directly into the brains of experimental animals, it reduces food intake. By contrast, a deficiency of leptin increases food intake. The reason these rodents had become obese is that a mutation had occurred in the gene that codes for leptin. Since then, disturbances of other brain neurochemicals have been found in other rodents that develop obesity.

However, the story of obesity is not so simple in humans. First, very few people have been found whose obesity was caused by a solitary defect in leptin, or, for that matter, any other brain chemical. Second, while it is known that the genes you inherit contribute to causing obesity, the population of the United States has become more and more obese over the past several decades. Clearly, genes don't change in such a short period of time, so cultural factors also appear to contribute to the problem. The cultural factors are not well understood and may be related to lack of exercise or eating too much junk food, but this remains uncertain. At this point, obesity appears most commonly to be a combination of genes (which ones remains unknown) and cultural and psychological factors. It is most likely that there are many different causes of obesity and that the proportion of the influence of genes and environment is different for each of us.

Recent research on sleep and dreaming reveals previously unsuspected links between this behavior and the other basic drives—a direct link to feeding and an indirect link to sexuality.

Animals that are deprived of sleep develop incapacitating and ultimately fatal disorders of temperature control, metabolic balance, and immune function. Sleep itself obviously saves calories. Being still is integral to deep sleep, and a still body uses less energy. Furthermore, a sleeping body in a bedroom (or a nest) and under cover (or feathers), especially snuggled beside a mate or offspring, does not radiate as much heat as it does out-of-doors. So in the short term we save in two ways: body heat and metabolic energy.

But that is not all: sleep somehow helps us restore our capacity to regulate both body heat and metabolism. After sleep we are better able to adjust to changes in the temperature around us so as to make efficient use of food. These facts emerged from long-term sleep-deprivation studies of rats. After about two weeks rats deprived of sleep begin to overeat, in spite of which they still lose weight. They seek sources of heat, but their body temperature falls anyway. These rats are like a wood stove with the draft open: all the heat (and nutritional benefit) goes up the chimney.

These changes lead to death within four weeks if a rat is totally deprived of sleep, or within six weeks if only the REM sleep is interrupted. Since REM sleep occupies only 15 percent to 25 percent of sleep, it would seem to constitute a supersleep state in terms of its efficiency in the maintenance of these thermoregulatory functions. If sleep is allowed, recovery is rapid and dramatic, but if deprivation is continued, the ensuing death may be associated with massive infection caused by bacterial invasion of the bloodstream from the animal's own digestive tract. This finding shows that immune functions also depend on sleep. While no such studies have been done on humans, unscrupulous interrogators have long known that sleep deprivation is one of the most powerful ways to break down a prisoner's will.

Learning is also highly sleep dependent, as recent experiments have clearly shown. Subjects who learn a visual discrimination task in which they are asked to detect a stimulus with different properties from the array in which it is embedded actually improve their skill on the next day's retest if they have ample NREM sleep in the first quarter and REM sleep in the last quarter of the night. If they are systematically deprived of sleep, they have to relearn the skill from scratch. This finding suggests that sleep not only consolidates new learning but may even improve it.

At a behavioral level, it is obvious that sleeping with another person provides regular mating opportunities. It is probably no accident that the vernacular phrase for sexual intercourse is "sleeping together." But there are deeper links as well. Major hormones essential to sexual development and reproductive capability are released on a schedule related to sleep. Body development, including the ratio of muscle to body mass, is regulated by growth hormone, about 95 percent of which is released in sleep. In some animals, sexual intercourse is immediately followed by sleep; lying still at this time may favor fertility. So sexual capacity, performance, and efficiency are all enhanced by sleep.

Differences and Disorders

All three basic drives are quite variable in their expression, both among individuals and be-

BRAIN TEMPERATURE AND COGNITION

Mammals are the only animals that regulate body temperature reliably, usually within a narrow range of .5°C (1°F) during good health. Why should they need to maintain so narrow a range of internal temperature? A speculative but compelling answer is that mammals' relatively large, complex brains cannot tolerate wider fluctuations of temperature. Human cognition, that powerful function that makes us unquestionably the king of the beasts, is particularly sensitive to body temperature. People's capacity to think rationally fails dramatically if their temperature rises above 39°C (102°F) or falls below 36°C (97°F).

Both eating and sleep have direct effects on the ability of our bodies to maintain a steady temperature. So it would seem that one important function of sleep is to maintain our capacity to keep our body and brain temperature within a narrow range in order to face the challenges of the day.

tween two people. Just as there are Jack Sprats who eat no fat and Mrs. Sprats who eat no lean, there are sexually uninterested and sexually insatiable individuals. There are adults who sleep as long as ten hours a day, or as short as four hours a day.

Eating

New information now suggests that alterations in brain chemistry may contribute to such eating disorders as anorexia nervosa. This disorder most commonly occurs in young women who see themselves as too fat, go on extreme diets, and become very thin. There is evidence that people with anorexia nervosa have too much activity of the neurotransmitter serotonin, which may increase anxiety and satiety. It may be that people with anorexia starve themselves because food restriction causes a reduction in tryptophan, an essential amino acid that we get only from food and that is the chemical which makes serotonin. This may be a mechanism whereby people with anorexia can reduce serotonin activity and make themselves less anxious.

Information is widely available about the ben-

eficial influences of a healthy diet and exercise. Such advice is often not followed, which may contribute to the high incidence of obesity and adult-onset diabetes in our culture. Whether this is related to some genetic influence in people that drives hunger or the difficulties people have in balancing short-term rewards (for example, too many appealing desserts) with long-term benefits (not getting diabetes 30 years in the future) is not clear. The current treatments for obesity, whether medication or some form of talk therapy, have limited success, and most people eventually relapse. A better understanding of these problems would thus be likely to result in more effective treatment.

Sex

Sexual functioning could be impaired in two ways: as a disturbance related to a particular phase of the sexual cycle, or as a disturbance involving unusual objects or activity. The first group, sexual dysfunctions, include sexual desire disorders (characterized either by a lack of sexual fantasies and desire for sexual activity or by aversion to or avoidance of genital contact), sexual arousal disorders (characterized by the failure to attain or maintain erection in men, and failure to attain or maintain lubrication in women), and orgasm disorders (recurrent delay or inability to achieve orgasm or, in men, inability to achieve ejaculation or ejaculating before they wish—so-called premature ejaculation). Other dysfunction may include painful sex. The second group, so-called paraphilias, involve unusual fantasies, urges, or practices (exposing oneself, sex with minors, sadistic sex, and so on). Homosexuality is not considered a dysfunction or abnormal behavior.

People may experience various sexual dysfunctions that may not have a detectable or obvious cause or that may result from various medical conditions (for example, diabetes mellitus, prostate surgery, trauma), substances (chronic abuse of alcohol and other drugs), medications (for hypertension, depression, heart conditions, and others), or psychological problems (conflict with partner, depression, anxiety).

Good sexual functioning requires good physical health and a good relationship with the partner. Obesity, lack of physical stamina, illnesses, chronic exhaustion, smoking, substance abuse, chronic conflict may be some of the causes of sexual dysfunction. Healthy diet and exercise, and a healthy lifestyle in general, help maintain a good sexual life. However, various misconceptions about sex could hamper sexual functioning further. The best approach to impairment of sexual functioning is to discuss it with a physician, as complete physical examination and laboratory tests may help reveal the underlying cause. It is not advisable to treat oneself with various over-the-counter substances, as these are mostly of unproven efficacy and could even be dangerous.

Sleep

As old age arrives, changes in sleep patterns often develop. A person's capacity for deep, refreshing, and prolonged sleep may deteriorate, with more frequent interruptions at night and a lingering sense of fatigue in the daytime. Old age has been justly characterized as more time in which to do less. Individuals can best respond to these biological changes by making deliberate and determined changes in their lifestyles.

Insomnia (or naturally diminished sleep capacity) is the leading complaint people bring to their physicians for remedy. Too often, doctors prescribe sedatives indiscriminately. While it may initially be effective, sleep medication is not physiological and may induce tolerance and dependency. Users need to be cautioned and should exercise both flexibility and restraint. The same counsel should be offered to those suffering from minor excesses and deficiencies of appetite, whether sexual or culinary. As with more problematic eating (**C27**) and sexual behaviors, disorders of sleep like narcolepsy (**C12**), sleep apnea syndrome, and periodic leg movement (**C11**), require a specialist's evaluation and treatment.

In all of these domains, brief psychotherapy can help inculcate a healthy, versatile, and philosophical attitude that walks the fine line between unrealistic optimism (the fountain of youth) and nihilistic despair (being old before one's time).

Movement, Balance, and Coordination

Reaching for a pencil, grasping a doorknob, skiing, and tightrope walking—to name but a few physical actions—all involve well-coordinated movements made with well-balanced postures. In fact, whenever we move the three basic functions of movement, balance, and coordination work in concert to produce graceful, purposeful motions of body parts. This is actually quite a feat, because moving is a complex process.

We hardly ever contract just a single muscle; practically all of our body motions involve several muscles working in sequence or at once. For example, walking is produced by contracting all the muscles of the legs in different intensities and at different times. Similarly, reaching movements are produced by contracting all the muscles of the arm, while grasping and manipulating objects require contracting many muscles of the forearm, hand, and fingers. In all of these cases, the result is a well-coordinated movement—that is, a movement of a body part that actually consists of many movements of joints, occurring in proper sequence and of appropriate extent, such that the resulting motion is smooth, straight, and directed to the object of interest. This is the essence of co-ordination, which applies equally well to muscles, joints, and whole body parts. Coordination is the essence of motor skill.

Superimposed on coordinated movements is our sense of body balance, which helps us keep our posture against gravity. In fact, the presence of gravity calls for balance. In outer space, there is no gravity and therefore no need to balance; bodies just float. Compared with other animals, humans face the especially difficult challenge of balancing on just two feet with a narrow base. Yet it is common for us not only to stand upright easily and apparently effortlessly, but also to perform many other actions—walking, reaching, dancing, and chewing gum—while keeping our balance.

We are hardly aware of how we maintain balance and coordinate our movements except when we learn new tasks. But it takes time and effort for a baby to learn to stand upright, to reach, and to manipulate objects. We usually forget the frustration and false steps of our early years. But later in life, we might learn the steps of riding a bicycle, driving a car, using a computer or other complex

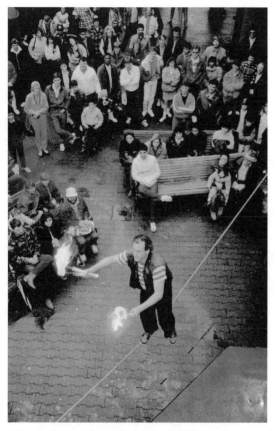

© Bob Daemmrich/Stock, Boston Inc./PictureQuest

machine, and, for a lucky few, walking a tightrope! For the first time in years, we are forced to *think* about how we are moving and to train ourselves to move and balance in new ways. It is no wonder that learning these tasks can make us feel as helpless as children.

We learn most of our basic motor skills during infancy and childhood and acquire different and more refined motor skills throughout adult life. Highly coordinated movements develop gradually from simpler components. For example, infants' reaching movements are initially composed of small, sequential, poorly coordinated movements.

These smaller movements gradually disappear and are replaced by larger movements that ultimately lead to smooth, single-component reaching movements several months after birth. Similarly, our initial unsteady toddling leads gradually to well-coordinated locomotion, and the same holds for other motor skills (manipulating objects, coloring within the lines, dressing, tying shoelaces, and so on). Most motor skills require good body balance, which develops gradually during the first year of life. Parents recognize the importance of balance when they applaud their babies' first steps. The most important factors in uniting movement, balance, and coordination into a tightly linked whole are practice, practice, and practice.

Movement and the Brain

Two important breakthroughs in understanding how our brains control movement occurred in the second half of the nineteenth century. First, John Hughlings Jackson in England made astute observations on how epileptics suffered seizures that spread in patterns through their bodies. He inferred that there must be a corresponding, orderly pattern in the brain representing movements of those various body parts. Then Fritsch and Hitzig in Germany were able to evoke movements in dogs' body parts by electrically stimulating the motor cortex area of their brains. Later, neurosurgeons evoked similar movements in humans who were awake on the operating table.

Scientists gradually developed valuable insights into the brain mechanisms behind coordination and balance, and specifically into the role

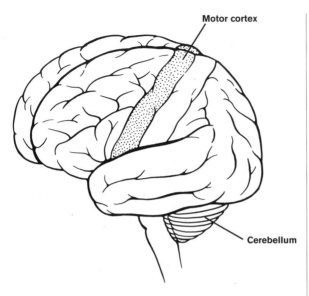

Motor cortex

Cerebellum

The motor cortex and cerebellum play the lead in co-ordinating movements. ILLUSTRATION © KATHRYN BORN

of the cerebellum in these functions, from observing humans in clinics and performing experiments with animals. There is still much to learn; research teams are actively investigating and debating the neural mechanisms underlying voluntary movement, coordination, and balance.

It is no exaggeration to say that most of our brain is geared toward action. Vast areas in the cerebral cortex, the basal ganglia, the cerebellum, the brain stem, and the spinal cord are intimately connected and cooperate in initiating, producing, and controlling coordinating movements and maintaining body balance. Although damage to a specific area usually results in a distinguishable motor disorder (**C71**), practically all of these areas interact in controlling motor function.

Here's how this system works when you set out to perform a particular movement, such as walking across a room. To begin with, the nerve cells in your body are always sending your brain information about your position: standing or sitting,

with your weight on one foot or distributed across both, and so on. Based on that information, your brain sends the appropriate messages to your muscles to step forward with one leg. These signals descend through the spinal cord and out the nerves to the proper muscles. Some muscles cause joints to flex, some cause them to extend, all in coordinated fashion. One leg moves while the other adjusts to maintain your balance.

Your spinal cord is not simply a conduit for these signals but a highly complex structure that organizes signals from the body's periphery (muscles, skin, joints) and center (brain). While spinal motor functions move your body, spinal sensory functions mediate not only the common sensations, such as touch, pain, temperature, and position, but also such powerful sensations as ticklishness, itchiness, bladder and bowel urgency, and muscle weariness. Autonomic functions control most of our internal organs, including bladder and bowel contractions, digestion, heart rate, breathing, and blood pressure.

The spinal cord is shorter than most people think. It starts at the base of the skull and stops a few inches below the lowest rib, typically a distance of about 20 inches in an average-size adult. The cord is encased in a tough membranous sheath called the dura, which also holds the cerebrospinal fluid that bathes the cord. The spinal cord lies in the middle of a marvelous articulated bony structure called the spine, which has 8 neck or cervical segments, 12 chest or thoracic segments, 5 lumbar segments, and 5 tail or sacral segments.

The spinal cord is connected to the body through nerve roots. Two pairs of these roots emerge from the spinal cord at each segmental level and run through openings in the spinal column between vertebral segments. Nerve fibers, or

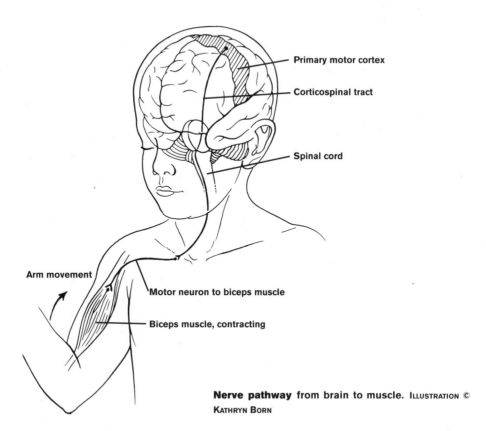

- Primary motor cortex
- Corticospinal tract
- Spinal cord
- Arm movement
- Motor neuron to biceps muscle
- Biceps muscle, contracting

Nerve pathway from brain to muscle. ILLUSTRATION © KATHRYN BORN

axons, that go from the spinal cord to muscles originate from motoneurons situated in the spinal cord and emerge from the cord in the roots toward the front. Axons carrying sensation to the spinal cord all come from a collection of nerve cells or ganglia adjacent to the spinal cord.

The neurons in the dorsal (toward the back) root ganglia are by far the largest cells known. These neurons send axons out to the body and to the spinal cord. The peripheral end of the neuron may go to the toes. The other end enters the cord and goes all the way to the brain stem. Depending on your height, the neurons may be several feet long. Large axons carry position and touch sensations while smaller fibers carry pain and temperature sensations.

About 20 million nerve fibers, or axons, are packed inside the human spinal cord. Some axons go from one part of the spinal cord to another while others connect the brain to the cord and vice versa. The spinal cord also contains many nerve cells that connect to muscles, called motoneurons (see figure above). Other spinal neurons receive signals from the brain or sensory signals from the body and then relay these signals to other neurons in the spinal cord or brain. These spinal neurons mediate reflexes and even complex behaviors such as walking. In addition, they filter incoming sensory signals and differentiate between normal and painful sensations. In fact, the spinal cord can support walking without the brain's involvement past the initial impulse to walk.

One major source of information sent to the

IT'S A REFLEX

Our spines direct certain body movements without needing instruction from the brain. We call these spinal reflexes. You might recall your doctor tapping your kneecap during a medical examination, and feeling the lower part of your leg jerk up. It usually takes less than a second for tendons in the knee to feel the tap's pressure and signal the spine that they are being stretched. The spinal neurons respond by cueing the thigh muscles to tighten, producing the movement. This signal system is in place to help us stand steadily. The system is faster and more efficient because it does not rely on processing by the brain.

Another useful set of spinal reflexes causes us to flinch away from something painful, such as a hot stove or an electric shock. If people's nervous systems are damaged so that their spines cannot cue these quick evasive movements, as in amyotrophic lateral sclerosis (**C53**), they are in danger of being burned, shocked, cut, or otherwise harmed.

One curious aspect of these spinal reflexes is that when a limb, hand, or foot jerks one way, the opposite limb, hand, or foot moves in the other direction. As one foot rises to get away from a sharp stone, for instance, the other foot extends or presses down. This reaction, called a crossed extension, is also controlled by the motor neurons in our spinal cords. The natural pairing of opposing actions comes in handy when we walk or swim. The programs controlling these movements appear very early in our fetal development, and probably show up in the way a fetus kicks in the uterus. For other animal species, such natural programming for opposite-limb movement allows babies to stand, walk, or swim very shortly after birth.

spinal motor centers is our antigravity system: the brain stem and those muscles in the neck, around the spine, and in the legs (the gastrocnemius muscles) that resist the downward pull of gravity. We depend on this system to maintain our upright posture. The antigravity nuclei in the brain stem mediate the reflexes that adjust our body position or muscle contraction slightly so that we do not fall. The cerebellum is heavily involved in this function; indeed, it is a cardinal sign of damage to the part of the cerebellum that controls balance when a person cannot stand upright, especially with feet close together and eyes closed.

Traditionally, we regard the motor cortex as the key structure in initiating movement. Our elaborate use of hands and fingers to manipulate objects seems to depend clearly on intact motor

cortical function. Following a stroke affecting the motor cortex or the signals from it, a person's hands usually remain clumsy after most other functions have recovered. At one point, neuroscientists thought that specific areas of the motor cortex controlled the contraction and relaxation of different muscles, just as specific areas of the sensory cortex organized the signals arriving from corresponding parts of the body. More recent research has shown that tightly interconnected neurons extend down in columns from the top layer of the motor cortex. Each column seems to control a group of related muscles.

Furthermore, many other areas of the brain are also involved in starting movements. The cellular mechanisms that promote motor function have been studied in detail by recording the impulse activity of single neurons in monkeys as they perform various motor tasks. Some clear results have emerged from such studies. First, many motor areas in the brain are activated concurrently when a movement is initiated, including the motor and premotor cortex, the cerebellum, and the basal ganglia. Therefore, generating a movement involves many competing areas, not just the motor cortex.

Furthermore, these studies have found that within a particular area individual cells can be more or less active during various movements (for example, moving an arm left, moving an arm right, and so on). Those movements therefore depend on the concurrent activation of groups of cells. Which cells in an area are activated determines the direction, speed, force, and other aspects of the movement. Finally, cell activity in various motor areas is almost constantly modulated by other factors, such as sensory stimuli in the environment and attention. Positron-emission tomography (PET) and functional magnetic resonance imaging (fMRI) studies of human brains have corroborated these findings and provided valuable information on how different areas are involved in motor function. This field is expanding quickly, and more discoveries will doubtless be forthcoming.

Movement Disorders

Losing too many neurons from the motor structures results in obvious disease. For example, severe alcoholism (C30) can lead to atrophy of the anterior lobe of the cerebellum and difficulty walking. Parkinson's disease (C41) involves loss of dopamine-producing neurons in the substantia nigra; it creates a variety of movement abnormalities such as akinesia (difficulty in initiating movement), rigidity, and tremor. Widespread cortical atrophy and a variety of motor defects characterize Alzheimer's disease (C67).

The most obvious motor deficits result from serious brain damage and are hard to miss. For example, strokes (C59, C60) often result in paralysis and spasticity of the arm and leg on one side (hemiplegia) due to damage of the internal capsule—the tract connecting the motor cortical outflow to the brain stem, cerebellum, and spinal cord. Lesions in certain areas in the parietal or frontal cortex can affect motor functions more insidiously. Such lesions frequently result in apraxias of various kinds (C71), meaning difficulty in performing motor skills a person has already learned (for example, how to dress, strike a match, and so on), copying shapes from a template or from memory, assembling objects from component parts, or imitating common gestures. Such difficulties will not become apparent until the person is asked to perform these actions.

Disorders of coordination and balance are more commonly the result of cerebellar damage. These diseases can interfere with the fine-tuning of muscular movement and result in coarse, uncoordinated movement. This type of condition is called ataxia (C46) and is easily seen in a person's jerky to-and-fro motion of the trunk and unsteady gait.

A very different class of motor abnormality comprises involuntary movements that a person cannot stop. These include:

- rather innocuous tics (C45)
- slow, writhing, well-coordinated movements of the arm (choreo-athetosis)
- rhythmic movements of the fingers (resting tremor; C43)

- involuntary movements of the face and mouth (tardive dyskinesia)

- wildly violent, throwing arm movements (hemiballismus)

Characteristically, almost all of these abnormal movements are the result of problems in the normal functioning of the basal ganglia. Some can be overlooked, while others intrude on people's lives.

Finally another motor disorder, called dystonia (**C44**), shows up as a continuous contraction of certain muscle groups, resulting in steady, strange, abnormal postures (for example, torticollis). These disorders, unlike those discussed in the previous paragraph, can hardly be missed. They are always present, and are very difficult to treat or alleviate.

In all cases of motor dysfunction, a person should consult with a neurologist about treatment.

Keeping the Body Moving

No two people are exactly alike, and that truism certainly applies to our movements. Indeed, how we move is an essential part of our individuality. That said, movement, coordination, and balance are very similar in men and women, as shown by how both sexes can excel in all kinds of sports. Women and men also share a common fate in that their motor systems change similarly with age. We may become wiser as we get older, but our motor skills tend to deteriorate. Movements take longer to start, they are slower and not as well coordinated, and keeping our balance becomes harder. These are manifestations of the cumulative loss of neurons with age.

To keep the motor system in good shape, it is important to live a healthy life. For example, a balanced, low-fat diet and regular exercise help reduce the risk of atherosclerosis and therefore the risk of strokes. People with high cholesterol, high triglycerides, or various lipid disorders should receive appropriate treatment for these problems. No one who wants to keep his or her brain healthy should smoke.

Exercise can add healthy and active years to your life. It is never too late to start exercising, and even small improvements in physical fitness can significantly raise the quality of your life. Resistance training is important because it is the only form of exercise that can slow and even reverse the decline in muscle mass, bone density, and strength. Adding workouts that focus on speed and agility are also useful, while exercises that increase flexibility can help reduce the stiffness and loss of balance that accompanies aging. Just as practice in our early years is the best way to make our movements smoother and more coordinated, practice helps us maintain those skills as long as possible.

Pain Perception

Pain is an unpleasant sensory and emotional experience usually produced by something that injures, or threatens to injure, the body. Pain begins with a stimulus, but is influenced by physiological and psychological factors before it becomes part of our consciousness.

Although pain is something that we invariably want to escape or to stop, it serves several very important functions. Pain protects us by triggering a reflexive withdrawal from something damaging before we can suffer further injury, such as when we drop a hot pan before we sustain extensive burns. It is also a warning system that lets us know when an injury is about to occur: the burning ache in our muscles during extreme exertion warns us to stop using them. Pain forces us to immobilize or protect an injured part, such as a broken ankle, thus giving it a chance to heal. Pain also lets us know when we need to seek medical help, and teaches us what behaviors to avoid in the future.

This section concentrates on acute pain, which occurs almost immediately upon tissue damage or injury and lasts only a limited time. When pain persists and cannot be avoided, it can

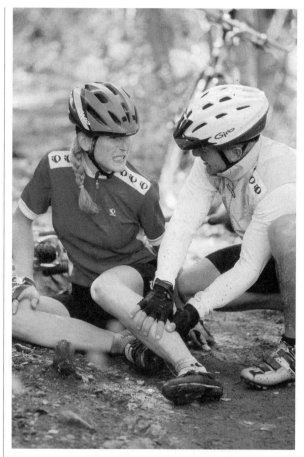

be quite destructive. In effect, it becomes a disease in itself. Pain that lasts for weeks, months, or years is called chronic pain and is a major source of suffering, disability, and economic loss (**C57**).

The Physiology of Pain

The nature of pain has intrigued philosophers for millennia. The ancient Greeks conceived of pain as an emotion. In the late nineteenth and early twentieth centuries, the view of pain as sensation became preeminent: it was seen as a direct response to a stimulus. From the mid–twentieth century to the present, these two views have been combined, so medical scientists who study pain now think of it as a subjective experience with distinct discriminative and emotional components.

Pain is associated with a variety of behaviors. A painful stimulus will arouse us, as in "Pinch me to see if I'm awake." It can focus our attention on the site of an injury: "I looked down at where it hurt and saw I was bleeding." It can cue us to try to escape from the cause of an injury or immobilize us so that we do not suffer further damage. In addition, pain causes changes in heart rate and blood pressure, and an endocrine response with elevated stress hormones. For each response elicited by the pain-producing injury, there is a unique central nervous system pathway.

In healthy individuals, the sensory experience of pain is usually triggered by events in the body that activate specialized nerve endings, called primary afferent nociceptors. Nociceptors are activated by any process that either causes damage or has the capacity to cause damage if continued or intensified. Most primary afferent nociceptors respond to a variety of noxious stimuli—extreme hot or cold temperatures, intense mechanical manipulations (pinching, pinpricks, cutting), increased tissue acidity, and other causes of injury. Nociceptors can also be activated by a variety of chemical agents released from cells that are damaged or responding to a foreign body such as a splinter or infectious agent (for example, a bacterium).

There are two types of nociceptors, and the differences between them can easily be understood. Let's say that you tripped and fell, landing hard on one knee. You would experience an acute, well-localized, painful sensation in your knee, followed by a dull and aching sensation. This reflects the two types of fiber systems that conduct pain from the periphery into the central nervous system. The first pain signals are carried by A-delta fibers, which are insulated with myelin and therefore conduct rapidly. The longer-lasting pain signals are carried by C-fibers, which are unmyelinated and conduct slowly.

Nociceptors from the body carry their message to the spinal cord, where they end in very specific areas. Those areas contain connections to the neuron pathways that conduct the message to the brain stem. Pain messages from the head arrive at similar groups of neurons in the hindbrain. The central nervous system neurons that receive the pain messages from all over the body target a variety of structures in the brain.

If significant tissue damage has occurred, or if there has been a prolonged or particularly intense activation of a primary afferent nociceptor, it will become sensitized. Sensitized nociceptors can be activated by moderate stimuli that normally do not produce pain. One common example of sensitized nociceptors is the agony produced by bath or shower water on sunburned skin. If you have arthritis, have "thrown out" your back, or have experienced a sports injury, you are also familiar with how you can be reasonably comfortable at

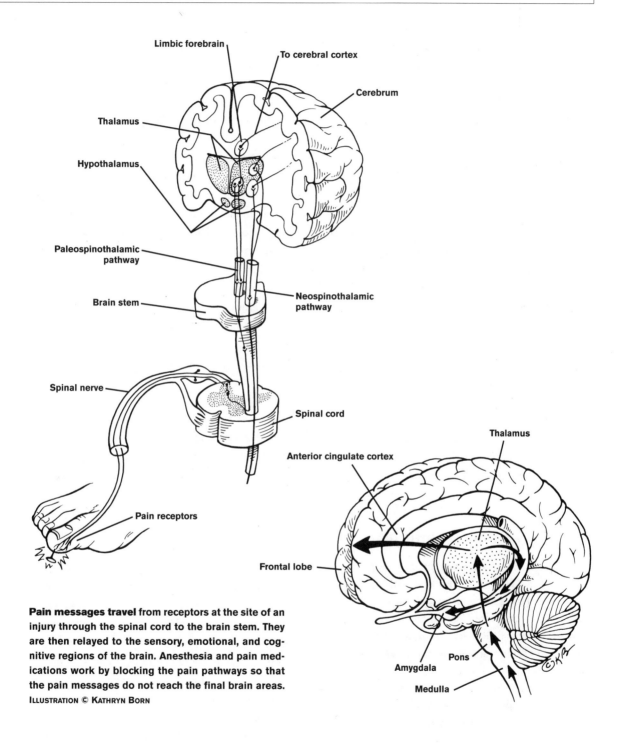

Pain messages travel from receptors at the site of an injury through the spinal cord to the brain stem. They are then relayed to the sensory, emotional, and cognitive regions of the brain. Anesthesia and pain medications work by blocking the pain pathways so that the pain messages do not reach the final brain areas.
ILLUSTRATION © KATHRYN BORN

rest but feel significant pain during normally innocuous movements. That is due to sensitized nociceptors in joints, tendons, and muscles.

Chemical agents that do not activate nociceptors can also produce sensitization. The best known of these agents are prostaglandins, which appear when tissues are inflamed by infection, arthritis, or other factors. Their synthesis depends on the enzyme cyclooxygenase. This enzyme is inhibited by many of the medicines that are used to treat pain: aspirin, acetaminophen, ibuprofen, and the new cyclooxygenase 2 selective drugs, celecoxib (Celebrex) and rofecoxib (Vioxx). These drugs are particularly effective for pain associated with sensitization and are better for tenderness than for continuous severe pain.

The central nervous system's pain transmission neurons can also become sensitized in a way similar to the primary afferent nociceptors. This process is called central sensitization, and it is set in motion by neurotransmitter chemicals released at the central terminals of nociceptors. Thus, when a person is injured, the subsequent activity of nociceptors produces a bigger and bigger response in pain transmission pathways; pain begets further

HOW ANESTHESIA WORKS

General anesthetics work by shutting down the forebrain regions whose activity regulates cycles of arousal and quiescence. There are several kinds of general anesthetics, but those most commonly used enhance or mimic the action of the inhibitory neurotransmitter gamma-aminobutyric acid (GABA). In contrast, a local anesthetic works by blocking the transmission of the pain message along a primary afferent nociceptor's axon. The message thus never reaches the central nervous system.

pain, even if the stimulus that triggered the response remains the same.

The Psychology of Pain

Another part of the brain is at work when we experience pain, integrating the physical sensation with psychological factors. Perhaps the most familiar example of the power of psychological factors on pain involves headaches (C54). It is almost a cliché that emotional stress can bring on a headache. Even our vocabulary of stress incorporates this concept: "This job is a real headache."

Memories, emotions, thoughts, and especially expectations are now known to have an enormous influence on how people perceive pain. A rough outline of the central nervous system pathways that mediate these psychological effects is beginning to emerge. In fact, the regions of the forebrain that are involved in emotion (the frontal and temporal lobes and the amygdala) are known to feed into a neural circuit in the brain stem that directly controls the pain pathways. Furthermore, the control exerted by this pathway is bidirectional, meaning that it can either reduce or enhance pain.

This pain-modulating pathway was discovered in the mid–twentieth century during an exploration of the brain stem using electrical stimulation. An area was found, called the midbrain periaqueductal gray, which, when electrically stimulated, produced a profound reduction of pain in both rodents and people with chronic pain. We now know that this area is part of a circuit that receives connections from the frontal lobe, the amygdala, and the hypothalamus and, in turn, connects directly to the spinal cord neurons that relay pain messages from primary afferent nociceptors. This pathway mediates the pain-relieving effect of powerful painkillers like morphine. In fact, the circuit has neurons that secrete morphine-like compounds, called endorphins and enkephalins. These chemicals interfere with pain-impulse transmission and can significantly lessen the perception of pain.

In animals, the pain-modulating pathway is most easily activated under conditions of threat, such as in the presence of a predator. The animal's system anticipates tissue damage, which would normally be painful, but being incapacitated by pain would lead to even greater injury; therefore, the animal has evolved the ability to dampen its perception of pain temporarily. It is not clear what situations activate this pathway in humans, but possible examples include athletes injured in the midst of competition, or soldiers wounded in combat; such people may not realize they have been hurt until after the stressful situation has ended.

In addition to its pain-suppressing actions, the same pathway can also enhance pain transmission. This raises the possibility that psychological factors that produce or exacerbate pain do so through this circuit. In fact, it has been shown that the anticipation of pain activates areas in the forebrain and midbrain that are part of this pain-modulating circuit, and that anticipation of pain can produce and enhance pain.

Studies have also shown that people can be trained to separate out the sensory intensity of pain from its unpleasantness, and to quantify each selectively. Imaging shows that two different parts of the brain are involved. Measuring the level of sensory intensity is associated with activity in the primary somatosensory cortex, whereas the unpleasantness is associated with activity in areas of the frontal lobe cortex usually associated with emotion (the anterior cingulate and insular cortices). In fact, certain surgical procedures, such as modified frontal lobotomies, can markedly reduce the suffering of severe pain without affecting its sensory intensity. This implies that the emotional aspects of an injury may be more significant than the extent of its physical damage in determining how intense we perceive the resulting pain to be.

Pain Treatment

In addition to the body's own mechanism, there are a variety of approaches to treating pain. The best approach, of course, is to identify the cause and remove it. This should always be the primary goal. Once you or your doctors have identified the cause of a pain and, if possible, treated it in the best way, that pain no longer serves its purpose and should be eliminated as quickly and completely as possible.

Pain relievers (analgesics) are the most common over-the-counter medications, and they are quite effective against most everyday pains. Some people are reluctant to use these drugs, feeling they should "tough it out" or use natural methods of pain relief, such as muscle relaxation. It is true that pain depends on psychological factors, and the experience can thus be affected by our attitudes and mental states. Nevertheless, pain is, by definition, not enjoyable. There is no reason to prolong it if it is interfering with your comfort, performance, or sleep.

Physicians can also prescribe more powerful drugs to counter pain due to a bad injury, surgery, cancer, or other causes. The most common mistake health workers make in treating someone in pain is to give an inadequate dose of these medicines out of fear that the person will become dependent on them. The treatment goal should be relief of pain. There is no reason to delay treatment for acute pain, and there are strong arguments for immediate treatment. First of all, because of the tendency of pain to increase with time and the fact that lower-intensity pain responds better to drug treatment, earlier treatment may require less medication and therefore cause fewer side effects. This is particularly important for intermittent pain that has the potential to become severe, such as in the case of a migraine headache (C55). For acute pain, there is no excuse for withholding powerful painkilling drugs such as morphine. If these drugs are used correctly, the risk of addiction is infinitesimal.

Consciousness

The meaning of *consciousness* can be quite varied, depending on who is using the word and in what context. At a basic level, to "lose consciousness" can mean to go to sleep, to faint, or to go into a stupor—which are all different states. We also use the word *conscious* to mean being aware of something in the present, as in, "I was suddenly very conscious of a large dog in my lap." And some people speak of a "level of consciousness" or "higher consciousness," meaning both a state of awareness and a state of being. Not all these uses of the word are scientific, but they are all related, and their range of meanings shows how fundamental and wide-ranging consciousness is.

In 1890 the psychologist William James defined consciousness as a person's "awareness of self and the environment." But that definition omits two critical words: consciousness is the *accurate* and *chronologic* awareness of self and the environment. Each of us, when mentally healthy, has a sense of who we are and what we are not—what parts of what we experience come from outside ourselves. Each of us also has a sense of time, especially the distinction between what we have experienced in the past and what we are experiencing now. The healthy, awake human brain never lets go of that consciousness. Consciousness reflects a person's inner and outer cognitive world. Like a brain-generated Mount Everest, it

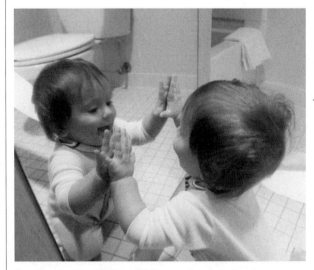

Growing up means becoming conscious of where our self stops and our world begins. This baby may still be wondering, "Am I seeing another baby, or another part of me?" PHOTO © BOB DAEMMRICH/STOCK, BOSTON INC./ PICTUREQUEST

towers over all the other remarkable functions of a person's body. Consciousness is thus the mental quality that identifies, measures, and expresses the quantity of the self.

Almost everyone with a healthy brain can describe consciousness if asked. Our descriptions may vary in detail or wording: "I'm awake and I'm here"; "I think; therefore, I am"; "I'm Jane Smith, and I know it!" Most educated people recognize conscious awareness as a continuously unfolding, automatic sense of being alive and filled with flowing thoughts, normal language, recent memories, and specifically expressed learned motor behavior.

Even the most educated people, however, rarely consider how their brains express their normal emotions, generate logical thinking, and produce a smooth flow of thoughts and deeds. "Now, how did I come to think of that?" is a question we might occasionally ask ourselves, but we rarely carry it into everyday conversation with others. Nor do people wonder what happens in their brains to make them daydream or take a daily walk. We are happy that these functions are largely automatic.

Ironically, even though our consciousness is founded on a sense of time, it is usually catching up to the activity in our minds. Many of our behaviors go through a "preconscious" stage—our brains actually start the process of acting or feeling a very brief time before the results are registered in our consciousness. When people instinctively jump out of the way of an oncoming vehicle, they don't stop to think. Only after they reflect on the danger they just encountered do they become consciously aware of their preconscious behavior and express an emotional response. When you converse, your mind preconsciously, explicitly formulated what you say a half second or more before you actually say it. Gerald Edelman recognized this necessary preformulation of thoughts and words when he ingeniously titled his book on consciousness *The Remembered Present*.

The Psychological Dimensions of Consciousness

Consciousness interweaves our outer perceptions, our inner memories, and our immediately occurring thoughts. Emotional feelings imbue our conscious awareness and sharpen our intentional actions. Memory, however, provides the foundation of consciousness (**B13**). Memory's qualities and quantities depend on the combination of a person's innate cognitive talents, subsequent schooling, and ongoing activities. All evidence indicates that the earlier people pursue learning, the greater their conscious mental and behavioral capacities will be. Indeed, many reliable studies indicate that the longer a person undergoes education and engages in occupations that require thought, the longer his or her mental and physical health will endure.

Several other distinct neuropsychological qualities accompany organized human consciousness. These include sensory perception (**B1**), attention and intention (**B10**), and instinctive awareness of spatial relationships (**B4**). Additional general traits include the chronological ordering of events, mood, and emotion (**B7**). Contributing to the special qualities of normal human consciousness are the symbolic abstractions of verbal, musical, numerical, and geometric languages (**B14**).

Normal consciousness reflects the product of at least three closely interdependent and often integrated aspects of awareness: behavioral intelligence, intellectual intelligence, and the emotional modulation of both.

Behavioral Intelligence

We can loosely define behavioral intelligence as "knowing how to move to accomplish certain things." This quality is expressed in several forms by the brain's two frontal lobes. Each lobe contains neural circuits that stimulate the conscious mind's intentions and attention, as discussed below. That preconscious quality of intention and attention rules almost all our daily behavior. We normally walk, run, and undertake other coordinated activities without specifically directing preconscious attention to those performances. Mundane, nonconscious undertakings can include walking at a routine pace, riding a bicycle, and even skiing a downhill slope. Practiced musicians, automobile drivers, and airplane pilots seldom apply continuous intentional consciousness to how they act unless they anticipate some difficulty.

Automatic motor performances are likely generated first in the frontal lobes, and are only partially recognized by the perception-generating neuronal circuits of the posterior lobes. Psychologists in the past have termed these primary frontal

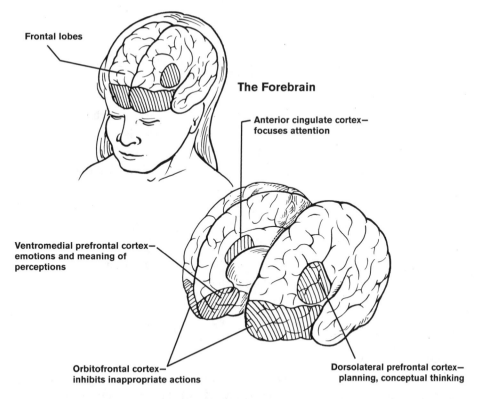

Frontal lobes

The Forebrain

Anterior cingulate cortex—
focuses attention

Ventromedial prefrontal cortex—
emotions and meaning of
perceptions

Orbitofrontal cortex—
inhibits inappropriate actions

Dorsolateral prefrontal cortex—
planning, conceptual thinking

Preconscious behavior refers to how our brains actually initiate action before we become conscious of taking that action. The frontal lobes store knowledge of how to perform tasks, which we often retrieve preconsciously. In contrast, the posterior lobes store knowledge we consciously retrieve: facts, ideas, events, language, and so on. Illustration © Kathryn Born

lobe–generated actions as reflecting "implicit" memory—in other words, directing actions before the mind presents conscious orders.

Intellectual Intelligence

What we classically consider intelligence depends almost entirely on short- and long-term stored memories of facts, ideas, time, events, language, and most other nonbehavioral knowledge. All of these specific functions are generated primarily from the posterior areas of the brain, including the parietal, occipital, and temporal lobes. Activity in these regions boils down all the stimuli our brains receive into what becomes our knowledge.

The normal, awake, conscious mind never ceases to scan its environment. Nor does it lose its memory of past events, thoughts, the expressed content of behavioral activities, the self, and its ever-growing knowledge. Only a few people report that they suffer from episodes in which their minds express no thought of self, memory, or intention. Serious psychiatric disease, certain illegal drugs (**C29**), and brief epileptic seizures (**C13**) may cause such episodes.

Even people with the best of minds, of course, sometimes become bored and lapse into daydreaming. Their minds wander listlessly. But this nonintellectual holiday can end in an instant because of an unexpected stimulus or an intruding thought. The healthy mind quickly returns to attention, once again aware of the world around it.

Emotional Effects on Mental Activity

Emotional states are noncognitive and nonsymbolic contributions to our overall experience of consciousness. They may affect both our behavioral and intellectual intelligence. They can ei-ther sharpen a person's performance by providing increased motivation or degrade it with excessive distractions, anxiety, fear, and other emotional states. If we are worrying about a family member's health, for example, we may experience the disruption as difficulty in concentrating on a book or sinking a free throw. Yet research has also shown that loss of these primitive states of emotional awareness leads to overwhelming failures of behavioral and intellectual intelligence.

The Neurological Underpinnings of Consciousness

A relatively simple brain map helps identify the cerebral areas that generate the behavioral intentions and psychological perceptions that express normal consciousness. The critical areas include the two cerebral hemispheres, each of which possesses approximately half of the cerebral cortex, the thalamus, and the basal ganglia. In the base of the skull, these structures connect with the large cerebellum and the arousal systems inside the brain stem. Discovering just how this network generates consciousness has become a major scientific effort.

The anatomical interconnections among the above areas are extremely complicated. During the last 20 years, about 30,000 published scientific reports have delved into just how this wiring in the brain generates human consciousness. We have learned a great deal but produced no fully satisfying answers. Nevertheless, these efforts are helping us to understand the general anatomy and workings of the conscious brain.

We have learned that nonspecific arousal, which is simply one's state of wakefulness or alertness, is generated largely in the brain stem and is indispensable to arousing consciousness. By itself, however, nonspecific arousal cannot formulate or express neuropsychological qualities. The brain mechanisms that govern sleep states and dreams overlap only partially with the circuitry of normal wakeful consciousness.

Our frontal lobes largely govern and express our behavior, both immediate and well learned. Their functions dictate consciousness and its generation of mood, behavior, and mind. The lobes' basal forebrain area has evolved from ancient mammalian brains and occupies most of the undersurface of the two frontal lobes. It participates in generating emotional feelings and social behavior (B7), as well as stimulating a person's intentional purposes. The lateral and medial prefrontal areas largely influence physical coordination (B4) and participate in volitional and cognitive aspects of attention (B10) and working memory (B13). The rearmost regions of the lateral and medial frontal lobe generate and regulate coordinated expressions of logical, cognitive language (B14), intentional eye movements, and ultimately, all coordinated, intentional behavior. When we perform complex, rapid activity, like skilled athletics or a well-practiced musical piece, we rely on those parts of the brain.

Examples of preconscious frontal lobe activity abound. Consider the experiences of a man who had recently had a close call on the road: "A car about 20 feet ahead of mine was going 30 miles an hour, and suddenly it braked. I swerved to the left and just slipped between that car and an oncoming driver. As I passed the rear door of the braked car, I suddenly felt perspiration. And for the first time, I felt scared." In this case, the driver's quick reaction to the danger posed by the stopped car in front of him was preconscious. His conscious and emotional reaction to the situation came about a half second *after* turning the steering wheel.

This driver's response to danger was more complex than the automatic reflex of jerking one's hand away from a flame. It required his knowledge of how to steer a car through a narrow gap. But his mind did not have to become fully conscious of the danger to react. Because this man had lots of practice driving, his brain was able to respond as quickly as needed. Most of our bodies' well-trained and frequently practiced behaviors perform their implicit, intended reactions without entering normal awareness. Such automatic expressions seldom reach consciousness unless we stumble. In that case, the conscious mind springs to the rescue and directs the brain's escape.

The posterior parts of the cerebrum, including the parietal, occipital, and temporal lobes, plus the thalamus, generate the contents of our thoughtful consciousness. They receive their initial commands of attention and intention from the frontal lobes and express their immediate demands. The occipital lobes receive the crude symbols sent by the eyes' retinas, and, in conjunction with the inferior temporal lobe, mature their associations. The temporal lobe also processes auditory stimuli. Our intellectually conscious knowledge relies on verbal, musical, mathematical, geometric, and pictorial languages; the left cerebral hemisphere dominates in expressing most of these cognitive contents.

Awareness of where we are in space arises from the lateral-ventral surface of each parietal lobe. As with language, the functional machinery behind that quality also has a dominant side, this time the right. Each parietal lobe normally pro-

ALTERED STATES OF CONSCIOUSNESS

SYNCOPE, commonly known as fainting, consists of brief unconsciousness caused by severe, acute reductions of blood flowing through the brain's arteries due to a sudden drop in blood pressure. Most fainting episodes are brief and benign. Some, because of blood loss or heart stoppage, are dangerous. Permanent brain damage may begin as little as two to four minutes after blood stops flowing to the brain completely—which would constitute a stroke (**C59**).

CONFUSION can be either temporary or permanent. Temporary confusion refers to disturbed memory and inexact orientation of time, place, or person. Awakening from deep sleep after moderate sedation, suffering the effects of excessive alcohol (**C30**) or street drugs (**C29**), or awakening in a strange room are typical examples. Chronic, waking confusion relates to sustained difficulties in identifying time, date, or environment, and the failure to recognize people one has known for a long time. In this case, confusion is a gentle term for dementia (**C69**).

CONCUSSION is an imprecise term for an acute traumatic brain injury (see **C61** for a more detailed classification of such injuries). In a classic concussion, such as when a boxer or football player gets knocked out, a person exhibits sudden confusion or relatively brief periods of stupor (see page 175) or unresponsiveness. The stupor usually lasts for less than an hour or so, but short-term amnesia (**C68**) may extend for several hours.

ABSENCE SEIZURES and **COMPLEX PARTIAL SEIZURES** both reflect brief, severe impairments of consciousness, accompanied by unique forms of behavior. People undergoing absence attacks (most often children) frequently lose all self-awareness, but they remain awake and usually continue vaguely purposeful behavior, such as fumbling with their hands or fluttering their eyelids. Those experiencing complex partial seizures lose their cognitive memories but may express a variety of pattern-learned behavior, such as chewing movements or unbuttoning. (See **C13** for more information on all sorts of seizures.)

DELIRIUM is generally perceived as an acute or semiacute temporary deficit of attention and working memory. One important component is temporal disorientation: not knowing what time it is. Delirium may follow moderately severe head injuries (**C61**), encephalitis (**C38**), bacterial meningitis (**C37**), exceptionally high fever, heat stroke, or withdrawal from chronic alcoholism (**C30**) or street drugs (**C29**). Elderly people suffering mild dementia often become delirious when they are physically ill or their surroundings change.

vides us with automatic knowledge of the functional state of the other side of the body and the space immediately around us. Serious damage to the vulnerable dominant right parietal lobe can erase all of a person's knowledge of the left side of the body and the left side of the surrounding world. This is an example of what is called focal unconsciousness—lack of consciousness about a particular aspect of life—which is a feature of several disorders (**C70, C71, C72**).

As stated above, normal integration of all these aspects of action and mind requires memory. Using the resources of many distributed cerebral regions, memory creates our reflective intelligence. In this way, memory is indispensable to consciousness.

Visual hallucinations or impaired perceptions often occur in withdrawal delirium, whereas auditory hallucinations appear more often, but not solely, in people with schizophrenia (C25).

DEMENTIA involves two different impairments. One is a permanent, sometimes fluctuating loss of short- or long-term memory. It can follow severe brain trauma (C61); a sudden, sustained loss of oxygen to the brain (C59); or the surgical removal of the front areas of both temporal lobes. The other is an insidious, gradual loss of memory—short-term first, and later long-term. This process results from the degeneration and death of nerve cells in the cerebral cortex and hippocampus. It is a hallmark of Alzheimer's disease (C67) and other conditions (C69).

STUPOR defines a condition of deep sleep or a state that looks much like it. A person in a stupor cannot be aroused except by vigorous and repeated stimulation from the outside; as soon as that stimulation stops, the person relapses into the unresponsive state. Most light cases of stupor are brought about by overdoses of soporific drugs (sleeping pills, narcotics; C29) or alcohol (C30). Deep stupor more often reflects severe pharmacological (C66), metabolic (C6), or traumatic injury (C61) to the brain.

COMA reflects a sleep-like, eyes-closed, totally unconscious and unarousable brain state lasting 24 hours or more. Coma can result from many causes: sustained therapeutic anesthesia, direct brain injury (C61), or various diseases affecting the brain's cerebral hemispheres and arousal systems (C6, C37, C38, C39). In most cases of coma, a person will awake spontaneously in a week or so. A very few of these wakeful patients will possess a minimal level of consciousness. Of these few, most will survive and have sleep-wake patterns every day; the majority, however, enter a vegetative state.

PERSISTENT VEGETATIVE STATE—in some patients who enter vegetative states, the mind may remain absent for many weeks, months, or longer, while physiologically active systemic organs, such as the heart, lungs, and intestines, continue to sustain life in the body. We use the term persistent vegetative state (PVS) to identify patients who remain psychologically unconscious for such an extended period, arbitrarily defined as at least a month. PVS patients have irregular sleep-wake patterns and must receive all their feeding and bodily care from external sources. They are alive, but totally unaware of self or the environment.

Why Consciousness?

Why does defining consciousness matter? The answer is that our consciousness equals our personhood. It confirms our existence and our individuality. "No man is an island," John Donne wrote, but in fact each of us lives on our own island of consciousness. Every spontaneous sentence, every unstated thought, every action is at least partially unique. Every human brain in one way or another expresses its conscious or behavioral actions differently from the brains of all other human beings on the planet. Even the shape of your brain is a little different from all others.

Our words and actions can be telephone lines from one island of consciousness to another, but they can convey only a portion of what's happening on the end of the line. Much of our human consciousness remains a mystery, and neuroscience is only beginning to understand how our brains generate this state. Even with advances that show us when and where the brain becomes active, and what neurochemicals and genes are at work, we suspect that science will never tell us exactly what is on someone else's mind.

CHAPTER 10

Emotions and Social Function

B7   Emotions   180

B8   Inhibition and Control   185

B9   Temperament   190

B10 Attention and Motivation   196

We humans are social animals, almost always living in groups. Our brains therefore perform many functions that help us get along with others. We can feel pleased, disappointed, bored, angry, and a wide range of other emotions—not simply physically full and intact, or needy and fearful. In addition, we can read other people's emotions, stay focused on important goals, and refrain from taking actions that might be harmful in the long run. No other animal has the wide range of emotional and social capacities discussed in this chapter.

Although we are programmed to be able to develop those capacities, human social behavior is far from instinctual. Our emotional responses and behaviors are molded by our experiences from infancy. We develop through an interaction between our genetic programming (nature) and environment (nurture). This process is lifelong. That is how each of us develops a unique and complex personality, and how our personalities continue to grow.

Emotions

Human emotion is an ancient system of pre-verbal communication that has common roots with the signaling systems employed by other mammalian species living together in social groups. Emotional expression evolved millions of years ago when our primal ancestors first began herding together for safety and the protection of their young. It is a system wired deeply into our heads. From the first moments of life outside the womb, long before we can talk, we employ emotional signals—of joy and despair, fear and disgust—to announce when we are hungry and want to be fed, discomforted, or frightened and in need of protection. And from those first moments we are sensitive to the emotional signaling of others. At once preprogrammed and shaped by experience, the human capacity for emotion is a brain system that has evolved in step with the growing complexity of our social interaction.

In Old English the word *emotion* was synonymous with a public commotion. Only later, in the nineteenth century, was it adopted as a psychological term meaning "to act emotionally or theatrically." This expression of the "instinctive affectations of the mind" was distinguished from those behaviors reflective of "knowledge and reason." Charles Darwin, the father of evolutionary theory, was very interested in emotion and was one of the first to recognize its importance as a link to understanding the common roots of behavior among animal species. In his popular book *The Expression of the Emotions in Man and Animals,* which was published in 1872 and became a scandal in Victorian England, Darwin provided lavish illustration that the emotions are the cornerstone of a stable social order. He established that human emotion is coded in facial expressions and is similar to the nonverbal signaling employed by other social animals, particularly the primates. Thus the facial expressions of anger and fear, disgust and surprise, joy and sadness—those emotions listed by the early philosophers as the primary passions—transcend variations in culture and language as a common means of human communication. The recognition and expression of these primary emotions is, for each of us, as innate and universal as the ability to identify the primary colors of red, yellow, and blue.

Emotions and Behavior

Our emotions are instruments of survival, adaptive behaviors that seek the best fit with prevailing environmental circumstances in the continuous service of preserving life and species. Thus in infancy crying entreats the parent to return, while in the adult, grief and sadness are designed to provoke sympathy and support. In both instances the goal of the emotional behavior is to solicit aid and ensure safety in the face of potential adversity. While in infancy the primary emotions dominate, as we mature into adulthood emotion becomes increasingly entwined with thinking and memory. The events remembered with particular clarity (moments that give meaning) are those about which we have strong feeling. Thus emotional expression becomes selective and idiosyncratic, and secondary emotions such as pride, shame, and guilt emerge as increasingly important in guiding our behavior. We are, however, herd animals. Our success as a species lies not only in our intelligence but also in our ability to work together in social groups. Thus social circumstance remains the most powerful regulator of emotion throughout life, with situations that promote intimacy, attachment, and security evoking in us expressions of emotional pleasure and happiness, while loss and threat engender the opposite.

Modern neuroscience has taught us that emotion (analogous to other complex behaviors, such as speech, vision, and hearing) originates from the coordinated and balanced activity of many brain centers. For emotion, these centers are located principally in the limbic system, or the old mammalian brain. Of special importance are the almond-shaped amygdalae, one in each temporal horn, which act as the fear centers of the brain and the sentinels of emotional awareness. Work-

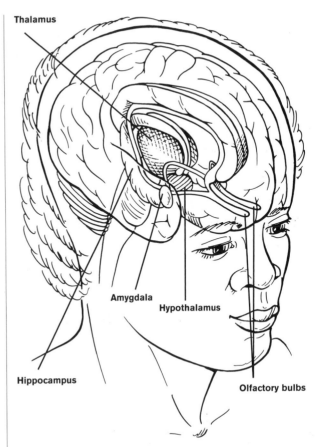

The limbic circuits are where emotions are regulated and processed in the brain. ILLUSTRATION © KATHRYN BORN

ing in close harmony with the amygdalae are the centrally located thalami, which serve together as the brain's telephone exchange, integrating the information coming from the senses and the body organs. New information is first coded in the two hippocampi (where short-term memory is processed) that wrap around the thalami and is then conveyed to the frontal lobes, where the memories of important events are placed in long-term storage for later retrieval and use in future planning. It is also via the circuits of the amygdala complex that the limbic system is wired into the muscles of the face (the vehicles through which we express our emotions to each other) and also to the tiny hypothalamus, at the base of the brain, which helps orchestrate the housekeeping functions of the body. It is because of this intimate linkage that during periods of turmoil, when our emotional balance is temporarily disturbed, the familiar daily rhythms of eating, sleeping, and sexual behavior are disrupted.

An important task of the emotional brain is to continuously integrate the environmental and bodily information gathered from our senses. An awareness of something interesting, novel, or threatening triggers a subjectively heightened state that we describe as feeling. (Actually, psychiatrists call this physiological arousal of the brain's emotional circuitry affective arousal—from the Latin *affectus*, meaning "completed action"—and it is the awareness or perception of the arousal that should more accurately be described as feeling.) Most of us are remarkably inept when it comes to characterizing these states of inner feeling. Our verbal descriptions are colorful but imprecise, which perhaps is something to be expected, given that human beings had feelings long before the invention of language.

Communicating Emotions

The words we use to communicate feelings are often descriptions of physical sensations. We speak of the thrill of surprise, the tingling sensation that goes down the back of the neck when something extraordinary happens; pangs of sadness and of hunger; twinges of guilt when an obligation is suddenly remembered, similar to a twinge of pain. In describing the throb of passion, we are comparing the experience with a wildly

beating heart. We speak of the gnawing of grief, hankerings, sinkings, chills, qualms, and so on. Our language suggests that feelings are tied closely to an awareness of the body's changing physiology. But the recognition of physiological "feeling" alone rarely has meaning. Personal interpretation is required, and that is where memory comes in. We string our memories and feelings together as personal stories, as emotional tales, that catalogue the significant moments that make each of us a unique person; these are the stories retold when we describe ourselves to others. Brought together as emotional experience, memory and feeling sustain individual identity, building for each of us unique strengths and unique vulnerabilities.

Individuals vary in the degree to which they experience and express emotion. These variations in the emotional tone are highly heritable and are called temperament, which means, roughly, an individual's "habit of mind." Thus some of us are born shy and some bold. As we grow, it is this temperamental predisposition that shapes our approach to others and to experience, helping mold, in turn, the way we are perceived. The shy, introverted individual for whom social interaction is a struggle, for example, and whose natural habit is to withdraw will find the world a difficult and sometimes frightening place. Such "introverts" become conscientious and meticulous workers—civil servants, accountants, diligent teachers, and managers of detail (who are the backbone of human social organization). On the other hand, the bold and impulsive "extrovert" engages the world at a run. Optimism and energy abound. Nothing is too much or too difficult. These are the versatile entrepreneurs who apply themselves successfully to business, to politics, and to adventurous pursuit.

In thinking about emotional behavior, it is important to distinguish among temperament, emotion, and mood. Temperament describes the habitual way in which an individual relates to the world; emotions, on the other hand, are mercurial. In everyday speech the words *mood* and *emotion* are often used interchangeably, but strictly speaking, mood is the consistent extension of emotion in time. An emotion is usually transient and responsive to the thoughts, activities, and social situations of the day. Moods, in contrast, may last for hours, days, or even months in the case of some illnesses. Thus the emotional state of grief, when extended in time, is called sadness; if it persists, unrelenting, for a period of weeks, the mood state is referred to as depression, or a disorder of "affect." Although we speak of affection—meaning fondness or love—*affect* is not a word we use now in everyday speech. It does appear, however, in the professional vocabulary of psychiatrists and behavioral scientists, where it provides the generic name for a family of illnesses (known as the affective disorders) in which a disturbance of emotional communication and mood regulation predominates. Depression, or melancholia, characterized by recurrent periods of sorrow, self-criticism, and social withdrawal, and its close cousin, mania, where euphoric irritability, overconfidence, creativity, and high energy predominate, are the principal members of this family of brain disorders.

Disorders of the Emotions

Eleven to 15 million people in the United States are afflicted with affective (or mood) disorders of some description, and of these, more than 2 million suffer the severe form of manic-depressive illness. However, fewer than one third of these millions ever receive treatment or even recognize that their misery could be relieved. This is a remarkable fact. Another intriguing statistic is that for those who do seek professional care, it may take up to ten years and three doctors to make the correct diagnosis. The usual justification for this extraordinary situation—so distinct from other serious medical illnesses—is a lack of public and professional education. But another major determinant of this collective blind spot lies in the nature of mood disorder itself. It stubbornly resists voluntary control. Thus, because moods develop from our emotions, and because emotional life lies at the very core of being a person, to accept that emotion and mood can be "dis-ordered" calls into question the very experience that most of us take for granted—the presence of a defined, predictable, and unique subjective entity that we fondly refer to as the intuitive "self." When emotion and mood are disturbed, it is the familiarity and stability of this personal being that is threatened. Fortunately, an understanding of how the brain works can be helpful here. It is now accepted knowledge that emotional communication, thinking memory, and the maintenance of the body's housekeeping are all intertwined and regulated by the coordinated activity of the limbic brain. It is this triad of behavioral activity (emotion, thinking, and the body's daily rhythms) that becomes disturbed in the affective disorders. When mood regulation, memory and decision making, and the rhythmic functions of the body are together persistently disturbed over an extended period, resulting in a profound disturbance of personal activity and social function, the probable explanation is one of illness, not a lack of self-control.

Compared with many other human ailments, such profound disorders of mood are common afflictions. Just how prevalent we consider them to be depends partly on how we define them, but by the diagnostic criteria of the American Psychiatric

Association they are common. By reasonable estimates 12 to 15 percent of women and 8 to 10 percent of men in America will struggle with a serious mood disorder during their lifetime. Their illness will impinge painfully upon family members and the many colleagues and friends with whom they share their daily lives. The economic impact on society is enormous—it has been estimated to exceed $40 billion each year in the United States alone, a social burden greater than that of heart disease. Adding to this, in the absence of treatment, is the common complication of addiction to drugs, alcohol, or both, which worsens mood disorders and compounds their social consequences. Of even greater significance is the extraordinarily high mortality of people who suffer mood disorders, whose suicide rate is 35 times greater than that of the general population. During periods of profound grief and in moments of unusual joy, we may each catch a glimpse of these states of disordered and disregulated mood. In their persistent form, however, mania and melancholia are moods that stand apart from common experience. They are serious medical illnesses that reflect a disregulation of the sentinel activities of the limbic brain.

Inhibition and Control

Our brains do more than tell us when to act or speak. They also tell us when *not* to do those things, and that function is just as important. Inhibition and control are fundamental components of our higher thinking processes and provide the underpinnings for several more complex and characteristically human faculties, including language (**B14**) and decision making, problem solving, and planning (**B11**).

Loosely defined, *inhibition* refers to the suppression of a reflexive, habitual, or otherwise highly compelling behavior that is disadvantageous or inappropriate for the context (for instance, the urge to tell someone, "Your hairdo is really ugly"). *Control* refers to the ability to direct mental function and behavior in accord with an intention or set of intentions. Clearly, control is closely related to inhibition—suppressing a statement that might offend someone else is an expression of the intention to be polite. However, control can also involve other functions, such as coordinating a sequence of behaviors needed to achieve a goal (for example, planning and carrying out a series of chess moves) or properly weighing alternative actions (eating now or waiting until your date arrives).

Our understanding of the brain mechanisms responsible for inhibition and control is still at a very early stage. For a long time, researchers were able to study such "high level" functions only by examining people with brain damage (lesion studies) or by recording the electrical activity of neurons in other animal species, such as nonhuman primates, our closest animal relatives. Such research suggested that an area at the front-most part of the brain—the prefrontal cortex—plays a critical role in inhibitions and control. For example, neurologists have long recognized that many patients with damage to this area exhibit what are referred to as frontal release signs: these are reflexes that infants or very young children display but that normally disappear as we mature. One example is the grasp reflex, which is useful for an infant in holding on to objects or its mother.

You can easily try out these reflexes yourself. The next time you are with an infant, try gently stroking his or her palm with your forefinger. The baby will reflexively grab your finger, a reaction sensibly called the grasp reflex. Try it on your adult friends: they will not exhibit the same response.

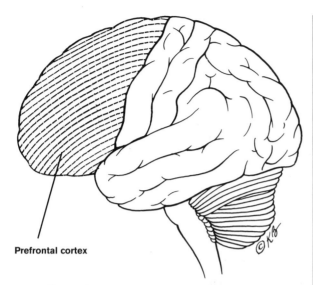

Prefrontal cortex

The prefrontal cortex acts as the chief executive of the brain, giving final say over whether or not to act on an impulse. ILLUSTRATION © KATHRYN BORN

However, a patient with damage to the prefrontal cortex may very well grip your finger. This suggests that the developing brain does not take away the reflex but rather suppresses it, since it is not needed in adult life, and that damage to the frontal cortex can "release" the old instinct. Thus, a healthy frontal cortex must play an active role in suppressing this unnecessary behavior, and probably many others.

The return of the grasp reflex is a common consequence of frontal brain damage, but not an especially debilitating one. However, consider the landmark case of Phineas Gage, described in chapter 1. He was foreman of a railway construction gang in Vermont in 1848 when an accidental explosion blew an iron bar through the front part of his head. The bar was over 3 feet (1 m) long and 1¼ inches (3 cm) in diameter. Remarkably, Gage recovered physically from his injury. But his behavior changed profoundly. Whereas before the accident he had been a highly capable and efficient foreman, after the accident his behavior was de-

scribed as "fitful, irreverent, and grossly profane, showing little deference for his fellows. He was also impatient and obstinate, yet capricious and vacillating, unable to settle on any of the plans he devised for future action." Reconstruction of Gage's injury from the wounds in his skull indicates that the bar was shot through his prefrontal cortex.

What this suggests, and what many studies have since confirmed, is that damage to the prefrontal cortex impairs people's capacity for cognitive control. These individuals are much less inhibited from performing primitive, often socially inappropriate behaviors, such as urinating in public or appearing not fully clothed. They also lose the ability to coordinate ordinarily routine behaviors, even though they can still execute each part of a sequence. For example, doctors observed one patient making a cup of coffee with sugar by pouring the coffee into a cup, stirring, and *then* adding sugar. This person obviously knew each individual bit of behavior but failed to execute them in the proper order.

This pattern of disturbance is often referred to as a dysexecutive syndrome, and it corresponds well with what we have learned from animals with damage to the prefrontal cortex. Like Phineas Gage, they become distractible, exhibit inappropriately aggressive or sexual behavior, and at times persist in seemingly useless actions. Studying animals with lesions of the prefrontal cortex has led to ideas about what functions different parts of this brain structure may serve. One notion is that the lower part of the prefrontal cortex (just over the eye sockets) is primarily responsible for inhibiting unwanted behaviors, whereas parts higher in the frontal lobes (behind the upper part of the forehead) are more involved in remembering goals and coordinating behavior. While this may be basically correct in humans as well, research has begun to suggest more complex possibilities.

The recent invention of methods for studying the brain activity of normal human individuals as they perform specific tasks has dramatically accelerated research in this area. Two of the most popular methods are functional magnetic resonance imaging (fMRI) and the recording of event-related electrical potentials (ERPs). These techniques have made clear that like most mental functions, inhibitions and control involve many brain regions, not just the prefrontal cortex. Although the prefrontal cortex is regularly activated in tasks that rely on inhibition and control, other parts of the brain also become active.

This finding has raised a fundamental question: Are there brain structures dedicated to inhibition and control, or do those functions arise from the interaction of many structures, no one of which can be credited exclusively as the "inhibitory" or "control" center of the brain? Although our brains are like computers in many respects, one dramatic way in which this is not true is that unlike most computers, brains do not have a central processing unit (CPU). If you remove the CPU from your desktop computer, it will grind to a complete halt and become only a rather expensive way of warming your office. In contrast, selective damage to the brain rarely if ever results in a complete loss of function. Rather, a person loses certain faculties (for example, vision, hearing, high-level reasoning), but often not completely, and most other abilities may remain. It appears that functions are distributed across the brain. This appears to be true for inhibition and control as well.

The CEO

One way to understand how control might be distributed across different structures in the brain is to consider an analogy between the brain and a large modern corporation, such as a car manufacturer, with many departments. The Research and Development (R&D) team might have come up with a great new design for a more efficient engine, or the folks in Market Research may have determined that there is a growing need for a particular type of vehicle. In an efficient corporation, one unit will transmit information directly to another rather than send everything to a CEO (or CPU) for redistribution. The R&D team consults with the market researchers to see if there would be any interest in the new design, or the marketing folks check with R&D about whether they can actually produce a car that would meet a market niche. As plans begin to take shape, other units weigh in on safety, costs, advertising and promotion, and so on. Eventually, as the plan takes shape, the CEO may be responsible for the final decision whether or not to go forward. But the full richness of the plan, its evaluation, and its execution involve many, if not all parts of the company. That is, even though we think of the CEO as the central executive of a company, planning and executing any new endeavor actually relies on interactions between a variety of different units within the company. Modern theories of how the brain functions are remarkably similar to this model.

Brain Tracks

Under one current view of how the brain executes its control function, the pattern of neural activity in the prefrontal cortex influences how information flows in the other parts of the brain that are responsible for actually carrying out a task. Another analogy might help. We can think of the frontal cortex as a switch operator for a complex system of railroad tracks. The brain is like a set of tracks (pathways) connecting various origins (for example, brain areas responding to particular sensory stimuli) to specific destinations (brain areas controlling behavioral responses, the retrieval of a memory, and so on). The operator's goal is to move the trains (neural activity carrying information about the sensory event) from each origin to its proper destination as efficiently as possible, avoiding collisions.

When the track is clear (that is, a train can speed from origin to destination without risk of running into any others), then no intervention is needed. Similarly, a behavior that is reflexive, or automatic, does not need the assistance of the frontal cortex. However, if two trains must cross the same length of track, then the railroad needs some coordination to guide them safely to their destinations. Neural activity in the prefrontal cortex can be thought of as a map that determines which pattern of "tracks" is used to solve the task. Note that this function need not be restricted to associating sensory stimuli to behavioral responses; it applies equally well to "routing" internal mental processes, such as the retrieval of a memory and the expression of an emotion.

This view accords well with the pattern of disturbances we see when a person's frontal lobes are damaged. If switch operators do not do their job, then the trains of the brain start to bump into each other, causing delays, confusion, and disorganized functioning. However, not all is lost. Trains that run on their own tracks, or simply happen not to be on a course that will cause them to collide with others, will run fine. This is the case for people with frontal damage. They retain the capacity for many behaviors (for example, pour-

ing coffee, knowing to add sugar, knowing that it is relevant to stir), even if they cannot execute them in a fully coordinated fashion.

Note that a critical function of the switch operator is to know exactly when to throw the switch: too early and a train will not make it onto the right track; too late and a collision may occur. Recent research has suggested that the neurotransmitter dopamine may play this critical role in the brain— telling the prefrontal cortex when to update its plans and switch the tracks in other parts of the brain. This may explain how disturbances in dopamine—thought to be a central player in psychiatric diseases such as schizophrenia (**C25**)— could lead to impaired frontal lobe function and corresponding deterioration of higher-level functioning.

The "brain track" analogy provides a useful view of how control may be exercised in the brain, but what does it tell us about inhibition? One of the easiest ways to see inhibition at work is the Stroop task, often used in laboratories. In this task, subjects are asked to name the color in which a word is printed. The twist is that the word itself names a color. To see how it works, try taking the Stroop test yourself; it is on page 13 of the brain primer, which is located after page xxxii. Take a moment to identify the colors of the words printed there.

You probably felt an instant of hesitation and confusion, perhaps even a sense that you were about to name different colors from the colors of the words themselves. When we see a word, we are more used to reading it than to naming the color in which it is printed. To prove this, show the words to friends, but don't tell them what to do: just ask them to respond however they wish. Almost certainly they will read the words and say, for example, "green" for the one printed in red. Reading the word is our "default," or prepotent, response. The reason you had trouble naming the color is that you had to suppress, or inhibit, this response in order to answer the question posed.

Some investigators believe that inhibition is a dedicated function of the prefrontal cortex, particularly the lower part. In the Stroop task, according to this model, the prefrontal cortex directly suppresses our tendency to read the word. However, another possibility—closer to that afforded by our "train track" analogy—is that the prefrontal cortex does not actually suppress word reading; rather, it gives extra "juice" to the effort to name the color. Since you cannot say "red" and "green" at the same time, these two responses are in competition. Without the assistance of the prefrontal cortex, the habitual word-reading response would win out (that is, saying "green"). However, with the assistance of the prefrontal cortex (switching the tracks so that color naming has the advantage), the color-naming response gets the edge and wins the competition. From this perspective, inhibition is a more distributed function, occurring at a more local level—that is, between the two verbal responses—and the role of the prefrontal cortex is simply to help favor the weaker one when that is needed.

The Influential Referee

We've described the prefrontal cortex as the managerial CEO and as the alert accident-preventing railroad switch operator. But this remarkable brain system is even more versatile; it is also a subtle influencer. To offer one final analogy, consider the two brain responses as if they were two boxers, and the prefrontal cortex as a referee who hopes to influence the fight. The view that the prefrontal cortex plays a central role in inhibition suggests that the referee tips the fight by slugging one of the boxers himself. Or, alternatively, the referee gives a bit of extra latitude to one of the boxers, who exploits this advantage to knock out the other. As yet, we do not know -for sure which image is a better metaphor for how inhibition is really carried out in the brain. However, this example shows how a function such as inhibition, which on the surface may appear centralized, could in fact be carried out in a more distributed way, involving close coordination between the prefrontal cortex and other areas of the brain engaged in performing a particular task.

While we have begun to gain insights into the brain mechanisms underlying inhibition and control, and how they can go awry because of injury or disease, we are not yet at a point where we can have a meaningful impact on these functions—either to enhance normal function or to repair damage. With deeper understanding however, and with the remarkable pace at which relevant technologies are developing, there is no question that we are moving toward this goal.

Temperament

Every baby behaves differently. Parents with two or more children are especially aware of this fact of life. One can often hear them comparing notes: "Sue was a fussy little thing, but her brother just sits and watches us for hours." "Vanessa crawls all over the place! Her sister didn't wear us out like that." "The day-care people say Shawn hardly ever cries when we leave, but he hardly ever smiles, either." Usually parents start to discern these differences in the first weeks of their children's lives, though an outsider may have to look hard to notice them.

Psychologists and psychiatrists use the term *temperament* to refer to the variations in how individuals consistently feel and behave in infancy and early childhood. Each of us seems to have some biases about how we respond to the world, natural leanings that are both biological and inherited. These psychological profiles involve variation in:

■ Activity: Does your infant squirm and reach for things, or lie still?

■ Smiling and laughter: How often does your baby show his or her happy moods?

■ Irritability: How easily upset is your infant?

■ Ease of being soothed: How long does it take to calm your baby down?

■ Fluctuations in mood: Can your child change emotions in an instant?

■ Fear or avoidance of novelty: Does your infant seek out new faces and activities?

■ Energy: Does your baby tire easily, or go all night?

■ Attentiveness: How long does your child focus on one object, person, or task?

As insulting as the proud parents of little Sue, Vanessa, and Shawn might find it, we can make an analogy between these temperamental biases and the behavioral and physiological profiles that distinguish different breeds of dogs: Jack Russell terriers being energetic, Saint Bernards being patient with children, and so on.

As soon as babies are born, however, their environments start to shape how these initial biases show up in their behavior. As a result, the psychological profile each person displays during childhood and adolescence is a combination of

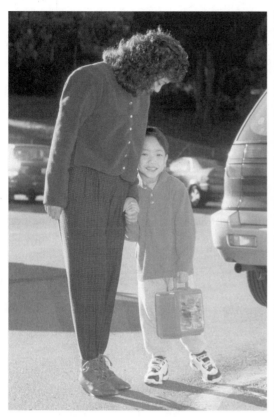

Separation anxiety is normal as young children adjust to spending time away from their parents. "High reactive" children seem more vulnerable to these fears, but the way parents respond to such situations can influence how well their children learn to handle separation. PHOTO © CINDY CHARLES/PHOTOEDIT/PICTUREQUEST

temperament and experience. Although each temperamental category exerts its influence throughout one's development, the personality that others see is always moderated by a person's history. For example, about 20 percent of infants are born with a temperamental bias that renders them vulnerable to becoming timid, shy, or eager to avoid unfamiliar people, places, and situations. If their parents accept their timidity while encouraging academic achievement, these children are likely to becoming introverted scholars. If, on the other hand, the parents encourage popularity and sociability, the children are less likely to develop into quiet, academically accomplished adolescents. They may even come to seem outgoing to their peers, though it is unlikely that they will ever be as adventurous as people who are born with a novelty-seeking temperament.

Where Temperament Comes From

Even in ancient Egypt and Greece, physicians recognized the importance of a person's biological character. The influential physician Galen of Pergamon, who lived in the second century A.D., identified four temperaments: sanguine, melancholic, phlegmatic, and choleric. He attributed them to the body's relative amounts of blood, yellow bile, phlegm, and black bile, which represented extremes of warm and cool, dry and moist. The balance of these four substances in a person's body determined his or her personality profile. Under this theory, the sanguine temperament, characterized by confidence and sociability, was assigned to the category warm and moist because of an excess of blood. The anxious, melancholic person was designated dry and cool because of too much black bile.

Medicine has long given up Galen's theory of the four humors, but we have once again started to identify substances that help determine people's personalities. These substances are not blood and bile but protein molecules at work in our brains. Contemporary scientists now believe that many temperaments are the result of different combinations of these chemicals, together with various densities of the brain's receptors for each molecule. Researchers have seen how the distribution of brain receptors influences animals' behavioral profiles in the difference between two strains of voles, small rodents resembling mice. One strain of vole bonds with its mate for life while the other strain does not. The two strains differ in the distribution of receptors in the brain for the chemicals oxytocin and vasopressin.

It is likely that scientists will discover that many human temperaments are the result of distinctive distributions of brain receptors for one or more neurochemicals. For instance, current research suggests that variations in the concentration and distribution of receptors for the chemicals serotonin, gamma-aminobutyric acid (GABA), opioids, and corticotrophin-releasing hormone are related to variations in children's tendency to avoid unfamiliar people and places. Because the brain contains over 150 different molecules, it is likely that researchers will discover many more temperaments than have so far been identified.

Each temperamental bias probably involves activity in many parts of the brain. For example, the temperamental traits of timidity and fearfulness seem to be related to receptors on the amygdala and its projections to the central gray (a region in the midbrain), the autonomic nervous system, the frontal cortex, and the hypothalamus. The temperament that predisposes a child to distractibility or hyperactivity probably involves the basal ganglia, ventral tegmentum, and dopaminergic tracts to the frontal cortex. Again, much remains to be discovered.

Differences

Some temperaments, like sociability or introversion, are common; others, such as an absence of any feelings of guilt, are rare. Shy, quiet, emotionally restrained children, called inhibited, and outgoing, relatively bold children, called uninhibited, represent two relatively common temperamental categories that have been studied in depth. One lesson we have learned from these studies is how consistent temperamental bias seems to be over a child's early life. Two-year-olds judged inhibited were more likely to have been babies who at four months of age consistently moved and fussed when presented with unfamiliar sights, sounds, and smells. This combination of movement and crying in reaction to unfamiliar stimuli implies a low threshold of excitability in the amygdala and its projections. We call this behavior high reactive. In contrast, the infants who would become uninhibited toddlers usually responded to the same stimuli with minimal activity and no crying, implying these brain structures had a higher threshold of stimulation.

As we accumulate more experiences in our lives, our observable behavior can deviate from the temperamental biases we were born with. Only 15 percent to 20 percent of the children in each of these temperamental groups remained consistently inhibited or consistently uninhibited from their first birthdays through late childhood. Nevertheless, not one high-reactive infant became a consistently uninhibited child, and only one low-reactive infant—less than 1 percent of the babies in the study—became a consistently inhibited child. This suggests that a person's temperament does not determine his or her later personality but does constrain the possibility of developing the opposite set of traits. Showing a high-reactive temperament in infancy reduces the likelihood that the child will become bold and extroverted; while having a low-reactive temperament limits the possibility that the child will become a fearful, anxious adolescent. It is easier

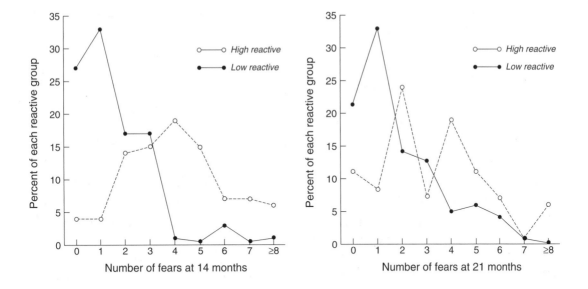

Temperament shortly after birth remains somewhat consistent as children grow but does not predict future behavior perfectly. Researchers watched how much 4-month-old babies moved and fussed in response to unfamiliar sights, sounds, and smells. Later, they observed those same children at 14 and 21 months and found that a higher percentage of "high reactive" infants were growing up to display more fears. GRAPHS COURTESY OF JEROME KAGAN, PH.D., DEPARTMENT OF PSYCHOLOGY, HARVARD UNIVERSITY. ADAPTED BY LEIGH CORIALE

to predict what babies will *not* become from knowing their temperaments than to predict the specific traits they will develop.

Variation in adolescent or adult personalities among people who were high- or low-reactive infants is due, in part, to family experience. Children with a high-reactive temperament raised by parents who encourage them to find ways to cope with fear are less likely to develop symptoms of anxiety (C21). Children with the same temperament living with parents who try to protect them from all stress are more likely to become anxious and timid. Parenting and home environment also influence other temperaments. A child who seems naturally driven to seek out new, exciting experiences might take bigger risks if his or her upbringing invites that behavior, or might learn the value

of safety from parents who persistently encourage and remind their child to think before acting.

Because of that family influence, adolescents do not necessarily behave according to the biological features that characterize their infant temperaments. One girl in a group studied over many years was a high-reactive infant and a fearful toddler. She lived in a supportive environment, however, and was academically accomplished. When this girl was observed at 10 years of age, she was relaxed, mature, and minimally anxious. From the perspective of brain science, this was especially interesting because measures of her brain function revealed several biological features characteristic of inhibited children. For example, her electroencephalograph (EEG) showed more activation in her brain's right frontal area than in its left, a trait that correlates with the brain's activity in anxious adults. Yet her behavior no longer seemed to reflect that biological inclination.

Culture also has a great influence on our personalities, and society's expectations for a child because of his or her sex, ethnic group, class, or other circumstances may work for or against an inherited temperament. At the same time, temperaments do seem to differ across sexes and ethnic groups. The bias against novelty-seeking is more common in girls. The temperament favoring high activity levels is more prevalent in boys. Low levels of reactivity in infancy appear to be more common among Asian infants than among Caucasians. It is important to understand how early environment starts to influence temperaments, and surprisingly, little cross-cultural research has so far been carried out on this question.

When Temperaments Spell Trouble

There are good reasons to believe that many psychiatric disorders are influenced, in part, by temperamental biases. For example, social phobia (**C22**), characterized by chronic avoidance of social gatherings and reluctance to meet strangers, is more common among inhibited than among uninhibited children. Panic disorder, characterized by a sudden onset of activity in the nervous system and an accompanying feeling of terror (**C21**), is likely to be a product of a different temperament. Psychopathy is more prevalent among uninhibited children, but only if they are raised in families and neighborhoods that are unduly permissive of aggression and other behaviors that violate the norm of the community (**C31**). Attention deficit/hyperactivity disorder (**C2**) is probably associated with a temperament that modulates dopamine function, while depression (**C20**) is probably linked to a temperament that influences the metabolism of norepinephrine in the brain. If a temperamental trait impairs a person's ability to work efficiently and to adapt to societal demands, psychotherapy or pharmacological interventions can be helpful.

At this point, however, our evidence is not robust enough to produce definite advice for individuals with particular temperaments. There is some basis for suggesting that in order to help their children conquer their vulnerability to fears, parents of high-reactive infants should not protect their toddlers from minor stresses. As the children recognize what constitutes actual danger or difficulty, they can face the uncertainties of normal daily life more bravely. This approach can be hard for the parents, especially if their own personalities lean the same way as their children's—if, for instance, they are also anxious about trying new things. But it helps for parents to be calm and firm. Similarly, parents of low-reactive infants should be consistent in discouraging antisocial and aggressive behavior. In general, understanding that children have different temperaments helps us to see each as an individual, not necessarily born to respond to the world in the same way as other siblings and parents.

In growing up, most people come to know themselves, what settings and activities make them comfortable and happy. Adolescents who are inhibited as children usually recognize they can feel uncertain or anxious when challenged by unpredictable situations. Some of these young people adapt by selecting activities and vocations that permit them to control encounters with unfamiliarity and unpredictability. For example, they might decide to become historians, scientists, computer programmers, or poets because these jobs require long periods of solitary activity and permit more control over the outcome of one's efforts. Other young people, knowing fairly early that they would find that sort of work boring or lonely, gravitate toward professions that involve meeting many people and having new experiences each day. Most of us have a mix of traits and interests. The temperaments rooted in our infant brains are an important factor in finding "the right fit" in life.

Attention and Motivation

Anyone who has lived with a pet has an intuitive sense that animals are devoid of the capacity for long-term, complex planning. Their behaviors are triggered by simple urges, like hunger and fear. By contrast, human behavior is not merely reactive; it is proactive. We formulate complex goals and intentions. This means that the human brain is capable of creating models of the world not only as it is but as we want it to be. The human brain is able to create models of the future. This is called intentionality. But merely creating a model of the future is not enough. We must have the ability to strive to change the world as it is into the world we want it to become. This ability is called motivation. Without motivation, no life challenge of any degree of complexity can successfully be met.

At any given time, the human brain performs numerous tasks simultaneously. At any given time, some of these tasks are more important than others. When circumstances change, cognitive priorities may change and different tasks become more important. Suppose you are watching TV while paying your bills. In all likelihood, your attention is on the bills (or at least it should be). Suppose then that the TV program is interrupted by a news announcement about an imminent tornado in your area, urging residents to take immediate precautions. Your attention will instantly be redirected to the news.

The ability to prioritize mental tasks, to focus on them, and to shift the focus to other tasks as

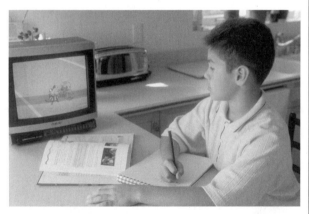

Recent findings have shown that the prefrontal cortex does not reach full maturity until about the age of 18. As a result, the immature brain has greater difficulty filtering out distractions, such as music and television noise. PHOTO © DAVID YOUNG-WOLFF/PHOTOEDIT/PICTUREQUEST

the need arises is critical to the success of every human activity. This ability is called attention. Attention is a complex function, and we distinguish between sustained attention, distributed attention, and other forms. Without attention, our life would become haphazard and chaotic. Motivation and attention are among the most advanced manifestations of brain function, reaching their fully developed form only in humans.

The Neural Basis of Motivation and Attention

Motivation and attention are controlled by the prefrontal cortex, which is to the rest of the brain what a conductor is to the orchestra. The functions of the prefrontal cortex are elusive but critical and are often referred to as executive functions. Damage to the prefrontal cortex results in severe disruption of motivation and attention. Human behavior becomes purposeless, chaotic, and impoverished, despite the relative sparing of specific cognitive skills, such as reading, writing, or the use of simple tools. The famous case of Phineas Gage, whose prefrontal cortex was damaged in an explosion that drove an iron bar through his head, is a case in point—his friends were forced to conclude that "Gage was no longer Gage."

The prefrontal cortex is the last part of the brain to mature. According to recent findings, it does not reach its functional maturity until the age of 18, or possibly even later. It has also been suggested that the prefrontal cortex is particularly vulnerable to the decline associated with aging. This suggests that the executive functions of the brain, while late to mature, are early to decline.

History

Neuropsychologists and neuroscientists have been studying the brain mechanisms of language, perception, and memory for many decades, but until recently attention and, particularly, motivation were regarded "off limits" for rigorous scientific exploration. The association of these complex mental functions with the prefrontal cortex was made only recently, within the last few decades. The advent of new technologies called functional neuroimaging, which enable us to examine patterns of physiological activity in the brain of a person engaged in a mental task, has been particularly important in advancing our understanding of the frontal lobes.

Looking for Personality Differences

Normal human brains are highly variable in morphology (overall brain size and the proportions of its parts) and biochemistry (the chemicals in charge of communications between the nerve cells). Neuropsychologists and cognitive neuroscientists are only beginning to study the biological basis of the normal variability of cognitive abilities and cognitive styles. The general public understands that differences among individuals in traits such as musical, literary, and mathematical abilities have something to do with the differences among human brains. But very few people seriously consider the possibility that differences in personalities (assertiveness as opposed to timidity, enthusiasm versus indifference, being a leader versus being a follower) are also related to differences among human brains. In fact, recent studies suggest that even such highly culture-dependent personality traits as morality depend on the integrity of the prefrontal cortex. An unusually high prevalence of frontal lobe damage or dysfunction has been documented in violent criminals and in people devoid of ethical insight (incapable of telling right from wrong in hypothetical situations). Certain types of patients with frontal lobe damage were referred to in the old neurological literature as pseudopsychopathic.

Disorders of Attention and Motivation

Attention and motivation may suffer in a wide range of disorders. Generally speaking, all these disorders involve damage to, or dysfunction of, the prefrontal cortex, certain structures particularly closely associated with the prefrontal cortex (for example, the anterior cingulate cortex, the neostriatum, the dorsomedial thalamic nucleus, and the ventral tegmental area of the mesencephalon), or their pathways. These conditions include traumatic brain injury (**C61**), various dementias (**C69**), schizophrenia (**C25**), autism (**C5**), Tourette's syndrome (**C45**), and others.

When the deficit of attention is relatively isolated, while other aspects of cognition are relatively intact, the diagnosis of attention deficit disorder, with or without hyperactivity, or ADHD (**C2**), is often made. It is important to keep in mind, however, that ADHD is a syndrome and not a distinct disease, and it may be caused by a large number of specific disorders. It may be caused by traumatic brain injury or viral encephalopathy (disease of the brain), and is known to be associated with Tourette's syndrome and other disorders.

When a previously highly motivated aging individual gradually loses his or her drive, the most common assumption is that the problem is depression (**C20**). With the common emphasis on memory loss, the general public and even many physicians and psychologists tend to overlook the fact that motivation and drive are among the first to suffer in most dementias, including Alzheimer's-type dementia (**C67**), cerebrovascular dementia, Lewy bodies dementia, Pick's disease, frontal lobe dementia, and others (**C69**). These conditions must always be considered whenever a decline in motivation and attention is noted in an aging person.

Changes in attention and motivation are also frequently observed in younger individuals recovering from the effects of traumatic brain injury suffered in, for example, a car accident or a job-related accident. These changes are often ignored or are attributed to something unrelated to the brain. But they are likely to be a direct consequence of the accident, since the prefrontal cortex and its pathways (particularly frontal connections with the brain stem) are particularly vulnerable in head trauma. The outcome of such injury is highly variable. Often considerable recovery takes place, sometimes even complete recovery, but in many cases long-term, or even permanent, impairment of attention and motivation takes place.

Advice and Intervention

Society has been slow to embrace the notion that diseases of the mind are diseases of the brain. It is still common for an individual whose mind is slipping, and for those around him witnessing cognitive impairment, to ignore this or to seek the help of everyone *except* a neurologist, psychiatrist, or neuropsychologist. Dysfunction of motivation or attention is particularly likely to be misattributed to some mysterious "extracerebral" factors, whatever they may be. The idea that persistent dysfunction of attention and motivation signifies brain disorder is still not well entrenched among the general public.

The situation is compounded by the fact that frontal lobe dysfunction, which affects motivation and attention, is also likely to produce lack of drive and inability to initiate behaviors, indifference, and anosognosia (lack of insight into one's own condition). Therefore it is particularly important to sound the medical alarm whenever you observe such a change in a family member or a friend, since the patient is not likely to do it for himself or herself.

Ironically, when the general public does recognize disorders of the mind, the recognition is often overly simple. Every case of cognitive decline associated with aging becomes "Alzheimer's disease," and every case of neurodevelopmental cognitive dysfunction becomes "ADHD." Even many professionals are guilty of this sin of sweeping oversimplification.

The bottom line is that deficits of attention and motivation may be caused by a wide range of neurological, psychiatric, neurodevelopmental, medical, and geriatric conditions. Careful, in-

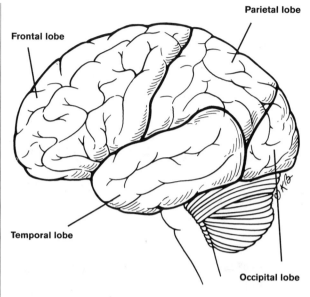

Attention and motivation are controlled by the prefrontal cortex. Problems in this area have been seen in a wide range of disorders, including dementia, schizophrenia, Tourette's syndrome, and others.
ILLUSTRATION © KATHRYN BORN

formed diagnosis is always better than a knee-jerk invocation of the diagnosis du jour. Precise diagnosis is becoming particularly important with the advent of increasingly targeted therapies—pharmacological, cognitive-rehabilitative, and others.

CHAPTER 11

Learning, Thinking, and Remembering

B11   Decision Making and Planning   201

B12   Intelligence   210

B13   Learning and Memory   217

B14   Speech, Language, and Reading   226

B15   Visualization and Navigation   232

B16   Creativity, Talents, and Skills   236

When we think about the brain, most of the time we think about thinking—the conscious manipulation of memories, knowledge, imagination, calculation, and other mental powers. Psychologists label these abilities and processes our cognitive functions. We also call them our higher functions because they set us off from other animals. They also happen to involve the upper parts of the brain: the cortex, which is so much larger in humans than in any other species.

One common feature of our cognitive functions is that we are usually aware (or cognizant) of when we use them. Despite that knowledge, these mental abilities are among the most difficult for us to understand. Most seem to rely on many parts of the brain, working in sequence or all at once. Brain researchers have to break down everyday thinking into very small steps in order to find a process simple enough to watch in action. But those abilities to imagine, communicate, judge, and learn, which seem so mysterious, are gradually enabling us to learn more about them.

Decision Making and Planning

One of the great unsolved mysteries of science is how the human brain, built from a myriad of small processing units (neurons) with no single one in charge, can support the complex, coordinated, and intelligent behavior of which we humans are capable. How can this hodgepodge of hundreds of billions of noisy cells organize itself to play a game of chess, write a novel, or plan the course of a career? More remarkable still is that each individual neuron operates at about one ten-millionth the speed of an average desktop computer.

As yet, we have relatively little insight into the answers to these questions. However, certain themes have begun to emerge, both from traditional behavioral and neuroscientific research and more recent studies using brain imaging technology. These findings are helping shape the way we think about the unique faculties of mind that make us human.

First, it is clear that the capacity for virtually all higher cognitive functions, such as reasoning, problem solving, and language, as well as decision making and planning, rely heavily on two fundamental functions discussed in section **B8**: inhibition and control. Searching for the solution to a complex problem, interpreting the meaning of a conversation, or formulating a course of future action are all forms of goal-directed activity. They rely on a person's ability to pursue an intended behavior even when more compelling but inappropriate alternatives are available. Classic examples of this include a teenager learning to study when he or she could be socializing, and a boss coaching employees gently rather than badgering them in order to create the most productive workforce. Our frontal lobes seem to play a critical role in this capacity for control and are therefore likely to play an equally important role in the higher faculties that depend on control.

Indeed, damage to the frontal cortex dramatically impairs the capacity for sensible decision making and planning. Recall the personality changes in Phineas Gage, the unfortunate railroad foreman who suffered damage to his prefrontal cortex. Originally considered to be thoughtful, responsible, and of sound judgment, he became "capricious . . . and unable to settle on any of the plans he devised for future action." Since the time of Phineas Gage, doctors have continued to observe similar changes in patients with damage to the frontal cortex, which often results in their inability to properly plan even the simplest of activities, such as cooking dinner.

More recently, brain imaging has shown increased activity in the prefrontal cortex when people engage in tasks that rely heavily on decision making and planning, such as playing chess, or in solving problems that require them to evaluate the outcome of a complex set of alternatives. These studies have not yielded any specific insights yet into precisely how the frontal cortex carries out these functions. Nevertheless, the opportunity presented by imaging machines to study the brain's normal workings noninvasively and with ever increasing detail promises, with time, to reveal critical information about our decision-making and planning processes.

Decision-Making Difficulties

Another important theme that has begun to emerge about our decision-making behavior is that we do not always—or even usually—conform to purely logical principles. This may not come as a surprise. We say with some pride that "we aren't computers," whose workings are based on mathematical logic. On the other hand, we humans also pride ourselves on our ability to reason. We believe that ability distinguishes us from our evolutionary ancestors, and we often hold rationality among our highest ideals. Indeed, the idea that human behavior is on average rational lies at the heart of traditional economic theory, which assumes that individuals seek to maximize their rewards in the best possible way. So ideally we should draw on those reasoning powers for every decision.

It is becoming increasingly apparent, however, that ordinary human behavior is often far from optimally rational. Both psychologists and economists have identified many situations in which people's thinking seems to be illogical or inconsistent—and consistently so! Furthermore, such deviations from optimality may not just be due to faulty reasoning, but may reflect specific adaptations of underlying neurobiological mechanisms. To explore how this might work, let us consider some examples of less-than-optimal human judgment and decision making.

In the 1970s the psychologists Daniel Kahneman and Amos Tversky started a remarkable series of studies examining human decision making, thus creating some of the most influential research in modern psychology. Kahneman and Tversky showed that humans systematically misestimate the probabilities of certain types of events and therefore make logically incorrect decisions. A common example is the general sense many people share that airplane travel is more dangerous than car trips. In fact, the reverse is true. Yet even though the real statistics have been widely publicized (not least by the airline industry), many people are still more afraid of flying than of riding in a car.

Kahneman and Tversky attributed this erroneous feeling of risk to the fact that people regularly overestimate the frequency of highly salient events like airplane crashes. That is, when an event is highly noticeable—it receives a lot of media attention, affects a large number of people all at once, and is emotionally arousing—it is more likely to "make an impression" on our memories. That event then influences people's future judgments and decisions out of proportion to its actual likelihood of happening again.

Another form of "wayward" reasoning occurs when people must decide between alternatives.

Notwithstanding traditional economics, this can be very difficult for the human brain. For example, in one experiment researchers asked people to choose between two objects that they could keep (for example, two types of pens); if they preferred not to choose, they would instead receive a small reward worth significantly less than either object. When one of the objects was clearly more desirable than the other, the choice was easy; virtually everyone chose the more valuable object. However, when the two objects were roughly comparable in apparent worth, people often decided not to choose and took the reward instead—even though it was the least valuable alternative.

Clearly such decision making was not optimal. Even if they could not tell which object was more valuable, completely rational humans would simply have chosen one or the other at random and come out ahead. Instead, people avoided the close decision. This behavior implies that the human brain is programmed to believe that deciding between apparently equally valuable alternatives has a cost. You may have experienced that phenomenon in your own life. Consider the difficulty of having to choose between two attractive plans for an evening, such as whether to go to a ball game or a movie. That situation seems better than having only one of the options, or neither. Yet the decision, paradoxically, can be more difficult. How often in such situations have you thought, "Oh, I'll just stay home"?

Evolution might explain that seemingly irrational form of decision making. Difficult decisions require time, and in the wild such time can be costly. An animal might do better to make a quick decision based on a simple rule, such as "A bird in the hand is worth two in the bush." Our brains may thus have evolved mechanisms that avoid uncertainty and lead to more assured, though less

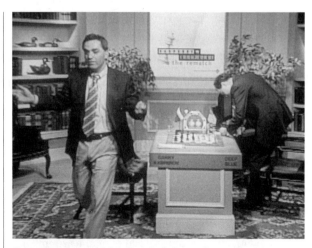

Garry Kasparov, highest-ranked chess player ever, became rattled when he faced Big Blue. According to game analysts, his emotional response to the unfamiliar challenge of playing against a computer led him to make uncharacteristically impetuous decisions. PHOTO © AP/WIDE WORLD PHOTOS

than optimal, results. This approach may no longer be as useful to us today, and therefore can appear illogical in particular situations. However, in the circumstances under which such a response evolved, it may have been quite reasonable. But that explanation is only speculative.

Both studies and everyday life also reveal the profound influence of emotions on our decision-making processes. Perhaps one of the most striking examples of this was the chess match between Garry Kasparov and the IBM computer Deep Blue. Kasparov was the human chess champion of the world, and Deep Blue was the computer chess champion. Many touted this as the ultimate intellectual showdown between human and machine: a contest to determine whether a device built from flesh and blood or from silicon could lay claim to the most powerful reasoning abilities on the planet.

Deep Blue surprised everybody and won, which

might have been taken as evidence that it possessed the superior capacity for the logic needed to play chess. However, chess pundits also reported that Kasparov was not playing at his best; in fact, he made several uncharacteristically impetuous moves. In interviews during the match, Kasparov seemed focused—even obsessed—with the fact that he was playing a computer. It appears that the champion may simply have "freaked out": the unusual situation evoked emotionally disturbing reactions that interfered with his ability to think clearly and play chess at his best. Thus, even a task that would seem to tap only pure, specialized human reasoning in a person who had most honed that ability was subject to emotional factors. In other words, emotions can insinuate themselves into our every thought and affect our every decision.

When Time Comes to Decide

Connecting complex behavior with mechanisms in the brain is difficult, and most studies of human decision making have relied on two approaches. First, as with many other brain functions, abnormalities can reveal as much or more than normal functioning. Studies often start with what we see when a part of someone's brain is damaged or the normal neurochemical balance is altered. Second, by posing a controlled, artificial challenge, such as a quiz or card game, to volunteers in the laboratory, researchers can observe their brains at work during the precise moment they are making up their minds.

Studies of patients with damage to the prefrontal cortex confirm the importance of this region in human decision making. Neurologist Antonio Damasio has reported the behavior of people with damage to a particular region of the

frontal cortex—the orbital frontal area, along the lower surface of the frontal lobes, just above the eye sockets, or "orbits"—in gambling tasks. His research team created a game that rewarded a conservative strategy over going for an immediate payoff. Most volunteers were able to play accordingly, but those with damage in the orbital frontal area had difficulty resisting the temptations of an immediate reward.

Observations of the brain in action seem to confirm that the orbitofrontal cortex plays a critical role in evaluating potential rewards. The first of these studies used direct recordings of animals' neurons in that area. Modern neuroimaging methods have begun to provide similar evidence in normal human brains as people play games very similar to those Damasio used to test his patients. Since parts of the prefrontal cortex are also crucial to our emotional processes, that suggests how emotions so easily affect the decisions we make. It also seems significant that the orbitofrontal cortex is largely guided by dopamine; the system for that neurochemical signal is hijacked when people abuse drugs (C29), which obviously affects their decision-making abilities.

Of course, the orbitofrontal cortex is not the only brain system involved in emotional processing. Both animal and brain imaging studies show that the amygdala—a specialized structure along the inner surface of the temporal lobes—plays a vital role in evaluating the emotional relevance of what a person's body is sensing. This is especially so for fearful stimuli, but may also be true for other types. Studies of the amygdala suggest that this structure may be especially important in detecting emotionally significant events (for example, events that should cause us to prepare for a "fight or flight" response), while other structures, such as the orbitofrontal cortex, may be more im-

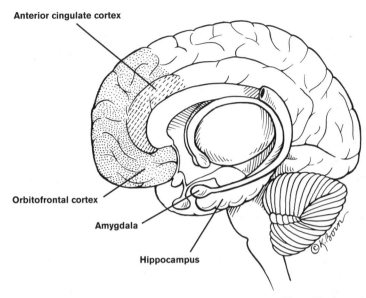

Anterior cingulate cortex

Orbitofrontal cortex

Amygdala

Hippocampus

Planning requires that many brain regions work in tandem. The orbitofrontal cortex helps us weigh immediate payoff against later rewards. The amygdala marks what is emotionally important. The anterior cingulate responds when we make mistakes. The hippocampus coordinates memories of past events. Much activity in planning takes place in the prefrontal cortex, which is not fully developed until late adolescence. ILLUSTRATION © KATHRYN BORN

portant for the careful or deliberative consideration of such events. When those other brain structures are damaged, the influence of the amygdala on decision making may become stronger.

Another brain structure that has attracted significant attention is the anterior cingulate cortex—a part of the frontal lobes that lies along their midline, just above the corpus callosum. Brain imaging studies have shown that in normal individuals this structure becomes active in response to pain and negative feedback, but it is abnormal in patients who suffer from anxiety (**C21**) or depression (**C20**). Recent studies have revealed that the anterior cingulate also responds when people make errors in simple cognitive tasks, and even when they respond correctly to a question but cannot be sure they are correct.

More generally stated, it appears that the anterior cingulate responds in situations associated with poor performance: uncertain decision making in challenging tasks, committing an error, receiving negative feedback, and experiencing pain (the ultimate consequence of poor performance!). This suggests that the anterior cingulate may monitor our internal decision-making processes for signs of deteriorating performance and the dangers that could ensue, much as the amygdala is thought to monitor the external world for signs of threats. Intriguingly, the anterior cingulate could be the evolutionary adaptation proposed earlier: the mechanism that keeps our brains from spending too much time considering a difficult choice. But, as stated before, that is just speculation.

A Glimpse of Higher-Level Reasoning

The brain systems just mentioned provide some insight into the apparent idiosyncrasies of human decision making and how these systems interact with emotional processes. It is a big step from these simple processes to the more complex areas of social interactions and higher-level reasoning. Neuroimaging studies are giving us our first glimpse of the brain systems engaged in such higher-level cognitive processes. For example, recent studies have examined the patterns of brain activity of people during a game that involves cooperation and trust, comparing those playing against a computer with those playing against another human being. Comparison of the two groups shows significantly different areas of brain activity, and many of the differences involve the areas that process emotions.

Moral reasoning is a field that we humans often consider our highest intellectual achievement. It is another area in which we exhibit patterns of behavior that have consistently puzzled philosophers and psychologists alike. It is not simply a matter of people holding different value systems, or of someone being "immoral." Even the same individual can reason quite differently when presented with dilemmas that appear different but are in fact similar. For example, consider the following scenarios:

- A trolley is headed toward five unsuspecting workers. A switch operator can avoid killing them all by moving the trolley to a sidetrack, on which there is only a single worker who will die.

- A trolley is headed toward five unsuspecting workers. There is a large man on a footbridge just above the trolley, and pushing this man off the bridge onto the track will cause the trolley to run over him and derail, saving the five workers.

Most people agree that it is morally justifiable, even imperative, to switch the train but impermissible to push the man off the bridge. Yet the logic of the two circumstances is the same: sacrificing one life will save five others.

There are many possible explanations for inconsistent choices in these two scenarios, and others researchers have imagined, but philosophers have failed to identify any general logical principles that can account for people's judgments under all the variants of those circumstances. This has led some to believe that people's moral judgments rely on a mixture of logic and emotion that varies with the specific nature of the circumstances. Thus, people may react more emotionally to the thought of physically pushing a man off a bridge to his death (even if it is to save five others) than they do to the thought of flipping a switch, which is an impersonal object.

As with simpler decision making, the paradox posed by these scenarios is reflected in the way the brain responds to each. A recent imaging study, described in the box to the right, has shown that the footbridge scenario activates emotional areas of the brain, whereas the switch scenario activates areas associated with more abstract processing. Again, our brains may have evolved to work the way they do because those adaptations were valuable in other circumstances. Perhaps our emotional reactions to directly harming people serve important social functions, prohibiting forms of aggressive or antisocial behavior that would challenge the species as a whole.

IMAGING MORAL JUDGMENT

The long-standing rationalist tradition in moral psychology emphasizes the role of reason in moral judgment. A more recent trend places increased emphasis on emotion. While both reason and emotion are likely to play important roles in moral judgment, relatively little is known about their pathways in the brain, the nature of their interaction, and the reasons for their respective behavioral influences in moral judgment.

In two functional MRI studies using moral dilemmas as probes, researchers applied the methods of cognitive neuroscience to the study of moral judgment. They argued that moral dilemmas vary systematically in the extent to which they engage emotional processing and that these variations in emotional engagement influence moral judgment.

The study participants were given many variants of life-or-death situations. In one, for example, a runaway trolley is headed for five people. The only way to save them is to hit a switch that will reroute the trolley to a different track where one person is standing. Should you turn the trolley to save five people at the expense of one? Most people say yes. In a second version of the dilemma, you are standing next to a stranger on a footbridge over the track, and the trolley is heading for five people. The only way to save them in this situation is to push the stranger off the bridge and into the path of the trolley. He will die, but the others will be saved. Should you push the stranger to his death in order to save the other five? Most people would say no. Why is this, and what happens in the brain when faced with these moral dilemmas?

The imaging results indicate that reasoning in some moral dilemmas activates brain areas previously associated with emotional processing, while reasoning in other dilemmas activates regions associated with working memory and logical problem solving, and that these differences align well with subjects' behavior in such tasks.

The results provide strong support for the idea that moral reasoning can engage emotional evaluation and that this can have an impact on the outcome of moral decision making. The results may shed light on some puzzling patterns in moral judgment observed by contemporary philosophers.

Planning Ahead

If deciding between options is an intricate brain action, planning is even more so. Planning is, in a way, an advanced form of decision making. It involves not merely making choices but also imagining what we want to do, what we need to accomplish that goal, and what might get in our way. It requires keeping those goals in mind over time. The function of consciously planning for the future instead of simply reacting to our environment according to instinct may be the most important ability we humans enjoy.

Once again, we have relatively little knowledge about the specific ways in which a human brain manages to plan a vacation, an election campaign, or any other complicated endeavor. However, we do know that this process relies heavily on the prefrontal cortex, most probably in close interaction with structures responsible for long-term memory and storage, such as the hippocampus (an area along the inner sur-

DECIDING WISELY

So far, our discoveries about human decision making have not led to new therapies to enhance that function or prevent its natural decline later in life. However, understanding the factors involved in how our brains process difficult problems may provide some insights into how to manage those decisions in our lives. Here are some things to consider:

- We cannot avoid having our emotions shape our decisions, sometimes in irrational ways. But knowing that emotions are part of the process can remind us to look at decisions from different perspectives.

- We all have capacity limits. Trying to do too many tasks at once may trigger the brain to ignore important new stimuli or to decide too hastily. One modern example of the danger of overloading the brain is talking on a phone while driving.

- Many brain diseases impair people's decision making, including depression (C20), schizophrenia (C25), late-stage Alzheimer's (C67), and such rare conditions as Pick's disease (C69). This underscores the connection between biology and the mind, and the importance of treatment where possible.

- Keeping the mind active also seems to preserve its higher functioning. In addition, there is evidence from neuroimaging and neuropsychological studies that physical exercise can help prevent a decline in prefrontal cortex functioning.

Finally, while our decision-making function seems to suffer a natural decline as we age, our life experience can continue to rise. Applying that wisdom to dilemmas in the real world may thus more than compensate for the natural decline.

face of the temporal lobes, very close to the amygdala).

These brain systems are responsible not only for allowing us to organize our behavior to deal with the complexity of daily life but for setting and pursuing long-term goals that can last a lifetime. Not surprisingly, these functions take a long time to develop to mature form. It is not simply an illusion that young children and adolescents have little sense of long-term planning; their brains are still developing that skill. In fact, with the prefrontal cortex not fully developed until late adolescence, children may not even be biologically ready for long-term planning.

Perhaps the most important aspect of planning is that it involves the ability to carry out actions well into the future, long past when we first conceive of them. For instance, a person may decide to earn an advanced degree in order to enter a new field, with an eye to eventually running his or her own business. That plan covers years, and it would be impossible for anyone to be actively working toward those goals every minute of the day. Indeed, there are long stretches in which the person will be engrossed in immediate tasks and not be thinking about his or her career plan at all. The ability to stick to a plan therefore depends on our brain's long-term memory. The prefrontal cortex maintains a mental representation of the goals of a person's current behavior (to balance the checkbook, to serve dinner), while the hippocampus and other parts of the brain invoke mental processes and actions related to career pursuits only when they are needed.

A simple example illustrates how the planning process may work in a much shorter time frame. Consider this situation: you wake up in the morning and go to the refrigerator to make breakfast, only to find that you are out of orange juice. You make a plan to stop at the grocery story on the way home from work. Obviously, you don't keep this plan actively in mind (that is, in your prefrontal cortex) all day long, repeating to yourself over and over, "I have to go to the grocery store at six o'clock." You devote your conscious thoughts to more immediate tasks, and to working on plans you've made as part of your work. Your ability to carry out Operation Orange Juice depends on its being stored in your mind and reactivated at the appropriate time.

Here's one model of how that reactivation may occur: when you make a mental note to stop at the grocery store on the way home from work, an association forms in your hippocampus between the steps of that plan (for example, turn left at the light rather than making the habitual right toward home, park in the store lot, and so on) and the circumstances under which it should take effect. Cues for activating the plan might include reading six o'clock on your watch, seeing the sun go down, and feeling your stomach growl. Whatever the association is, it allows you to put the plan "out of mind" (that is, to deactivate its representation in the prefrontal cortex). The day goes on, and you don't think about it. Then six o'clock rolls around, the sun goes down, and your stomach growls. Because these cues are linked with your plan to buy orange juice, they activate the representation of that plan in your prefrontal cortex, and you think to yourself: "Gotta go to the grocery store." Activation of this plan also ensures that you make the left turn at the light rather than the default right turn home.

We do not know for sure that these interactions are what actually happen in the brain when you make a plan, nor whether similar interactions occur when you make and follow even longer-term plans, such as for a family vacation or a new career. However, we do know that complex behaviors like planning are likely to involve intimate interactions between different brain regions, each of which contributes critical and complementary functions. This model of interaction between the hippocampus and the prefrontal cortex provides an example of the hypotheses about brain function that are beginning to drive research in neuroscience and psychology. Using the tools now available to test such theories, such as brain imaging, we can develop new understanding of the brain mechanisms underlying some of our highest and most cherished faculties.

Intelligence

Intelligence has been defined in many different ways. In this section we use the word to refer to individual differences in cognitive abilities, such as the capacity to reason, to solve problems, to think abstractly, to understand new material, and to learn from past experiences. By this definition, we are not including wisdom, creativity, or acceptance of the moral standards of one's society. The term *intelligence quotient* (IQ) refers to a way of comparing one individual's or group's intelligence with the average on specific tests of cognitive intelligence.

Historically, there has been a furious debate over whether intelligence is a single thing or reflects a cluster of specialized abilities. After a century of controversy on this topic, the answer is becoming clearer. Evaluations of cognitive ability virtually always have a positive correlation, meaning that an individual's scores on a variety of cognitive tests usually cluster around the same measurement. This and other evidence suggest that there is an underlying dimension of mental competence, a "general intelligence," that is reflected in a wide number of cognitive activities.

There are two important qualifications to this statement. First, visual-spatial reasoning, which is the ability to solve problems that involve manipulating visual representations and understanding the space around one, varies somewhat separately from verbal and logical problem solving. Second, the degree to which cognitive performance reflects separate abilities or a single general intelligence depends on the level of the performance. With some exceptions, low levels of mental performance are almost always pervasive: people who have very low scores on a verbal test are likely to have similarly low scores on a nonverbal one. High levels of performance tend to be much more differentiated; very high performance on a verbal test is not necessarily indicative of a similarly high level of performance on a nonverbal test, although high scores in one area virtually never indicate low scores in another.

Testing Intelligence

The tests for cognitive competence range from brief evaluations of reading samples to the

Six Examples of Simple vs. More Complex IQ Test Items

Directions	Simple item	Complex item
1. Compute	60 x 3 =	Sarah drove 3 hours yesterday at an average speed of 60 miles per hour. How many miles did she drive?
2. Define	Conceal	Encumber
3. State one similarity	Dog — Lion	Praise — Punishment
4. Give the next 2 numbers	3, 5, 7, 9, __ , __	10, 9, 8, 9, 8, 7, __ , __
5. Reproduce pattern with blocks whose sides are ☐, ■, ◣	Use 4 blocks:	Use 9 blocks:
6. Complete the pattern		

IQ test questions are devised to test people's ability to process complex information regardless of their cultural background. These questions cover verbal, mathematical, logical, and visual-spatial reasoning. COURTESY OF LINDA S. GOTTFREDSON, PH.D., UNIVERSITY OF DELAWARE

solving of abstract puzzles. Examples are the Wechsler Adult Intelligence Scale, which is the most widely used individually administered intelligence test, the Raven Progressive Matrices Tests, which are commonly used to evaluate intelligence without relying on language, and personnel screening examinations, such as the Scholastic Aptitude Test (SAT), which is required by many colleges and universities, and the Armed Services Vocational Aptitude Battery (ASVAB). Most testing is done in schools, especially to predict success in higher education, but businesses, the government, and the military also use tests of cognitive competence on occasion. Generally, people's results on these tests correlate with a number of measures of success in life, such as academic or business achievement and the resulting improved salary and rank. In fact, in what we might consider the ultimate test, studies have found that children with high intelligence-test scores grow up to have lower mortality rates than those with low test scores and that the advantage extends into late adulthood. Of course, not every individual fits into this general pattern.

Mental test scores are not as useful in determining a person's ability to do a specific task, because intelligence is not the same as competence in solving problems within a specialized occupation or situation. Experience is a major factor in establishing competence, and test scores are likely to underestimate how easily an individual can work in a familiar setting. Studies of expertise have shown that within-field competence is very much affected by practice. Thus there are strong trade-offs between initial competence and amount of training. On the other hand, mental test scores do predict the time it will take to achieve a given level of expertise. This has been demonstrated in studies ranging from university course work (the correlation between grades and test scores, and the correlation between test scores and graduation rates) to studies of on-the-job performance by military enlisted personnel.

Test scores are affected by age. After reaching a peak in early adulthood (age 20 to 35), test scores show a gradual decline until the mid-60s, and sharp declines thereafter. Again, there are very important qualifications to this statement. The first is that evaluations of mental competence that permit a person to use his or her knowledge show much less change than tests that require the solution of new or unusual problems. Second, verbal measures are more resistant to age-related decline than nonverbal measures. Finally, there are very large individual differences in the age-related decline. The top scores of people in their 60s and 70s are only slightly below the top scores of people in their 20s. The bottom scores show major declines with age. It is not clear what contributes to the increase in variance with age, although changes in health and personal lifestyle do make a contribution.

With one exception, there are absolutely no differences between men and women on intelligence tests. The exception is visual-spatial problems that require reasoning about imagined or visual motion. In this case men will, on the average, score higher than women.

The Biology of Intelligence

Francis Galton, who did important work on intelligence in the nineteenth century, believed that differences in general mental competence were due to individual differences in the efficiency of the nervous system as a signaling device. According to modern studies, Galton was right, in principle. We know that measures of cognitive competence are related to a person's ability to keep track of several things at once and to focus on the aspects of a situation relevant to the problem that needs solving. These abilities are generally subsumed under the title "working memory." Other work has related intelligence to the speed with which a person can access information in his or her long-term memory.

These findings suggest that indicators of intelligence may in part reflect individual differences in brain functioning. Behavioral genetics studies provide further evidence that this is so. A great many studies, using a variety of designs and tests, have shown that IQ scores, especially for measures of general intelligence, have a hereditary component. In fact, genetic inheritance is a larger influence on intelligence, at the population level, than any known social or physical environmental influence. More recent quantitative genetics stud-

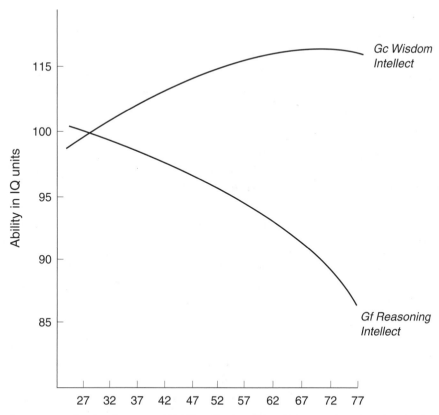

As one ages, the development of fluid intelligence ("the ability to solve new problems") drops off, and crystallized intelligence ("the ability to apply past knowledge to the current problem") continues to increase. FIGURE ADAPTED WITH PERMISSION FROM *ADVANCES IN THE PSYCHOLOGY OF HUMAN INTELLIGENCE,* © 1986 LAWRENCE EARLBAUM & ASSOCIATES

ies indicate that intelligence is partly a multigenetic trait. Some individual genes have been implicated in the development of intelligence, but a definitive list of the genes for intelligence has not yet been obtained.

Given this evidence, it is natural to ask just what structures in the brain might be related to intelligence. Over the years a number of investigators have asked whether or not intelligence was related to overall brain size. This resulted in considerable debate, caused in part by our inability to measure the size of the live brain. There are major problems with measurement and interpretation of data based on pathological or even archaeological analysis, or on such measures as skull size (which Galton used in his studies). Modern medical imaging techniques have resolved some of these questions. There is a reliable positive correlation between brain size and test score, but the closeness of the correlation is in question because brain imaging technology is too expensive for studies of large groups.

IQ SCORES AND ETHNICITY

Within industrial societies, there are substantial differences in test scores among ethnic groups. Historically, immigrant groups have tended to test lower than the norm when the group first arrives, but by the second and third generations their descendants have scores indistinguishable from the average scores in the country. This fact alone indicates that intelligence, as evaluated by the IQ test, has a substantial social component.

In the United States, Asian Americans have test scores slightly higher than all other ethnic groups, especially on tests that have a substantial visual-spatial reasoning component. The median test score for Caucasian Americans exceeds the scores of roughly 80 percent of African American examinees. The Caucasian American–African American gap in a variety of tests of cognitive performance narrowed from 1950 until the 1980s, and since then has remained fairly constant. Hispanic American scores are somewhat higher than those of African Americans but on the average are lower than those of non-Hispanic Caucasians.

There is no evidence that the tests are unfair in the sense that they are inaccurate predictors of performance for minority group members. The validity of the tests within various ethnic groups is virtually identical. Whether various tests are unfair in the sense that minority group members do not receive enough preparation to take them is an issue of social equity rather than a reflection on the tests themselves.

There have been a great many heated assertions about why ethnic group differences appear. The only defensible statement is "We do not know." The data we have now do not rule out purely social effects, a combination of social and physical-environmental effects (for example, poorer people living in areas that suffer from concentrations of toxic chemicals), or purely physical effects, such as differences in genetic inheritance.

A more useful approach than correlating test scores and brain size is to examine the role that specific parts of the brain play in establishing intelligence. Here imaging techniques are extremely helpful, and we have learned a good deal by analyzing the behavior of brain-damaged patients. These studies have implicated three areas of the cortex. The dorsolateral frontal cortex is selectively activated when people attempt tasks that are good indicators of general intelligence, such as the Raven matrices tests mentioned earlier. Visual reasoning tasks activate many of the areas of the brain associated with visual perception. Finally, the hippocampus is involved in committing information to long-term memory, a vital building block for intelligence, and is also involved in the ability to reason about geographic routes.

Influences on Intelligence

Many disorders can produce losses in intelligence. A variety of genetic disorders, as well as perinatal disorders, which occur primarily five months before and one month after birth, produce profound loss of mental competence. These include genetic abnormalities, such as Down's syndrome, Turner's syndrome (which is one of the few syndromes that produces a specific effect, in this case loss of spatial-visual reasoning), and Williams syndrome (**C3**). Following birth, virtually any injury to the brain may produce a drop in intelligence. Situations that produce prolonged coma, such as severe closed head injury, are particularly dangerous (**C61**). Profound losses of intelligence are associated with some diseases that involve neural degeneration. Alzheimer's disease (**C67**) is one of the most common and best publicized, but a similar loss of reasoning ability is often associated with the latter stages of other diseases, such as Pick's disease, dementia with Lewy bodies, and frontotemporal dementia (**C69**), that affect the central nervous system.

Certain specific environmental and lifestyle influences can produce smaller effects on intelligence. By far the most common of these is alcoholism (**C30**). In adults, high alcohol consumption is generally associated with lowered intelligence-test scores, but whether this is a cause-and-effect relationship is difficult to discern. However, alcoholism carried to the point of unconsciousness is clearly not a good idea, both for its effect on intelligence and for many other reasons. Heavy alcohol consumption by pregnant women may produce fetal alcohol syndrome in the child. Environmental toxins, especially atmospheric lead, have also been shown to have deleterious effects on intelligence, but these effects are so small that they only appear in fairly large studies (**C66**).

There is some evidence that social withdrawal and general lack of intellectual engagement can produce lowered test scores in adults. For instance, people who read widely appear to be considerably better problem solvers than people who do not. But while it would be nice to think that maintaining an active intellectual life protects one from the general decline associated with advanced age, the cause-and-effect relationships are very hard to untangle.

Dynamic Intelligence

Because intelligence appears to have a substantial genetic component, there has been a popular tendency to regard intelligence as fixed, but this does not follow, either logically or in fact. Test scores of mental performance that approximate samples of everyday cognitive behavior, such as the Scholastic Aptitude Test, virtually all respond to education. In fact, test scores in industrialized countries rose steadily from 1925 through 2000. The reason is not clear, but it is hard to believe that near-universal public education was not partly responsible. In addition, studies have found that individuals in the bottom 20 percent of the population, the below-normal to educable-retarded group, can often be productive citizens if they live in a well-structured environment with orchestrated social support.

It is extremely unlikely that an "intelligence pill" will be discovered in the near future. On the other hand, it is conceivable that researchers will discover therapies for some of the major causes of abnormally low intelligence, including the neural degeneration associated with Alzheimer's disease and changes in brain structure or function that are associated with the genetic mental diseases.

If you wish to maintain your intelligence until

great old age, there are really only two pieces of advice:

■ Maintain an active intellectual life.

■ Avoid things that can injure the brain. In particular, do not drink large doses of alcohol, abuse drugs, or expose yourself to situations that are likely to result in brain injury, ranging from reckless driving to unnecessary exposure to environmental toxins.

We cannot do much about our genes, or our vulnerability to other people's actions, but we can increase our chances of enjoying our intelligence for a long time by using that intelligence to avoid needless risks.

Learning and Memory

When we speak of a person with "brain-power," we often refer to the ability to take in new information and to recall it quickly. The value of such memory skills goes well beyond television quiz shows. Our ability to learn and retrieve knowledge is crucial to recognizing friends, following directions, and even turning a doorknob smoothly. Most of how we interact with the world has been shaped by our experiences, whether or not we remember them. Compared with other animals, our instincts tend to be a less important influence on our behavior. Being able to acquire new knowledge has allowed humans to remain biologically the same for several hundred thousand years yet build the civilization we know today. That is the power of memory.

The Many Modes of Memory

Memory is not in fact a single function but a collection of mental abilities that depend on different systems within the brain. Careful studies can isolate memory from perception and other intellectual abilities and examine each kind of memory separately.

The most important distinction between forms of memory divides our conscious recall of facts and events (declarative memory) from various skills, habits, and reactions we remember without conscious effort (nondeclarative memory).

Declarative Memory

Declarative memory is our storehouse of detailed information about the world and our experience of it: a story, an image, a mathematical relationship, and so on. Memory researchers group the information in declarative memory into two categories:

- Episodic memory, for specific experiences in our lives (your first kiss, last night's dinner, where you found this book)

- Semantic memory, for facts (when the Declaration of Independence was signed, where your supermarket stocks cooking oil, $12 \times 12 = 144$).

Episodic memory always includes information about where, when, and how you experienced an

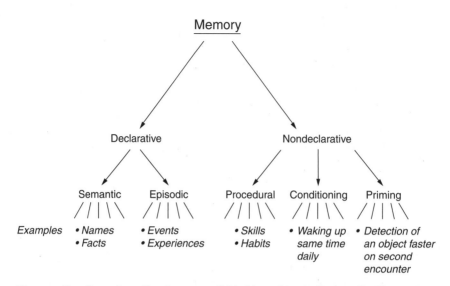

Memory "tree": a schematic of memory divided by subtypes. In everyday life, we draw on all these memory systems in tandem to learn and remember. GRAPH © LEIGH CORIALE

event ("The first time I met Aunt Millie's dog"). In contrast, you may not recall when and how you learned about a fact in your semantic memory, but nevertheless you feel sure of the fact ("That's Aunt Millie's dog").

Declarative memory is fast, specialized in learning things quickly. It makes connections among different stimuli, helping us model the world around us: what things are, how they work, what events we have personally observed or participated in. The capacity for declarative memory takes a while to develop, which is why it is rare to truly remember experiences from before the age of 3 or so.

Amnesia (**C68**) is an impairment of declarative memory, affecting the ability to retrieve past memories, the ability to form new memories, or both. A memory loss affecting someone's knowledge of what he or she once knew is called an agnosia (**C72**).

Nondeclarative Memory

When we use nondeclarative memory we are remembering reflexively, but this is not the same

as instinct. We had to learn the information stored in nondeclarative memory at some point, although, like instinct, nondeclarative memory is responsible for a great range of automatic human behavior. Nondeclarative memory handles three types of memory activity that we need in order to function from moment to moment:

- Procedural memory, or knowing *how* to do something, is the most important task of nondeclarative memory. It is the basis of our mental and physical skills. We usually acquire such skills gradually over time. Though we may experience sudden breakthroughs, repeated practice is key.

- People with amnesia usually retain most of their skills: they may not recall where they bought their shoes, but they remember how to tie those shoes. Amnesic patients can also usually learn new skills. Those facts underscore how declarative and procedural memories rely on different systems within the brain.

A person who has lost the knowledge of how to perform particular acts is said to have an "apraxia" (**C71**).

■ Conditioning is the process of acquiring the kind of information that the brain sends to the body for an automatic response. The information and response are generally the same every time this form of memory is triggered. That is, a particular stimulus—a bell, in Ivan Pavlov's classic experiments with dogs, or the sight of a clock's hands approaching lunchtime—cues a physical reaction. A conditioned response can occur through our involuntary autonomic nervous system (faster heartbeat, salivation, and so on) or our voluntary muscles (getting up from our desks).

■ Priming is the nondeclarative memory function that improves the brain's ability to detect, identify, or respond to a stimulus that it has processed recently. For instance, it takes about .8 seconds for the average person to name each object in a series of drawings, but only .7 seconds for a drawing he or she has seen shortly before.

■ People with difficulty forming new declarative memories still display the phenomenon of priming. They can, for example, read material aloud more quickly if they have seen it before, even though they do not remember having seen it.

Emotional Memory

An example of emotional memory is a phobia. This kind of memory depends on the amygdala. The amygdala also modulates declarative and nondeclarative memory. Thus we remember arousing (declarative) events better than boring ones.

Experiences that are novel or emotionally affecting are especially memorable, and emotions (**B7**) can color all forms of memory. Emotional meaning gives more weight to particular details or episodes. Conversely, strong emotion can cause difficulty in recalling certain episodes or facts. Sometimes an emotional memory can produce a feeling, such as fear, even when a person cannot dredge up from his or her declarative memory any reason to be frightened; in extreme cases, this can become a phobia.

In everyday life, we draw on all these memory systems in tandem to learn. A basketball player preparing for a game, for example, mentally replays previous games (episodic memory), reviews facts about the upcoming opponent (semantic memory), and practices the coach's new plays with other team members (procedural memory, conditioning, and priming). Especially if the game is a big one, the player's practice may be associated with thoughts of excitement or apprehension, due to previous experiences stored in memory.

The Stages of Memory and Learning

Not only do we constantly take in and store new information, but to help do so, we retrieve, use, and re-store existing memory information. For example, you overhear a coworker introducing a new employee, a tall, thin woman with red hair, as "Sheila." Your declarative memory says she resembles Sheila who carpooled with you to school in fifth and sixth grade. You go over to shake hands, asking if she is the same person, and then store the new information that she grew up in another city. In a large firm with many employees, you may remember her better because of this momentary link to your past. In an example like this, you called on

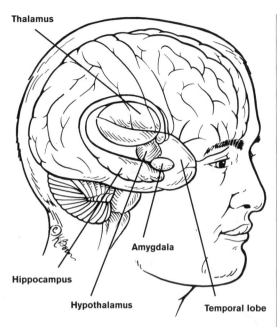

Thalamus

Amygdala

Hippocampus

Hypothalamus

Temporal lobe

The major brain regions and structures involved in memory. ILLUSTRATION © KATHRYN BORN

both declarative (childhood experience) and non-declarative (the handshake) memory functions, here with an emotional (nostalgia) overlay. (Conditioning being what it is, you might also find yourself wondering for a few mornings how she is getting to work.) These memories, both new and old, seem to go through short-term and long-term stages, though they rely on different systems.

Sensory Memory

When information enters our eyes, ears, or other sensory channels, the nervous system creates a very brief but thorough record of all those stimuli. This sensory memory can hold a great deal of information, but only for a short period. Our visual systems seem to retain images for about a tenth of a second, while our hearing retains sounds for one or two seconds.

One study that demonstrated the power of sensory memory involved showing volunteers 12 letters, arranged as three rows of four. A researcher flashed these rows on a screen and asked the volunteers to report the letters they had seen; typically, people recalled about 40 percent. Then the researcher told the volunteers they would hear a high, medium, or low tone to indicate which single row they should try to remember. The tone sounded just as the letters disappeared, so the volunteers could not focus their attention on the single row while the letters were still visible. Despite that timing, most people named at least three of the four letters—more than 75 percent—in the designated row. The volunteers' sensory memories must therefore have held the information about *all* the rows, enabling the volunteers to retrieve the designated row when they heard the tone.

Sensory memory gives the brain's cognitive areas time to choose which parts of the stream of incoming information are worthy of further processing. This choice relies on what the brain identifies as important. For example, the areas responsible for attention (**B10**) may be looking for the information, those responsible for pain (**B5**) may register it. In the case of the new employee, Sheila, her resemblance to a childhood acquaintance prompted the brain to get more information.

Short-Term Memory

The next stage of the learning process is short-term memory, which we can also think of as working memory. Our brains temporarily store the information we need at the moment, whether we are reading a sentence, solving a problem, or planning an action. Short-term memory handles both new information, such as a telephone number someone has just given you to call, and old information, retrieved to compare with something new ("Is this the same person I went to school with?"). Short-term memory is powerful but not infinite, and limits to its capacity can cause us to feel overwhelmed with information.

There are, in addition, different forms of short-term memory, determined by the data being processed and thus the parts of the brain involved. A sort of sketch pad called the visuospatial loop stores images and patterns, speech-based information travels the phonological loop, and so on. Indeed, some research suggests that each of the brain areas that process specialized information might have its own working memory system.

Long-Term Memory

Learning information for longer than a few minutes means encoding it in a stable way somewhere in the brain. We humans have a vast capacity for such long-term memory, but retrieving information in a useful and timely manner depends on how it is stored.

During the storage phase, the mind performs two essential actions that make learning more efficient. First, it does not attend to some of the data the brain has processed. To learn valuable information, we usually have to grasp the gist of an experience, or its most important aspects, not every detail. To recognize patterns in various objects or experiences, we need to set aside their differences. If we didn't exclude extraneous information, our minds might easily become crowded, like an e-mail in-box.

The second important phase of storing new information is consolidation: organizing the new material alongside what the mind has already remembered. To store all the data usefully, our brains organize material into networks based on conceptual categories. Your memory of how to use an eggbeater is probably linked to your knowledge of other kitchen utensils, memories of particular recipes, recollections of learning to cook, and so on. That style of organization explains why people who suffer injuries to small parts of the brain can lose very specific knowledge: of animals, for instance, which are often learned about by knowing how they look, but not of tools, which are often learned about by knowing how they are used.

Consolidating a memory also involves stabilizing the information, which can take several years. During that time, new data can cause a memory to change, strengthen, or grow weak and confused. Once a memory has been consolidated, it becomes robust and difficult to revise. That does not mean, however, that a consolidated memory is complete, or completely accurate. Memory does not work like a video camera, capturing every detail of an experience. Rather, it seems to retain snatches of our experiences, enough to allow the mind to reconstruct events when needed. When our minds try to "make sense" of our memories, they sometimes fill in or alter details. Retrieving a memory is seldom exact, therefore, and the act of retrieval itself can even change what we remember.

The Anatomy of Memory

Learning a fact, skill, or habit depends on making structural changes in the brain. That does not mean each new memory creates new neurons. Rather, the process of forming a memory changes the way existing neurons connect and communicate with each other.

MAKING THE MOST OF MEMORY

We would all like to learn more easily, to retrieve useful facts more quickly, and to enjoy our memories as long as possible. But there is no "memory pill" or other simple solution, unfortunately, although a number of pharmaceutical firms have research programs aimed at finding one.

Maintaining an intellectually stimulating lifestyle seems to be the best—and most enjoyable—way to ease learning and preserve memory. This has been shown by studies that ranged from tracking individuals over their lifetimes to finding that rats placed for a time in environments enriched with toys and other rats are better at navigating complex mazes than rats exposed to less stimulating environments.

As for learning specific material, that task is usually easier when we can relate the new information to what we already know. Patterns are also important. People with expertise in a particular field do not rely on any general memory ability, but rather on a specialized and gradually acquired ability to encode and organize the information most useful to them, such as a chess master, who is able to envision all the ways pieces can move across a board.

Learning information under the same conditions and with the same methods that a person will have to use to remember it enhances the memory process. Studies have also found that learning information over several sessions is better than doing so in a single long session. Theories suggest that a longer period of learning, and pauses between sessions, help the brain process and store the information a person wants to retain. It has also been suggested that sleep, and specifically dreaming, is crucial for this process (B3), but like much regarding learning, that has yet to be conclusively demonstrated.

As most college students know, caffeine and other substances can enhance memory and other cognitive performance for a while. These substances act primarily by boosting arousal, however, not by improving memory as such. Over time, a healthy body and a stimulated mind are still the best program for a powerful memory.

Short-term memory involves temporary changes in neurons' electrical activity and the chemicals that they exchange through their synapses. Depending on what a person has experienced, specific connections become stronger or weaker. Animal studies indicate that the process of forgetting can involve weakening of the synapses between cells.

To store information in long-term memory, the brain must make more permanent changes, which take two forms:

- Nerve cells can extend their axons, thus allowing more connections to other cells.

- Cells can increase their ability to release chemical neurotransmitters through their synapses, thus increasing the power of each connection.

What determines the "content" of a memory is the location in the brain where synaptic changes occur.

The brain stores information about various

aspects of the world in the same parts of the cortex that process that information when it first arrives. Thus, one part of the brain deals with smells, another musical sounds, another faces, and so on. If we think of memories as perceptions that the brain has chosen to store, it makes sense for them to be encoded in the areas that deal with similar new experiences. Usually the memory of an event, or even the memory of an object, is broken into component parts and stored in several areas of the brain at once. Thus, when the brain processes new stimuli in any of these areas, the record of what a person has already learned is nearby.

The crucial step of transforming a perception into a long-term memory occurs not in the cortex, however, but in other parts of the brain. Declarative memory depends on the medial temporal lobe (parahippocampal cortex, entorhinal cortex, perirhinal cortex, and the hippocampus) and the diencephalon. The various regions of the frontal lobes contribute the crucial information about an event, including information to link the experience with a time and place. Information from all these structures is distributed to the appropriate networks in the cortex for storage.

Different long-term storage systems are involved in learning skills, priming, and conditioning. To learn habits, for example, we depend on the caudate nucleus and putamen. Emotional memories—recollections of fear, sadness, pleasure, and other states—involve the amygdala.

Learning thus causes significant, permanent changes in the brain, even in areas once believed to be immutable. For instance, scientists have long known that we all have representations of our bodies in the sensory cortex. Research has shown, however, that learning can alter how much of that

band of brain tissue is devoted to the various parts of the body. If people learn to use the ring finger on the left hand unusually often, as violinists do, the corresponding area in the cortex expands. That effect is especially notable when people start such learning early in life.

Memory, Aging, and Disease

Our memory functions decline naturally as we age, usually starting in our mid-30s. Common memory problems in normal aging include trouble recalling where or when we learned something or in what order events occurred and difficulty remembering the need to do particular tasks at scheduled times. Sometimes we may not even perceive a problem with memory as such.

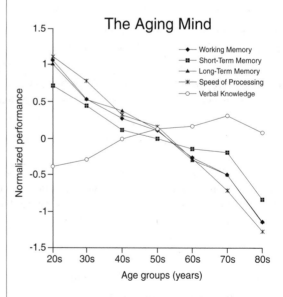

As the brain ages, different forms and aspects of memory (working, short term, and so on) decline at different rates. GRAPH COURTESY OF DENISE C. PARK, PH.D., CENTER FOR APPLIED COGNITIVE RESEARCH ON AGING, UNIVERSITY OF MICHIGAN

THE MAN WHO COULD NOT REMEMBER

In 1953 a man underwent surgery to treat epilepsy that was interfering drastically with his life. Doctors removed part of the medial temporal region of his brain—a section about 2 inches (5 cm) long from front to back in both hemispheres. The surgery stopped the disabling seizures but, unfortunately, impaired his brain in an unexpected way: he became unable to store new declarative memories, a form of amnesia.

Over the following decades the man, known publicly as "H.M.," helped researchers reveal some fundamental facts about our memory system. He continued to score above average on intelligence tests, to display normal short-term memory, and to remember his childhood and early life. Yet he was unable to learn new facts. Each time he met the researchers who studied him, he would greet them as new acquaintances. When those scientists asked H.M. to remember the words *salad* and *nail,* he quickly described a mental picture of a nail sticking into a salad. But after a few minutes of conversation on another topic, H.M. could not remember the salad, the nail, or his mental image.

H.M.'s capacities showed how procedural memory is separate from declarative memory. He could acquire new motor skills even though he could not remember the process of learning them. For instance, he was given the following learning test: he was told to stand a small mirror on one end beside the figure of a star like the one below. Looking only at the mirror image, he was asked to try to draw a pencil line quickly between the inner and outer borders of the star. Like most people, H.M. found this difficult but improved at staying within the borders from day to day. Yet each day he had no recollection of having done the exercise before. Thus, though the surgery had crippled his declarative memory, H.M. could still learn this skill.

H.M.'s case showed that the medial temporal lobes are not necessary for short-term memory or procedural memory but are absolutely essential to our ability to acquire long-term episodic and semantic memories. H.M. could process perceptions and perform other intellectual activities but retained no enduring record of them. Canadian psychologist Brenda Milner's first paper on H.M. became as much a landmark in how we understand memory as Phineas Gage's case was in how we understand inhibition, judgment, and emotional control.

Star test: Looking only at a mirror image of this star, try to draw a pencil line quickly between its inner and outer borders. Like you, a person with amnesia will learn to do it, but he or she won't remember learning. ILLUSTRATION © LEIGH CORIALE

Older people often report difficulty following conversations in noisy rooms and assume the problem is hearing loss, but studies indicate that usually the real challenge is mentally sorting the most significant information from all the other sounds flowing into their ears.

These ordinary memory slippages seem to be related to anatomical changes. As we age, we tend to lose neurons in the dentate gyrus and subiculum, which are connected to the hippocampus. Fortunately, most people can compensate for these problems in daily life. Furthermore, individuals retain a wide range of abilities. On some standard memory tests, 20 percent of septuagenarians outscore the average 30-year-old.

It is important to distinguish normal age-related memory loss from that caused by injury or illness. For example, the neurons in a particular portion of the hippocampus called CA1 remain intact as we age, but this region is especially vulnerable to damage from loss of blood (ischemia) during surgery or stroke (**C59**). Damage to the CA1 region disrupts the flow of information into and out of the hippocampus, thus causing amnesia and other memory problems. In addition, an early hallmark of Alzheimer's disease (**C67**) is the death of nerve cells in CA1 and the nearby entorhinal cortex, which impairs the brain's input and output for long-term memories. And losing part of our memories or our ability to remember means, in some profound ways, losing part of ourselves.

Speech, Language, and Reading

Language is one of the pillars of human intellect. It is the principle way we formulate thoughts and convey them to others. It plays a role in how we analyze the world, reason, solve problems, and plan actions. It lets us convey memories of the past and beliefs about the future, engage others in thinking about events that have not taken place, and express the relationships we perceive between events.

Language is also an indispensable part of human culture. Without it, our systems of jurisprudence, commerce, science, as well as other human endeavors, could not exist in the forms we know, if at all. Without language, each person's discoveries would die with him or her; language makes it possible for the achievements of one individual to be transmitted to the rest of the human species. Language skills are also vital to a person's success in society. Without language, most individuals are unable to function normally in their families and communities. We celebrate when children learn to speak and read, and feel distress if a person loses these abilities because of disease or injury.

Our Understanding of Language

Before exploring how our brains deal with language, it is useful to understand what language is. Modern linguistics has taught us that language, in its essence, is a special kind of code. An ordinary code, such as those used by spies or computer programmers, consists of a set of symbols that people in the know can connect to the words and phrases in their language. When we crack such a code, we understand the encoded messages because we can translate them into a language we understand. Natural language is a different sort of code because its forms are directly related to meanings in our minds, not to another language.

The forms of language are grouped into several levels: simple words, words formed from other words, sentences, and discourse. Each of these levels of the language code pairs a certain form with some meaning. Words consist of elementary sounds: phonemes (such as a long *a* or a hissing *s*), syllables (*fa*, *ing*, and so on), tones (rising, falling, flat), and stress patterns (what syllables or sounds a speaker accents). Words refer to objects, actions, properties, and logical connections. Some words are formed by combining other, elementary words with such affixes as the sign for the past tense (usually *ed* in English); these words also refer to objects, actions, properties, and logical connections. Sentences consist of words grouped and organized to relate their meanings to each other to depict events and states in the world. Discourse consists of sequences of sentences, with relations between words and sentences defined in ways that tell us what the topic of the discourse is, what information is new and what is old, how the sentences relate to each other in logic and in time, and so on. We can convey these aspects of meaning using the positions of words in sentences, intonation and stress, and other structures of our language. Discourse also relies on inferences based on language users' knowledge of the real world, including the context of statements.

Language is an intricate code, with all these types of representations interacting to determine the meaning of everything we say. That intricacy is also why language can communicate so powerfully. The same sounds appear in "You brought the cats," "You caught the brats," and "The ewe trots back," but our knowledge of words tells us these statements have completely different meanings. Similarly, intonation and context help us discern what people mean when they say, "We bought a car" or "We bought a *car!*" or "*We* bought a car?"

Humans usually produce language aloud, for someone else to hear. Speech is an intricate process because each level of the language code affects the sounds that a person produces when speaking. We select our words according to what we want to talk about and whom we're addressing.

We choose a syntax to relate the words to each other, and an intonation to convey that syntax and the discourse structure. For instance, we say the word *fire* differently if we want to produce an exclamation ("Fire!") or a question ("Fire?"). When we set out to voice a long sentence, we start by taking a deeper breath and speaking with a slightly higher pitch than when we start a short sentence. Thus, as soon as we begin to say a word or sentence, we both activate its form and fit that form into the discourse we intend to produce.

Our brains translate all this outgoing information into movements of the mouth, jaw, tongue, palate, larynx, and other articulators, regulating them on a millisecond-by-millisecond basis. On average, we produce about three words per second, or one sound every tenth of a second. The process of perceiving speech is equally complex because the hearer must extract all the levels of the language code from the signal, based on very subtle acoustic cues. Despite that complexity, speech is very accurate: we make only about one sound error per thousand sounds, and one word error per thousand words in speaking.

Though we usually use language in spoken form, there are other ways to use language. Many deaf individuals learn language in gestural forms, known as signing, and in fact most people who speak aloud also use some gestures in linguistic fashion. These two modes of using language develop without explicit instruction. Most babies naturally start to babble in the middle of their first year, playing with the sounds their mouths can make. Babies raised by parents who communicate through signing "babble" in sign language, trying out simple hand movements in the same way. With the encouragement of their parents and other caregivers, infants acquire more and more

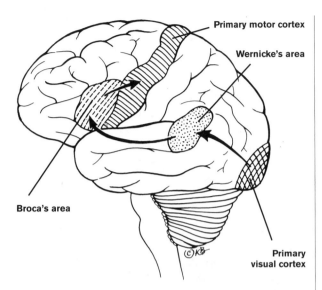

Primary motor cortex

Wernicke's area

Broca's area

Primary visual cortex

©KB

When you say a word that you read, the information about the word travels from your primary visual cortex to Wernicke's area, which recognizes the word's meaning, to Broca's area, which is involved in formulating spoken language, to the primary motor cortex, which enables the movement of muscles to let you say the word aloud. ILLUSTRATION © KATHRYN BORN

communication skills. Learning language is part of the cognitive development of every normal human being exposed to an adequate linguistic environment.

In addition to these two "naturally" occurring ways of using language, humans have developed written forms. Writing systems represent words: sometimes with symbols that correspond more or less to the sounds within words (as in English), sometimes with symbols that correspond to syllables (as in Japanese kana), and sometimes with symbols that correspond to entire words (as in Chinese). Written language requires instruction and conscious practice to master. It is therefore likely to have a different neurological basis from spoken and signed language. For us humans, writing serves the critical function of leaving a long-

lasting and portable record of the language that a person has produced.

Language and the Brain

Scientists have made systematic investigations for more than a century of how the brain learns, stores, and processes language. The task is difficult because there are no animals who have symbol systems as rich as ours. Therefore, for a long time, information about how our brains processed language could come only from studying the effects of neurological diseases. Scientists had to wait to examine the brains of language-impaired patients until after they died. This was how the nineteenth-century doctors Paul Broca and Carl Wernicke each connected an area of the brain to an element of speech. In the past decade, exciting new techniques have allowed us to picture the normal brain at work processing language. What used to take decades to learn we can now approach in months using positron-emission tomography (PET), special analyses of electroencephalograms (EEGs), functional magnetic resonance imaging (fMRI), magnetoencephalography, and other tools. (For more about these tools of brain science, see chapter 2.)

As is true for every other function, particular parts of the brain specialize in language. The brain has two roughly identical halves—the left and the right hemispheres—but we now know there are small differences in the sizes of some regions in those two halves. These differences may form the basis for the first major brain specialization for language—one hemisphere handles most of this function, a phenomenon called "lateralization."

In about 98 percent of right-handers, the left hemisphere manages most language-processing functions. For non-right-handers (including both left-handed and ambidextrous people), language functions are far more likely to involve the right hemisphere. There is some evidence that lateralization differs in males and females: men's brains tend to solve problems verbally in the left hemisphere, while the equivalent activity in women's brains extends across both temporal lobes. There is also evidence that a person's nondominant hemisphere is most involved in the next step beyond relating a word or sentence to its literal meaning; these advanced language functions include determining the emotional state of a speaker from his or her tone, and appreciating humor and metaphor.

Within the typical person's left hemisphere, only a relatively small part of the cortex is responsible for language processing. Most of this region lies around the sylvian fissure and consists of advanced cortex. This area appears to be responsible for sign language as well as spoken language, but the way a person communicates exerts some effect: written language probably involves areas nearer the visual cortex, and sign language may recruit areas close to those related to our ability to locate objects in space. Very recent studies have also provided evidence that other parts of the left hemisphere may be involved to a lesser extent. These include regions in the inferior and anterior temporal lobe, the basal ganglia and thalamus, and motor-planning regions (the supplementary motor cortex). A part of the brain outside the cerebral hemispheres—the cerebellum—may also be active. Language is, after all, a complex, important, and wide-ranging function.

Can we be even more specific about exactly where in the brain particular language operations are carried out? Where do we activate the sounds of specific words, or compute the meaning of a

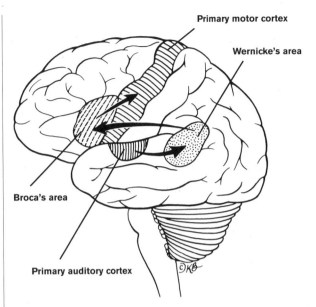

Repeating a word you hear involves a slightly different pathway. Your auditory cortex processes the word's sound. Information then travels through Wernicke's area, Broca's area, and the motor cortex, until you speak aloud. ILLUSTRATION © KATHRYN BORN

sentence? Since the earliest investigations, some scientists have thought that the language region works more or less as a unit. Others have sworn by the idea that individual language operators are localized in specific parts of this region: one area generates what you say, another area processes what you hear from others, and so on. There are suggestive studies that pin specific language representations and processes to small parts of the brain, but for almost every study that supports this view, there are others that disagree. We can therefore say that it is clear that the entire brain is not involved in all language functions, and that each individual has some small regions in the brain's language area that are involved in particular operations. But the jury is still out on the question of whether a specific function is always carried out in the same brain region for everyone.

Language Disorders

Although being deprived of any brain or body function is difficult, diseases that affect language are especially devastating to humans. Not being able to communicate thoughts efficiently can cut us off from our livelihoods and families. It can have immense effects on our emotional states and social positions. Such disorders of language can arise as part of otherwise normal development, as happens in dyslexia (**C1**). They can appear gradually, as a consequence of degenerative brain diseases such as Alzheimer's (**C67**) and Parkinson's disease (**C41**), or suddenly, as in acute brain injuries (**C61**) and strokes (**C59, C60**). Language abilities also change with age, but these changes are much more mild than those caused by disease or injury.

For more than a century, researchers and clinicians tended to classify language disorders into a small number of syndromes that were characterized by how fluently people spoke, how accurately they could repeat statements, and whether they suffered from disturbed comprehension. We are now able to go far beyond these syndromes—to make highly specific diagnoses of what language processors are affected in a particular disorder. Language disorders can be extensive, affecting virtually all language-processing operations, or highly selective. For instance, some stroke patients have lost the ability to find the words for specific types of objects, such as fruits and vegetables, but have no problem with the words for animals and man-made objects. Others can give definitions for abstract words, but cannot list common objects' physical features, such as the long neck of a giraffe. These isolated problems can affect any aspect of language, including reading. Some people after strokes cannot read irregular words (*pint*—as opposed to mint, hint, lint, etc.) but can read complex nonsense words (*bleferate*); others have the opposite problem. By identifying language problems more specifically, we can better help people recover from them or work around these disabilities. Studying such disorders also helps us understand normal language processing.

Parents occasionally wonder if their infants are learning to speak "on schedule." There is in fact a wide time range within which babies learn their first words, speak their first sentences, and so on. These landmarks differ according to a number of variables, including the child's temperament, environment, and general health. Emotion is one key to acquiring language skills; when infants hear the adults they love speaking with emotion in their voices, they seem to sense the importance of this activity and want to participate. Children can also suffer from a slow or deviant development of part of their language-processing system. Sometimes parents notice a toddler has trouble hearing sounds or discerning the separate sounds in words. This may be the sign of a hearing problem, or of a need for more structured help. A fairly common disorder appearing among school-age children is dyslexia, which affects the ability to read or write with little relation to other cognitive development. Working with special teachers can usually help a child overcome dyslexia, usually with excellent outcomes.

Because language is so much a part of our lives, a problem in communicating is usually apparent. Many adults suspect that a language problem means they or someone they know well has a disorder of the brain, but that isn't necessarily so. The most common of these problems is difficulty finding words. This difficulty increases naturally with age, and there is a wide range of normal performance in this area. Testing by a psychologist or speech pathologist can determine whether someone's ability to name things matches his or her age and education; only if this is not the case do those tests suggest the need for neurological investigation. Other language impairments, such as when a previously literate individual has obvious trouble reading or repeating words accurately, are relatively uncommon and demand attention.

When a person experiences a language disorder, therapy can be effective. The plasticity of our brains often allows them to work around injured areas, creating new circuits to perform the same important functions. Recent work shows that targeting specific impairments can improve language functioning. Advances in augmentative communication aids, such as specially designed computers, have allowed many patients with severe speech disorders to communicate. Even in cases in which families can expect little progress, therapy can help a person maintain and use the language he or she has. (Specific therapies are discussed in the appropriate sections of Part IV.)

As with every skill, exercising our language faculties leads to greater proficiency. We cannot say exactly what effect practice has on the brain—that is, what parts of our language-processing system benefit from use and how—but there is clear value in keeping the system in top shape. The language function is one of the greatest gifts of our brains.

Visualization and Navigation

Our visual system is the primary means by which we learn about the world, and we receive more information visually than by any other means. Most people would say that the organ of vision is the eye, but in fact the eye is only the beginning of the visual system.

The processing of visual information takes place in a network of areas throughout the brain, with different functions performed in different regions. Seeing color and motion; recognizing shapes, such as printed words, objects, and faces; finding our way around our environments; and imagining an appearance from memory are among the vital and complex functions our brains perform.

The ultimate goals of vision can be divided into two very general categories:

■ to recognize what we see

■ to navigate through space

These categories of visual function are carried out by largely separate systems, each one of which involves multiple stages of visual information processing.

One consequence of this networked arrangement is that disease or damage in the brain may affect our vision in different ways, depending on what parts of the brain are harmed. Strokes (**C59, C60**), injuries (**C61**), and brain tumors (**C10, C64**) can all damage particular regions while leaving others intact. Damage to certain parts of the temporal lobes can impair visual recognition, while

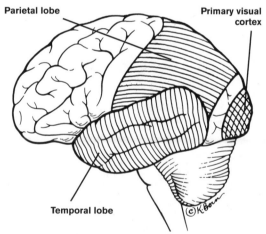

Visualization requires more than seeing. The primary visual cortex recognizes and processes information from our eyes, but areas of the temporal lobe are necessary for recognizing what we see: objects, faces, and so on. Areas of the parietal lobe process information about moving through the space we see. ILLUSTRATION © KATHRYN BORN

damage to certain parts of the parietal lobes can impair visual-spatial functioning.

What We See

The first part of the cerebral cortex to which the eyes and optic nerves send visual information is called, appropriately enough, the primary visual cortex. It is situated at the very back of the brain in the occipital lobes and plays a crucial role in the early stages of processing signals for form, motion, and color vision. Damage here causes cortical blindness, as opposed to forms of blindness caused by damage to the eyes or optic nerves. Partial damage causes only partial blindness, as when problems in just one occipital lobe cause a person not to be able to process information, and thus see, one side of space (**C15**).

From the primary visual cortex, the brain's representation of the visual world is split into many specialized processing pathways. Damage to these pathways can affect vision in very specific and sometimes surprising ways. For example, our brains appear to process color and motion in distinct areas. People sometimes lose the ability to see color while retaining all other aspects of vision. This is different from inborn color blindness, which results from defects in the retina and usually lets a person perceive at least some colors. People with cerebral color blindness describe the world as looking like a black-and-white movie. A person's ability to see motion can also be disrupted, so that he or she sees only a rapid sequence of still images when looking at objects in motion.

Impairment of visual recognition is termed visual agnosia and takes different forms depending on the brain areas affected (**C72**). One area of the temporal lobes is devoted to recognizing faces, presumably because of the crucial importance of face recognition to our functioning and survival. Damage here can result in a relatively isolated but still troubling loss: individuals suffering from what is called face agnosia report that while faces continue to look like faces, they also look too similar to tell apart. One man with this condition described the experience of coaching his son's soccer team and not knowing which boy was his son when they were in uniform.

Visual agnosia can affect how people recognize everyday objects as well, causing tremendous difficulty. People can see the sizes and shapes and colors of the things around them, yet not know the identity of these things. Because the damage is usually confined to the visual areas of the temporal lobe, such people will often put their intact touch areas to work. They will pick up an object and feel it in order to identify it.

Printed words constitute a very special category of visual object for literate humans, and it seems that our brains develop specialized areas for the recognition processes of reading (**B14**). Accordingly, it is possible to sustain damage to this area alone and lose the ability to read. This form of visual agnosia is usually called pure alexia because it is a relatively isolated loss of the ability to recognize words. At first, pure alexics may feel that they need new glasses or better light for reading. Unfortunately, the problem is not external and will not be solved by large print or good light. Instead, an internal bottleneck has developed in their visual processing, allowing them to read only slowly, often letter by letter or with many errors.

Navigating Through Space

Just as the temporal lobe recognition system comprises specialized subsystems, so does the parietal lobe spatial system. One of the most fundamental spatial functions of the brain is the allocation of spatial attention to objects and locations in the visual field. Thanks to this system, we can focus our visual attention on the book in front of us, yet still notice and look up if someone walks into the room.

When a lesion to one paretial lobe disrupts this allocation, the result is "hemispatial neglect." In this syndrome, individuals fail to pay attention to one side of space. The magnitude and persistence of this attentional impairment may astonish friends and family. After a right parietal lesion, for example, a person may fail to dress the left side of his or her body, leave food on the left side of a plate and complain about the hospital's stingy

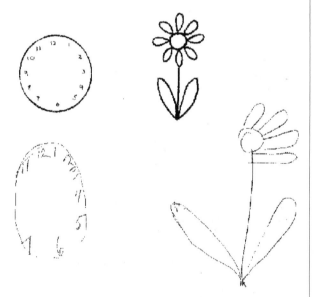

Examples of "hemispatial neglect." Damage to the parietal lobe can cause people to process information from only half their visual fields. A volunteer with this problem was asked to draw the clock and daisy at the top and produced the results below, missing details from the left side. Courtesy of Marlene Behrmann, Ph.D., Psychology & Center for the Neural Basis of Cognition, Carnegie Mellon University

portions, and simply ignore anyone who approaches from the left. Suggesting that the person orient to the left has little effect. Clearly, hemispatial neglect puts a person at risk for injury from walking into unnoticed objects on the affected side.

Bilateral damage to the parietal lobes can cause an even more severe loss of spatial attention, known as simultanagnosia. People with this disorder have trouble shifting their attention in any direction, left or right, and as a result see only one object at a time. In many ways, this condition is as disabling as blindness.

The visual areas of the parietal lobe are also important for guiding human action in space. This is true for small-scale spaces, where actions may include reaching for an object with the appropriate arm movement without knocking over other objects. It is also true for large-scale spaces, where actions may include moving toward destinations that may be distant and even out of sight while avoiding collisions along the way. With these functions the brain once again employs a divide-and-conquer strategy. Thus, the tasks of reaching for objects at nearby locations and of moving to distant objects are processed in different parts of the brain. Indeed, the process of navigating can itself be broken down into different components with different brain bases.

Each navigational process can therefore be disrupted separately by damage to different locations. The spatial-perception problems of simultanagnosia will impair a person's sense of orientation within the large-scale environment. A more specific form of environmental spatial impairment can follow damage to the posterior cingulate gyrus, located in the evolutionarily older limbic cortex of the brain. In this case, the individual cannot perceive and remember the spatial relations among landmarks in the environment, or his or her orientation relative to them.

A person's ability to navigate through the environment can also be disrupted by damage to the temporal system for recognizing objects described earlier. Such a person cannot recognize landmarks. In some cases, people become agnosic primarily for landmarks such as buildings, monuments, squares, and so on. This suggests the existence of yet another specialized processing system.

Visual Memory

The primary function of the cortical visual system is perception, but we also rely on it to represent visual and spatial information in the absence of external stimuli—in other words, to remember or imagine things. When we imagine the appearance of an object or the layout of a scene from memory, we are using some of the same mechanisms in the occipital, temporal, and parietal lobes that are used when we recognize and localize physically present and visible stimuli.

There are many reports of both imagery and perception being impaired after brain damage, which suggests that these functions are related. For example, people with acquired cortical color blindness frequently say that their mental images are devoid of color, and they have trouble answering questions that rely on creating mental images, such as, "What color are the stars on the American flag?" Individuals with agnosias of certain types, such as for faces, also report impaired imagery for that category.

Hemispatial neglect may also extend to mental images. Researchers first demonstrated this with people living in Milan, who were very familiar with the large central square known as the Piazza del Duomo. When asked to describe the piazza viewed from the steps of the cathedral, those with hemispatial neglect affecting the left side of perceived space mentioned the buildings on the right side of the vista they were imagining and omitted the ones on the left. To show that this was not simply due to one side of the piazza's being more memorable than the other, the scientists then asked the individuals to imagine the square from the opposite end. The people then described the buildings they had previously omitted, and neglected those they had mentioned before.

When a person's perception is intact but his or her imagery abilities are impaired, the underlying problem must lie somewhere other than the visual representations that are shared between perception and imagery. In some cases, the disruption appears to lie in the "image generation" process, by which we use long-term visual memory knowledge to reconstruct a visual mental image. Researchers have long noted such impairments, usually after damage to the visual areas of the left hemisphere.

Current research on vision and the brain is using functional brain imaging to confirm and extend what has been learned by studying neurological patients. In the future we are likely to see these methods combined, allowing researchers to image the brains of patients at different stages of recovery from visual-spatial impairment. Such an approach will teach us much about the development of vision beyond childhood, and may suggest new avenues of treatment to facilitate recovery.

Creativity, Talents, and Skills

For years, Einstein's brain has been a prized object of research that only a few scientists have been allowed to study, so it was national news in 1999 when some of those researchers reported finding a physical difference between the great physicist's brain and others. The difference was the absence of a particular groove (a "sulcus") in the cortex in an area of the brain that we generally use in mathematical thinking. The finding suggested that lacking the groove probably allowed Einstein's brain to devote more neuronal connections to his mathematical abilities.

Einstein's brain seems remarkable to us because of the way we think about creativity, talents, and skills. Most of us consider ourselves fortunate to have one or two of these attributes, and we believe that only a few lucky people have all three in combination, which adds up to fame. The good news is that this popular belief is wrong. Our brains are constructed for creativity, talents, and skills; some combination of all three is the rule, not the exception.

The Brain Basis of Talents and Skills

Looking at the brain allows us to appreciate the subtle differences among creativity, talents, and skills, as well as the way in which these attributes both overlap and stand apart.

Skills

Skills—the things we learn to do well—may be the most thoroughly studied, partly because they present a high profile in the brain and partly because a variety of disorders can impair them. Brain imaging studies in particular have shown that the development of a skill leads to differences in either brain anatomy, neural processing, or both. These differences have been observed, for example, in the way a highly skilled person uses memory (**B13**). Brain imaging studies comparing expert chess players with amateur players recently confirmed a longtime theory that expert players are able to "chunk" complex configurations into quickly discernible amounts of information for easy retrieval from memory. Researchers estimate that it takes 50,000 chunks (patterns of information) and approximately ten years to make an ex-

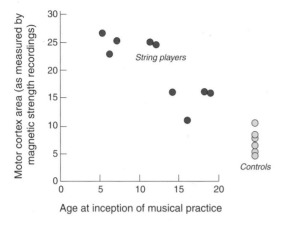

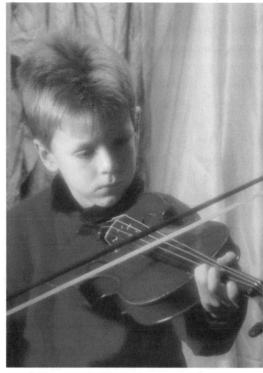

Learning a skill increases the amount of brain area devoted to the skill, as more neuronal connections form in the areas of the brain that the skill calls on most. One study found more motor cortex area devoted to the fingers in trained string players than in untrained people. It also found that the younger the person was at the start of musical training, the greater the area devoted to the skill. GRAPH © LEIGH CORIALE. ADAPTED WITH PERMISSION FROM *SCIENCE*, OCTOBER 13, 1995

© SUNSHINE INTERNATIONAL/ESTOCK PHOTOGRAPHY/PICTUREQUEST

pert. Studies of people with professional-level skill on a stringed musical instrument showed that, in the motor cortex, which is responsible for movement (B4), the areas devoted to finger movement had grown larger than in people who did not play. Other data analyzed in the study showed that this difference was greater the younger the musicians had been when they started their studies.

Talents

Talents, by contrast, and despite Einstein, are harder to pick out in the brain. The evidence of the brain's role, while intriguing, is indirect and warmly debated among researchers. For example, another study that looked at musicians found that the auditory association cortex (a left-hemisphere area of the brain that recognizes sound) was larger

in musicians with absolute pitch than in musicians without it and in nonmusicians. But it was impossible to say if this difference was inborn or a result of the way they listen. Because results like these run head-on into the argument over nature versus nurture, a more promising way to explore talents may be studies that focus on two types of children—gifted children and savants, both very different from other children at unusually young ages. Gifted children are striking for developing adult-level skills, often in music or language, but also in mathematics and spatial interests, such as geography, and frequently in more than one domain. They reach impressive levels of achievement rapidly, almost spontaneously, beginning as early as preschool. Savants, too, show unusual musical, linguistic, or artistic gifts as small children, but their talents dwell side by side with profound mental retardation (C3) or, sometimes, autism (C5). One of the key insights that child savants offer is how little general intelligence (B12) has to do with talent.

One interesting study of gifted individuals suggested that unusual talents in one area might represent the brain's response to problems in another. In this study, the researchers noticed that the personal histories of their subjects who were gifted in right hemisphere domains had more than the expected number of instances of dyslexia (C1) and other language difficulties, which are considered to be related to the left hemisphere. This led the investigators to ask if the right-hemisphere-oriented gifts could represent a compensatory development. Somewhat similarly, a recent study that looked at visual performance after one-sided brain damage offered the idea that weakness in one hemisphere could reduce the competition for the other. In other words, the hemispheres might typically be in a kind of tension or equilibrium that, if disturbed, can free the unaffected side to act more vigorously, with better results.

The nature-nurture debate over talents won't be settled anytime soon, but an area of research that seems to tip the scales slightly in favor of nature is behavioral genetics, particularly the findings of twin studies. The high heritability of certain talents is suggested by the findings that identical twins who were reared apart tend to be remarkably similar in their talents.

The main point brought home by studies of skills and talents in the brain is that we can set out to develop these attributes with confidence that our brains will cooperate, at least in the mechanical sense. Whether we end up satisfied with our efforts, however, may depend more on bringing a positive attitude and temperament, especially as we age. In general, the skills we use to develop our talents may work better if they are trained in youth (see chapter 6).

Creativity

Creativity may be notable for how often people deny having it. We tend to say, "I'm not creative; I can't write (or paint, or sing)." We may further limit our view of creativity to that which achieves formal recognition: for example, painting well enough to be shown in a gallery, or winning prizes for writing. But this common view, giving creativity a capital C, owes more to social or perhaps economic perspectives. From the standpoint of the brain, creativity is not only a distinct form of mental activity, it is also ubiquitous in human beings.

Everyday Creativity

Psychologists studying creativity put it in two categories, everyday creativity and eminent creativity. Everyday creativity is defined in terms of two criteria only—originality (something new) and meaningfulness (communicates something to others). Such creativity occurs widely across the activities of daily life, at work and at leisure. Everyday creativity can, of course, involve producing something "from scratch," such as writing or drawing, but it also includes accomplishments that use clever and original ideas to deal with tasks such as settling a problem at work, handling a difficult child, getting out of the woods when lost, starting a stalled car, or producing a meal from a skimpy larder. In other words, it's not what you do, it's *how* you do it, whether you're an entrepreneur, a parent, a home hobbyist, or a gourmet cook.

We tend not to realize that this is creativity; we may call it coping, making do, know-how, or savvy. Creativity, however, is a particularly human capability and perhaps a cognitive style. It is one that may be seen as essential to life, a fundamental survival capacity. Everyday creativity involves the suppleness of thinking that allows us to adjust to changing circumstances or to alter those circumstances when necessary. Research has suggested that everyday creativity is not only necessary in our response to our environment but also has an ongoing role in our health. Numerous studies of aging identify flexibility, improvisation, and the ability to take new perspectives and think for oneself—all characteristics of everyday creativity—as qualities associated with longevity. Other research has found that creative activity improves health. Hundreds of studies show successful healing provided by art therapy, music therapy, drama therapy, dance therapy, and writing therapy. For example, in one set of studies subjects who wrote about their traumatic experiences made fewer doctor's visits, reported increased feelings of well-being, and had elevated levels of two biological markers of immune function. By contrast, feelings of helplessness, an inability to think of a "way out," and paralysis of action—the loss of everyday creativity—are the hallmarks of depression **(C20)** and its debilitating effects on mental and physical health.

The evidence is plentiful that creative work can contribute to the healing of psychological problems. For many years research has found that creative people tend to have a number of positive characteristics for mental health, including a high level of autonomy, motivated goal setting, a wide range of interests, and originality. Creativity may be used as a way to help resolve internal conflicts or as protection against the disorganizing and immobilizing potential of such conflicts. Creative capabilities can help individuals tolerate ambiguity and uncertainty and enable them to reshape their world at a higher level of organization.

Eminent Creativity

In contrast to the importance to individuals of everyday creativity, eminent creativity is activity that a culture elevates as meaningful, formally recognizing it through monetary reward, prizes, and honors. We can say an eminent creator is an everyday creator who is a special case because his or her creativity has achieved social recognition and serves a wider social purpose. Eminent creativity also offers many ways for researchers to explore the underlying features of creative mental activity.

A longtime question in this regard has been about the significance to creativity of the brain's distribution of processing to either the left hemisphere or the right hemisphere. Starting in the 1960s, when this distribution was first recognized, researchers theorized that the right side of the brain was primarily responsible for creative activity, whereas the left side was more linear and mathematical. This led to a popular stereotype of people being right-brained or left-brained. However, improved electroencephalographic (EEG) measurements and functional brain imaging technology subsequently showed this division to be much too simplistic. For example, EEG studies clearly indicate that solving complicated creative verbal tasks involves both the left and right sides of the brain. Other research using brain scanning has found that when we listen to music, which is supposedly a right-brain activity, our auditory association cortex and language areas, both usually located mainly in the left hemisphere, are highly active.

Another way to get at creativity is through the study of intelligence. Neuropsychological studies *may* indicate that intellectually advanced individuals are mentally less active during problem solving than average individuals. (This is still speculative but is interesting and important in exploring the way the brain functions during the process of problem solving.) Two possibilities may explain why this occurs. Some researchers propose an "efficiency" hypothesis, suggesting that irrelevant areas of the brain aren't used during problem solving. Use of task-relevant areas may cause this. Another possibility is that the lower mental activity may define the ability of good problem solvers to bring order into their thoughts and operations.

Although expertise may fit more into the category of skill than creativity, experts and eminent creators appear to share a common specialty in their use of memory. A good example in experts is the chess master's facility in "chunking" some 50,000 patterns in memory, mentioned earlier. In highly creative people, memory also probably differs from the norm, storing information in patterns that more easily allow insight, analogical transfer of knowledge, and access to unusual, remote associations. Experts also develop protocols, which have been studied by having them think aloud. For example, a chess expert recalls potential moves and then plays them out mentally, making adjustments as necessary. Eminent creators may also make use of such tailored rules for their actions. Once expertise is achieved, however, highly creative individuals will carry their involvement a step further and attempt to make a novel contribution to their area by studying and analyzing the work of masters in their field.

Eminent creativity is not just a matter of the brain's ability to manage a prodigious amount of the information related to a particular art or science. Other requirements, such as flexible thinking and originality, are also required for creativity. From these requirements, research has found, emerges an unusual connection, the only one of its kind that seems to apply to mental life: an advantage for creativity from the presence of mental illness.

Creativity and Mood Disorders

The popular belief in a connection between creativity and psychological disorder may indeed have a basis in truth—but it may be a little more complicated than Dryden said in *Absalom and Achitophel:* "Great wits are sure to madness near allied/And thin partitions do their bounds divide." Eminent artists show very high rates of mood disorders, particularly bipolar disorder, or manic-depressive illness (C24). For example, in one set of studies of eminent writers, as many as 80 percent had experienced at least one episode of clinical depression (C20), and more than half had bipolar disorder. Eminent nonartists (such as social scientists and physicists, for example) present a healthier profile.

Efforts to understand this phenomenon go back more than a century. Freud saw creativity as a way of solving the basic conflict involving sex and aggression. The struggle to solve these conflicts, if unconscious material is not disguised and transformed through creative activity, may emerge as neurosis. One difficulty with this was always that, as friends and family of mood-

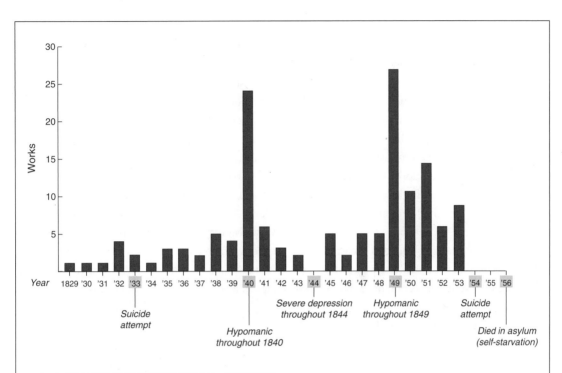

Year: 1829 '30 '31 '32 '33 '34 '35 '36 '37 '38 '39 '40 '41 '42 '43 '44 '45 '46 '47 '48 '49 '50 '51 '52 '53 '54 '55 '56

Suicide attempt

Hypomanic throughout 1840

Severe depression throughout 1844

Hypomanic throughout 1849

Suicide attempt

Died in asylum (self-starvation)

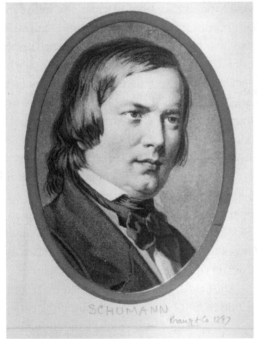

The composer Robert Schumann (1810–1856) probably suffered from bipolar disorder. During his manic periods he created many works, though not necessarily his best. During his depressed states, Schumann produced little and repeatedly tried to end his life. PHOTO COURTESY OF THE LIBRARY OF CONGRESS. CHART COURTESY OF K. R. JAMISON, WITH PERMISSION OF S. KARGER AG, BASEL; ADAPTED BY LEIGH CORIALE

disordered artists can testify, neurosis may continue despite creative activity.

Jung saw less abnormality in the manifestations of mood disorders by highly creative people, maintaining that we are all born with a collective unconscious that includes dreams, visions, religious experiences, and myths. Still another perspective, Janusian theory, proposes that creativity consists of holding two opposite thoughts simultaneously so that something new is conceived—a use of mind perhaps made easier by the help of a disorder.

Superficially, the link between creativity and mood disorders may appear to be one of style: a depressed poet writes sad sonnets; a manic playwright gives the world a slapstick comedy. Indeed, the experience of a mood disorder may provide rich material for the artist. But at the level of the brain, the link is much more basic. A disorder's possible effects involve thought, affect, and motivation—or, to put it another way, creativity and these disorders share similarities in how the mind works.

Modern cognitive science has sorted out several characteristic features of creativity: the bringing together of unusual material or connections through intersecting frames of reference, discrete remote associations, a more generally "overinclusive" cognitive style that allows richer associative networks in the brain, and chance configurations in creativity, in interaction with social and historical forces. Another feature, which researchers have called flow, or being in the moment, is considered the creative brain's facilitator for creative activity including analogies, metaphors, dreams, visualization, and meditation.

Some of these characteristic features of creativity are reminiscent of the mind in a hypomanac (or mildly mood-elevated) phase of bipolar illness, particularly overinclusiveness, extremely rapid thought, and a sense of great and profound insight. Both eminent creators and everyday creators suffering with these disorders report to researchers that they can receive benefits from their disorder in three areas: thought (freer associative process), affect (richer experience), and motivation (confidence and energy)—up to a point. These reports are so common that the phenomenon has come to be called the creative advantage. Many studies have tried to pin down exactly where, along the spectrum of mental states, a disorder's effects may serve a creator's goals. The evidence seems to show that, within varied mood states, a state of mild mood elevation is particularly conducive to varied phenomena, including unusual associations, overinclusion, and creative problem solving.

Studies of noneminent creators that investigated the occurrences of creativity and mood disorders among those with manic-depression and their biological relatives have turned up very interesting findings. The creative advantage has also been seen with psychiatrically normal relatives of patients with bipolar disorder, suggesting that suffering the pain of the disorder may not be necessary to have the effect. In addition, depressive persons with a family history of bipolar disorder may also show the effect, compared with people with depression without a bipolar family history. This is important, because creative people who have bipolar disorder have more relatives with unipolar depression or milder dysthymias than relatives with bipolar disorder.

The field of genetics may one day make a contribution to this issue: the question is why these mood disorders are so prevalent and so persistent down through the generations. The fact that family members who do not have bipolar disorder

CREATIVITY AND LIABILITY FOR SCHIZOPHRENIA

A variety of observations and studies link creativity with another mental illness, schizophrenia (C25). Two of the twentieth century's most creative figures in their fields, Albert Einstein (science) and James Joyce (literature), both had children who were treated for schizophrenia, while John Nash, a Nobel laureate in economics, was diagnosed with schizophrenia after he had completed his most creative work. A 1992 study reviewing the biographies of many of the twentieth century's most influential avant-garde writers and artists concluded that many had a type of personality disorder that may be genetically related to schizophrenia. Such studies have led to the suggestion that a tendency toward psychoticism, when present to a milder degree, might actually be conducive to creativity. In a recent study testing these predictions, a questionnaire measuring proneness to psychosis was filled out by professional artists and control subjects, nonartists similar in age and education. The artists scored significantly higher. Another study had college students take personality tests as well as paper-and-pencil tests of creativity. This study found that the students who appeared to be more creative by paper-and-pencil measures scored significantly higher on scales of proneness to psychosis.

Several other studies compared the creativity of biological relatives of people with schizophrenia with that of control subjects, as measured by third-party judgments of how creative the individuals had been in their jobs and hobbies. For example, a study in Iceland found that the biological relatives of those with schizophrenia were significantly more likely than other people to be listed in *Who's Who* as having distinguished themselves in a creative profession. A meticulously designed study examined the creativity of the work and hobbies of Danish adoptees who were born to either parents with schizophrenia or control parents with no history of psychiatric hospitalization. Both groups of adoptees were placed with adoptive parents at an early age. In the study, evaluators, who were not told the adoptees' personal and family histories of psychopathology, assessed the creativity of the adoptees' activities. The scales used to rate creativity were designed to reflect creativity not just in the fine arts or sciences, but in a wide variety of job and hobby activities. The hypothesis was that the greatest creativity would be found in individuals who had schizotypal traits because, while not psychotic, they would be more likely to carry genes for schizophrenia. These genes would tend to predispose them to unusual styles of thinking and perceiving, which in turn would be conducive to creative ideas. As predicted, adoptees who did not have full-blown schizophrenia but *did* have multiple schizotypal signs (such as odd speech, recurrent illusions, or magical thinking) were rated as showing greater creativity in their jobs or hobbies than adoptees who had one or none of these signs.

enjoy the creative advantage suggests that understanding the genetics of the disorder offers the possibility of protecting and fostering the cognitive style involving features such as "overinclusion." Thus the openness to the outside world and one's inner states that are typical of this style—and are physically as well as psychologically healthy—could be sustained while treating the harmful and debilitating effects of the disorder.

It is critically important that mood disorders not be romanticized: the rate of suicide for untreated persons with bipolar disorder is 20 percent.

Moreover, the disorder in its full-blown state is not conducive to creativity but detrimental to it. Only along the road to that misery, when the disorder passes through the stage of mild mood elevation, do creators report any benefit. Most important, not only are these disorders highly treatable, but treatment appears to enhance rather than detract from creativity. (Remember, family members who are not ill also demonstrate the creative advantage, so it must not be necessary to be ill first.)

Creativity and Psychopathology: Some Practical Implications

Findings linking creativity to psychopathology have potential practical implications for fostering both mental health and creativity. First of all, the associations between creativity and liability for schizophrenia or bipolar disorder may apply not simply to a few psychotic geniuses in the fine arts, but also to *non*eminent or "everyday," levels of creativity in a wide variety of fields of endeavor in the general population. The results suggest that the association may also extend, not only to the millions of individuals who have a diagnosis of outright schizophrenia or bipolar disorder, but also to the much larger group of individuals who carry genes that predispose them to the disorders. Knowing that the genes that carry risk for these disorders may actually have a *beneficial* aspect, or "silver lining," could help boost the morale of patients and their families, as well as combat the stigma that is often associated with these illnesses.

Finally, it bears repeating that the studies have found the greatest creativity, on average, not in individuals who suffered from full-blown forms of these disorders, but rather in individuals who had mild psychiatric symptoms—or even none—but who *were* biologically related to a patient with bipolar disorder or schizophrenia. That underscores the importance of treatment: to realize the potential creative advantages that may be associated with genetic liability for these disorders, one need *not* pay the price of the suffering that is often associated with them.

PART IV

Conditions of the Brain and Nervous System

CHAPTER 12

Conditions That Appear in Childhood

C1   **Dyslexia**   248

C2   **Attention Deficit/Hyperactivity Disorder**   254

C3   **Mental Retardation**   259

C4   **Cerebral Palsy**   265

C5   **Autism**   270

C6   **Metabolic Diseases**   278

C7   **Neurofibromatosis**   284

C8   **Hydrocephalus**   288

C9   **Spina Bifida**   293

C10 **Tumors of Childhood**   298

Our nervous systems develop in crucial ways in the womb and during the first years of life, as chapters 5 and 6 explain. Babies arrive unable to hold up their heads or control their limbs, and after a year they are usually moving around on their own. Parents watch for a child's first step and first word, and pediatricians and child psychologists have identified many similar landmarks in our first years. Children do not exhibit these abilities according to a strict timetable. Nevertheless, when a young child's development seems unusually delayed, or he or she appears to be losing abilities once learned, parents and doctors have reason for concern. Those events might be the signs of a developmental disorder or a physical condition affecting the brain.

In many cases such disorders arise from a child's genes; often, therefore, genetic testing can verify or rule out certain explanations. Rarely do such disorders stem from an event during a child's early months. Sometimes children benefit from surgery or medications and resume developing like other children. In other cases, the disorder is a lifelong condition that might require physical assistance, special education, or other aid. No matter what their condition, young children are capable of further development with their families' support and love.

Dyslexia

Dyslexia is a brain disorder that primarily affects a person's ability to read and write. In fact, the word's Greek roots simply mean "language problems." Dyslexia is the best known of the specific learning disabilities—problems with mastering particular types of information, such as numbers or spatial relations, rather than low intellectual performance in general. Dyslexia is also the best defined of these problems, and the best understood. Although these disorders originate in the brain, they are not medical problems in the sense that a physician or surgeon can cure them. Instead, the accepted treatment for dyslexia and similar conditions consists of specific, structured forms of training.

In rare cases, a person starts to suffer dyslexia because of a stroke (**C59, C60**) or injury affecting particular parts of the brain. Much more often, dyslexia appears as a developmental disorder in childhood. Some toddlers have difficulty learning to speak: a delay occurs in normal speech development between two and three years of age, or the children frequently mispronounce words. These children seem to be at higher risk for developing dyslexia, and parents should watch their progress carefully so that they can receive appropriate education as soon as they enter school. Usually, however, parents have no clues about their child's possible dyslexia before he or she first encounters reading and writing.

Most children easily learn the basics of how to read in kindergarten or first grade, but dyslexics do not. Schoolteachers and parents can often tell that a child is having difficulty as soon as reading lessons begin. It is important to help these children from the very start and to track their progress closely. However, it is unreasonable to label a child at that level because many children who start reading slowly will catch up with most of their peers within two years.

To make a diagnosis of dyslexia, most specialists look for a discrepancy between a child's chronological age and his or her reading age, with a two-year gap being the most common indicator. Children usually begin to read in kindergarten or first grade, when they are 5 or 6. In theory, therefore, the problem cannot be spotted until children reach age 7 or 8, in the second or third grade. An 8-year-old dyslexic would be reading at a first-grade level or below.

Another important indicator that a child might have dyslexia is whether members of his or her family have been diagnosed with the disorder or have a history of reading problems. As many as 50 percent of children from families with dyslexia will exhibit the learning disability during the school years. However, in previous generations, schools recognized dyslexia much less often; a parent or other relative may therefore not be aware of the root of his or her own frustrations with reading. Sometimes uncomfortable memories of school affect how parents react to the possibility that their child is dyslexic; some resist such "labeling" and the special lessons that go with it. In other families, learning that a mysterious problem has a history and a name actually comforts parents and makes them more eager to help their child overcome it.

There are no brain markers for dyslexia, so ordinary computerized axial tomography (CAT) scans, magnetic resonance imaging (MRI), or electroencephalograms (EEGs) are no help in diagnosing it. A physiological test called event-related potentials (ERPs), which clinicians can do as early as infancy, has been shown to predict which groups of children are more likely to develop dyslexia, but this test cannot forecast the course of an individual child's development.

Misconceptions and Realities

A diagnosis of dyslexia implies nothing about a child's intelligence, emotional makeup, neurological health, or cultural and educational potential. Some bright children have dyslexia; so do some children who are mildly retarded in overall learning. Sometimes children with dyslexia suffer emotional problems, either because of their frustration in school or because of other factors. These students' feelings can make it harder for them to deal with the language problem and learn ways around it, but their emotional states do not cause or worsen the disorder.

Culture plays a role in dyslexia, of course. The condition could not be identified in an illiterate society. Furthermore, the language a child grows up using affects how hard it is to overcome the disorder. English is problematic for dyslexics because it contains many inconsistencies between sounds and their written symbols. In contrast, modern Italian is more uniform in spelling and pronunciation, and fewer young Italians seem to have problems with dyslexia. Nonetheless, there is no evidence to support the notion that such cultural factors as different ways of teaching children to read cause dyslexia.

In every major culture today, being able to read and write well is a gateway to further education and success. Dyslexics often lose out on opportunities because of their disability. Many trickle to the bottom of the socioeconomic ladder, and more than a fair share even take to criminal behavior. Low self-esteem and its many psychiatric complications are common. These problems are not due to anything inherent in dyslexics' brains but to a lack of adequate educational interventions when they were young. Recent research and publicity have increased public awareness of dyslexia, and common misconceptions that these children are lazy and irresponsible—that they just aren't trying to learn—have begun to fade.

Today the controversies surrounding dyslexia usually involve scarce resources and perceptions of fairness. In many communities, school budgets and teachers' time are stretched thin. How much of those precious resources, people ask, should be devoted to special education? Should a child who has dyslexia but few other difficulties receive extra time and attention? If a child has trouble reading along with other cognitive problems, such as attention deficit/hyperactivity disorder (ADHD; **C2**) or poor memory, what is the most appropriate way to assist him or her? Does identifying some children as dyslexic label them as inferior and unlikely to catch up with their peers? Would it be better for these children's self-esteem and education to say they have a "learning difference," not a "disability"? Semantics aside, our society seems to have reached a consensus that schools should help all children learn to their full potential, even if some need special attention more frequently than others. (We all need special attention sometimes, after all.)

Another flash point is the flexibility some dyslexics request on assignments, standardized tests, and other classroom challenges. Is it fair for a dyslexic student to have extra time to read an exam or write an essay, or assistants to take notes and read textbooks aloud? Some people speak of dyslexia as a "fancy label for unsuccessful rich kids," even though all socioeconomic classes are touched by the problem. It is important to realize that dyslexia is not a catchall term for trouble in school, or even trouble with reading; it is a diagnosis of a brain condition based on specific, scientifically based criteria. Simply because dyslexic children look like most of their peers and exhibit a wide range of aptitudes doesn't mean that they aren't all working to overcome a real problem.

Forms of Dyslexia

For most dyslexics, the disorder involves the ability to understand the sound structure of their native tongue. To learn to read and to acquire new written words throughout life, we must match a visual symbol (a grapheme, such as a letter) to a speech sound (a phoneme). As we speak or comprehend what others say, we are not conscious of the individual sounds that make up words, even though we must have representations of these sounds in our minds. But to learn to read, we must become aware of which individual sounds correspond to which letters. Reading involves seeing the correspondence between the sights and sounds of language.

Dyslexic children most often have problems consciously recognizing the sounds of their native language. This form of the disorder, known as phonological dyslexia, can be revealed by various challenges: rhyming, decoding pig Latin, breaking words into segments, identifying words after the removal of one phoneme. Dyslexics of this sort also have trouble reading pseudowords like *cattigen, teepress,* and *berticks* because they cannot map individual letters to the sounds they correspond with. Known words are easier to recognize because we can assemble clues: a familiar visual feature, the word's general shape, its context. Such pointers probably help all of us recognize words, but for dyslexic readers they are crucial. (In fact, some children with dyslexia become very adept at such skills and at otherwise masking their difficulties with reading and writing.)

Autopsy studies of phonological dyslexics indicate that the brain areas involved in language processes can develop minor malformations during the fetal period. Imaging studies of such people using language or performing other cognitive tasks show dysfunction in the parts of the cerebral cortex that are involved in phonological processing and auditory-visual association. All of this points to phonological dyslexia as an innate, constitutional problem that arises during early brain development and becomes apparent only when a child is exposed to reading.

In contrast, some dyslexics (probably a small proportion, but the exact numbers are not known) have no unusual problems handling speech sounds. They can read pseudowords with ease. These dyslexics have trouble only with irregular words, such as *enough, yacht,* and *naive.* This form of the disorder is known as surface dyslexia. In stroke and brain injuries, the site of the lesion that produces problems with reading irregular words is different from that causing problems with pseudowords. It should therefore be the case that the two forms of developmental dyslexia, phonological and surface, have separate brain mechanisms. This, however, has not yet been proven.

An even rarer form of the disorder is called deep dyslexia. This type of reading disorder can appear after diffuse brain injury or in conditions such as Alzheimer's disease (**C67**). It consists of reading words as other words related to them in meaning—for instance, *chair* for *table.* Deep dyslexia is rare in the West, but may be more common for children learning to read languages like Chinese, where the visual forms of words with related meanings may be quite close to one another.

Dyslexics may also have problems with processing rapidly changing sounds not involved in language. It is not clear how many people have this difficulty, however, or how it affects learning to read.

Little is known about the biological factors that increase the risk for developmental dyslexia. There is no evidence to support the idea that dyslexia results from a pregnant mother's ingestion of toxins or from direct injury to the fetus. On the other hand, there is certainly a genetic component, as the condition tends to run in families. Several studies have implicated genes on chromosomes 15, 6, 1, and 2, each occurring in different families. This suggests that there are probably several independent genetic causes of dyslexia. It is also possible that different genes are associated with different types of the disorder—a gene on chromosome 6 with the phonological form, for instance. No specific gene or genes have been identified, however.

Getting to the biological roots of dyslexia is difficult because the disorder is so complex. We expect that genetic research will lead to improvements in classifying dyslexia into different types, each of which will respond to a different treatment. Even based on what we know today, there is no reason to expect that one educational program will work for all dyslexics. Discovering early markers for a high risk of developing dyslexia will also allow educators to intervene earlier and probably produce better outcomes for students.

Helping a Child Overcome Dyslexia

The treatment of dyslexia is seldom medical. Rather, it is most often treated educationally, with specially designed tutoring that relies heavily on phonological training. If, however, a student is also suffering from ADHD (**C2**), depression (**C20**), anxiety (**C21**), or epilepsy (**C13**), a physician may treat these conditions to improve the child's general cognitive function and thus increase the benefit of the educational program.

The treatment should begin soon after specialists confirm the diagnosis of dyslexia. Most states define special-education procedures by law as a way to ensure that every child in public schools can benefit. Schools start by alerting the student's parents to the situation and proposing a program of lessons tailored to help the child over-

WHEN READING IS HARD ON THE EYES

The reading problems of some dyslexics may stem from, or include, difficulty processing rapidly changing visual images. A part of the visual system called the magnocellular pathway stabilizes images as our eyes move across a page. If the magnocellular pathway is impaired, a person may feel eye discomfort while reading. This is different from the eyestrain that develops from reading intently for a long time, which usually goes away with rest.

Judging from autopsy studies, functional MRI (fMRI), and experiments in which people look at flashing geometric figures or moving pictures while researchers measure their event-related potentials (ERPs), the areas of the brain involved in this condition are different from the language areas. These findings point to a brain region known as the thalamus, which includes sites related to hearing and seeing, and the visual and auditory cortices.

That these visual deficits affect a person's ability to read is not widely accepted, but they could contribute to a reading problem. Specialists have used tinted lenses or eye patches to deal with this obstacle, with variable and unclear results. Debate therefore continues about the usefulness of these approaches, but when a dyslexic child complains of such visual symptoms as distortions, eye fatigue, or double vision, it's reasonable to consider them.

come his or her specific difficulties. Educators can take no special steps without the parents' approval, but parents cannot dictate every detail of their children's education; teachers and families need to work together. There is usually a regular schedule for evaluating the child's progress and revising the program as needed.

Dyslexia treatments almost always consist of structured lessons in language use and especially in reading. These usually require students to work for at least part of the school day with a teacher alone or in a small group, away from the distractions of a larger class. Students' reading strategies change with practice and maturity. The letter-by-letter approach that is crucial when a child is just beginning to read becomes less important later. As students grow older, they also become more aware of what's most difficult for them and how they can manage those reading challenges.

A more recent approach to dyslexia involves training children to recognize rapidly changing sounds; this is based on the finding that many dyslexics experience difficulties with such sounds. However, the jury is still out on whether this treatment helps with reading. The best evidence indicates that no matter what other treatments are employed, dyslexics still need specific reading instruction.

The improvement of a child's dyslexic symptoms depends on the severity of the problem, his or her general intelligence, the age when treatment begins, and the parents' support. Early recognition is an important factor. Unfortunately, fiscal considerations often determine how early and to what extent children can receive appropriate help. As ongoing research discloses what portion of reading problems relate to perceptual deficits, visual and auditory, and

ABCs OF DYSLEXIA

Dyslexia is difficulty with language. Intelligence is not the problem; the problem is language. People who are dyslexic may have difficulty with reading, spelling, understanding language they hear, or expressing themselves clearly in speaking or in writing. An unexpected gap exists between their potential for learning and their school achievement.

- **DYSLEXIA:** a language-based disability, in which a person has trouble understanding words, sentences, or paragraphs; both oral and written language is affected.

- **DYSCALCULIA:** a mathematical disability in which a person has unusual difficulty solving arithmetic problems and grasping math concepts.

- **DYSGRAPHIA:** a neurologically based writing disability in which a person finds it hard to form letters or write within a defined space.

- **AUDITORY/VISUAL PROCESSING DISORDERS:** disorders in which a person has difficulty understanding language despite normal hearing and vision.

Source: *Basic Facts About Dyslexia: What Every Layperson Ought to Know,* copyright © 1993, 2nd edition 1998, The International Dyslexia Association

what part is cognitive and linguistic, specialists will introduce newer and more effective treatments.

Most people with dyslexia can eventually read at near normal levels with good comprehension. They may always have problems with spelling and learning foreign languages. Often continued difficulties or a return of the problem after a period of improvement can be linked to changes in demand (for example, college suddenly requires much more reading) or other problems (inadequate sleep, depression, anxiety, abuse of alcohol, and more). Overcoming these separate challenges can put young people back on track for progress with reading. Adults with dyslexia have succeeded in many fields, including finance, film, politics, art, and even creative writing, so the condition does not have to limit a person's accomplishments.

Attention Deficit/Hyperactivity Disorder

The label "attention deficit/hyperactivity disorder" (ADHD) refers to a family of chronic neurobiological disorders that interfere with people's capacity to attend to tasks, regulate their activity, and inhibit their behavior in ways appropriate to their ages and circumstances. There are actually three subtypes of ADHD:

■ Inattentive type—characterized principally by difficulty paying attention to tasks.

■ Hyperactive-impulsive type—characterized by being overly active and impulsive.

■ Combined type—the most common form, characterized by *both* inattentive and hyperactive-impulsive symptoms.

All children have occasional trouble paying attention or suppressing their impulses. ADHD is a chronic condition, however, and its main symptoms have a larger effect on people's lives.

Inattention. People with ADHD often have a hard time keeping their minds on one thing and may get bored with a task after only a few minutes. Focusing conscious, deliberate attention to or-ganizing and completing routine tasks may be difficult. However, the problem may not be uniform across all settings: a child or adult with ADHD may focus very well on some activities that require different forms of attention, such as video games or highly stimulating experiences.

Hyperactivity. People with the full syndrome of ADHD (combined type), particularly boys in the elementary school years, usually seem to be in constant motion. They can't sit still; they may dash around or talk incessantly. For them, sitting through a lesson can be impossible. They may roam around the room, squirm in their seats, wiggle their feet, touch everything, or noisily tap a pencil. The motor hyperactivity tends to decrease with age. Adolescents and adults with ADHD may report feeling intensely restless without actually having to move so much.

Impulsivity. People with ADHD often seem unable to curb their immediate reactions or to think before they act. As a result, they may blurt out answers to questions, make inappropriate comments, or run into the street without looking. In the case of children, their impulsivity may make it hard for them to wait for things they want or to take turns in games. They may grab toys from other children or hit when they are upset.

ADHD is the most commonly diagnosed disorder of childhood, estimated to affect 3 percent to 5 percent of school-age children. On average, about one child in every classroom in the United States needs help for this disorder. Parents or preschool teachers often notice the first manifestations of ADHD in a child who cannot sustain attention on a level comparable to his or her peers. Parents and teachers may be concerned that this child "can't sit still," "can't pay attention," daydreams, or needs repeated reminders to stay on task, finish household chores, or do schoolwork. At times, the child's difficulties with attention may be more subtle or masked by other activities, such as acting the "class clown" or being overly social and talkative.

ADHD occurs three times more often in boys than in girls. Furthermore, because girls tend to display fewer obvious problems with motor hyperactivity, they are often not diagnosed, or are diagnosed two to three years after boys. Likewise, very bright children with ADHD may be missed because they are "getting by," but they often significantly underperform in comparison with their intellectual abilities.

Life is often very difficult for children and adolescents with ADHD. They face challenges sitting still and paying attention in class, at home, and even in the playground. As a result, they often may be in trouble at school, cannot finish games, and have difficulties making friends. They may spend hours each night struggling to keep their minds on their homework, then forget to bring it to school.

Complicating these problems, young people with ADHD often experience negative consequences of their behavior: being scolded, doing poorly on tests, or being shunned by classmates. Their difficulties can increase family conflict. Adolescents with ADHD are at increased risk for having automobile accidents, using tobacco, becoming pregnant, and doing poorly in school.

Approximately 60 percent to 80 percent of children will continue to experience significant symptoms of ADHD in adulthood. As adults, people with ADHD face a higher risk of lower vocational attainment, marital problems, and injuries of all sorts and an increased likelihood of substance use or abuse (C29). However, those poor outcomes are far from definite, and many people with ADHD have recognized their problems with inattention and impulsivity and found successful ways of coping.

Mechanisms of ADHD

Though we still do not know the exact brain mechanisms underpinning ADHD, imaging studies have linked the condition with specific structures of the brain. Using magnetic resonance imaging (MRI), a number of teams in the United States and abroad have examined the prefrontal cortex, basal ganglia, and cerebellum in children with ADHD. The results of these studies indicate that in children with ADHD, the size of these structures is 5 percent to 10 percent smaller than in ordinary children. These same structures, especially the prefrontal cortex and basal ganglia, are rich in dopamine receptors. And since such medications as methylphenidate (Ritalin) work on dopamine receptors, these findings support the hypothesis that one underlying problem for children with ADHD involves disturbances in the dopamine-signaling system.

Researchers have used functional brain imaging to compare children with and without ADHD. These studies initially used single-photon-emission computed tomography (SPECT) and positron-emission tomography (PET) to estimate where blood flows in a child's brain. In general, these studies showed lower than normal blood flow into the brain areas already implicated in ADHD. The PET studies in particular have shown that the reduced blood flow is related to the severity of ADHD symptoms. In the past several years, a number of investigators have used functional magnetic resonance imaging (fMRI) to further document the relatively low blood flow in specific brain regions, and these findings have generally confirmed the earlier SPECT and PET studies of ADHD children and adults. Most recently, two PET studies have found that administering methylphenidate to ADHD children appears to increase blood flow to these brain areas.

Similar studies have not always yielded consistent findings, but all together they are providing promising results, and the methods continue to improve. At this time, imaging is still not appropriate for diagnosing children with ADHD or screening them for it.

Factors in ADHD

One of the difficulties in researching the possible genetic aspect of ADHD is that the diagnosis can be overapplied. Studies must start by rigorously identifying people with the disorder using standard, reliable assessment procedures. When that is done, ADHD appears to be highly heritable. However, there have been few studies on the normal development and regulation of attention; since we do not know all the basics of this brain function, we may not know all that can go wrong with it. Furthermore, there may be nongenetic forces involved in turning supposedly "fixed" genes off and on. Therefore, we must be cautious about assigning an immutable role to genetic factors in the onset and development of ADHD.

Geneticists are following two major approaches to identify genes associated with ADHD. The first, called whole-genome scanning, relies on obtaining DNA from large groups of affected family members (usually siblings). The research team tries to find links between specific chromosomal markers and ADHD disorder traits. The second method involves focusing on what is termed a candidate gene. Using this strategy, investigators typically examine people for the frequency of various forms of specific genes known to be of possible interest in understanding the source of the disorder.

A number of candidate genes have been investigated by researchers in the last five years. A particular form of the dopamine transporter gene (DAT1) has been found to be associated with ADHD, and another candidate gene under study is dopamine D4 receptor (DRD4). Unlike similar studies involving other neuropsychiatric disorders, more times than not independent laboratories have been able to replicate the original findings of these studies, indicating that the work is on the right track. Investigators are also exploring other candidate genes involved in the dopamine and noradrenaline signaling systems, with promising results.

There are also nongenetic factors in the development of ADHD. Mothers of affected children are more likely to have had complications during pregnancy, such as toxemia, lengthy labor and delivery, excessive nausea, and undue weight loss or gain. High-quality care before and just after birth may therefore forestall the development of ADHD in children who would otherwise be vulnerable.

Some environmental toxins have been implicated in the development of ADHD: alcohol and nicotine in the fetal brain, and lead in growing children. Much more attention has been paid to the supposed role of food additives, sugar, and possible food allergens, but few rigorous studies of these substances have been replicated, and their possible effects remain controversial. Though studies of possible toxins and other chemical factors are intriguing, findings generally indicate that they account for relatively few cases of ADHD. Many children are exposed to comparable levels of these substances without developing the disorder. That fact indicates that combinations of trauma, toxic exposure, and subtle forms of brain injury, along with a certain pattern of susceptibility genes, are required for the full syndrome of ADHD to emerge.

Diagnosis and Treatment

Physicians and other health care practitioners can identify ADHD reliably using well-tested diagnostic interview methods. Checklists can be useful as screening devices, but doctors should

---

ADVICE FOR PARENTS OF CHILDREN WITH ADHD

Living with and helping a child diagnosed with ADHD is challenging and sometimes overwhelming. Here are some tips on how to be an effective parent:

- **Do research. Scientists are learning more about ADHD all the time, and the Internet offers numerous sites with updates on research.**

- **Seek professional evaluation and treatment. An assessment of your child's strengths and weaknesses can help both you and the doctors develop an effective treatment plan.**

- **Join a support group. Networks of other parents dealing with the same issues are an invaluable source for information, guidance, and support.**

Parent training from a qualified mental health professional can teach you strategies and techniques to change behavior and improve relationships between parent and child. Some of these include:

- **providing clear expectations and limits**

- **setting up an effective discipline system**

- **assisting your child with adjustments to different social situations**

- **setting aside daily time for your child**

Adapted from www.chadd.org (Children and Adults with Attention-Deficit/Hyperactivity Disorder); additional resource: www.add.org (National ADD Association)

not rely on them as diagnostic tools. Using check-lists alone tends to identify far more children as having ADHD than careful interviews—up to two or three times more. The most reliable diagnoses are based on careful history and observable behaviors in the child's or youth's usual settings. Ideally, a health care practitioner should obtain information from parents and teachers.

Children usually do not recognize their ADHD symptoms. Adults with ADHD appear to be more accurate in describing their behaviors and feelings, however.

Treating ADHD usually involves medication, specific forms of psychotherapy or training in social skills, and often a combination of these strategies. They are effective in different ways.

Medication Strategies

By far the most widely researched and commonly prescribed treatments for ADHD are psychostimulant medications, including methylphenidate (for example, Ritalin, Concerta, Metadate), amphetamine (Dexedrine and Adderall), and pemoline (Cylert). Many studies have demonstrated their short-term efficacy compared with placebos in improving both core ADHD symptoms and associated features. These investigations have used a wide variety of assessment methods, including ratings from parents and teachers, direct observations of children in natural and laboratory settings, and performance on objective laboratory tests. Controlled studies of stimulants have shown them to be effective in reducing interruptions in class, activities not relevant to schoolwork, and overt and covert aggression and in improving performance on spelling and arithmetic tasks, sustained attention and compliance, making friends, short-term memory, and parent-child interactions. There have been studies showing that stimulants improve a child's attention during baseball.

These short-term benefits are limited by several important considerations. First, treating ADHD with medication alone does not always help a child attain normal behavior or improve in all domains of functioning. In addition, most investigations of stimulant efficacy have been quite brief, covering only weeks or months, though there have been recent clinical trials of one or two years' duration.

Mental Retardation

The term "mental retardation" covers a wide range of conditions. People with these conditions have an equally wide range of functioning: some live independently, others live in structured environments, and still others need constant care. It is impossible to discuss all these conditions here in detail, but we can describe what they have in common.

There are two definitions of mental retardation. The most commonly used, from the American Psychiatric Association, requires:

- intellectual functioning significantly below average—an IQ of approximately 70 or below on an individually administered test

- problems in meeting standards the person's cultural group expects for his or her age (referred to as deficits or impairments in adaptive functioning) in at least two of these areas: communication, self-care, home living, social/interpersonal skills, use of community resources, self-direction, functional academic skills, work, leisure, health, and safety

- onset of these problems before the person turns 18

The American Association on Mental Retardation (AAMR) also focuses on adaptive functioning but differs in how it defines significantly low intellectual function. Because of the variability of IQ measurement, the AAMR endorses a more inclusive definition, with IQ extending as high as 75. This may seem like a small difference, but because those scores fall on the steeply rising slope of a bell curve, the shift doubles the number of people with mental retardation.

Mental retardation affects a person's ability to reason. It limits an individual's ability to think from the concrete to the abstract, from the specific to the general case. In everyday life, mental retardation affects judgment, socialization, education, and work. More severe cases of mental retardation may affect a person's safety, ability to perform everyday activities, and communication.

Sometimes a family knows that a child is mentally retarded when he or she is born, perhaps even before. Using amniocentesis and chorionic villi sampling, we can now detect Down's syndrome, which involves an easily recognized chromosomal abnormality, while a child is still in the mother's womb. Babies born with this condition also have recognizable physical traits, including eyelid and palm folds. However, people with Down's syndrome (and other forms of mental retardation) have a wide range of intelligence and abilities, not to mention diverse personalities. Thus, a family cannot know how their baby will learn and behave until he or she actually starts to grow up.

Other forms of mental retardation are not as obvious at first. Usually parents become aware of their child's slow acquisition of skills when comparing him or her with other children of the same age. Most toddlers with mental retardation are relatively slow in acquiring language. They may or may not have behavioral difficulties. Delays in gross motor abilities, such as difficulty in crawling or walking, may be associated with mental retardation, but in the absence of other delays, they usually point to other brain impairments, such as neuromuscular (**C51**) and metabolic (**C6**) disorders. Variances among very young children may not be obvious, but they become more apparent as time passes—especially to parents—and are evident by age 2 or 3. Families usually consult their pediatricians when they decide the delay is significant.

A family can also learn that a child is mentally retarded when doctors evaluate him or her for other brain dysfunctions. For example, parents may bring an infant to a pediatrician because he or she is having seizures (**C13**), and the doctor might diagnose tuberous sclerosis, with accompanying mental retardation.

Other cases of mental retardation result from brain disorders that are obvious and dramatic. For instance, a child may have a bad case of meningitis (**C37**), which interferes with the brain's development. Brain trauma (**C61**) at an early age can also slow a child's mental development permanently.

In most cases, we do not know why people are born with mental retardation. Despite this, parents often feel guilty when they learn about their child's condition. They fear that they are responsible. Frequently families focus on insignificant events that they think might have been the cause, such as a cold during pregnancy, one glass of wine, or the choice to use low forceps. Such worries are unfounded.

A New Understanding of Mental Retardation

Over the years our understanding of mental retardation has grown in several important ways. First, we have identified many biomedical conditions associated with it. For instance, we know that a pregnant woman drinking significant amounts of alcohol creates a greater chance that her child will be born with fetal alcohol syndrome (**C30**). The past two decades have also seen an explosion in our knowledge of genetics and metabolism. Whole new classes of metabolic disease have been identified that are associated with mental retardation. Most are rare, but some are treatable, with the result that some mental retardation can be prevented. Newer genetic techniques allow us to determine causes of mental retardation that were unknown five years ago. The completion of the sequencing of the human genome holds promise for tremendous growth in determining the causes of mental retardation.

Second, by better understanding the natural history of mental retardation, we have found ways to lower the risk that children will be born with or develop the condition. To decrease the number of cases of fetal alcohol syndrome, public health ini-

HOW MENTAL RETARDATION MAY BE APPARENT AT DIFFERENT AGES

AGE	AREA OF CONCERN
Newborn	Physical abnormalities (dysmorphisms) Major problems in such physical activities as eating and breathing
2 to 4 months	Failure to interact with the environment, which might prompt questions about sight and hearing impairments
6 to 18 months	Delays in gross motor skills: sitting, crawling, walking
2 to 3 years	Language difficulties or delays
3 to 5 years	Language difficulties or delays Behavior difficulties, including play Delays in fine motor skills: cutting, coloring, drawing
Over 5 years	Slow academic achievement Behavior difficulties (attention, anxiety, mood, conduct, and so on)

tiatives warn pregnant women about the risks of drinking. Statewide screening programs routinely test all newborns for phenylketonuria (PKU) and many other metabolic disorders for which early treatment may prevent mental retardation. Government initiatives such as removing the lead from gasoline have decreased mental retardation caused by lead poisoning. Seat belt laws and accident prevention campaigns have lowered the frequency of trauma (C61). Immunization programs have greatly decreased the rate of measles, *Hemophilus influenzae,* and rubella, consequently reducing the cases of mental retardation due to encephalitis (C38), meningitis (C37), and congenital infection.

We expect similar results from programs designed to lower the rate of teenage pregnancy, maternal smoking, and alcohol use, all of which raise a child's risk of being born with mental retardation. Intensive prenatal care of "high risk" mothers attempts to lower rates of premature birth, which is another risk factor. Intensive care of newborn infants and such programs as WIC, Medicaid, EPSDT, and CHIP improve access to health care. All women who might become pregnant are also urged to take folic acid supplements, which reduces the risk of spina bifida (C9).

Our third area of progress has been in recognizing that people with mental retardation can be integrated effectively into the larger society and be valuable, productive family members and citizens. The intellectual limitation may not prove handicapping. Individuals with mental retardation have increasingly been accepted as functioning members of society—many live in community settings, are competitively employed, and are accepted for their abilities. This may be the most important change in the field.

Education has reemerged as the dominant discipline in the care of children with mental retardation. Education is directed toward maximizing function in community settings. The growth of community programs has helped families maintain their children at home and allowed adults to participate in society.

We have also come to understand that mental retardation may not be a lifelong disorder. Children's IQs can change as they mature. Some seem to plateau, with their IQs declining in later childhood. Children with Down's syndrome sometimes follow this pattern; they continue to learn, but lag farther behind their peers. But other individuals who are diagnosed with mental retardation during their school years develop sufficient adaptive behavior abilities that they no longer fit the diagnosis as adults. In fact, very young children may show intellectual functioning significantly below average but improve so much that they are not considered mentally retarded by the time they start school. This has led some authorities to defer diagnosing mental retardation until a child is 3 years old, and raises the possibility of altering the severity of people's conditions through early intervention.

Mechanisms and Factors

There are approximately 7 million Americans with some form of mental retardation. About 2 million of these children and adults need ongoing services and supports. At least 5 million more people will be identified as having mental retardation at some point in their lives.

It is clear that mental retardation can result from many causes. We see so many different types of cognitive dysfunction in mental retardation that it is unlikely they all stem from a single mechanism in the brain's development. For example, people with Down's syndrome have a relative weakness in language abilities compared with their visual-spatial abilities, while those with Williams syndrome have the opposite pattern. Furthermore, because most forms of mental retardation affect cognition while sparing other brain functions, they probably do not result from a broad-ranging mechanism.

Studies of brain structure have revealed that most people who have mental retardation have normal-looking brains. Investigations of brain chemistry have not yielded a testable hypothesis. That means the primary area of research into the mechanism of mental retardation remains focused on how people learn. Researchers have studied brain plasticity, memory, attention, language, and perception, learning useful things about particular conditions but leaving much more to discover.

Overall, mental retardation is more common in boys than in girls, which may point to susceptibility genes on the X chromosome. Girls have two X chromosomes, so they can compensate for an abnormal gene on one, but boys have only one copy. Even more than chromosomal abnormalities and single-gene disorders, mental retardation seems to cluster in families. However, the condition can arise in many ways.

Diagnosis and Treatment

Assessing the cognitive development of infants and young children requires considerable experience. Mental retardation may mimic such conditions as a language disorder, attention deficit/

EXAMPLES OF MENTAL RETARDATION FROM DIFFERENT CAUSES

TYPE OF DYSFUNCTION	EXAMPLES
Developmental	Premature birth
	Hydrocephalus (**C8**)
	Migration errors by neurons
Degenerative	Adrenoleukodystrophy
	Tay-Sachs
	Ceroid lipfuchinosis (Batten's disease)
Genetic	Down's syndrome
	Fragile X
	Prader Willi
	Williams syndrome
Hypoxic/Ischemic	Placenta abruptio
Immunologic	Hyper IgE syndrome
Infectious	Meningitis (**C37**)
	Infection at or before birth by syphilis (**C38**), HIV (**C35**), cytomegalovirus, toxoplasmosis, rubella
Metabolic	Hypothyroidism
	Phenylketonuria (PKU)
Nutritional (iodine deficiency)	Cretinism (**C65**)
Oncologic	Neurofibromatosis (**C7**)
Toxic	Lead (**C66**)
	Maternal alcoholism (**C30**)
	Maternal anticonvulsant syndromes
Trauma (**C61**)	Motor vehicle accidents

hyperactivity disorder (**C2**), deafness (**C16**), schizophrenia (**C25**), and autism (**C5**), or a child with mental retardation may have any of those conditions as well. Mental retardation may also be a component of neurodegenerative diseases.

Pediatricians are usually the first professionals to detect mental retardation. Psychologists diagnose it by administering a standardized measure of intellect (for example, Bayley, WPPSI, WISC, or WAIS) and a standardized measure of adaptive behavior. The tests must be individually administered and be appropriate to the person's language. Psychologists may supplement their test findings by asking parents or teachers about the child.

Early diagnosis gives families more time to adjust to their children's needs and abilities. It enables early intervention, heads off behavioral and emotional disturbances, and allows long-term planning. Diagnosis allows families to enter a system of services that, at their best, provide coordinated, continuous, and individualized care. Support groups help parents better understand their child's disorder; provide practical information on management, entitlements, and rights; and serve as a resource to identify professionals who "do a good job." Our primary way of helping children with mental retardation is special education.

At present, there is no medical treatment for mental retardation. Most people with the condition have the same health needs as the rest of us. However, they have a higher than average risk of such neurological problems as seizures (**C13**) and cerebral palsy (**C4**); behavior/emotional disorders such as autism (**C5**), depression (**C20**), anxiety (**C21**), and adjustment disorders; and impairments in vision (**C15**) and hearing (**C16**). Medical treatment or therapy is available for these associated impairments.

Some forms of mental retardation are associated with medical conditions that require special care. People with Down's syndrome have an above-average risk of thyroid, heart, blood, orthopedic, and gastrointestinal disorders. There are neurodevelopmental pediatricians, geneticists, neurologists, and psychiatrists who specialize in caring for individuals with mental retardation.

The prognosis for people with mental retardation depends on the severity of their condition, any associated impairments, and the extent to which their community can help them maximize their abilities.

In the future, noninvasive functional neuroimaging technology holds promise that we will better understand the nature of mental retardation. Even more promising is analysis of how various genes express themselves, made possible by the human genome project. We also anticipate the new pharmacological and behavioral interventions will help people with mental retardation improve their abilities and adaptive functioning.

Cerebral Palsy

erebral palsy (CP) is the term for a group of lifelong neurological disorders of varying severity that alter body tone and impair movement. CP results from genetic or acquired medical conditions affecting brain formation and development, rather than from conditions primarily affecting nerves or muscles themselves. These conditions, most of which begin before labor, disrupt developing networks of neurons (brain cells) that control movement, and the myelinated fibers (brain white matter) that connect them to the spinal cord. In most cases, affected individuals have primary limitations in mobility and hand use, but they may have or develop associated problems with speech; seizures; eye movements; swallowing; bone, muscle, or joint structure; and cognitive processing. People with CP may have normal intelligence despite their speech-generating problems, and many overcome their physical disabilities and live fulfilling lives.

Symptoms may appear soon after birth or during early childhood. Infants with markedly increased or decreased body tone, or difficulty with head control, are at increased risk. Other early signs of concern include delays in rolling, sitting, crawling, standing; and becoming right-handed or left-handed before twelve months of age. However, children with specific genetic disorders may develop signs of cerebral palsy later in infancy or early childhood. For example, children with a condition called glutaric aciduria, a metabolic disorder, develop normally until an acute metabolic stress such as a viral illness leads to a sudden, dramatic loss of motor function and the subsequent finding of cerebral palsy.

It is important to recognize that the manifestations of CP may change and that the symptoms sometimes progress over time. For example, infants who are hypotonic (floppy) in the first one to two years of life may develop hypertonia (stiffness) later in childhood. Adults may develop signs of spinal cord injury with loss of extremity function as a result of repeated, long-standing abnormal body movements. These changes highlight the need for lifelong care by experienced professionals.

Classifying Cerebral Palsy

In determining the type of CP and specifics of rehabilitation, medical and rehabilitative specialists look for particular neurological signs and assess limb involvement and severity of functional impairment. Depending on the neurological findings, CP may be classified as spastic, extrapyramidal, or mixed. In *spastic* cerebral palsy, motor pathways descending from the brain to the spinal cord send abnormal signals, resulting in increased muscle tone. This produces a resistance to movement similar to the feeling of opening a pocketknife. Functional impairment is generally greater in the legs than in the arms. Because of the abnormal pull of muscles around joints, deformities of joint (orthopedic), including hip dislocation, scoliosis (curvature of the spine), and deformities of the foot, ankle, and arm, may develop.

Extrapyramidal (also called *dyskinetic*) forms of CP involve increased or reduced body movements in association with muscular rigidity or hypotonia. The term *extrapyramidal* (meaning outside the pyramidal tract) refers to abnormalities in brain areas including the basal ganglia, thalamus, and cerebellum, which regulate motor function. This is distinct from the pyramidal motor pathways directing movement, which are made up of large myelinated bundles of white-matter fibers that may be affected in spastic CP. In extrapyramidal CP, the arms are usually more affected than the legs, with less risk for orthopedic deformities. Movement abnormalities may include chorea (dancelike movements of the hands), athetosis (slow, writhing movements of the extremities), and dystonia (fixed, twisted postures). It is important to note that while speaking may be impaired, understanding of language may be normal in extrapyramidal CP.

Other terms also help carefully define the disorder for purposes of planning care and treatment. Affected individuals may be described as having diplegia, quadriplegia, or hemiplegia. *Diplegia* refers to the greatest involvement being that of the lower extremities; *quadriplegia* describes four-limb involvement; and *hemiplegia* refers to the involvement of one side of the body. Rehabilitation therapists may also classify cerebral palsy according to the ability to walk, or "ambulate." For example, in some people ambulation is limited to the home or rehabilitation facility, while others may freely move in a community setting. This description is further refined by the nature of any assistive devices required (for example, cane, walker, or wheelchair).

In most individuals with CP, structural brain abnormalities are seen using magnetic resonance imaging (MRI) or computed tomography (CT). White-matter pathways from the cortex to various brain structures and the spinal cord are vulnerable in premature infants (24 to 34 weeks) who later develop spastic forms of cerebral palsy. This can be seen by MRI as periventricular leukomalacia (PVL), the term used to describe this white-matter injury. As the fetus approaches term, vulnerability shifts from white matter to neurons in the motor cerebral cortex and basal ganglia, with the common clinical presentation of extrapyramidal CP. For example, acute perinatal injury often has a characteristic imaging pattern of abnormal signaling in the basal ganglia (putamen) and thalamus.

Causes of Cerebral Palsy

The cause of CP has been controversial for more than a century. Sir William Little, an orthopedic surgeon in Great Britain in the mid-1800s, attributed CP to problems with birth. Alternatively, Sigmund Freud, who spent the early part of his career as a neurologist, favored a prenatal origin for the disorder. Sir William Osler, the noted Johns Hopkins physician, contributed a book on CP at the turn of the century, highlighting the role of infection. The National Collaborative Perinatal Project, which was sponsored by the National Institutes of Health (NIH) and studied more than 54,000 mothers and their infants born between 1959 and 1966, provided the most comprehensive information about the causes of CP. The study found that most CP is caused by prematurity, infection, genetic syndromes, and developmental brain malformations. Fewer than 20 percent of cases are thought to result from trauma or lack of oxygen associated with labor and delivery.

Disorders involving energy production may affect the brain at birth or during infancy. Many of these disorders, including kernicterus (yellow jaundice) and pyruvate dehydrogenase deficiency (mitochondrial disorder), target specific regions in the basal ganglia and also lead to extrapyramidal CP. Genetically based developmental brain malformations can cause CP as well—for example, lissencephaly, an abnormality in brain cell migration that leads to a smooth brain surface, or holoprosencephaly (where the front part of the brain doesn't divide into two halves, which should occur at two to four weeks gestation). It is important to identify children whose CP has a genetic cause because some have medically treatable disorders. Furthermore, some of these disorders have specific recurrence risks for future pregnancies, which is important information for families.

Diagnosis

History and neurological examination remain key components to diagnosis. A medical specialist will review the family history for possible relevant genetic disorders and will observe the infant or child's movement and motor abilities, such as rolling, sitting, crawling, and standing. Once the child is comfortable, a detailed neurological examination will be conducted to determine what type of CP is present, which is of great benefit in determining medical therapies, including drug therapy and surgical interventions.

When CP is suspected, a brain scan should be obtained. Depending on the situation, this may be an ultrasound scan of the head, a CT scan, or an MRI. Of the three, MRI often provides the most useful information. The changing vulnerability of different parts of the brain to insults occurring during early development results in distinct imaging patterns. For example, there are often relatively specific findings for spastic and extrapyramidal types of CP. A careful interpretation of each scan is important for diagnosis and treatment, as well as establishing the recurrence risk for future pregnancies.

Treatment

Like the progress in understanding the causes of CP, advances in medical care offer improved treatment options. Most medium-to-large medical centers in countries around the world have experienced clinicians, including neurodevelopmental pediatricians, neurologists, orthopedists, physiatrists, nurse-practitioners, nurses, and therapists, to help individuals with CP and their families. These professionals are trained to

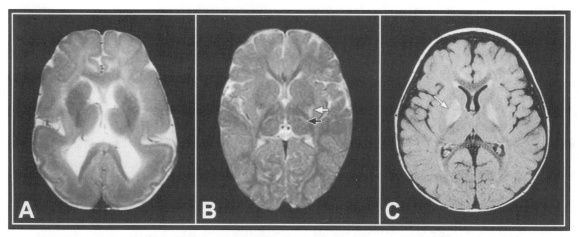

These brain MRI scans, selected from three children with extrapyramidal cerebral palsy, demonstrate distinctive patterns that can be used to improve diagnosis and management. **A** shows the smooth surface of the disorganized cortex in the genetic disorder lissencephaly; **B** shows the specific pattern seen in acute perinatal distress, with injury in the putamen of the basal ganglia and thalamus (arrows); **C** shows the genetic metabolic disorder methylmalonic acidemia, with injury in another basal ganglial nucleus, the globus pallidus (arrow). COURTESY OF ALEXANDER HOON, M.D., M.P.H., AND MICHAEL JOHNSTON, M.D., KENNEDY KRIEGER INSTITUTE, BALTIMORE

select and carry out optimal therapies at the appropriate time in the child's, adolescent's, or adult's life. Modern rehabilitation offers a wide range of effective treatment approaches. The overall purpose is to improve motor abilities, develop communication and independence skills, and address any associated problems. Physical, occupational, and speech therapies are the mainstays of treatment, serving to promote development and foster independence.

When spasticity affects motor development, oral drugs including baclofen and valium are often used, with injections of botulinum toxin (Botox) into specific muscles as required. These treatments are used to decrease spasticity and improve motor abilities. For more severe degrees of spasticity, procedures called selective dorsal rhizotomy and intrathecal baclofen have been effective. Selective dorsal rhizotomy involves cut-

ting a small number of nerves at the base of the spinal cord that affect foot and leg movements. Cutting these nerves diminishes spasticity and may improve mobility. In intrathecal baclofen, a pump placed under the skin in the abdomen delivers a continuous dose of baclofen to the spinal cord through a catheter. This treatment is often very effective in reducing spasticity and at times improving functional abilities.

If skeletal deformities progress to the point at which either function or the activities of daily living (for example, dressing or bathing) are significantly affected, orthopedic surgery is often required. Frequently soft tissue procedures are performed first, where tendons are lengthened, or contracted muscles cut, for example, to reduce toe walking or decrease hip dislocation. If the deformities continue, surgery on affected bones may be required. It has not yet been clearly established that drug therapy, rhizotomy, or intrathecal baclofen reduces the need for orthopedic surgery.

Extrapyramidal forms of CP with disorders of movement may respond to one or more oral medications, with some types also responding to intrathecal baclofen. Another type of surgery, stereotactic neurosurgery, is more frequently being considered in highly specialized medical centers for those for whom more conventional therapies have not worked. In stereotactic surgery, lesions or fine electric wires are strategically placed in the thalamus or basal ganglia to decrease unwanted movements. Long-term studies of this surgery are currently not available.

Affected people and their families often consider alternative therapies when conventional ones fail to achieve desired effects. Acupuncture, energy therapy, massage therapy, water therapy, and horseback riding have all been reported to be of benefit. Recently, therapy by means of high-oxygen environments, termed hyperbaric oxygen therapy, has been employed for a wide range of medical conditions, but there is little evidence that it is successful. To date, theoretical concerns that high oxygen could cause oxidative damage to developing brain pathways have not been substantiated.

In summary, CP is a chronic disease that affected individuals and their families need to learn to manage. Federal law, contemporary medical practice, and parental input have combined to improve medical and rehabilitative care for affected children, adolescents, and adults with CP. However, families still face financial barriers in gaining access to equipment, therapies, transportation, and housing that would serve them best. The psychological challenges of raising children with disabilities, as well as the problems faced by the individuals affected, can be daunting. Furthermore, adults with CP still face obstacles with respect to the workplace, housing, medical care, and opportunities for social interaction.

Recent advances in diagnosis and management are cause for optimism. A number of techniques are being developed to more accurately image the brain, and promising therapeutic strategies are being developed, including intrathecal drug administration and stereotactic neurosurgery. For parents of a child with cerebral palsy, early identification and intervention services provide parents with the guidance and encouragement needed to optimize their child's potential and to intervene in medically treatable disorders. These advances will lead to further improvements in care and lifestyle.

Future Challenges

The wide range of conventional and alternative therapies available serves to point out the need for improved classification and more objective measurements of outcome. Using these tools, careful studies can then be done so that the best form of rehabilitation is selected for each person with CP. It is encouraging that researchers around the world are currently addressing these challenges.

Autism

Autism is a disorder in brain development that becomes apparent in earliest childhood. It is defined by problems in three areas:

- severe impairments in how children relate to other people

- delays or abnormalities in how they communicate

- restrictive, odd, and repeated (stereotyped) behavior

Autism is the best known of the pervasive developmental disorders (PDDs). Others include childhood disintegrative disorder (CDD) and pervasive developmental disorder not otherwise specified (PDD-NOS), covering individuals whose impairments do not meet all the clinical criteria for autism (because of when the impairments developed or what behaviors emerged). The treatments and prognoses for these conditions are the same as for autism, and because people show a wide range of functioning within each, we consider them all to be within an "autistic spectrum" in this book. Also among PDDs are Asperger's syndrome and Rett's disorder, discussed in the sections that follow.

PDDs are much less rare than we once thought. It is reasonably certain that at least 20 of every 10,000 individuals have such a disorder. About one fourth of these cases meet the criteria for autism, with about an equal number of cases of Asperger's and PDD-NOS. Rett's disorder is much rarer. The ratio of males to females with all PDDs is more than 3 to 1, except for Rett's disorder, which only girls develop.

Manifestations of Autism

Autistic individuals differ greatly in the type and severity of symptoms they may exhibit. At least two subgroups in the range of autism appear to exist, defined by their degree of intellectual and social impairment: high functioning and low functioning. Many people with autism make considerable progress in various life skills, though most retain clear and disabling limitations.

Social Behavior
Some parents recall their child in infancy showing unusual social behaviors: being content to lie in

ASPERGER'S SYNDROME

Asperger's syndrome ranges from mild to severe. Children with the disorder have average and, in some cases, above-average, intelligence, develop language skills normally, and remain curious about the world around them. Many develop very large vocabularies, even at a young age. However, they tend to use that language very literally, have difficulty with nonverbal communication, and often violate other people's expectations of personal space. They are usually physically clumsy and have difficulty concentrating, which has led some to be diagnosed with attention deficit/hyperactivity disorder (C2). Most people with Asperger's prefer routine and dislike change. Some develop obsessive habits or interests. They are often very sensitive to sounds, sights, smells, and tastes, and perhaps need to wear soft clothing.

Compared with children with autism, many with Asperger's are very high functioning. Nevertheless, they do not experience the world as other children do and can therefore be naive, socially clumsy, and easily teased or bullied. Bright children with Asperger's can learn social skills from their parents, teachers, and therapists, but this does not come naturally to them; what other children pick up in early life they must learn, almost as if they were learning a technical skill, such as cooking or playing a musical instrument.

the crib staring at inanimate objects, crying less than usual, not seeming to crave being held or cuddled. Often, they also report that an infant makes little or no eye contact, does not imitate gestures or facial expressions, and does not "coo" back and forth with adults as most babies do. Other autistic infants are remembered as colicky and irritable, and crying inconsolably, yet resistant to being held and comforted. However, many parents do not notice anything unusual until their child reaches age 2 without responding to spoken language.

From the age of about eight months to three years, autistic children display other social deficits not seen in children developing normally. Autistic toddlers generally fail to use eye contact to check for parents' approval or attention. Instead of pointing to an appealing object (a complex, coordinated act that involves making eye contact and guiding the caretaker's gaze), they may take someone's hand and attempt to use it as a tool to grasp the desired thing.

Autistic children's social skills and behavior lag well behind other children's, but they often do progress as they grow older. A 2- or 3-year-old autistic child might consistently treat a parent like any adult stranger. A school-age autistic child, in contrast, might selectively prefer being with his or her parent but remain isolated from peers at school. An autistic early adolescent might wish to relate to peers but not know how.

At one extreme among children with autism, a low-functioning 8-year-old might appear completely detached, avoid closeness with others, and seem totally absorbed by a few inanimate objects. At the opposite extreme, another 8-year-old autistic child might show active interest in other children at a playground but express this interest in odd ways—for example, by running around at a distance from the group.

General Intelligence

The range of general intelligence within the autistic population is wide. Approximately 70 percent to 80 percent have IQs consistent with men-

RETT'S DISORDER

In Rett's disorder, babies (almost all of them girls) have normal development for 6 to 18 months but then start to lose such physical skills as walking and moving. Parents next see a loss of mental abilities, speaking, and reasoning. The babies' early hand skills are replaced by repetitive, meaningless gestures, especially a constant motion like wringing or washing their hands. By their fourth birthday, children with Rett's disorder have measurably smaller heads than their peers. During the onset of this disorder, children often lose interest in social interaction, but in many cases this interest returns later. However, their language skills are severely impaired. Compared with autism and Asperger's, Rett's disorder is quite rare.

tal retardation (**C3**). These children show the fewest developmental gains as they age. About 20 percent of autistic individuals have average or superior intelligence. They are most likely to speak by age 6 and eventually attain language skills.

Some autistic individuals appear cognitively deficient in some areas, yet may be remarkably superior in others. Such "savants" may display advanced skills in reading (hyperlexia), mathematics and counting, memory, art, and music, or acquire incredible knowledge in restricted areas. Thus, some children with autism have islands of average or excellent intellectual ability ("splinter abilities"), yet cannot adapt this intelligence for general use. This implies that the crucial cognitive deficits in autism involve the brain's executive functions.

Language and Communication

All young autistic children show some delay in language, as well as a lag in becoming aware of communication itself. Often parents suspect the problem is deafness, the most common fear that first brings families with autistic children to a pediatrician. However, the children usually have even more difficulty with nonverbal communication; infants and toddlers almost always have problems processing other people's gestures or facial expressions of emotion and appropriately using such gestures or expressions themselves.

Overall, the way in which people with autism attain and use language varies greatly. Most autistic children never develop speech or use only a few words and gestures. Substantial numbers attain partial, restricted, and highly deviant communication skills. For example, they may speak mostly in seemingly meaningless repeated phrases, though sometimes caregivers can learn to decipher these vocalizations in context. Very high functioning autistic children may, by age 2, have some words for greeting, identifying caregivers, or stating a few specific requests. By age 6, these children can attain some receptive and expressive verbal language, and eventually acquire normal or near-normal vocabulary and syntax. Yet even they retain subtle deficits: poor comprehension of abstract ideas and the vocabulary of emotions, inferences, intuition, and metaphors. They may have difficulty generalizing information beyond the immediate context in which they learned it. Even the most high-functioning people with autism have problems with the nonverbal aspects of communication, such as body language, and providing enough contextual information for others to understand what they are talking about.

Imaginative Play

Most low-functioning autistic children develop little or no imaginative play, a feature of normal child development. At 4 years of age, an autistic child might pick up a toy car and put it in his or her mouth, or turn it upside down and spin its wheels in fascination for several minutes. A high-functioning 4-year-old might gather many toy cars in a corner and make imitation car sounds, showing awareness that the toys represent real cars—but do that over and over and resist letting anyone bring another toy car to interact. Only the highest-functioning autistic children develop true imaginative play.

Unusual Patterns

Younger autistic children are likely to engage in repetitive behavior, sometimes referred to as self-stimulation, such as flapping their hands excitedly, rocking back and forth, or spinning. Also common are clutching or flapping a favorite object, even if it is simply a piece of plastic trash bag. In general, such behaviors seem to increase when the child is excited or under stress. Related behavior includes fascination with spinning wheels and fans or opening and closing window blinds. However, a sizable minority of autistic children either never exhibit any of these sensory obsessions or grow out of them.

Unusual perceptual problems are also a common feature, particularly in younger children. They may not be able to tolerate bright lights, certain sounds, or sensing some fabrics against their skin. Often the same youngsters may have a greatly elevated pain threshold. These unusual sensory patterns are not considered diagnostic of autism, but they occur often enough to suggest a dysfunction in the way the brain processes information from the senses.

In some low-functioning autistic individuals, self-stimulation can veer toward compulsive self-inflicted injury by hitting, biting, banging their heads on the floor or walls, or other actions. Such behavior is frightening and frustrating for parents. It constitutes a psychiatric emergency. Self-injurious actions are not unique to autism, however; some severely mentally retarded individuals also display them.

Some autistic people show a preference for highly structured, predictable, and repetitive routines, which at times is essentially indistinguishable from obsessive-compulsive behavior (**C23**). Many autistic individuals become very distressed when their customary routines are disrupted, or when they must change activities. Others insist that all objects in a room remain in the same positions at all times.

Many people with autism have behavior problems, often quite severe, that are common in the nonautistic population. Treating these problems separately, even though they may derive from the same underlying neurodevelopmental pathology, is one of the most helpful ways to intervene in autism. The most common of these are attention deficits and impulsive, hyperactive, and distractible behavior (**C2**). Anxiety and panic disorders (**C21**) and mood disorders (**C20, C24**) are also widespread.

Causes

Whether autism is present at birth or arises after normal early development is still unsettled. About 20 percent of parents with an autistic child report that he or she developed normally for one or two years, although in many of these cases the parents may have overlooked the condition's subtle early signs. Nevertheless, some autistic people appear to have developed normally in infancy. In fact, there are rare reported cases of autism starting after age 3. Late-onset cases do not seem to differ in their clinical features or prognosis for improvement, however.

Very strong evidence suggests that autism has a genetic basis. About 20 percent of cases occur in association with illnesses we know are inherited, most commonly fragile X syndrome and tuberous sclerosis (though only a minority of people with these conditions develop autism). Phenylketonuria (PKU) is an inherited metabolic disorder that, when untreated, leads to autism and severe mental retardation; fortunately, most babies are tested at birth for this condition, and a medically regulated diet prevents the severe brain damage.

About 80 percent of autism cases are idiopathic (caused by unknown mechanisms), but there is still evidence that most cases are inherited. When one identical twin has autism, the odds of the other having it range from 60 percent to 90 percent. In contrast, the concordance rate found for fraternal twins and siblings ranges from 2 percent to 5 percent—and even that rate is 50 to 100 times higher than the rate in the general population. Recent research has shown that siblings, parents, and other close relatives of people with autism have an unusually high rate of learning disabilities, language delays, and impaired social skills.

After several large genetic studies, only a few genes have been weakly associated with autism, which strongly implies that several genes in combination must produce the disorder. The preponderance of males with PDDs compared with females raises suspicion that the X chromosome, of which males have only one copy while females have a "backup," contains high-susceptibility genes. However, genetic research has not borne this out. There may actually be several different genetic types of autism.

The evidence for brain abnormalities underlying autism is impressive. Eighty percent of people with autism are also mentally retarded, reflecting neurodevelopmental defects or brain damage. Many of these have very severe intellectual impairment. By adulthood, between 20 percent and 35 percent of people with autism have experienced seizures, much more than in the general population. Imaging studies (most recently using magnetic resonance imaging, or MRI) have supplied more evidence of brain abnormalities in autism. Most studies find that autistic individuals have larger overall brains than other people, especially in the posterior regions. The rear portions of the corpus callosum (the main connecting fibers between the two sides of the brain) are smaller in autistic people. These findings have caused researchers to propose that autism involves failures in the neurons' migration or in pruning before birth or in the early months of life. Many cases of autism are also associated with specific brain lesions (certainly the case for tuberous sclerosis) and other malformations, but we do not know the significance of these in how autism develops.

Diagnosis

Diagnosing autism and other PDDs early, in the preschool period, is crucial for providing children with the intensive early intervention they need to improve their functioning. While there is still no cure for autism, we have made much progress in helping children with PDDs develop, learn, and adapt to the world.

There are really two stages to diagnosing PDDs. First, child psychiatrists or clinical child psychologists who have received specialized training must recognize and confirm the condition. This requires systematically obtaining information from parents, caregivers, and perhaps teachers and interviewing the child. There is no biological test to confirm a PDD diagnosis (except for the rare case of Rett's disorder). However, a physician may request laboratory tests to check for associated genetic disorders or seizure disorder (C13).

Recently, psychiatrists have made considerable progress in creating short and convenient screening tests for autism and other PDDs. These are essential in helping pediatricians identify autism in very young children. The most extensive comprehensive interview in widespread use is the Autism Diagnostic Instrument (ADI), a detailed review based on interviewing parents about all symptoms and behaviors associated with autism.

The second stage in diagnosing PDDs is determining exactly how a child is affected and how severely. Every child has different abilities, and it is important to recognize those in order to help him or her make the most of them. Recommending ways to help the child often requires the collaboration of the child's psychiatrist, pediatrician, or pediatric neurologist, cognitive and behavioral psychologists, speech and language specialists, and occupational therapists. A diagnostic report on a child with autism has enormous practical significance. Parents and public agencies rely on it in making major decisions about early intervention, school placement, special education, and access to community services. A child should have individualized treatment and education, not a "one size fits all" plan.

Treatment and Teaching

Drug therapy has a role in treating autistic behavioral problems, but no evidence shows it affects underlying autism. The greatest obstacle to effective drug treatment in autism is the mistaken assumption that all behavioral problems that autistic people have are part of the disorder. Parents should be aware that autistic children have an increased likelihood for abnormal responses to medications. For example, while selective serotonin reuptake inhibitors (SSRIs) are often effective in reducing anxiety, repetitive behavior, and tantrums, much anecdotal evidence exists that for some people they actually increase the behaviors. Sedatives seem more likely to provoke what is termed a paradoxical reaction, of silly or out-of-control behavior, while other medications produce sedative side effects, which can interfere with a child's attention and learning.

Parents of autistic children face extraordinary challenges: managing their child's difficult behavior, spending extra time assisting him or her in self-care routines, maintaining composure when their child displays odd behaviors or tantrums in public, accepting that he or she cannot express normal affection, and advocating for their child's education, often in underfunded, resistant school systems. One major advance in the treatment of autism has been the rise of strong, well-organized parent advocacy groups offering a range of support services.

Early-intervention programs involving intensive one-on-one behavioral lessons for 10 to 40 hours each week have shown considerable success with many autistic preschoolers, particularly those who are higher functioning. Using positive reinforcement, the trainer first teaches a child to follow verbal or gestural instructions, then trains him or her in a graded series of communication, thinking, and social skills.

Very encouraging data also support the efficacy of specially designed preschool programs

THERAPIES USED FOR AUTISM

Parents with children recently diagnosed with autism face a bewildering array of information about the disorder. While there is currently no cure for autism, and the underlying causes are poorly understood, a variety of therapies have been developed to help each autistic person adapt to the challenges of his or her environment. Here are a few of the many kinds parents may discuss with specialists:

- **Auditory training may be used with individuals who are oversensitive to sound. Different sound frequencies are tested to evaluate the individual's impairment.**

- **Behavior training focuses on positive techniques to encourage or discourage different behaviors of the individual.**

- **Communication, including speech therapy (either oral or sign language, depending on the needs of the individual), electronic communication methods, picture communication methods, and other techniques, may be used by a speech language pathologist.**

- **Diet modifications and vitamins may be helpful treatment adjuncts for the individual with autism, since some autistic persons have low tolerances for or allergies to certain ingredients.**

- **Medications: Though there is no medication to specifically target autism, some medications may be used to treat symptoms the individual may have, such as aggression, seizures, hyperactivity, or anxiety.**

- **Music therapy may help some individuals with autism learn cognitive, motor, and daily living skills.**

- **Social skills training can help the autistic person recognize facial expressions and emotions. This training also helps individuals with autism communicate and behave properly in different social situations.**

NOTE: There is no *one* treatment that is effective for every individual with autism. Parents and professionals must examine the unique needs and potential of each person with autism and match them to the treatments that will be most effective. This can be an intensive process, and individuals with autism may undergo a variety of treatment options in tandem so as to achieve maximum results.

Adapted from www.autism-society.org (Autism Society of America); additional sites: www.naar.org (The National Alliance for Autism Research); www.cureautismnow.org (Cure Autism Now Foundation)

that foster communication and social skills. Other, more psychotherapeutically oriented programs rely on intensive parent-child interventions, such as training parents in extensive floor play with their young preschoolers; these programs have resulted in less scientific documentation of improvement. Many of these programs demand major time commitments in a child's critical pre-school years, and parents must evaluate them carefully because the time and expense may effectively rule out other approaches.

Language and communication therapy includes training in everyday communication through individual and small-group therapy. Use of sign language, pictures, and both manual and computer-assisted communication boards creates rewarding ways for nonverbal children to communicate. While many low-functioning autistic children will probably always have severe communication deficits, some can learn to point and make simple requests, greatly improving their own and their families' lives.

A variety of educational interventions are in use. One widely used model involves specially designed classrooms and predictable, behaviorally reinforced lessons. All children with autism should have their schooling planned and reviewed through the individualized educational program (IEP) defined by law.

Most advances in psychotherapy and drug treatments for autistic children target their very common behavioral problems, including disruptive behavior disorders, anxiety and phobias, obsessional rituals, tantrums, mood swings, and self-injurious behaviors. These disorders often affect family life more than the direct symptoms of autism. In some communities behavioral therapists are available to go into homes after school to assist parents in developing improved behavior management strategies and to reinforce training in self-care skills. Very high functioning older autistic children and adolescents can sometimes benefit from individual psychotherapy. Such individual therapy usually emphasizes counseling for more effective socializing, as well as direct modeling and role-playing to increase social coping skills.

Metabolic Diseases

The word *metabolism* refers to how our bodies process the food we ingest to make the many chemicals we need to live. Our brains are uniquely sensitive to disturbances in this body chemistry. The brain needs amino acids to make and then break down neurotransmitters, and many specialized structural and catalytic proteins. Because of the brain's specialized role in generating electrical impulses, it requires a flow of such ions as sodium, potassium, and calcium. It also needs lipids to form the myelin sheaths that insulate axons connecting cortical nerve cells with other parts of the nervous system.

Any disturbance in the brain's chemical environment can lead to a metabolic disorder. Such a disease can take many forms. The lack of an enzyme or vitamin necessary for a specific chemical reaction in the body can cause a deficiency of an essential metabolic product (called a metabolite). That lack may impair brain development (as with cholesterol in Smith-Lemli-Opitz syndrome), cause seizures (as with copper in kinky hair disease), or have other harmful effects. Slowed chemical reactions can also cause the buildup of a compound that would otherwise be metabolized.

The stored material may become toxic, as with lactic acid in the case of a mitochondrial disease, which in turn can lead to loss of nerve cells and breakdown of brain white matter. Some metabolic disorders produce mental retardation (**C3**), cerebral palsy (**C4**), and seizures (**C13**).

Metabolic dysfunction can also be the result of an external factor, such as a toxin (**C66**) or a nutritional deficiency (**C65**). It can be the effect of disease in the liver, endocrine glands, or other organs. The fetal brain may be harmed by the mother's alcohol abuse (**C30**), thyroid deficiency, or phenylketonuria. This section is primarily concerned, however, with metabolic disorders that arise from a child's genes.

A Spectrum of Symptoms

The symptoms of a genetic metabolic disorder can appear at any age, even in adulthood. Sometimes a child's brain can be seen to have developed abnormally even before it is born, as in Zellweger's syndrome, Smith-Lemli-Opitz syndrome, and other disorders.

Symptoms of neurometabolic disease apparent just after a baby is born include seizures and lack of normal consciousness, muscle tone, movements, reflex activity, vision, breathing, sucking and swallowing. Some newborns with diseases known as lysosomal storage diseases exhibit generalized accumulation of fluid, a condition called nonimmune fetal hydrops. Unusually shaped facial features and limbs may suggest a chromosomal defect but can also arise from a metabolic disease.

Doctors begin to suspect a metabolic problem if a young infant fails to progress developmentally, exhibits severely weak muscle tone, is too easily startled, lies or sits abnormally, or suffers recurrent episodes of respiratory distress, vomiting, or lethargy. An abnormal odor of the body or urine, eye defects, a persistently small head, and seizures may also prompt investigation.

Toward the end of a baby's first year, metabolic brain disease can cause more delays in development or even regression from skills the child has learned. Older infants may also show difficulty walking, twitching and seizures, skeletal abnormalities, and enlargement of the liver or spleen. In some cases, parents may see abnormalities of their child's skin and hair. Often a child with a metabolic disorder responds poorly to going without food or having a fever because his or her metabolism is so fragile. The metabolic problem may thus be most apparent when a child is sick.

Toddlers, too, may have developed normally but then encounter problems. Again, these might appear as developmental delays or the loss of previously acquired skills. Children's walking may become unsteady (ataxia), and their muscle tone increased (spasticity) or decreased (hypotonia). Other possible symptoms include visual problems, poor coordination, a disturbance in speech, and jerking muscles. If a child develops an unusually large or small head while showing signs of developmental delay or regression, doctors should investigate.

Generally, the later the onset of metabolic brain disease, the slower it progresses. However, an unrelated illness or other stress can bring about an acute health crisis with acidosis, coma (**C61**), and seizures (**C13**). This is often how the disorder glutaric aciduria appears.

Mechanisms and Causal Factors

Metabolic disorders have long been known to run in families. Archibald Garrod first proposed the concept of an inborn error in 1909, and that path of inquiry led to the idea "one gene, one enzyme." Each gene in our bodies determines the expression of a single protein, many of which (but not all) are enzymes. If a defect or mutation in one gene disrupts the structure and function of its corresponding protein enzyme, that leads to a particular metabolic disease. (Many of the neurodegenerative diseases that begin in later life involve similar defects in nonenzymatic, structural proteins.)

Two people can have mutations of the same gene without suffering the same health problems because each variant of the gene can produce a different clinical picture. One child might be obviously and severely ill at birth and die soon afterward, while another might be only mildly affected by symptoms appearing later in life.

We now know of more than a thousand gene defects, of which at least 30 percent affect brain function. Since there are probably more than 30,000 genes in the human genome, we are likely to discover many more inborn errors of metabo-

CLASS OF DISEASE	EXAMPLES
Amino acid disorders	Phenylketonuria
	Maple syrup urine disease
Organic acid disorders	Glutaric aciduria
	Proprionic acidemia
Urea cycle disorders	Argininosuccinic aciduria
Disorders of purines and pyrimidines	Lesch-Nyhan disease
	Adenine deaminase deficiency
Lactic acidemias	MELAS
	Pyruvate dehydrogenase deficiency
Disorders of glycogenolytic and glycolytic pathways	Acid maltase deficiency
	McArdle's disease
Lysosomal diseases	Tay-Sachs disease
	Metachromatic leukodystrophy
Peroxisomal diseases	Zellweger's syndrome
	Adrenoleukodystrophy
Membrane transport disorders	Glucose transporter deficiency
	Kinky hair disease
Cofactor deficiency diseases	Pyridoxine dependency seizure disorder
	Molybdenum cofactor deficiency
Fatty acid oxidation defects	Medium-chain acyl-CoA dehydrogenase deficiency
	Carnitine palmitoyltransferase deficiency

lism. The frequency of inherited metabolic diseases varies widely, from greater than 1 in 3,000 children for common disorders to less than 1 per million for rare conditions. The table above lists the major classes of inborn errors causing neurological disease, and some examples of each, but it obviously cannot list the hundreds of genetic brain disorders we know about.

The vast majority of inborn errors of metabolism are inherited in an autosomal recessive manner. This means that both parents carry an abnormal DNA sequence for the same gene on one of a pair of nonsex chromosomes. Since each parent also carries one chromosome with the normal gene sequence, he or she produces half of the normal protein—which is usually enough to remain healthy. However, if both parents pass on the abnormal gene sequence to their child, he or she will be unable to make any of the normal protein and will have the disease. Thus, each child of such parents has a 25 percent chance of being affected.

Because most metabolic conditions are inherited as recessive traits, their prevalence is higher in families in which relatives intermarry. Particular ethnic groups may have developed a genetic predilection for certain diseases, as is the case with Tay-Sachs disease and type 1 Gaucher's disease among Jews of Eastern European ancestry. In these circumstances, it is hypothesized that a single ancestor passed along a mutation that remains within a relatively small population that is geographically or culturally isolated and thus more likely to intermarry. Alternatively, the mutant gene may confer some specific environmental advantage on its carriers that helps them have more offspring, even if those children are at greater risk for disease. For example, sickle-cell patients may be resistant to malaria, which would explain the sickle-cell trait's continuing presence in a population.

In the case of diseases carried on the X chromosome, males are more severely affected because they have only one copy. Females who have one X chromosome with the gene defect and one without may or may not develop symptoms. Normally only one of a female's two corresponding genes on her X chromosomes is expressed as a protein, so chance helps determine the severity of her disease. Examples of X-linked conditions with mild symptoms in women include adrenoleukodystrophy (a peroxisomal disease) and Fabry disease (a lysosomal disorder).

People also inherit diseases of mitochondrial DNA (mtDNA) from their mothers. MtDNA encodes a number of proteins involved in the production of energy by mitochondria, which are the

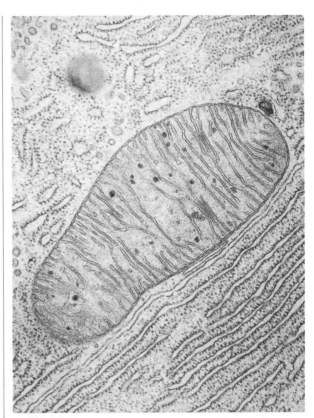

Mitochondria float inside cells, providing energy by processing sugar and oxygen. They contain their own DNA, which is known as mtDNA and is separate from the cell's chromosomes. Defects in mtDNA can damage a person's metabolism. IMAGE © K. R. PORTER PHOTO RESEARCHERS, INC.

powerplants of the cell. Mitochondria are also very important during development and after brain injury because proteins released from mitochondria can trigger programmed cell death. An individual's total complement of mtDNA normally comes from the egg from which he or she grew, and that egg came from the mother alone. Disorders of mtDNA may affect both males and females, but only women will pass on the genetic defect. MELAS (which stands for mitochondrial encephalopathy, lactic acidosis, and stroke) is inherited in this way.

SCREENING TESTS

In recent years researchers have identified many genetic mutations that lead to specific metabolic disorders. Individuals or couples can choose to be tested for these genes, especially if these diseases or other neurological or developmental disorders run in their family. That gives these prospective parents more information about the likelihood that their children will develop such diseases.

Medical ethics preclude doctors from screening all babies for the genetic markers of a disorder unless there is some treatment for those children. One such disorder occurs when newborns are missing a particular gene that helps metabolize the amino acid phenylketonuria (PKU). The accumulation of dangerous levels of PKU, and the resulting brain damage, can be prevented with a strict diet. To give these children a chance to stay healthy, most states mandate PKU testing for all newborns, and this compulsory testing has greatly reduced the damage from this relatively common metabolic abnormality.

Diagnosing metabolic diseases as soon as possible has other benefits in addition to prompt treatment, if it is available. Early identification can also minimize the amount of testing a child has to undergo, and can provide parents, therapists, and teachers with a clearer picture of what to expect in the future. For these reasons, many health departments maintain programs that test newborns for metabolic disorders.

In the future we may be able to screen newborns for many more diseases, letting doctors start more treatment before a child has suffered symptoms and brain damage. Similarly, genetic tests for carriers should enable more couples to be aware of genetic risks to their offspring, and permit prenatal diagnosis.

Diagnosis and Treatment

If a child shows the symptoms of a metabolic disorder, physicians must often perform many tests to confirm the cause. They may examine urine for metabolites. Blood studies might include a complete blood count and measurement of cholesterol, electrolytes, ammonia, uric acid, lactic acid, pyruvic acid, acylcarnitines, and blood gases. Doctors can sample cerebrospinal fluid for its content of glucose, protein, lactic and pyruvic acids, amino acids, and neurotransmitter metabolites.

A magnetic resonance imaging (MRI) scan is especially helpful in looking for a congenital malformation in the brain, cortical atrophy (shrinking), or leukodystrophy. Doctors may also take a specimen of skin, using electron microscopy to rule out a storage disease and culturing cells for tests of the body's enzymes and DNA.

In the metabolic brain disease, an electroencephalograph (EEG) shows slower-than-normal background electrical activity. Seizures often produce a particular wave pattern. Evoked-potential studies can show whether certain pathways in the brain are impaired because of lost myelin or axons. Doctors perform electromyogram (EMG) and nerve conduction studies to assess whether peripheral nerves and muscle are involved.

Once physicians identify the biochemical abnormality of a child's nervous system, they can design appropriate therapy. To reduce the amount of a toxic metabolite, they might prescribe a restricted diet or add a substance that joins with the offending material to neutralize it and facilitate its elimination. Another approach is to block the reaction producing that toxic product.

When a child's system is not generating an essential metabolite in healthy quantity, large amounts of the right vitamins can often activate the dysfunctional enzymes enough to overcome the defect. Enzyme-replacement therapy has been used successfully in Gaucher's disease and is now being tried in several other lysosomal storage diseases. For several of the inherited leukodystrophies, a bone marrow transplant before the symptoms have progressed far usually minimizes the damage; however, this approach has not proven effective in diseases involving nerve cell storage.

When metabolic disorders produce mental retardation, cerebral palsy, or seizures, doctors must treat those conditions along with the underlying problem. Therapies include anticonvulsants for seizures and muscle relaxants for spasticity. Supports and braces can help children sit and move more easily. Physical, occupational, and speech therapy can help them learn particular tasks. Some children may require tube feeding because they have difficulty swallowing. Others need basic help to maintain adequate nutrition, prevent contractures, and avoid infection. Quality of life is far better for people who can both understand and express themselves through language, so therapists often focus on helping children learn to communicate, if necessary through a picture board, computer, or sign language.

Unfortunately, no definitive therapy is yet available for the vast majority of people with inherited neurometabolic diseases. Indicators of a particularly severe prognosis are a small head that is not growing, blindness, absence of speech, and the inability to sit, stand, and walk. Intractable seizures and severe hypotonia or hypertonia are also unfavorable prognostic signs.

Researchers are developing animal models of more and more human diseases, making it possible to develop new therapeutic strategies, especially using bone marrow transplants. Recombinant DNA technology is facilitating the large-scale production of proteins that we may be able to use in enzyme-replacement therapy. Gene therapy is also a theoretical possibility for metabolic disorders; it has restored enzyme activity and improved symptoms in several animal studies of the storage diseases.

Neurofibromatosis

Neurofibromatosis consists of two different genetic disorders: neurofibromatosis 1 (NF1) and neurofibromatosis 2 (NF2). Both forms cause tumors to grow along the nerves and also affect nonnervous tissues, such as the skin. Some NF2-associated tumors may be fatal; fatal tumors are less frequent in NF1 but can occur. There are other similarities between the two, but NF1 and NF2 are distinct entities caused by mutations of different genes.

NF1

NF1 affects about 1 in 3,000 people. It is caused by mutations of the neurofibromin gene (designated *NF1*) on chromosome 17. We do not completely understand the function of neurofibromin, but it is probably involved in regulating cell growth. The disease can be passed on from parent to child; each child of an affected person has a 50 percent risk of inheriting the disease. Half of NF1 cases arise as new mutations and, therefore, occur in individuals whose parents are unaffected. The other half of individuals with NF1 inherit the disease from an affected parent.

The first signs of NF1 are usually changes in the skin, which may include multiple café au lait spots (light brown, the color of coffee with cream) and freckling in skin folds as well as on areas exposed to sunlight. Most affected people develop neurofibromas, which are firm, noncancerous tumors of the nerve sheaths. These growths appear as lumps in or under the skin. Neurofibromas can range in diameter from three hundredths of an inch to more than half an inch and tend to increase in number and size as people age. Older adults may have hundreds or thousands of skin neurofibromas. Their impact is often only cosmetic, but they may cause pain or affect the function of adjacent structures.

In addition to café au lait spots and skin neurofibromas, the other most common features of NF1 are:

- mild shortness of stature

- learning disabilities (of varying severity, but usually with normal intelligence)

- macrocephaly, or an abnormally large head

- scoliosis, curvature of the spine

■ large neurofibromas that can affect almost any part of the body.

In addition, about 15 percent of people with NF1 develop optic nerve tumors; these usually do not cause any symptoms and do not become progressively worse. Other central nervous system tumors may also appear. All the symptoms of NF1 and their severity can vary greatly, even within affected members of a single family.

About 5 percent to 10 percent of people with NF1 develop malignant, or cancerous, peripheral nerve sheath tumors. Brain tumors (C64), seizures (C13), long-bone pseudarthrosis (bending and fracturing of a long bone, usually in the leg), pheochromocytoma (a tumor of the adrenal gland), and vascular disease are less common but potentially serious complications. Many people with NF1 never develop any of these severe features, but it is hard to predict who will.

Diagnosis and Treatment

Doctors generally make a diagnosis of NF1 based on physical findings. The café au lait spot is the hallmark of the disorder and is often the only feature apparent in young children. Many people have one or two small spots of this sort, but adults with six or more café au lait spots greater than half an inch in diameter are likely to have NF1. (For children, doctors look for six or more spots one fifth of an inch in diameter.) Multiple café au lait spots can also occur in other conditions, so a confident diagnosis of NF1 requires the presence of at least one other characteristic feature as well.

Other signs of NF1 include freckling in the armpits (axillae) or in the groin; at least two neurofibromas of any type, or at least one large neurofibroma that involves a more extensive area

than the typical skin tumor (a plexiform neurofibroma); a distinctive bony lesion that shows up on X rays; and two or more clumps of pigment on the iris (Lisch nodules). Thus, a doctor may take X-ray or magnetic resonance imaging (MRI) scans of an affected site, examine the eyes, order a biopsy of skin lesions, perform a black light test, and do other analyses.

Most symptoms of NF1 do not appear until people with the disorder are older, and doctors cannot make the diagnosis in some young children even though they may have the NF1 gene. A gene test has been developed, but it is not widely available and usually is not needed to establish the diagnosis.

Specialists who see people with NF1 include medical geneticists, neurologists, dermatologists, ophthalmologists, and orthopedic surgeons. Some major medical centers have neurofibromatosis clinics that bring together physicians from these many disciplines. Early diagnosis of NF1 permits increased vigilance in monitoring complications and allows patients and their families to consult genetic counselors about the possibility of children inheriting the disease.

No specific treatment for NF1 is available. We do not know how to prevent the onset or progression of particular symptoms. Treating serious symptoms by surgery or otherwise is often possible, however. Malignant tumors or tumors that cause pain or loss of function are removed on an individual basis.

The life expectancy for people with NF1 is reduced by about 15 years from the norm, on average. Most of these deaths result from malignant tumors or vascular disease. NF1 is extremely variable in its manifestations, however, and the cause of this variability is unclear. One area of active research is the role of neurofibromin in the control of cell growth and tumor development.

NF2

NF2 affects about 1 in 40,000 people. It is caused by mutations in the merlin (sometimes called schwannomin, or *NF2* gene on chromosome 22. The function of merlin is poorly understood, but it appears to be involved in regulating cell structure and growth. The NF2 protein has some structural similarities to a class of proteins known as erlins. "Merlin" is a play on the word *erlin*. The disease is transmitted genetically from parent to child, with a 50 percent risk that it will be passed on to any child. It can occur sporadically as a result of new mutations. Many people with NF2 inherit the disease from an affected parent, but it may also arise as a new mutation in an individual whose parents are unaffected.

For most people with NF2, the first symptom they notice is ringing in the ears or hearing loss (**C16**) as a result of schwannomas (benign tumors) of the vestibular nerves. Seeking medical help for the hearing problem can lead to diagnosis of a person's NF2. Although vestibular schwannomas are not infrequent in older adults who do not have NF2, these tumors tend to occur at a much younger age, sometimes even in childhood, in people with NF2. The diagnostic feature, however, is that schwannomas usually involve *both* vestibular nerves in NF2, and this rarely, if ever, occurs in people who do not have the condition.

Most symptoms of NF2 are caused by compression of neural structures by schwannomas or other tumors of the cranial nerves, the spinal nerves, or the central nervous system. Meningiomas (tumors that grow on the membranes that enclose the brain and spinal cord) may also occur, often several at a time. A variety of neurological symptoms can result, depending on the structures affected by tumors. Localized weakness, loss of sensation, and seizures are the most common symptoms arising from tumors of nerves other than those of the ears.

NF2 is progressive, with worsening neurological problems as the tumors increase in size and

---

NEUROFIBROMATOSIS

There are many things one can do to help manage NF. Here are some suggestions.

■ **Seek a physician for evaluation and follow-up care who is knowledgeable about the disorder and its complications or is willing to learn about it.**

■ **Include a family history and a family tree in the medical evaluation.**

■ **Individual or family counseling by a social worker or psychotherapist is often helpful.**

■ **Genetic counseling provides individuals and families with information on the nature, inheritance, and implications of genetic disorders to help them make informed medical and personal decisions.**

Adapted from www.nf.org (National Neurofibromatosis Foundation); additional site: www.nfinc.org (Neurofibromatosis, Inc.)

number. The age at onset and rate of progression vary in different families, but the course tends to be similar in affected relatives. The average age when people are diagnosed is in the early 20s, and some individuals are much more severely and quickly affected than others.

Doctors usually diagnose NF2 using an MRI to confirm the presence of vestibular nerve tumors. Spotting the disease in people who do not have these tumors but have other symptoms is more difficult, and several sets of diagnostic criteria have been proposed. There is a gene test for NF2, but it is of limited value clinically. Its use is generally limited to presymptomatic diagnosis in the offspring of affected individuals. Neurologists, otolaryngologists (who diagnose and treat disorders of the ear, nose, throat and nearby parts of the head and neck), and medical geneticists are often involved in caring for people with NF2. Early diagnosis of the disorder permits doctors to watch carefully for tumor development and associated complications. Regular neurological assessment and hearing tests are important to determine whether the problems are getting worse and to permit early treatment of complications. Treatment options for vestibular schwannomas and other tumors include surgery and radiation therapy.

On average, people with NF2 die from their tumors at about 36 years of age, but this prognosis varies substantially from family to family. Researchers are seeking ways to improve treatments for NF2-related tumors, as well as to determine the role of merlin in tumor development.

Hydrocephalus

Hydrocephalus, from the Greek words meaning "water" and "head," is caused by excess cerebrospinal fluid (CSF) in the spaces within and surrounding the brain. Most cases of hydrocephalus occur in infants and children, at a rate of 3 in every 1,000 live births. However, people can also suffer hydrocephalus later in life in association with brain tumors (**C64**), intracranial hemorrhage (**C60**), head injury (**C61**), or meningitis (infection of the meninges covering the brain; **C37**). We do not know exactly how common hydrocephalus is in adults, but adult cases account for approximately 40 percent of the total.

In the healthy brain, the choroid plexus produces CSF at a rate of approximately 1 pint per day. The fluid is secreted into the ventricles of the brain and subsequently flows into the spaces surrounding the brain and spinal cord. The average volume of CSF within the skull at any given time is about 5 fluid ounces.

CSF acts as a cushion to protect the brain and spinal cord. It also supplies the brain with such nutrients as minerals and proteins, and carries away the waste products of metabolism. Normally the body reabsorbs CSF through specialized channels that connect the ventricles with the superior sagittal sinus, a large vein that returns blood from the brain to the heart. This removal balances the rate of fluid production, producing a healthy equilibrium.

For hydrocephalus to develop, one of several factors must upset the normal flow of CSF:

- The brain produces too much CSF.
- Outflow from the ventricles is blocked, a condition called obstructive hydrocephalus.
- The bloodstream is unable to reabsorb CSF, leading to a relative excess of fluid, referred to as communicating hydrocephalus.

Each of these factors results in a buildup of fluid within the skull. In infants whose cranial sutures (the fusion joints between skull bones) have not yet closed, the extra fluid causes the head to expand. For older children and adults, whose skulls are already hardened, hydrocephalus produces increased pressure within the skull, and this increased pressure on the brain creates neurological

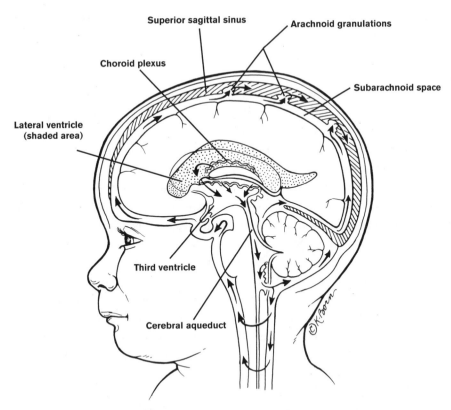

Superior sagittal sinus

Arachnoid granulations

Choroid plexus

Subarachnoid space

Lateral ventricle
(shaded area)

Third ventricle

Cerebral aqueduct

Cerebrospinal fluid normally flows from the choroid plexus through the ventricles and around the outside of the brain and spinal cord, cushioning these vital organs. The body reabsorbs the fluid through the superior sagittal sinus, a vein leading to the heart.
ILLUSTRATION © KATHRYN BORN

symptoms. Some adults may exhibit swollen ventricles with no increase in pressure (referred to as normal-pressure hydrocephalus).

Because the skull of an infant can expand until the cranial sutures close, the most frequent sign of hydrocephalus in infancy is rapid head growth, associated with a bulging anterior fontanel ("soft spot") when the infant is held upright and not crying. The cranial sutures may be separated and the skin overlying the skull may appear thin and transparent, with scalp veins clearly visible. In more advanced cases, the infant's eyes may be di-rected downward, with the white of the eye visible above the iris—an appearance known as the setting sun sign. In babies with hydrocephalus, this sign is often accompanied by crossed eyes or abnormal involuntary eye movements. Parents should be aware, however, that both an enlarged head and the setting sun sign may appear in infants without hydrocephalus, so a pediatrician must consider various possibilities. If an infant with hydrocephalus is left untreated, over time he or she will lose developmental progress, including verbal and motor skills.

In children, hydrocephalic symptoms result from the effects of increased intracranial pressure. The most common acute symptoms are headache (**C54**), vomiting, and lethargy (changes in consciousness). Chronic increases in pressure within the head will show up as intermittent, progressive headaches with nausea and vomiting, abnormal eye movements, and poor appetite. Eventually, continued brain damage will lead to behavioral changes and deteriorating performance in school.

Hydrocephalus in childhood has many possible causes. Prenatal hydrocephalus most commonly arises from genetic or sporadic developmental abnormalities that block the outflow of CSF from the ventricles. It can also result from maternal infections and disorders of the blood vessels. Problems appearing after birth include tumors or other masses (cysts, abscesses, and blood clots) that obstruct CSF flow; meningitis; hemorrhage; or blockage of the drainage channels into the bloodstream. In many cases, however, the cause is unknown.

Treated hydrocephalus has a very good prognosis: most children attain normal intelligence with few or no physical limitations. In some cases, a degree of neurological impairment may remain, such as a learning disability. But if the condition is untreated, it is debilitating and eventually lethal in 50 percent to 60 percent of cases. Prolonged delay in treatment, particularly in children, will cause irreversible brain damage.

In adults, the symptoms depend on the type of hydrocephalus. High-pressure symptoms include headache (**C54**), nausea, abnormal gait (**C46**), and visual disturbances (**C15**). Symptoms of normal-pressure hydrocephalus include dementia (**C69**), abnormal gait (**C46**), and urinary incontinence; the result may resemble Alzheimer's disease (**C67**).

Diagnosis and Treatment

Many cases of hydrocephalus are first diagnosed by pediatricians. A sudden increase in head growth can alert an infant's doctor to possible hydrocephalus even before the head becomes very enlarged. Confirmed cases are referred to neurosurgeons for evaluation. Prompt diagnosis and treatment are extremely important, especially in children. Early relief of the increased pressure prevents the permanent developmental and neurological consequences that will otherwise occur.

Confirmed diagnosis is based on the history of the illness in combination with the doctor's physical examination of the person and X rays. In infants, transfontanellar ultrasound—scanning the soft spot where bones have not yet fused—provides a simple and noninvasive diagnostic technique but is often not enough to make a definitive diagnosis. A computed tomography (CT) or magnetic resonance imaging (MRI) scan of the head is the best diagnostic test.

While the nature of hydrocephalus has been recognized for several centuries, successful surgical treatment was not possible until the twentieth century. Neurosurgeons knew that draining the fluid from the skull would be a useful treatment but were frustrated by technical impediments. Metal, plastic, and rubber tubes to divert the fluid, called shunts, caused severe tissue inflammation. A major boost was provided during World War II with the development of silicones, originally used as insulation in bomber spark plugs. Silicone elastomer (Silastic™) proved to be an excellent material for shunts because it did not inflame the tissues it touched. Another problem was over-shunting, or removing too much fluid. In the 1950s, John Holter, an engineer with a hydrocephalic child, designed a pressure-sensitive valve

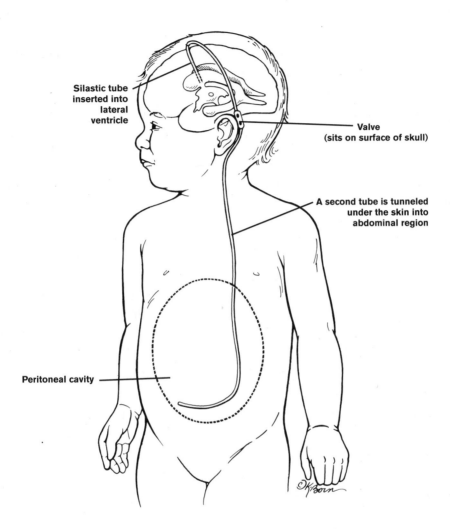

Silastic tube inserted into lateral ventricle

Valve (sits on surface of skull)

A second tube is tunneled under the skin into abdominal region

Peritoneal cavity

This schematic shows how a ventriculoperitoneal shunt relieves chronic hydrocephalus. Surgeons insert tubes that let the cerebrospinal fluid drain out of the brain into the abdomen, where the body reabsorbs it. These tubes, hidden under a child's skin, can prevent brain damage. ILLUSTRATION © KATHRYN BORN

that made it possible to control CSF drainage as needed.

Currently, the most widely performed treatment for hydrocephalus is to drain the excess fluid from the brain through a shunt into the abdomen's peritoneal cavity, where the body can reabsorb it more easily. This operation is called a ventriculoperitoneal shunt, meaning a diversion from the ventricle to the peritoneum. One end of a flexible Silastic tube is inserted into a lateral ventricle of the brain. The other end is attached to a valve on the surface of the skull, which is connected to a second tube tunneled under the skin into the abdominal region, where its free end is tucked into the peritoneal cavity. Some shunts are fitted with on-off valves or other devices to regulate the drainage of CSF.

The ventriculoperitoneal shunt operation itself is generally straightforward. However, shunts can, and often do, become infected, blocked, or otherwise nonfunctional, especially in growing children. While some individuals need only a single shunt placement, others have to have multiple operations. The average number of replacements is about two per child. People with hydrocephalus and their caregivers should be aware of symptoms of increased intracranial pressure that could indicate that a shunt is malfunctioning, in which case they should notify a physician promptly. Children and adults with shunts for hydrocephalus should also avoid rough contact sports.

Surgeons can also alleviate some cases of obstructive hydrocephalus with endoscopic procedures that avoid shunt placement. The doctor inserts a small fiber-optic instrument (endoscope) into the ventricular system of the brain and relieves obstructions that impede CSF flow.

Medical treatment of hydrocephalus with drugs to retard the production of CSF is generally only a temporary measure, being ineffective in the long term.

While some researchers aim to perfect CSF shunts, the common malfunction of these devices suggests that other cures will ultimately be better. At present, approximately 25 percent of cases can be cured without shunt placement. This number should increase with more widespread use of endoscopic procedures and the development of specific drugs. In cases of hydrocephalus without a known cause, further research using animals that develop similar conditions should lead us toward a more satisfactory cure.

Spina Bifida

Spina bifida is a birth defect in which one or more of the vertebrae (the small bones that form the spine) fail to form properly in the fetus during the first trimester of pregnancy. Spina bifida is one of the more common birth defects; in different parts of the world, it occurs between 1 and 5 live births per 1,000.

There are several causes of spina bifida, including:

- low levels of folic acid in pregnant women
- chromosomal abnormalities
- an unusually high body temperature during pregnancy
- some drugs, such as valproic acid, taken during pregnancy

The disorder affects girls more often than boys, and there seems to be a slight genetic factor. If you have had a child with spina bifida, the risk that a subsequent baby will have the disorder is 5 percent, climbing to 10 percent to 15 percent for a baby with two older siblings affected. Mothers who had spina bifida have a 3 percent chance of giving birth to a child with the condition. The effects of this disorder can range from no disability at all to permanent and serious disability.

The disorder is traditionally divided into two main types: spina bifida occulta and overt spina bifida.

Spina Bifida Occulta

Spina bifida occulta is the more common of the two types; it is often very mild and rarely causes disability. For most infants, it involves a failure of one vertebra in the lower back to fuse properly. Spina bifida occulta is often either largely or completely hidden from sight (hence the term *occulta*). Frequently it is not even discovered until doctors take an X ray of the child's lower back for an unrelated problem.

For a very few infants, however, spina bifida occulta is much more serious. This form can be marked by a visible sign on the skin, such as a red or brown birthmark, a very deep dimple or sinus (a tiny opening in the skin that extends deeply toward the spinal canal), a tuft of hair, or a soft lump or mass of fatty tissue (lipoma) under the skin, which may extend toward the spinal canal. In rare cases, the spinal membranes and cord will protrude through the gap in the vertebra; this can cause the same problems as overt spina bifida, described below.

In other infants, spina bifida occulta is associated with the spinal cord being tethered to the backbone. When this happens, the cord does not slide up as the child grows, as it normally should, because it is held in place by surrounding tissue. This can sometimes result in nerve damage. Symptoms may not appear until adolescence or even early adulthood. They commonly include an inversion of the feet (usually one before the other), and impaired bladder and bowel control.

A skin "marker," an X ray, or an early change in foot posture or bladder function should alert a physician to the possibility that a child has one of the complicating anomalies of spina bifida occulta. X ray, ultrasound, computed tomographic (CT) scanning, magnetic resonance imaging (MRI), and at times myelography (in which an opaque material is injected into the cerebrospinal fluid to outline the spine structures for X rays) are all used to confirm the diagnosis. Doctors should scrupulously examine infants and children with meningitis **(C37)** for small sinus defects in their skin; these may have served as pathways for the bacteria that have invaded the children's bodies.

Overt Spina Bifida

Overt spina bifida, which used to be called spina bifida cystica, is much more apparent than spina bifida occulta because of the presence of a sac or cyst on the infant's back. There are two forms of overt spina bifida. The first, called meningocele, occurs in about 10 percent of cases. It involves a defect in the vertebra, and in the soft tissues overlying that portion of the spine, so that the coverings of the spinal cord protrude through the opening in the vertebrae but are nevertheless well covered by skin.

The second, more common type of overt spina bifida is called myelomeningocele. Here the sac or cyst includes not just the coverings of the spinal cord but also the cord's nerve roots, and often the cord itself, the whole bulging out and often not covered by skin. In these cases the children are virtually never able to control their bladder and bowel and often suffer loss of sensation or paralysis below the damaged vertebrae. If those vertebrae are very low, sometimes only the feet and bladder are affected, and the child will be able to walk. The higher up the spinal cord the problem appears, the more of the body it affects.

The larger majority of infants and children with meningomyelocele also suffer hydrocephalus **(C8)**, a condition in which cerebrospinal fluid (CSF) does not drain properly from the head. That symptom is usually apparent shortly after birth, but occasionally appears in early childhood. This is particularly true when a simple myelomeningocele has been surgically repaired—presumably because the cyst that doctors removed was serving as a reservoir for the CSF and thus reducing the pressure inside the head. In infancy, hydrocephalus is made apparent by a rapidly growing head, while in childhood, symptoms include headache **(C54)**, unsteadiness, vomiting, and lethargy.

Virtually all children with myelomeningocele and hydrocephalus have a problem known as the Arnold-Chiari malformation, in which the brain stem, cerebellum, and lower cranial nerves are pushed downward through the opening of the

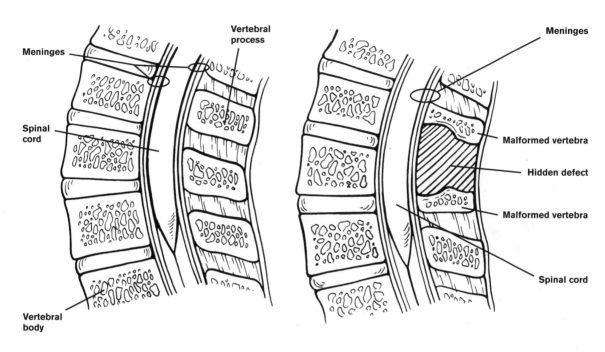

Normal spine (no defect)

Spina bifida occulta: no sac or protrusion of spinal cord

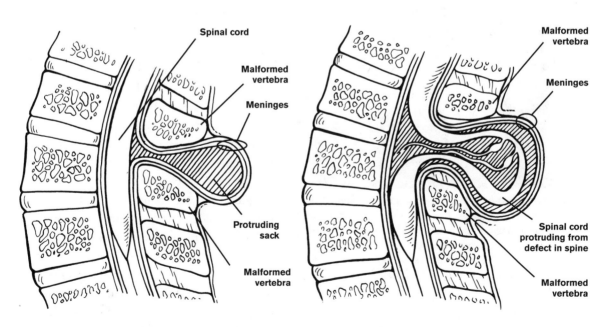

Meningocele spina bifida: spinal cord stays within spinal canal, but meningeal sac protrudes

A. Myelomeningocele spina bifida

ILLUSTRATIONS © KATHRYN BORN

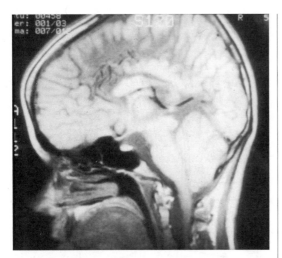

Normal lateral view of MRI of the brain. Normal position of cerebellum and brain stem.

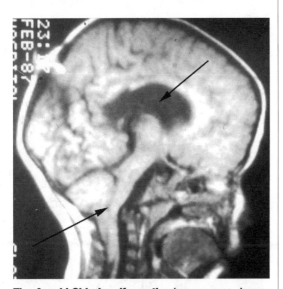

The Arnold-Chiari malformation is a common danger from hydrocephalus. This image shows the downward displacement of the cerebellum and brain stem (lower arrow), with cerebrospinal fluid build-up expanding the ventricle at the center (dark area, higher arrow). SCANS COURTESY OF ABE CHUTORIAN, M.D., PEDIATRIC NEUROLOGY, CORNELL UNIVERSITY MEDICAL COLLEGE, NY

skull (the foramen magnum) into the upper neck region (the cervical region). This compression of neural tissue can cause its own symptoms: difficulty swallowing, respiratory problems and stridor (a harsh, high-pitched sound made while breathing in or out), and abnormal eye or facial muscle movements. Timely surgery can relieve hydrocephalus and all of the symptoms of the Arnold-Chiari malformation.

Prevention and Treatment

Women of childbearing age should take a daily dose of 400 micrograms (mcg) of folic acid to prevent spina bifida beginning *before* they become pregnant. Taking folic acid *after* you have missed your first menstrual period does not prevent spina bifida, because the problem arises so early in pregnancy.

Pregnant women are routinely offered a prenatal test that screens their blood for alpha-fetoprotein (AFP), a protein from a fetus with an open neural tube defect that leaks into the amniotic fluid and thence into the mother's blood. AFP detects spina bifida with 90 percent accuracy. Two additional tests, ultrasound and amniocentesis, are usually recommended to confirm any AFP test that suggests a fetus has spina bifida. (For more on prenatal tests, see chapter 5.)

Spina bifida occulta usually requires no treatment. If a child has a tethered cord and surgery is performed shortly after the symptoms begin, he or she will often recover.

Children with overt spina bifida may need the cooperative efforts of neurosurgeons, orthopedists, genitourinary specialists, pediatricians, and pediatric neurologists to address the various po-

SPINA BIFIDA

Birth defects can happen in any family. Many things can affect a pregnancy, including family genes and substances women may come in contact with during pregnancy. Recent studies have shown that folic acid taken before and during early pregnancy is one factor that may reduce the risk that a baby will have a neural tube defect.

Taking folic acid cannot guarantee having a healthy baby, but it can help. Here's what you can do:

- Take a vitamin with 400 micrograms (mcg) folic acid every day.

- If you have a child with spina bifida, have spina bifida yourself, or have a history of pregnancy affected by a neural tube defect and you are thinking about becoming pregnant, you may need a higher dose of folic acid. You should take 4,000 mcg of folic acid by prescription for 1 to 3 months before becoming pregnant.

- Plan your next pregnancy. Speak with your health care provider about your personal risk of having a baby with a neural tube defect. You may need to get a prescription for folic acid before you try to become pregnant.

Adapted from www.sbaa.org (Spina Bifida Association of America)

tential complications of the disorder. Meningocele can be repaired surgically by replacing the sac internally and using skin grafts to cover it. There are usually no lasting effects.

If a baby has the most severe form of spina bifida, doctors usually operate shortly after birth to reposition the spinal cord and cover it with muscles and skin. This surgery helps prevent infection and additional nerve damage but cannot reverse the nerve damage that has already occurred. For children who have some degree of paralysis, physical therapists can assist with leg braces, crutches, or, in the most severe cases, wheelchairs. With treatment, children with spina bifida can usually become active individuals. With early treatment of hydrocephalus, most children with myelomeningocele have average cognitive function and survive well into late adult life.

Tumors of Childhood

The word *tumor* simply means a growth. If a tumor grows rapidly beyond the body's normal control system, disrupts healthy tissue, or spreads (metastasizes) to other parts of the body, it becomes a cancer. All cancers seem to arise from a defect in the critical cells' genes; put simply, either a growth-causing gene goes too far, or a growth-halting gene stops working. Some cancerous tumors grow more slowly or compactly than others, and treatment for each case is determined by the quality and location of the tumor.

There are several significant differences between tumors that appear in childhood and those that appear in adulthood (**C64**). To begin with, cancer is more common in adults than in children. This may be because failure of control mechanisms is more likely as the body ages. While people can inherit an increased risk for certain cancers, the mutated genes in childhood cancers seem in almost all cases to be confined to the abnormal cells. Thus, children are unlikely to pass on the disorder if they grow up and have children of their own.

About 1 in every 350 U.S. children will be diagnosed with cancer before the age of 20. Fortunately, over 70 percent of these children live for at least five years after treatment; that is a better survival rate than for adults, and it continues to improve. The most common form of cancer in children is leukemia, which arises from white blood cells and accounts for about 30 percent of all cases. The second most common form (19 percent) is tumors of the brain. (In contrast, brain tumors make up less than 2 percent of cancers in adults.)

Dealing with Childhood Brain Tumors

Tumors growing inside the skull produce a wide range of symptoms, depending on their characteristics and the age of the child. Very young children may not be able to express their difficulties in words, of course. Slow-growing tumors may cause symptoms to appear gradually, so children and their parents do not initially connect headaches, school difficulties, or clumsiness with a growth in the brain. Pediatricians may also suspect that particular symptoms are caused by sinus infections, intestinal problems, viruses, or other illnesses much more common in childhood than cancer. On the other hand, some brain tumors announce themselves through seizures (**C13**) or other dramatic symptoms that send a family to a hospital immediately. (Tumors account for less than 1 percent of all childhood seizures, however.)

One of the more common ways tumors can harm the brain is by blocking the drainage of cerebrospinal fluid from the head, producing hydrocephalus (**C8**), whose symptoms can show up in a variety of ways. In an infant whose skull bones have not fused, the head can become visibly swollen. In older children, the most common effect of hydrocephalus is headaches (**C54**); a regular headache on getting out of bed that is relieved by vomiting is an especially important sign. Other signs include unusual irritability, loss of appetite, and loss of motor or intellectual abilities.

Tumors can also invade or push against structures of the brain, disrupting particular functions. For instance, a cancerous growth in or around the brain stem can cause problems with balance and coordination, abnormal speech, and weakness in a portion of the face. A tumor in the cortical areas can produce headaches (**C54**), seizures (**C13**), weakness in one limb or side of the body, and subtle changes in personality and thinking. Tumors affecting the visual pathways can cause loss of sight, quickly or gradually, completely or partially (**C15**).

A pediatrician's initial response will focus on any acute symptoms, especially making sure hydrocephalus does not permanently damage the child's brain. If doctors suspect the underlying problem might be a brain tumor, they recommend a variety of further tests. Computed tomography (CT) and magnetic resonance imaging (MRI) scans detect nearly all brain tumors and also help determine whether a cancer has metastasized to other parts of the nervous system. A lumbar puncture (spinal tap) may also be necessary to check for abnormal cells in the cerebrospinal fluid. A neurological exam may be useful, depending on how well the child can cooperate. To determine the exact nature of the tumor, however, it is usually necessary to obtain a sample of its cells and study them in the lab—the process called biopsy. For growths inside the skull, biopsy requires surgery because there is no other way to reach the tissue.

If a child has been diagnosed with a cancerous brain tumor, there is still hope. As stated above, well over half of children diagnosed with cancer today live for at least five years. Still, fighting and recovering from cancer is a difficult challenge for children and their families. Some diagnostic or treatment procedures are painful or exhausting. Some side effects can also be difficult in both short term and long term: chemotherapy and radiation may cause adolescents to lose their hair when looking good seems most important. And of course, any threat to the life of a young person is sad and frightening for everyone involved. Often the prospect of death is more emotionally devastating for parents and other adults than it is for children. Parents may also have the responsibility of looking after siblings of the child with cancer, helping them through their worries and making sure they don't feel neglected.

On top of the emotional impact, families must deal with a complex system of names and treatments for different types of tumors. The remainder of this section will briefly discuss the three main forms of cancer treatment and then various tumor types and the best treatment for each. However, every child's prognosis and treatment depends on his or her particular condition, so families should work closely with their doctors when making any treatment decision.

The Treatment Triad

The goal of all cancer treatments is simple: to remove or disable the harmful cells while leaving normal cells as healthy as possible. Children with cancers are generally more resilient than adults in the same situation, who often have other health problems. This means that doctors can treat childhood cancer a little more aggressively (with the exception of radiation, discussed below) than adult cancers.

Most children diagnosed with brain tumors or other types of cancer receive care through specialized cancer centers. These facilities provide the widest range of treatments and expertise; dealing with brain tumors often requires a team that includes cancer specialists (oncologists), pathologists, neurosurgeons, nurses, nutritional counselors, and others. Cancer centers also provide valuable support services for children and their families: psychological counseling, discussion groups, even the chance to make friends with other children dealing with the same experiences.

Surgery is the treatment of choice for most brain tumors in children. Neurosurgeons try to remove all the cancerous tissue, or as much as possible, without hurting the surrounding structures—a tricky challenge when dealing with an organ as vital as the brain. MRI helps in this task by letting surgeons see the growth area more clearly. Very young brains show more plasticity than older ones, so children are more likely than adults to recover from the loss of brain tissue and achieve normal functioning again. Often a surgeon must also deal with the hydrocephalus a tumor has caused, inserting a tube (shunt) in the head to drain excess cerebrospinal fluid.

Chemotherapy involves using medications to kill the cancerous cells in a person's body. Again, the challenge is not to allow the same drugs to do too much damage to a person's healthy growing cells. Brain tumors are more difficult to affect by chemotherapy than tumors in other parts of the body because of the blood-brain barrier, which keeps poisons in the blood out of the brain. The choice of medications and their schedule (before, during, or after other treatments) depend on the nature of the tumor.

Chemotherapy in high doses can kill a child's bone marrow along with the cancerous cells; both types of tissue produce new cells quickly, but the red blood cells created by bone marrow are crucial to healthy life. In treating leukemia, doctors often prepare for that problem by removing and saving some of the child's own marrow tissue or stem cells—replacing them in the child's body after the chemotherapy is over. This is called autologous bone marrow rescue and allows for more aggressive chemotherapy. The same technique offers promise for treating brain tumors.

Radiation is another way to attack cancerous cells without physically invading a child's body. This type of therapy poses more dangers for children, especially infants, than it does for adults because the same energy that can stop harmful cells from spreading can also affect other cells' normal growth and development. As a result, young children who have had radiation therapy show a higher risk for delayed intellectual development (**C3**) and pituitary deficiency. With stereotactic radiosurgery, the radiation beam can now be shaped to focus on particular parts of the brain without penetrating other regions. In general, however, oncologists still use radiation less often for children than for adults, and even less often for children under 2.

In addition to helping doctors detect and operate on brain tumors, advanced MRI techniques are also useful in tracking the effect of treatments. Imaging can show tissue growth or shrinkage with great accuracy and help detect any spread or recurrence of the disease. Children who have had a brain tumor often return for periodic MRI scans months after treatment to confirm that no sign of cancer remains.

Gliomas

Gliomas are tumors that grow from the glial cells that support the brain's neurons. They are the most common form of brain tumor in children, accounting for half of all cases, and can start anywhere in the brain. Low-grade gliomas generally grow slowly and rarely spread. In contrast, high-grade gliomas (about 20 percent of all gliomas) grow aggressively, sometimes over only a few weeks, and often metastasize to other parts of the brain.

The lowest grade of glioma, found only in children, consists of pilocytic astrocytomas. Pathologists recognize these growths because their cells appear almost normal. They can occur in the optic nerves, hypothalamus, brain stem, and possibly the cerebral or cerebellar cortex. If such a tumor is accessible to a surgeon, completely removing it should allow the child to live a long and normal life. If not, the best way to manage such a low-grade growth is biopsy and observation, to catch it quickly if it becomes more dangerous.

The slightly higher-grade fibrillary astrocytomas also grow slowly but pose more of a threat to a child. When such an astrocytoma appears in an easily accessed area—for example, the cerebral hemispheres—the best treatment is surgical removal. But when doctors find a low-grade astrocytoma where it would be dangerous to operate,

they often consider radiation first. Astrocytomas are termed anaplastic and moved up one grade if they are invading brain cells. Surgery is often useful, but not enough on its own; radiation attacks the cancer that has spread.

The highest grade of glioma is termed glioblastoma multiforme, and it can be devastating in both children and adults. It is characterized by cell death (necrosis), a proliferation of blood vessels feeding the tumor, and markedly abnormal cells. The usual treatment is to remove as much of the growth as possible through surgery and then to use radiation on the tumor and for a short distance (three quarters of an inch) around. Chemotherapy is sometimes added but does not have a striking success rate. Survival is usually one to three years.

Another important variable among gliomas is where they appear. Tumors may thus be classified as optic nerve, hypothalamic, brain stem, hemispheric, and so on. The location often affects treatment. Gliomas of any grade in the brain stem are particularly difficult to remove surgically because of the high density of vital nerves there. Gliomas on the pons are usually high grade and have a bad prognosis, but about 30 percent of brain stem tumors are low grade, with much better long-term survival rates. There is a similar discrepancy between the two types of gliomas on the cerebullum, depending on how they have spread and affected the surrounding region:

- Type A tumors have a ten-year survival of 94 percent.

- Type B are more deadly, with a 29 percent ten-year survival in one study.

Low-grade tumors in the area of the neck and medulla (cervicomedullary tumors) should be removed; even aggressive removal of brain tissue in this area has surprisingly few adverse effects. Gliomas on the optic nerves may be biopsied to determine the type of cells involved but probably do not need further treatment unless the child's vision deteriorates, in which case radiation is the best treatment.

Other categories of gliomas are defined by the type of cells that make up the tumors. Cell characteristics help determine a child's prognosis and treatment, so a biopsy is crucial in identifying these tumors:

- Xanthoastrocytomas are glial tumors with giant cells, often filled with fat. They have a better prognosis than most astrocytomas.

- Gangliogliomas involve cancerous growth by both neurons and glial cells, usually in the temporal or frontal lobes. They are rare in adults, less so in children. Often they cause seizures (**C13**). Removing as much of the tumor as possible in surgery is the procedure of choice. Long-term survival is not unusual.

- Oligodendrogliomas arise from the cells called oligodendrocytes, which wrap myelin around neurons. Pathologists recognize these cells because they are small and regular, with an open "fried egg" structure beyond the nucleus. Surgical removal is the best course. Radiation therapy appears to add little. A genetic test helps predict how effective chemotherapy will be.

- Ependymomas (less than 10 percent of all childhood brain tumors) arise from the ependymal cells in the brain's innermost lining, usually in the posterior fossa in children. They often produce hydrocephalus (**C8**). The

best treatment uses microsurgical techniques to remove the tissue and perhaps place a tube to drain cerebrospinal fluid. Radiation is important in treating ependymomas, but chemotherapy has limited effect.

Finally, some children develop tumors of mixed sorts, with components of oligodendroglioma or ependymoma along with astrocytoma.

Embryonal Tumors

About a third of all childhood brain tumors are termed embryonal, defined as containing small, round, uniform cells that appear blue when examined by microscope after staining. It is quite possible that these tumors arise from nervous system stem cells in which something has gone wrong. They generally grow quickly over weeks or months, spreading through the cerebrospinal fluid to other parts of the brain and spinal cord. In about 40 percent of children diagnosed with embryonal tumors, the cancer has already metastasized.

The most serious form of embryonal tumors are medulloblastomas, which arise in the cerebellum. These are quite harmful, both because of their aggressive growth and because they commonly cause hydrocephalus. In recent years it has become clear that the amount of medulloblastoma tissue a surgeon removes is important to a child's outcome. Doctors once used radiation of the head and spine as a routine initial treatment for medulloblastomas; now MRI can provide clues as to whether a tumor has actually spread along the spine. As an alternative for children aged 2 and under, several cancer centers have tried chemo-

NEUROBLASTOMAS—TUMORS OF THE SYMPATHETIC NERVES

Neuroblastoma is the type of cancer most often diagnosed in infants in their first year, accounting for about 8 percent of all childhood cancers. These tumors grow from the cells of the sympathetic nervous system, which regulates heartbeat, blood pressure, and other automatic processes.

In about half of all cases the tumor appears in the abdomen, with an adrenal gland (sitting atop a kidney) as the most common starting point. The growth can also begin in the chest or neck. Sometimes doctors can see or feel the tumor from outside the child's body as a hard, painless mass. Or they may notice the growth on X rays taken to check another problem. If the cancerous cells have spread, they might produce such symptoms as a limp, leg weakness, or Horner's syndrome (drooping eyelid, dilated pupils, and no sweating on one side of the face). Doctors usually recognize neuroblastomas while a child is quite young; the average age for diagnosis is 2.

This type of cancer can easily spread, especially to lymph nodes, bone marrow, the liver, and other sites. In about 75 percent of cases, the tumor has already metastasized by the time it is spotted. The earlier that a neuroblastoma is recognized and treatment begun, the better the child's odds for survival. Infants seem to have an unusually high rate of survival, and sometimes in such young children the cancer regresses spontaneously for reasons we do not understand. Treatment for neuroblastomas usually starts with surgical removal of the tumor if it has not already spread. Chemotherapy is often effective; over 80 percent of infants recover with a simple combination of two drugs. Most neuroblastomas are sensitive to radiation, as long as they have not metastasized widely.

---

therapy using procarbazine, CCNU, and vincristine; in one study the two-year survival rate after this treatment was 96 percent.

Most other embryonal cancers are called primitive neuroectodermal tumors (PNETs). These can occur in the cerebral hemispheres and are treated by surgical removal as vigorously as possible, followed by radiation.

Other Types of Childhood Tumors

Retinoblastomas are malignant tumors of the retina, the inner layer of the eye. Usually these growths begin before a child is born and are recognized sometime during the first year, often because of a telltale white spot in the eye. Only about 200 cases are diagnosed in the United States each year, but the children involved usually lose sight in the affected eye(s). As long as the cancerous cells have not spread to the optic nerve, however, these children are almost certain to survive.

Choroid plexus papillomas are rare tumors arising from the small blood vessels and membranes that project into the brain's ventricles. They may be malignant or benign. Surgical removal is the major method of treating these growths, but the operations are complex because the tumors are so closely connected with the brain's blood supply.

COMMON PEDIATRIC BRAIN TUMORS BY LOCATION

Cortex or thalamus	Astrocytomas
	Anaplastic astrocytomas
	Glioblastomas
	Dysembryoplastic neuroepithelial tumors
	Primitive neuroectodermal tumors
	Oligodendrogliomas
	Gangliogliomas
	Xanthoastrocytomas
	Mixed tumors
Ventricles	Ependymomas
	Choroid plexus papillomas
	Medulloblastomas (fourth ventricle)
Suprasellar region	Optic or hypothalamic gliomas
	Craniopharyngiomas
	Dysgerminomas
Pineal region	Intrinsic pineal tumors
	Dysgerminomas
	Hamartomas
	Astrocytomas
Cerebellum	Medulloblastomas
	Ependymomas
	Astrocytomas
	Gangliogliomas
Brain stem	Gliomas

Craniopharyngiomas develop at the base of the brain, around the pituitary gland. They are benign tumors, usually treated by surgical removal and radiation. These steps must be taken with care, however, because the treatment has an unusually high rate of such harmful side effects as visual loss, low pituitary function, and behavioral difficulties.

Tumors near the pineal gland can be roughly divided into two sorts:

■ Germ cell tumors are often very sensitive to radiation; indeed, some doctors recommend trying radiation treatment first to see if they respond. They may be detected by increased alpha-fetoprotein (AFP) in a child's cerebrospinal fluid, obtained through a spinal tap.

■ Pineal parenchymal tumors require a biopsy and, if that test suggests there has been any change in tissue structure, probably excision.

Finally, children with neurofibromatosis of either type (**C7**) are at higher risk for brain tumors. These disorders cause other nervous system tumors as well, usually of less consequence. Optic nerve tumors appear in about 15 percent of people with neurofibromatosis 1, but this type of growth rarely spreads or produces harmful symptoms. Similarly, neurofibromatosis 2 is often associated with acoustic neuroma, a benign tumor most often found on the auditory nerve.

CHAPTER 13

Disorders of the Senses and Body Function

C11   Sleep Disorders   307

C12   Narcolepsy   315

C13   Epilepsy and Seizures   319

C14   Dizziness and Vertigo   327

C15   Seeing Problems   332

C16   Hearing Problems   341

C17   Smelling and Tasting Problems   347

C18   Autonomic Disorders   352

C19   Chronic Fatigue Syndrome   357

This chapter addresses some of the disorders that occur when our brains' basic regulatory functions do not work properly. Among our brains' most important tasks is governing when and how much we sleep. If that system breaks down, or if emotional tension or physical problems interfere, a person may be unable to enjoy healthy sleep or to remain awake at appropriate times. Epilepsy is a separate condition that causes individuals to lose consciousness. That problem does not involve sleep regulation, however, but an abnormal electrical discharge in the brain. Such discharges can also cause convulsions or involuntary movement, again unregulated.

The chapter next discusses difficulties with our major senses: balance, sight, hearing, and smell and taste, which are closely linked. Such difficulties are symptoms, which have many possible causes. Physicians must usually identify the underlying disorders before addressing the problem.

The chapter's final sections address disorders in how the body maintains itself through the autonomic nervous system (heartbeat, blood pressure, perspiration, and so on), and in a person's ability to maintain sufficient energy to get through the day.

Sleep Disorders

Sleep is essential to our lives, and it's one of the few activities we do for large parts of the day from infancy through old age. Many people, however, suffer some form of sleep disturbance troubling enough to send them to their physicians. The most common complaints involve getting too little sound sleep, feeling excessively sleepy, or having disturbances or difficulties during sleep, such as sleepwalking (somnambulism). These are not trivial problems. If you have ongoing disorders of sleep and wakefulness, you are clearly at risk for poor health and impaired occupational, social, and psychological functioning.

The symptoms of insomnia and excessive daytime sleepiness can arise from several different disorders, each of which requires specific evaluation and treatment. Before discussing these possibilities, however, we will describe how people normally sleep.

The brain has three major states of activity and function: wakefulness, rapid eye movement (REM) sleep, and non-REM (NREM) sleep. It's during REM sleep, identifiable because the sleeper's eyes can be seen shifting quickly below his or her eyelids, that we have our most vivid dreams. In this state, your brain becomes electrically and metabolically activated; in fact, electroencephalographic (EEG) readings during REM sleep would be somewhat similar to those recorded when you are awake. At the same time, the brain automatically stills your muscles. Even though you may be dreaming vividly, you cannot normally react to that mental activity.

Healthy sleep consists of recurring cycles, 70 to 120 minutes long, of NREM and REM sleep. Typically, a sleeping person proceeds from wakefulness through the four stages of NREM sleep until reaching the first REM period. The sleeper then returns to NREM sleep, and the cycle begins again. In healthy adults, the deepest stages of sleep—NREM stages 3 and 4, or "slow-wave sleep"—occur predominantly in the first two cycles. The REM periods in the first half of an adult's sleep period are brief; they get longer in later cycles. Ideally, you should be able to sleep well through these cycles on a regular basis.

Evaluating Sleep Disorders

Diagnosing conditions that affect how a person sleeps starts with taking a thorough medical and psychiatric history. The doctor should look into what that individual experiences over the entire 24-hour day, not just during the nighttime. The impact of disrupted sleep on daytime mood, fatigue, muscle aches, attention, and concentration may be significant. Often doctors ask people to keep a two-week log recording their sleep-wake patterns; napping and activity during the day; use of stimulants, hypnotics, or alcohol; diet; number of times they wake during the night; how long they think they have slept; and how they perceive their daytime mood and alertness.

Only about 4 percent to 5 percent of the general population complains of being too sleepy during the day. A much larger percentage complains of insomnia, or not being able to fall asleep at night. Nevertheless, over half of the people referred for formal sleep studies have symptoms of excessive sleepiness, especially a propensity to nod off. The severity of this problem is called mild if a person falls asleep during a sedentary activity, such as watching television; moderate if a person drifts off during mild physical activity, such as driving; and severe if sleep occurs during a physical activity that requires moderate attention, such as talking or eating. Obviously, falling asleep at the wheel of your car is much more hazardous than falling asleep during a conversation, and doctors take that symptom very seriously. But nodding off while talking actually indicates a more severe disorder because that activity engages more of your brain at once.

Doctors usually ask sleepy individuals about such symptoms as morning headaches; cataplexy (loss of muscle strength triggered by strong emotions); hallucinations during drowsy periods; sleep paralysis; finding one has done tasks during sleep without remembering them; and feeling confused or disoriented during the transition between sleep and being awake (called sleep drunkenness). Doctors also often interview bed partners about behavior that a sleeping person cannot perceive, such as snoring, respiratory

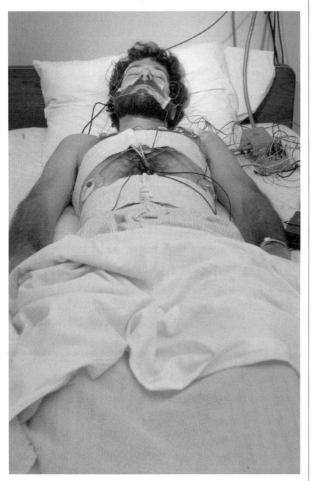

All-night sleep recordings, or "polysomnography," in a lab provide data on an individual's periods of uninterrupted sleep, REM and NREM stages, breathing patterns, oxygen levels, heart rhythm, and movements. PHOTO © DAN MCCOY/RAINBOW/PICTUREQUEST

pauses longer than ten seconds, unusual body movements, and sleepwalking. If you complain of disturbances during sleep, expect questions about nocturnal incontinence, sudden episodes of troubled breathing, headaches, jaw clenching or teeth grinding (bruxism), talking in your sleep, and sleepwalking.

All-night sleep recordings, or polysomnography, remain the principal diagnostic tool in the field of sleep medicine. A thorough test provides data on an individual's periods of uninterrupted sleep, REM and NREM stages, breathing patterns, oxygen levels, heart rhythm, and movements. Doctors may also want to monitor body temperature and whether a man has erections while asleep. This test usually requires spending one night in a sleep clinic. If you are excessively sleepy, polysomnography is well justified given your high risk of having sleep apnea or narcolepsy (**C12**). Doctors may also use polysomnography for anyone with other problems they suspect are related to sleep apnea or nocturnal seizure disorder (**C13**). Polysomnography is generally not used to evaluate chronic insomnia except when doctors suspect the root cause is an undetected, or occult, sleep disorder like sleep apnea or nocturnal myoclonus, or involuntary muscle contractions.

Primary Insomnia

Primary insomnia is the medical term for difficulty falling asleep, remaining asleep, or waking up feeling unrefreshed for over a month. By definition, primary insomnia must result in significant daytime impairment and not be connected to another sleep disorder.

For some people, this condition lasts a lifetime. These individuals have a constitutional predisposition for fragmented sleep. We do not know the reason, but the condition probably stems from a neurochemical or structural disorder involving the neural networks that govern our sleep-wake states. People with this disorder are extremely light sleepers, easily perturbed by noise, temperature fluctuations, and anxiety.

Some people develop primary insomnia following a period of severe stress. For these individuals the difficulty going to sleep lingers after the source of stress has been removed because they have adapted new behaviors that disrupt sleep. Often they have come to associate cues in their sleeping environment, such as clocks, with being awake, thus reinforcing the sleep disturbance. This disorder can persist over many years and cause chronic fatigue, muscle aches, and mood disturbance.

Treatment for insomnia often involves education about healthy sleep practices and an examination of behaviors that may interfere with sleep. Individuals may be instructed to improve their sleep hygiene by maintaining a regular bedtime, avoiding alcohol and caffeine, getting regular exercise, and avoiding stressful activity before retiring. Such relaxation therapies as meditation, deep breathing, and progressive muscle relaxation can be helpful. It is often beneficial for people to modify their behavior so they don't spend much time awake in bed. This allows them to associate lying down in bed with sleeping. These are all effective treatments for insomnia that do not involve the use of sleeping pills.

Treating chronic insomnia with sleeping medications remains controversial, particularly for the elderly. Sleeping medication should be considered only after doctors have thoroughly assessed the possible causes of the insomnia that may be treated in other ways, and after sleepers have tried to improve their sleep through behavioral changes. If those steps are unsuccessful, then doctors may prescribe hypnotics, starting with very low doses for short, limited periods. Sleeping medications such as zolpidem, zaleplon, and short and intermediate half-life benzodiazepines are safe and effective in treating transient insomnia in people who have not had problems with substance abuse.

Sleep Apnea

People with sleep apnea frequently stop breathing during sleep. This makes the oxygen levels in their blood drop, and they may wake up gasping loudly and thrashing. Though EEG readings would show these people's brains reach a wakeful state, they usually return to sleep quickly and do not remember the interruption. They sim-

A. Obstructive sleep apnea

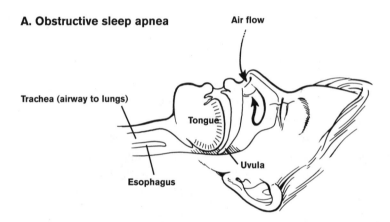

B. Continuous positive airway pressure opens airway

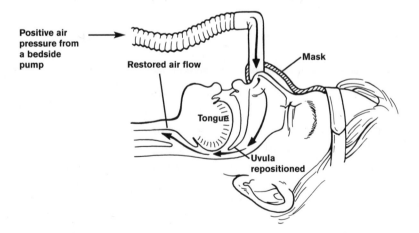

A continuous positive airway pressure (CPAP) device prevents the airway obstruction that causes sleep apnea. Illustration © Kathryn Born

ply feel a lack of refreshing sleep in the morning. Often, alarmed bed partners alert people with sleep apnea to the problem, and their observations of the sleeping subject are very useful to doctors. Although it occasionally causes insomnia, sleep apnea is typically an occult disorder that causes daytime sleepiness, impaired concentration and intellectual functioning, and morning headaches. Sleep apnea is associated with obesity and loud snoring, and it seems to be connected to high blood pressure, irregular heartbeat, and early death. Sleep apnea is also related to age: it affects approximately 24 percent of people over the age of 65 and 42 percent of the elderly living in nursing homes.

There are a variety of treatments for sleep apnea. People often benefit from losing weight, abstaining from sedative-hypnotic drugs, and learning to avoid sleeping on their backs. Mechanical approaches include devices to hold down the tongue or pull the jawbone forward, both of which help keep the airway clear. Continuous positive airway pressure (CPAP) is the treatment of choice for moderate to severe sleep apnea. The sleeper wears a device over his or her nose and mouth that blows air into those orifices, causing the mouth and throat to remain open for every breath. For severe cases, surgical techniques to increase the size of a person's airway include reshaping the inner structures of the mouth and throat (uvulopalatopharyngoplasty), shifting the bones of the jaw area (maxillomandibular and hyoid advancement), and chronic tracheostomy.

Circadian Rhythm Disorders

The timing of our daily sleep-wake cycle is mainly under the control of the suprachias-matic nucleus in the hypothalamus, which establishes a daily, or circadian, rhythm. This rhythm can be disrupted by external demands on us to be awake at particular times. Circadian rhythm sleep disorders show up as either insomnia or excessive sleepiness, depending on when a person's body thinks it is in the sleep or wake cycle. Travelers flying across multiple time zones and rotating shift workers can experience fatigue, gastrointestinal upset, and other physical symptoms because of disruptions of their circadian rhythms. Some studies have shown that people with disrupted circadian rhythms also think less effectively and less quickly.

The treatment for many circadian rhythm disorders involves realigning a person's sleep-wake schedule by manipulating or augmenting the external environmental cues our bodies rely on. One example is bright light therapy. Many studies have shown that exposure to bright light can shift and realign people's circadian rhythms.

Some individuals have circadian rhythm disorders related to a diminished capacity to respond to environmental cues about when to sleep, especially the natural daily cycle of light and dark. People with the delayed sleep-phase disorder seem to have an innate preference for beginning to sleep in the late hours of night and staying in bed until late morning or early afternoon. If such "night owls" can find work and social life that fit that schedule, of course, their preference stops being a disorder.

Nocturnal Myoclonus and Restless Legs Syndrome

Nocturnal myoclonus, or "twitching at night," is characterized by periodic leg movements

COMMON SLEEP DISORDERS

ADVANCED SLEEP-PHASE SYNDROME

A disorder in which the major sleep episode is advanced in relation to the desired clock time, resulting in symptoms of compelling evening sleepiness, an early sleep onset, and an awakening that is earlier than desired.

Synonyms & keywords: phase advance, stable asynchrony relative to typical environmental patterns, evening somnolence and early-morning wakefulness, extreme larkishness.

CENTRAL SLEEP APNEA SYNDROME

A syndrome characterized by a cessation or decrease of ventilatory effort during sleep, usually associated with oxygen desaturation.

Synonyms & keywords: central apnea, nonobstructive sleep apnea, Cheyne-Stokes respiration.

DELAYED SLEEP-PHASE SYNDROME

A disorder in which the major sleep episode is delayed in relation to the desired clock time, resulting in symptoms of sleep-onset insomnia or difficulty in awakening at the desired time.

Synonyms & keywords: phase lag, phase delay, sleep-onset insomnia, morning sleepiness, stable asynchrony relative to typical environmental patterns.

INSOMNIA

Difficulty in initiating or maintaining sleep.

NARCOLEPSY

A disorder of unknown etiology that is characterized by excessive sleepiness and that is typically associated with cataplexy and other REM-sleep phenomena, such as sleep paralysis and hypnagogic hallucinations.

---

that interrupt a person's sleep. People are usually unaware of this disorder except as morning leg cramps and a sense of insufficient sleep. They may complain of either insomnia or daytime sleepiness. Nocturnal myoclonus is a relatively common disorder that frequently appears in association with sleep apnea, narcolepsy (C12), uremia, diabetes, and a variety of disorders affecting the cortex, brain stem, and spinal cord. Typically, however, it has no obvious cause and no link to larger problems in the central nervous system.

Restless legs syndrome is another disorder that prevents people from falling asleep. A person feels discomfort in his or her calf muscles and an urge to keep the legs in motion. This condition is associated with uremia, anemia, and pregnancy, as well as with nocturnal myoclonus.

The most common treatments for both nocturnal myoclonus and restless legs syndrome involve medications. Specifically, physicians prescribe benzodiazepines, dopaminomimetics such as L-dopa and bromocriptine, or other drugs that increase the brain's supply of the neurotransmitter dopamine. Other medications cur-

Synonyms & keywords: excessive sleepiness, abnormal rapid eye movement (REM) sleep, cataplexy, sleep paralysis, hypnagogic hallucinations, nocturnal sleep disruption, positive human leukocyte antigen (HLA)-DR2 or -DQ1, genetic component.

OBSTRUCTIVE SLEEP APNEA SYNDROME

A syndrome characterized by repetitive episodes of upper airway obstruction that occur during sleep, usually associated with a reduction in blood oxygen saturation.

Synonyms & keywords: sleep apnea, obstructive apnea, upper airway apnea, mixed apnea, hypersomnia sleep apnea syndrome, adenoidal hypertrophy, cor pulmonale syndrome.

PERIODIC LIMB MOVEMENT DISORDER

A disorder characterized by periodic episodes of repetitive and highly stereotyped limb movements that occur during sleep.

Synonyms & keywords: periodic leg movements (PLMs), nocturnal myoclonus, periodic movements in sleep (PMS), leg jerks.

RESTLESS LEGS SYNDROME

A disorder characterized by disagreeable leg sensations that usually occur before sleep onset and that cause an almost irresistible urge to move the legs.

Synonyms & keywords: restless legs syndrome (RLS), disagreeable sensations in legs.

Source: International Classification of Sleep Disorders, American Academy of Sleep Medicine

rently under investigation include opioids and anticonvulsants.

Parasomnias

Parasomnias are adverse events or behaviors that occur during sleep. Sleepwalking and sleep terrors both involve incomplete awakenings that generally occur when individuals are in the deepest stages of NREM sleep: stages 3 and 4. Sleepwalking and night terrors are normally experienced by young children, though in some cases these problems may persist into adulthood.

Sleepwalkers become partially aroused and start to move around their homes. They are typically difficult to fully awaken and do not remember their activity. They are frequently clumsy and occasionally hurt themselves during these episodes.

Sleep terrors involve the emergence during sleep of intense fear and its normal autonomic symptoms—sweating and increased heart rate, for instance. The people who suffer these terrors are inconsolable, difficult to fully awaken, and unable

HOW TO MANAGE YOUR SLEEP DISORDER

- Avoid caffeine within four to six hours of bedtime.

- Avoid the use of nicotine close to bedtime or during the night.

- Do not drink alcoholic beverages within four to six hours of bedtime.

- Avoid large meals before bedtime.

- Avoid strenuous exercise within six hours of bedtime.

- If you are unable to fall asleep or stay asleep, leave your bedroom and engage in a quiet activity elsewhere. Do not permit yourself to fall asleep outside the bedroom. Return to bed when—and only when—you are sleepy.

- Maintain a regular arise time, even on days off work and on weekends.

- Avoid napping during the daytime. If daytime sleepiness becomes overwhelming, limit naptime to a single nap of less than one hour, no later than 3 P.M.

- Don't bring any work to bed! Leave paperwork, bills, and other chores at your desk! Try to keep your bedroom for sleep and relaxation.

Adapted from www.aasmnet.org (American Academy of Sleep Medicine)

to recall the specific thoughts or images that made them anxious. In contrast, children (or adults) who suffer nightmares are usually able to remember their anxiety-provoking dreams in vivid detail.

Normally our muscles do not work when we are in REM sleep, but in rare cases that off switch does not work. The term REM behavior disorder refers to prominent motor activity during dreaming. Several dramatic cases have involved patients who suddenly assaulted their bed partners in response to frightening dreams. REM behavior disorder can appear during periods of drug intoxication or withdrawal, or be a chronic condition, most typically in people with a clear neurological disease.

Treatment for parasomnias is directed toward reducing sleep deprivation, stress, and anxiety, all of which are known to exacerbate these disorders. When families can identify sources of stress or anxiety, psychotherapy is usually helpful. Children may also benefit from changing their behavior (maintaining regular sleep hours, perhaps including naps) or from more specific behavioral techniques (such as hypnosis, or awakening the child at appropriate times to preempt episodes). In extreme cases, low-dose benzodiazepines are effective. For patients with REM behavior disorder, doctors have found that benzodiazepines, such as clonazepam, and the anticonvulsant carbamazepine are useful in reducing the troubling episodes.

Narcolepsy

The most visible symptom of narcolepsy is daytime sleepiness. We all feel sleepy sometimes, of course. But people with narcolepsy can suffer frequent and overwhelming sleep attacks, forcing them to nap often during the day. They or their families may interpret this pattern as indicating fatigue or depression (**C20**). Such sleepiness can cause people great trouble at school or work and is usually what brings them to their doctors.

Narcolepsy's other prominent symptom is cataplexy, a brief and sudden loss of muscle strength triggered by strong emotions. It is very important in diagnosing narcolepsy because it does not show up in any other disorder; however, not all narcoleptics experience cataplexy. Typically, people feel weak in the knees and have to sit down when they are emotionally excited. Any strong emotion can cause this reaction, from laughing at a funny joke to getting angry. Other attacks of muscle weakness may affect the head (head dropping), jaw (jaw dropping), face, or arms. Cataplexy is frequently mild. It may occur only a few times per month or several times a day. Strong attacks may escalate to complete body paralysis lasting a few minutes. Cataplexy may be confused with epilepsy (**C13**) or other neurological and psychiatric problems, but people remain awake and conscious during cataplexy. Cataplexy can also be confused with catalepsy, a symptom characterized by increased muscle tone and body rigidity, most often in the context of schizophrenia (**C25**).

Other symptoms of narcolepsy include sleep paralysis, hypnagogic hallucinations, and insomnia. But people with other sleep disorders (**C11**) can have these experiences, too, as do normal individuals on occasion. Sleep paralysis is an inability to move when waking up or falling asleep; the first episode is often frightening, but the feeling always ends after a few seconds or a few minutes. Hypnagogic hallucinations (*hypnagogic* means "when falling asleep") are dreamlike visions or perceptions of noise that occur when patients are tired or actually falling asleep. People with vivid dreamlike hallucinations have occasionally been misdiagnosed as schizophrenic (**C25**).

Contrary to popular belief, people with narcolepsy do not typically sleep more than others. Rather, they fall asleep easily many times during the day and night but have great difficulties staying asleep at night. In other words, they are unable to stay either awake or asleep for long periods of time. Insomnia is thus common for people with narcolepsy. But their total amount of sleep across the 24-hour day is usually normal.

As you would guess, a child who easily falls asleep at school often has trouble following the lessons and receives little sympathy from teachers who do not realize the true problem. Falling asleep on the job is equally troublesome. Less careful observers might assume a narcoleptic has been drinking (C30) or taking drugs (C29). Narcolepsy can thus be socially isolating. Unfortunately, it usually takes many years for the disorder to be diagnosed—14 years from onset is the typical lag. Early detection and treatment can help children receive appropriate schooling and adults function more normally in their daily lives.

Causes and Mechanisms

Narcolepsy typically starts when a person is between 15 and 25 years of age, but it may affect children before puberty and older adults as well. Once established, it is a lifelong condition; genuine remissions are exceptional. In the West, approximately 1 person in every 2,000 has narcolepsy with cataplexy, and many more may have narcolepsy without cataplexy. Most cases of narcolepsy are nonfamilial, but first-degree relatives (parents, children, and siblings) of people diagnosed with the disease have 20 to 40 times the risk of developing it.

Many of the symptoms of narcolepsy are due to abnormal transitions from wakefulness to rapid eye movement (REM) sleep. Normally people enter REM sleep 90 to 120 minutes after they fall asleep and return to that state periodically all through the night. Normal REM sleep is associated

THE KEY TO NARCOLEPSY MAY LIE IN MAN'S BEST FRIEND

In 1999, researchers at Stanford University in California announced that after a decade-long search, they had identified a gene that causes the sleep disorder narcolepsy. The research team, led by Emmanuel Mignot, M.D., Ph.D., isolated the gene in two breeds of dogs: Doberman pinschers and Labrador retrievers. Dogs are one of the few species besides humans known to develop narcolepsy.

The researchers suspected that humans with narcolepsy carry the same defective genes, and in September 2000 they confirmed that people with the sleep disorder have a breakdown in the same molecular pathway as that observed in canines. Specifically, they found that a small protein—or peptide—present in the brain cells of normal people was absent in every narcoleptic brain they studied. Armed with this information, researchers now have a specific target for which to develop drug treatments.

Narcolepsy, whose most recognizable symptom is sleep attacks, is not exclusive to humans. This dog is in the midst of a narcoleptic attack, asleep with a ball in his mouth. Studying narcoleptic dogs has helped researchers gain understanding of the disorder, including the role of genes that may be involved. PHOTO COURTESY OF EMMANUEL MIGNOT, M.D., PH.D., CENTER FOR NARCOLEPSY, STANFORD UNIVERSITY SCHOOL OF MEDICINE

with vivid dreaming, rapid eye movements, and complete muscle paralysis. It normally occurs in the middle of the night. People with narcolepsy experience abrupt transitions from wakefulness to REM sleep, often before they are completely asleep. This problem produces "dissociated" states in which a person is half awake and half in REM sleep. For example, in sleep paralysis a person is conscious, but his or her muscles are still paralyzed. In hypnagogic hallucinations a person is awake but dreaming as if in REM sleep. Cataplexy is considered similar to REM sleep paralysis but occurs when the brain is excited by an emotion.

Narcolepsy-cataplexy is most often due to a lack of the brain hormone called hypocretin, or orexin. The hormone is synthesized by approximately 20,000 cells in the hypothalamus that help control sleep. Most narcoleptics have lost these cells, so their sleep is not normally regulated. How these crucial cells have been destroyed is still unknown, but most researchers believe an abnormal immune response is involved. In other words, people's immune systems have mistakenly attacked cells in their own brains. If this hypothesis is confirmed, narcolepsy will be classified as an autoimmune disorder like multiple sclerosis (**C33**) or juvenile-onset diabetes mellitus.

Diagnosis and Treatment

The diagnosis of narcolepsy is usually made by sleep specialists, generally neurologists in a sleep laboratory. If you are seeking such an evaluation, look for laboratories accredited by the American Academy of Sleep Medicine and physicians board certified in sleep medicine; they usually have more experience with the condition. After listening to a person's experiences, a special-

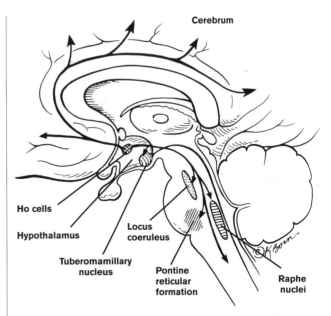

Lack of a brain hormone called hypocretin, or orexin, is believed to cause narcolepsy. Hypocretin is manufactured by cells in the hypothalamus, which helps control sleep. Most people who suffer narcolepsy have lost these cells, possibly because of an abnormal immune response. ILLUSTRATION © KATHRYN BORN

ist arranges for him or her to sleep in the lab for a night. Observing sleep can exclude the possibility of sleep apnea and other sleep disorders (**C11**).

The next day the specialist performs a multiple sleep latency test. This starts with asking the patient to nap four to five times for 20 minutes every two hours. The doctor measures how fast the person falls asleep and notes the presence or absence of REM sleep, using scalp electrodes. Normal individuals either do not fall asleep in these short periods or sleep for a long time, though not long enough to enter REM sleep. In contrast, people with narcolepsy generally fall asleep for short periods and often experience REM sleep in these short naps. The criteria for diagnosing narcolepsy are naps that occur on average less than eight minutes, with two or

LIVING WITH NARCOLEPSY

The goal of treatment is to keep the patient as alert as possible during the day and to minimize any recurring episodes of cataplexy, using a minimal amount of medication. Two methods are used:

■ **Drug therapy**

■ **Nap therapy (2–3 short naps during the day)**

Regardless of the type of treatment, continuing doctor-patient communication is recommended to successfully manage symptoms. Educating one's family and friends about narcolepsy is equally important, as is contact with a support group of others who have or who are familiar with narcolepsy.

Adapted from www.narcolepsynetwork.org (Narcolepsy Network)

more REM episodes occurring in the four or five naps.

Physicians may also run a test to look for the human leukocyte antigen (HLA) in a person's blood, searching for specific types. HLA is only weakly predictive of narcolepsy, however. Another possible test is a lumbar puncture (spinal tap) to measure hypocretin levels in the person's cerebrospinal fluid (CSF); the result of this test demonstrates narcolepsy very specifically, but it is more invasive and uncomfortable, and doctors usually perform it only when they are doing research on the disorder.

Some people with narcolepsy find their conditions improve when they make changes in their lifestyle, such as napping on schedule and avoiding specific foods. These steps are rarely enough to control the problem, however. Most patients are prescribed medications for their symptoms:

■ stimulants (modafinil and amphetamines) for sleepiness

■ antidepressant compounds for cataplexy, sleep paralysis, and hypnagogic hallucinations

■ sleep-inducing agents for insomnia

These medications help control the symptoms of narcolepsy but do not treat the cause of the disease. They have many side effects and are often only partially effective. Support groups such as the Narcolepsy Network are very helpful for people dealing with the condition.

New treatments aimed at replacing the missing hypocretin hormone are being developed and will probably become very effective. Additionally, researchers are exploring the destruction of the hypocretin-containing cells in the brain. We must understand this process before we can truly prevent or cure narcolepsy.

Epilepsy and Seizures

A seizure is a sudden, brief attack caused by an abnormal electrical discharge in the brain. People experience it as altered awareness (losing consciousness, for instance), involuntary movements, or convulsions. During a seizure, a person's brain cells "fire" uncontrollably, temporarily affecting the way he or she behaves, moves, thinks, or feels. This abnormal firing may involve the entire cerebral cortex (primary generalized seizure), or it may begin in one brain area and affect only a limited region (a partial, or focal, seizure).

Many conditions can trigger a seizure, including injury or trauma to the head (**C61**); brain tumors (**C10, C64**); infections, especially meningitis (**C37**) and encephalitis (**C38**); genetic conditions; and structural abnormalities in the brain's blood vessels (**C60**). Seizures may also result from high fever (called febrile seizures) or heatstroke, severe sleep deprivation, diabetes (if blood sugar levels become too low or too high), alcohol or drug withdrawal (**C29, C30**), or a reaction to medications (**C66**). Some people may have a single unprovoked seizure for no discernible reason. Others will have repeated seizures, again without explanation despite doctors'

best efforts to establish a diagnosis. Although seizures, these examples are not necessarily epilepsy.

Epilepsy is a condition of spontaneously recurring seizures that are typically unprovoked and usually unpredictable. It can arise from a variety of underlying conditions and mechanisms, but the majority of cases in both adults and children have no known cause. Forty-five million people worldwide have epilepsy, and each year 125,000 to 150,000 people are newly diagnosed with the condition in the United States. About 30 percent of these are children.

A person's lifetime risk of experiencing at least one unprovoked seizure is about 4 percent, and the likelihood of experiencing a seizure of any sort, including those brought on by fever or acute illness, rises to at least 9 percent. The risk that a person will develop epilepsy is about 3 percent. Although genetic diseases account for only 1 percent of epilepsy cases, inheritable factors are important in a much higher percentage, especially in children. As a general rule, however, even children born to a parent with epilepsy have no more than a 10 percent chance of developing the disorder.

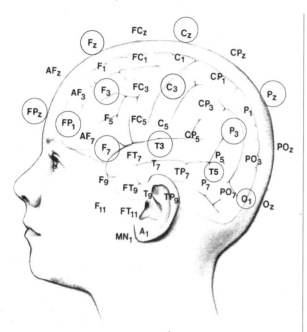

An electroencephalogram (EEG) is the most important diagnostic test for epilepsy. It is able to show specific patterns of brain waves, helping a doctor determine the precise type of seizure. This schematic shows the locations where EEG leads are placed to record brain waves. The circled positions are always used; the other positions are added when necessary to clarify or localize an abnormality. Even-numbered electrodes are placed on the right side of the head. Readouts, on the next page, from the circled positions show the pattern of brain waves in different types of seizures. ILLUSTRATION COURTESY OF TIMOTHY A. PEDLEY, M.D., NEUROLOGICAL INSTITUTE, COLUMBIA-PRESBYTERIAN MEDICAL CENTER

Types of Seizures

As mentioned above, there are two major types of seizures: generalized and partial. In generalized seizures, abnormal firing of brain cells begins on both sides of the brain at about the same time. There are four common types of generalized seizures, each producing different symptoms.

Generalized tonic-clonic seizures are also called grand mal seizures. During such an episode, a person abruptly loses consciousness and falls to the ground. All body muscles can contract at once in a sustained fashion (tonic), or they can contract in a series of shorter rhythmic contractions (clonic), or both. Loss of bladder control is common, while loss of bowel control is rare. The seizure episode typically lasts for about 90 seconds and is followed by a brief period of deep stupor, then a longer period of lethargy and confusion. Many people experience headaches (C54), muscle aches, lack of energy, inability to concentrate, and mood changes for up to 24 hours after the seizure.

Absence (petit mal) seizures occur mainly in children. They are characterized by sudden, momentary lapses in awareness, staring, rhythmic blinking, and often a few small jerks of the hands or arms. Most last for less than ten seconds. Because behavior and awareness return immediately to normal, a person usually has no idea that a seizure has occurred. Absence seizures can occur hundreds of times a day.

Myoclonic seizures are characterized by rapid, recurrent, brief muscle jerks. These jerks can range from small movements of the face or hands to massive spasms that can affect the head, arms, legs, and trunk of the body at the same time. The person does not experience a loss of consciousness. Although myoclonic seizures can happen at any time, they are most likely to occur shortly after a person wakes up or while falling asleep.

Atonic seizures, also called drop attacks, are characterized by a sudden loss of muscle tone, which may occur in one part of the body (such as a head drop) or be more generalized, which usually results in the person falling. Sometimes atonic seizures are preceded by a brief myoclonic seizure or a tonic spasm, which can add force to the fall.

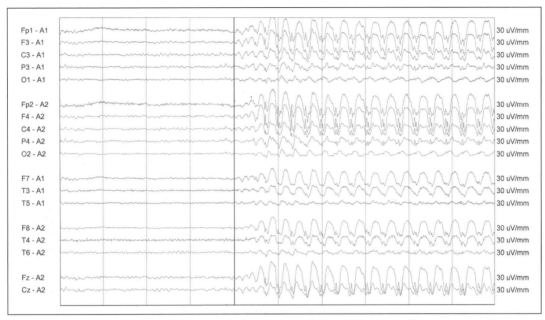

Fp1 - A1	30 uV/mm
F3 - A1	30 uV/mm
C3 - A1	30 uV/mm
P3 - A1	30 uV/mm
O1 - A1	30 uV/mm
Fp2 - A2	30 uV/mm
F4 - A2	30 uV/mm
C4 - A2	30 uV/mm
P4 - A2	30 uV/mm
O2 - A2	30 uV/mm
F7 - A1	30 uV/mm
T3 - A1	30 uV/mm
T5 - A1	30 uV/mm
F8 - A2	30 uV/mm
T4 - A2	30 uV/mm
T6 - A2	30 uV/mm
Fz - A2	30 uV/mm
Cz - A2	30 uV/mm

Absence seizures, sometimes called petit mal seizures, cause a momentary interruption of normal brain function. Brain waves to the left of the heavy vertical line on the graph are normal; to the right, the change is obvious. The seizure discharge begins in all areas of the cortex in the fifth second of recording. During this discharge, the patient, a child, stared and was motionless and unresponsive. This is one kind of "generalized onset" seizure.
ILLUSTRATION COURTESY OF TIMOTHY A. PEDLEY, M.D., NEUROLOGICAL INSTITUTE, COLUMBIA-PRESBYTERIAN MEDICAL CENTER

People experiencing this type of seizure are more apt to injure themselves.

In partial or focal seizures, the abnormal firing of brain cells originates in only one region of the brain. This results in seizures that are categorized as either simple or complex. In addition, some partial seizures can evolve to affect the whole brain at once, a condition called secondarily generalized seizures.

Complex partial seizures are the most common type of seizures in adults. A person loses awareness of his or her surroundings, becoming unresponsive or only partially responsive. Some individuals may smack their lips, swallow repeatedly, or engage in other random and inap-propriate activity, called automations. After the seizure the person may remain confused and disoriented for several minutes.

In **simple partial seizures,** the seizure-related discharge remains very localized, sometimes exquisitely so, and the person remains awake and aware. Symptoms vary greatly depending on the specific brain area involved. A person may perceive abnormal smells (C17) or a distorted environment, feel ready to throw up, experience feelings of unreality or detachment, have jerking movements in one area of the body, or experience unexplained emotions such as fear and rage. People come to recognize their seizures' characteristic aura.

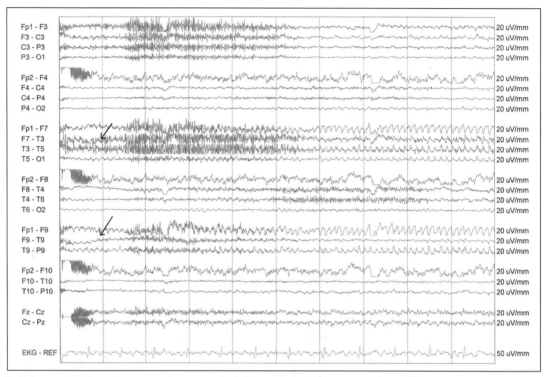

Left-temporal-lobe seizures produce a marked change in brain wave recordings. The seizure discharge can be seen beginning in the left-temporal electrodes. During this electrical abnormality, the patient stared, had chewing movements of the mouth with lip smacking, and made rubbing movements with the left hand on her thigh. Afterward, the patient was briefly confused and, after recovery, had only a vague memory of having had a seizure. This is termed a complex partial seizure, which is a seizure that begins locally in a particular brain region and is associated with altered consciousness. ILLUSTRATION COURTESY OF TIMOTHY A. PEDLEY, M.D., NEUROLOGICAL INSTITUTE, COLUMBIA-PRESBYTERIAN MEDICAL CENTER

Doctors classify types of epilepsy as well. The major divisions depend, first, on whether the seizures are partial or generalized, and second, on their causes. Subtypes are defined by the person's age and by the anatomic area in which the seizure originates. Other helpful data include the individual's medical history, findings of neurological examinations, and results of electroencephalograms (EEGs), brain imaging studies, and other tests. Defining seizures within these epileptic syndromes helps doctors evaluate and treat people more specifically.

There are dozens of these epileptic syndromes. Some of the generalized epilepsy syndromes include infantile spasms (West syndrome), childhood absence epilepsy (petit mal), Lennox-Gastaut syndrome, and juvenile myoclonic epilepsy. Localized epilepsy syndromes include benign focal epilepsy of childhood ("rolandic epilepsy"), temporal lobe epilepsy (the most common type in adults), frontal lobe epilepsy, post-traumatic seizures (**C28**), and epilepsia partialis continua (unremitting seizures on one side of the body).

WHEN SOMEONE IS HAVING A SEIZURE

It can be frightening the first time you see a loved one experience a seizure, especially if that person is a child. Here are some steps to take to ensure the best possible outcome:

■ Protect the person's head from hitting anything hard.

■ Make sure the person's breathing passage remains open. Clear the nose and mouth if necessary, and pull the head back slightly to straighten the neck. Artificial respiration is rarely necessary.

■ Do *not* try to force anything into the person's mouth, either medicine or an object meant to keep the airway open or to stop tongue bites (which are actually rare). Such action can cause much worse damage than it prevents.

■ If the person has a high fever, try to lower his or her body temperature with sponging. *After* the seizure is over, you may administer acetaminophen or other fever medication.

As a person recovers from a seizure, he or she probably feels confused and frightened, on top of any physical symptoms such as grogginess. Offer reassurance and help finding a doctor.

About 50 percent to 70 percent of people who develop epilepsy are eventually able to keep the disorder under control to their satisfaction. On the other hand, severe seizures that resist treatment, especially those that appear in early childhood, are associated with a shortened life span, risk of intellectual impairment, and a sharply reduced quality of life.

Diagnosis and Treatment

When doctors treat a person who has had a seizure, they have three goals:

■ determining whether the person has epilepsy, or whether the seizure has some other cause that requires treatment

■ classifying the seizure and type of epilepsy

■ identifying, if possible, the underlying cause

A doctor first takes a medical history, which should include a detailed description of the person's seizure. The doctor will also ask about relevant risk factors for epilepsy, such as a family history of seizures, severe head trauma, encephalitis, meningitis, or recent infection with fever. Most people with epilepsy have normal results on a physical examination, but in some the examination may uncover underlying neurological or systemic problems, of which the seizures are a symptom.

An EEG is usually the most important diagnostic test for epilepsy. An EEG can show specific types of brain wave patterns, helping physicians determine the precise type of seizure. Sometimes doctors need to do multiple tests to actually record a seizure while it happens.

In addition to the EEG, brain imaging studies, especially magnetic resonance imaging (MRI), can aid in the diagnosis. Some people may benefit from the other types of brain scans as well, including computed tomography (CT), positron-emission tomography (PET), or single-photon-emission computed tomography (SPECT). Other basic laboratory tests may include blood tests, a lumbar puncture (spinal tap) if physicians suspect meningitis or encephalitis, and toxicological screens for possible drug use or poisoning.

Treatment depends on the cause of the seizure. For those with a known cause (such as an infection, a blood vessel malformation in the brain, a brain tumor, or a severe chemical imbalance in the blood), the condition can often be corrected with medication or surgery.

Treating unprovoked seizures can be a bit trickier. About 25 percent of people with unprovoked seizures come to a doctor after a single attack, nearly always a generalized tonic-clonic seizure. Only about a quarter of these people later develop epilepsy. Providing medications to head off future seizures carries a risk of adverse effects, which approaches 30 percent after the initial treatment. Treating children with antiepileptic drugs raises additional issues because we do not know their long-term effects on brain development, learning, and behavior. Therefore, physicians do not treat many people after a first seizure. After a second seizure, however, a person's risk of further seizures rises to 80 percent, and drug treatment is usually recommended.

There is no treatment currently available that can cure epilepsy. The treatment of epilepsy therefore has three main objectives:

- eliminating seizures, or reducing them as much as possible

- avoiding drug-related side effects

- helping the person restore or maintain a normal lifestyle

Of people with epilepsy, 60 percent to 70 percent achieve satisfactory control of their seizures with antiepileptic drugs, but fewer than 50 percent of adults achieve complete control without drug side effects.

Drugs used to suppress partial and secondarily generalized seizures include carbamazepine (Tegretol), phenytoin (Dilantin), and new medications such as oxcarbazepine (Trileptal), levetiracetam (Keppra), lamotrigine (Lamictal), topiramate (Topamax), and zonisamide (Zonegran). Valproate has been the drug of first choice for generalized-onset seizures, but many patients now have the option of taking lamotrigine or levetiracetam as well. All of these drugs can produce side effects, the most common of which are dose-related and typically occur when the drug is first given or when the dose is increased. These side effects include nausea, sleepiness, mood changes, mental dulling, and dizziness. Other side effects indicating too high a dose include blurred or double vision, dizziness, slurred speech, and incoordination. Individuals and their doctors should be alert to these possible problems when starting a new dosage. All of these effects go away when the dosage is lowered. Side effects unrelated to the dosage, such as allergic reactions, can be severe but are rare.

Some people continue to have seizures despite drug treatment. When medication fails to control a person's seizures, surgery is an option—but not a risk-free one. The decision to perform surgery depends on many factors, including the frequency and severity of seizures, the risk of brain damage or bodily injury from frequent seizures, the likelihood that the operation will control seizure episodes, the seizures' effect on quality of life, and the person's overall health. The most common type of epilepsy sur-

EPILEPSY SAFETY MEASURES

Try these simple suggestions to make your home as safe as possible.

- Hang bathroom doors so they open outward instead of inward (so that if someone falls against the door, it can still be opened).

- Keep water levels in the tub as low as possible, and set water heaters at a temperature low enough to prevent burns.

- Use plastic dishes and cups with lids.

- Use a microwave oven for cooking.

- Use heavy pile carpeting on your floors, with thick padding underneath.

- Pad sharp corners of tables and other furniture.

- Don't smoke or light fires when you're by yourself.

Adapted from www.efa.org (Epilepsy Foundation)

gery is focal cortical resection: removing the small part of the brain in which the seizures originate so that the remaining portions can operate without disruption. People with focal seizures whose attacks cannot be controlled with drugs may benefit from this. Another surgical approach involves cutting the corpus callosum, thus disconnecting the brain's two hemispheres; this does not cure a person of seizures but limits how the seizures can affect the whole brain and thus lead to injury.

Living with Epilepsy

Many people who take medication for epilepsy never experience another seizure. In fact, 60 percent to 70 percent of people with epilepsy will not have a seizure for five straight years at some point within ten years of being diagnosed. About half of these individuals eventually become seizure-free. A seizure-free period of three or four years may indicate that it is possible to reduce an individual's medications. Some people may be able to eliminate them altogether. For others, however, seizures cannot be eliminated. The risk of continued seizures is higher for those who have partial seizures, an abnormal EEG, or associated mental retardation (C3) or cerebral palsy (C4).

The episodic nature of the disease—periods of wellness punctuated by unpredictable attacks—can make epilepsy difficult to live with. Infrequent seizures may not severely restrict people's lifestyle; you do not necessarily need to restrict work, school, and recreational activities. However, serious injury may result if a seizure occurs while a person is driving or operating dangerous equipment, so people with poorly controlled seizure disorders should not perform these activities. Accidental death, especially by drowning, is also more likely in people with epilepsy. Avoid factors that increase the likelihood of a seizure's occurring, such as lack of sleep, use of alcohol and other drugs, and stress.

Despite dramatic scientific advances, we have many unanswered questions about seizures: why they begin, how trauma can produce them years later, how genetic factors influence seizures, and what factors make brain cells susceptible. Research to provide answers to these questions is under way and may lead eventually to the cure.

Dizziness and Vertigo

When we experience dizziness—an often confusing and difficult-to-describe sensation—it is because we are no longer certain of our position or motion in space, something that we ordinarily take for granted. To know where we are in space and how we are moving depends on accurate, reliable, and rapid perception by five senses:

■ Vision, which uses the horizon and vertical objects for coordinates.

■ Vestibular sensations from the inner ear, which perceive both *angular* acceleration, as when we turn our heads rapidly, and *linear* acceleration, such as gravity or the motion of a car as it gains speed.

■ Touch and pressure sense, which identifies our weight pressing on the soles of our feet or the seat of our pants.

■ Proprioception, which detects the movements of our limbs and neck.

■ Hearing, which orients us to sound-emitting and sound-reflecting objects.

Our brains integrate these sensations to give us a complete picture of where we are and how we are moving. We rapidly and continually repeat the process of perceiving our environment, integrating the sensations, and moving appropriately. With this feedback of information, and appropriate motion in response, we can walk, run, cycle, or skate smoothly (**B4**). As infants, we develop this process in our first years until it becomes so natural that we are rarely aware of it, or need to make conscious adjustments. When this "feedback loop" is disrupted for any reason, however, we can experience dizziness—due to our uncertainty of position or motion in space—and we may feel unsteady and light-headed, move awkwardly, or lose our balance.

When people say they feel dizzy, their symptoms can be of four quite distinct types:

1. True rotational vertigo—a spinning sensation.
2. A feeling as if you are about to faint, called presyncope.
3. Disequilibrium, or unsteadiness of gait and balance without abnormal feelings in the head.

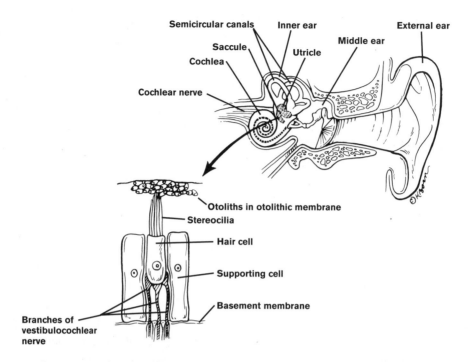

Our sense of balance depends on tiny structures in the inner ear. Fluid in the semicircular canals flows back and forth as we move our heads. Nerve cells attached to specialized "hair cells" sense the changes in flow and pass that information to the brain. One type of dizziness is caused when "otoliths," tiny calcium carbonate crystals that float in a gel above the hair cells, move from the part of the inner ear where they are normally present to a part where they are not. ILLUSTRATION © KATHRYN BORN

4. Light-headedness—a vague, abnormal head sensation other than types 1–3.

Dizziness can be a spontaneous sensation, occurring without relation to position or motion, or it can be triggered by standing or certain movements, positions, or situations.

What Causes Dizziness?

Dizziness is either a complaint or a symptom, like pain or fever, and it has many possible causes. In fact, more than 60 different disorders can cause dizziness, including many conditions involving the brain, inner ear, heart, blood vessels, lungs, and other organs. In this section some of the more common neurological causes are discussed.

We start with two disorders that affect the inner ear and cause vertigo. They can occur at all ages.

Benign Paroxysmal Positional Vertigo

Benign paroxysmal positional vertigo (BPPV) is one of the most common conditions causing vertigo, and certainly the most easily treated and cured. A person with BPPV experiences vertigo—

a sensation of rotation—on changing position, especially when lying on one side, rolling over in bed with the affected ear down, or reaching up to put something on a high shelf. The vertigo of BPPV is often described as spinning and may be violent; it usually lasts 30 to 45 seconds and can be accompanied by nausea or vomiting. If a person changes, then resumes, the provoking position several times, the vertigo diminishes on subsequent movements, but the susceptibility to vertigo returns after a short rest interval.

BPPV is due to the movement of tiny calcium carbonate crystals (otoliths) from a part of the inner ear where they are normally present (the utricle) to a part where they are not (the posterior semicircular canal). This condition can be easily cured in less than ten minutes with the "Epley canalith repositioning maneuver": a physician trained in the maneuver moves the person through a series of four positions in order to roll the otoliths back into the utricle.

Ménière's Disease

Ménière's disease is due to the excessive accumulation of the normal endolymphatic fluid in the inner ear, usually on one side only. Three symptoms occur with Ménière's disease: vertigo, hearing impairment (**C16**), and tinnitus (ringing in the ear). Typically, attacks of vertigo recur several days to several years apart, while hearing often fluctuates but declines over time.

To relieve the vertigo, a doctor can prescribe medications that suppress peripheral (inner ear) or central (brain stem) vestibular function, such as meclizine and some benzodiazepines. Three medications also cause drowsiness, and methylphenidate is helpful to reduce that side effect. A variety of surgical procedures can relieve the fluid pressure but are not consistently effective. Some

people with Ménière's disease benefit from steroids. If the attacks of vertigo become frequent and disruptive, a physician can stop all vestibular function in the inner ear (and therefore all vertigo arising from that ear), without further damaging hearing, by injecting certain aminoglycoside antibiotics (gentamicin) into the ear canal.

Multisensory Dizziness

Many elderly patients, especially those with diabetes, experience multisensory dizziness due to a combination of visual impairment (**C15**), peripheral neuropathy (**C48**), arthritic changes (especially in cervical joints), and often impaired inner ear function and hearing (**C16**). When we lack the necessary sensations to know precisely where we are, or how rapidly and in what directions we are moving, we may experience dizziness when in motion, and feel much more stable when sitting, lying, or leaning against a stationary object.

Treatment for multisensory dizziness involves helping a person learn to use the senses that are intact more effectively. People who have been wearing bifocals can benefit from using single-vision distance glasses so they can look down for orientation. Using a cane that is dragged rather than lifted can provide additional balance clues. If cervical arthritis is a contributing factor, a soft cervical collar can help by limiting neck movements. Physical therapy with gait training, and other exercises to improve balance, can also be useful.

Orthostatic Hypotension

When people with orthostatic hypotension stand up, their blood pressure falls, resulting in insufficient blood flow to the brain, and they may feel faint. This can be due to multiple system atrophy (also known as Shy-Drager syndrome; **C42**), which is a disorder involving the autonomic nervous system (**C18**). Other symptoms of multiple system atrophy include Parkinsonism (**C41, C42**), unsteadiness of gait, impotence, and peripheral neuropathy (**C48**). Physicians can treat the low blood pressure with fluorohydrocortisone or midodrine. Occasionally symptoms improve with nonsteroidal anti-inflammatory drugs (NSAIDs).

Strokes

Strokes (**C59, C60**) may cause vertigo when they involve the areas of the brain stem to which the inner ear sends signals—the vestibular nuclei. Nearly all people with this problem also have additional neurological symptoms and signs, such as facial numbness or weakness, clumsiness, or weakness of a limb, and so on. In transient ischemic attacks, in which blood flow to a part of the brain is diminished or stops temporarily, the same symptoms may last minutes to hours, then disappear. That experience is a warning that one is at risk for a stroke. Strokes are more easily prevented than treated; see section **C59** for preventive steps, such as controlling blood pressure, reducing cholesterol, and not smoking.

Psychological Disorders

Among young adults, panic state, agoraphobia, and hyperventilation syndrome (**C21**) are common causes of dizziness. Panic state and agoraphobia produce severe nonrotational dizziness, often in crowded places (supermarkets, cocktail parties, elevators, and so forth). This problem can lead people to avoid these settings, becoming reclusive. The disorder can be treated with certain benzodiazepine tranquilizers; some of the antidepressant selective serotonin reuptake inhibitors (SSRIs), such as paroxetine; and behavior modification. Treatment is often quite successful.

Hyperventilation refers to breathing too deeply or rapidly, thereby reducing the normal amount of carbon dioxide in the body. People who hyperventilate are usually anxious (**C21**) or depressed (**C20**), or may have panic attacks. They are rarely aware of hyperventilating, however; typically they sigh deeply and frequently. The loss of carbon dioxide causes their cerebral blood vessels to constrict and produces a feeling of type 4 dizziness—that is, light-headedness without vertigo. While the effects of hyperventilation can be frightening, most people can learn to recognize their onset and take preventive steps (including rebreathing into a small plastic bag) when an attack begins.

Dizziness can also result if a person is excessively aware of normal sensation. Our five senses are capable of perceiving and accurately reporting a broad, but limited, range of physical experiences. When this sensory capacity is exceeded, we normally experience dizziness—for example, on the tilt-a-whirl in an amusement park, or while watching a car chase in a wraparound movie theater. Some people are more sensitive than others to brief, everyday sensations of dizziness and may regard these momentary uncertainties as possibly pathologic. Small doses of methylphenidate can reduce this symptom for some individuals, but most benefit just from understanding that the feeling is normal.

Other Causes

Other possible causes of dizziness include:

- Irregular heartbeat; anemia; hypothyroidism.

- Certain neurological disorders, including multiple sclerosis (**C33**), Parkinsonism (**C41**), and diseases involving the cerebellum or frontal lobes.

■ Many medications, especially those with sedative or other central nervous system effects (**C29, C66**).

Treating the dizziness that accompanies these medical problems should always begin by identifying the underlying disease and treating it directly (for example, irregular heartbeat or hypothyroidism).

Diagnosis

To determine why a person feels dizzy, the physician must start by taking a detailed neurological and medical history and performing a physical examination focused on the particular causes of dizziness.

Four questions in particular help with the diagnosis:

1. How old are you? Certain conditions typically occur at young or old ages: for example, strokes and multisensory dizziness occur in the elderly, while hyperventilation, panic states, and agoraphobia are most common in young women; multiple sclerosis usually affects young adults. Thus, a person's age suggests some of the most likely explanations for dizziness.

2. Do you feel as if you're spinning? True rotational vertigo indicates a disorder of the inner ear or its brain stem connections.

3. Do you feel as if you're going to faint? Faintness suggests a cardiovascular cause.

4. Do you feel unsteady on your feet even though your head is clear? Disequilibrium of this sort is common in patients with neurological disorders affecting balance and coordination.

A person whose complaint is light-headedness may have hyperventilation or a psychiatric disorder, or may have a limited form of one of the other types of dizziness. Because many people have difficulty describing their symptoms accurately, however, the doctor may use a Dizziness Simulation Battery of eight maneuvers that reproduce these varied symptoms, allowing a person to choose the best match for his or her complaint.

Routine laboratory studies for diagnosing the cause of dizziness include a complete blood count, a chemistry survey, thyroid function tests, an electrocardiogram (ECG) with a rhythm strip, an electronystagmogram (inner ear test), an audiogram, and the MMPI, a psychological screening test. Specialized tests that may answer specific diagnostic questions (but are *not* routine) include an MRI/MRA (magnetic resonance imaging/magnetic resonance angiography) scan, a Holter monitor to evaluate cardiac rhythm, a five-hour glucose tolerance test for hypoglycemia or diabetes, a tilt-table (which monitors whether a person can keep a stable blood pressure when tilted from a horizontal to a vertical position), an electroencephalogram (EEG), and a battery of psychological tests.

Seeing Problems

The ability to see is one of our greatest gifts. Most of us never have a problem with our sight, other than having to wear glasses. We can see minute objects, experience color, and take in vast panoramas without a thought that something could go wrong. Unfortunately, a number of medical conditions can affect your vision. The eye itself may cause visual disturbances, as in cataracts (clouding of the lens) and glaucoma (rising pressure within the eyeball). This section will not discuss those problems, nor injuries to the eye, but rather the neurological conditions that affect sight—those involving the optic nerve system or the parts of the brain that process visual information.

Your retina acts like the light sensor in a digital camera: its photodetector neurons, the rods and cones and the other retinal neurons to which they connect, convert the light that flows into your eyeball into electrical signals. These neurons and their synapses then feed that information into the eye's optic nerve, which sends it on to your brain. Some of the optic nerve fibers cross in what is called the optic chiasm, at the base of the brain. The result of the crossing is that the brain can process all visual information about the right half of the world in the left occipital cortex and all information about the left half of the world in the right occipital cortex:

Many conditions occurring along this pathway can affect your ability to see. Diagnosis of a particular problem usually starts with identifying the type of vision loss, how quickly it came on, how long it lasted, and whether any other symptoms appeared at the same time. Often people experiencing a sudden loss of vision assume that they have had a stroke, and that is indeed a possibility. In fact, one out of seven people in the United States will have some type of stroke during his or her lifetime, and most of those strokes will have some effect on the visual system. But other conditions can cause the same symptoms. Recognizing the type of vision loss may help you receive early and effective therapy if you need it, and prevent greater or permanent losses in your ability to see.

Whatever turns out to be the cause of a vision problem, it is a serious problem that demands quick medical attention. Here are some basic rules for responding to this symptom:

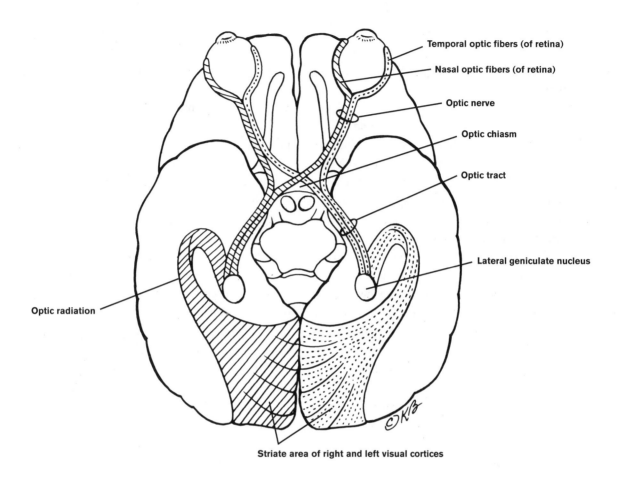

Visual pathways of the brain. Illustration © Kathryn Born

If a person has also suffered loss of consciousness, weakness, immobility, or some form of impaired thinking, the problem is a medical *emergency*. That holds true even if the symptoms are unilateral, meaning that they affect one eye or one side of the body, and a person feels fine otherwise.

A person suffering a sudden visual problem and no other symptoms should nonetheless contact an ophthalmologist immediately. If the eye doctor finds nothing physically wrong with the eye, he or she may refer the person to a neurologist for further diagnostic tests.

Common Neurological Causes of Vision Loss

Four types of conditions or accidents are the most common neurological causes of vision loss. They are impaired blood flow to the retina, damage to the optic nerve, pressure on the optic chiasm, and impaired blood flow in the brain. People's risk for each varies; each has different symptoms, and each is diagnosed and treated differently.

Impaired Blood Flow to the Retina

A number of conditions within the retina may affect vision in only one eye at a time. The most serious is a transient ischemic attack (TIA) that briefly clogs one of the retinal blood vessels. In this case, you would notice an abrupt change in vision in one eye, often a sudden loss of part of the visual field or an effect like a window shade coming down in a few seconds. Fortunately, the unilateral vision loss in TIAs lasts just a few minutes.

Vision loss because of a TIA may be mimicked by migraine headache (**C55**). However, in contrast to TIAs, migraines usually produce colorful, scintillating patterns in part of the visual field.

The usual cause of TIAs is small particles of cholesterol and other material from arteries in the neck that travel through the blood vessels to the eye area, get stuck, and block blood cells from supplying oxygen to the retina or optic nerve. This causes a temporary or, in rare cases, permanent area of vision loss in that eye. Other symptoms of TIAs, such as numbness or weakness on the *other* side of the body from the affected eye, would support the diagnosis: something is interfering with the flow of blood to one part of the head. This is not an ischemic stroke of the brain, but it means a person is at higher risk for that life-threatening problem (**C59**).

Your risk for TIAs of all kinds goes up if you have hypertension or high cholesterol levels, if you smoke, or if you are over 40. For people under 40, retinal TIAs may be due to certain clotting disorders in the blood. Multiple TIAs of the eye could, if untreated, eventually lead to single-eye, or monocular, blindness.

DIAGNOSIS AND TREATMENT

Anyone who may have suffered a retinal TIA should be evaluated by a neurologist specializing

SYMPTOMS	PROBABLE SOURCE
Sudden loss of a portion of the vision in one eye, or temporary loss of vision in one eye	Retina suffering a transient ischemic attack (TIA)
Sudden loss of vision in one or both eyes, accompanied by a scintillating visual "aura"	Migraine headache due to vascular spasm (C55)
Loss of vision in one eye, accompanied by pain as the eyes move	Optic nerve affected by multiple sclerosis
Narrowing field of sight, a condition called tunnel vision	Pituitary tumor pressing on nerves at the optic chiasm
Sudden loss of vision on one side, accompanied by weakness or immobility in one side of the body	Ischemic stroke in the prefrontal cortex (C59)

in visual problems, such as a neuro-ophthalmologist. It is very important for doctors to make an early diagnosis in order to prevent future TIAs or strokes.

In addition to cholesterol particles, a possible cause of TIAs is emboli, or blood clots, produced by disease in a carotid artery. Physicians can evaluate this possibility with an ultrasound scan of those arteries and perhaps an arteriogram.

One treatment for TIAs caused by blood clots involves taking anticoagulation medicine to prevent clots from forming so easily. The medications usually prescribed for this condition include aspirin, drugs known to affect platelets (Plavix and Ticlid), and blood thinners such as warfarin (Coumadin).

If you have had a TIA, it is important to treat the accompanying risk factors: hypertension and high cholesterol. People can improve these conditions by dieting, avoiding salt, and, if necessary, taking medications.

Damage to the Optic Nerve

Overall, the most common cause of a vision loss in a single eye in a person under age 50 is optic neuritis, and the most common cause of optic neuritis is multiple sclerosis (MS; **C33**). The usual first symptom of MS is loss of vision in one eye, accompanied by pain, particularly when the eyes move. Sometimes these eye movements create little flashes of light called photopsias. An individual's vision usually decreases over a matter of hours, and the loss may last for weeks. Most people have an initial recovery but can suffer later attacks in which they lose their vision totally.

This type of vision loss is brought about by an

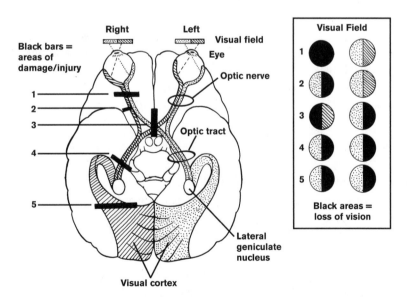

This schematic shows how many problems of seeing arise from impairments along the brain's visual pathways, particularly along the optic nerve, in disorders such as transient ischemic attacks (TIAs), which can interrupt the blood supply to that nerve. ILLUSTRATION © KATHRYN BORN

acute demyelination, or loss of the fatty covering, of the optic nerves. It is therefore called demyelinating optic neuritis and is one of the hallmarks of MS. The process may affect other portions of the brain as well, producing double vision, numbness, weakness, imbalance, or facial pain. Some people also experience loss of bladder control. When a person suffers unilateral visual loss and, either at that time or within a few weeks, unilateral numbness or tingling, MS is the most likely cause.

The usual age when people develop MS is in their 20s or 30s, and the incidence is three times higher in women than men. Early in the twentieth century, epidemiologic studies revealed that people in the northern parts of the United States and of northeastern European ancestry had a higher risk of this condition. Recent studies also indicate that there is a clear genetic tendency toward susceptibility to MS. The disorder affects about 57 people out of every 100,000 people in the United States.

DIAGNOSIS AND TREATMENT

The best test to diagnose multiple sclerosis is a magnetic resonance imaging (MRI) scan. It is extremely important to make a diagnosis early because there are now treatments that may prevent new attacks.

For an acute attack of MS, particularly those involving optic neuritis, doctors prescribe intravenous steroids in the form of methylprednisolone. This hastens recovery and protects the individual from attacks over the next year. Eye discomfort is treated with pain medication so the person can obtain enough rest.

When optic neuritis is the first sign of MS, 90 percent of women and 50 percent of men develop other symptoms of the condition during the next 20 years. These subsequent attacks affect other parts of the nervous system, causing such problems as weakness and numbness on one side, or weakness in both legs when the spinal cord is affected. But at least a third of the people with MS are fortunate in having a very benign course to the disease.

There is no surgical treatment for MS, but new medications called interferons help in reducing, by about a third, the occurrence of new episodes or attacks, both in the optic nerve and elsewhere in the brain. Interferons also reduce areas of demyelination, or MS plaques, over time. The most practical steps that people can take once they contract MS are to lead a healthy life, get regular exercise, and avoid exposure to excessive heat.

Pressure on the Optic Chiasm

The optic chiasm is where your optic nerves cross. The most common cause of visual difficulty in this area is a tumor in the pituitary region pressing on those nerves. This condition produces tunnel vision, making you unable to see anything at the edges of your visual field.

Because the tumor continues to grow, a person's tunnel vision can become steadily worse. If the tumor grows large enough, it may also affect the temporal lobes of the cerebral cortex on either side, producing seizures, or the hypothalamus, causing disorders in appetite and control of the sodium and potassium in the body. Other symptoms of pituitary dysfunction may appear as well, such as fatigue or, in the rare cases when the tumor secretes growth hormone, increasing hand and foot size.

Pituitary tumors account for approximately 1 percent of all tumors that occur inside the skull, so it is an uncommon condition. There is no known specific cause; neither age, sex, nor ethnicity seems to play a role. Moreover, there seems to be no specific genetic prediction toward developing a pituitary tumor.

DIAGNOSIS AND TREATMENT

Over time, we have learned the growth patterns of pituitary tumors. Physicians can diagnose them early by testing a person's levels of hormones that may be affected, such as growth hormone and prolactin. Further tests then determine what sort of tumor is causing the problem, and how large it has grown.

The majority of these tumors secrete no substances and are therefore known as nonsecreting pituitary tumors. They manifest themselves mainly by pressure on the chiasm, causing the tunnel vision. It is extremely important to find these tumors early and treat them, either medically or surgically, to prevent permanent loss of vision.

Some pituitary tumors secrete prolactin, a hormone that causes loss of a woman's menstrual cycle and lactation, or discharge from the breasts. In this case, the drug bromocriptine may be useful in stopping the symptoms and reducing the tumor size. Doctors must watch the tumor carefully with repeated MRI examinations to make sure it is shrinking.

If the tumors are large, surgeons should remove them, usually by performing an operation through the nose. Afterward, a person will need hormone replacement therapy because the pituitary gland will no longer be available to control the production of hormones in the body (B2).

The defect in the outside portions of the visual

COPING WITH BLINDNESS

Coping with the loss of vision is an overwhelming change and stressor in a person's life. There may be partial loss of vision or total loss, severely affecting the person's ability to function in ways he or she had in the past. There are many resources and supports for the person living with visual loss. Safety in the home is of the utmost importance, and adjustments can be made with the help of visual specialists and home-care nurses.

- The agency for the rehabilitation of the blind in your state is your resource for services available to you or your loved one.

- The blind or partially blind need specific instructions as to where objects are.

- Objects should not be moved unless the blind person is told.

- Increased lighting and glare reduction will help the partially sighted.

- A referral to the state agency for the blind may help in obtaining audiobooks, accessing classes in Braille, and obtaining a guide dog, health care funding, and transportation services.

Additional Web sites: American Foundation for the Blind, www.afb.org; Guide dogs for the blind, www.guidedogs.com

MACULAR DEGENERATION

Age-related macular degeneration (AMD) is progressive, incurable, and responsible for some 250,000 new cases of severe vision loss, sometimes called low vision, each year. About 2.5 million people are diagnosed with macular degeneration annually. Screening is conducted in a primary care doctor's office, using a checkerboard pattern or Amsler grid. AMD has begun if wavy or broken lines appear in the center of the patient's vision while viewing the grid. Macular degeneration occurs in two forms, "dry" and "wet." In the most common, dry form, the gradual destruction of the macula, the most sensitive and central portion of the retina, is associated with increasing amounts of a yellowish waste substance called drusen (the connection between this material and AMD is unknown). About 10 percent of AMD cases are "wet," and involve leaking retinal blood vessels. Laser treatment may temporarily halt the degenerative process, but without restoring normal vision. In this treatment, a medication called Visudyne is injected into the patient's arm and travels to the eye. A mild laser light is shone into the patient's eye, activating the drug and destroying leaky blood vessels in the retina that threaten sight. The procedure costs about $2,000 and may need to be performed several times before it works.

Recent research has begun to decipher AMD. It has been found that a genetic immune mechanism plays a role in wet AMD. Deficiencies in genes called *Fas* and *FasL,* which are important for controlling immune cells in the retina, appear to allow increased growth of leaky blood vessels. Efforts to discover more of the genetic causes behind vision diseases could soon yield benefits for sufferers of macular degeneration.

Another, rarer, degenerative vision disorder, retinitis pigmentosa (RP), is also incurable and is untreatable. RP is a genetic disorder for which several genes have been identified. These findings offer hope that treatments to prevent the progress of the disorder may eventually be developed. AMD, RP, and a few other eye diseases are all part of a family of allied genetic diseases that cause functional problems in the retina.

field caused by a pituitary tumor is severe and irreversible. If you have tunnel vision, you must always be aware that you do not see to the sides as you once did. You must move your eyes and head to scan your environment on either side to make up for your loss of vision.

Impaired Blood Flow in the Brain

After information from either of your optic nerves reaches the lateral geniculate nucleus inside your brain, it is relayed to the many appropriate neurons in the visual cortex. Any problem in this system can produce seeing problems, usually affecting one half of a person's field of view. This symptom is different from being able to see only out of one eye. No matter which eye you use, you would see only half of the world, or half of an object. The problem is not in your eyes, but in the part of the brain processing the eyes' information.

The most common cause of these same-side visual defects is a stroke. (Strokes can also affect

Researchers are investigating several possible treatments. One is substances that protect nerve cells—for example, ciliary neurotrophic factor and basic fibroblast growth factor—which might be delivered to vulnerable tissues in the eye via gene therapy. Another approach is prosthetic; in July 2001, surgeons implanted the first experimental artificial retinas made from silicon chips into the eyes of three patients who had lost almost all their vision to retinal disease. The artificial retinas were silicon microchips about one tenth of an inch in diameter and one thousandth of an inch thick, each containing about 3,500 microscopic solar cells that convert light into electrical impulses. The chip is an attempt to replace damaged photoreceptors, the light-sensing eye cells that normally convert light into electrical signals within the retina, and thus restore some degree of vision. At the time this book went to press, the results of the operations had not yet been released. A third possibility is the use of neural stem cells, which have shown promise for retinal disease in animal experiments.

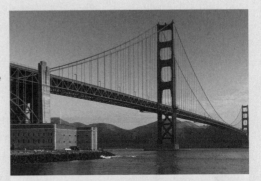

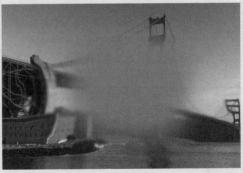

Simulation of low vision resulting from the "wet" form of age-related macular degeneration. Normal vision (*top*); the center of the visual field is lost from degeneration of the macula of the retina (*bottom*). PHOTOS COURTESY CIBA VISION AND ADAIR-GREENE COMMUNICATIONS

the retina and optic nerve fibers, in which cases they affect all vision through one eye rather than vision to one side.) The usual first sign of a stroke affecting the visual pathway is a sudden loss of vision on one side. You may also feel numbness of the face, arm, or leg, or weakness on one side of your body. If you have difficulty seeing to the left and have left-sided facial, arm, and leg numbness or weakness, the problem is probably on the right side of the brain—specifically, in the cerebral cortex.

The risk factors for strokes include hypertension, smoking, high cholesterol levels, diabetes, and a variety of clotting disorders. Increasing age also brings a higher incidence of stroke. When the damage is due to lack of blood supplying part of the brain, usually because of a clot blocking a blood vessel, it is called an ischemic stroke (C59). When a blood vessel bursts in the brain, the problem is called a hemorrhagic stroke (C60). These types of stroke are treated differently, so swift and accurate diagnosis is vital.

A person may also experience a brief, temporary loss of vision in one side of space. This is often caused by a TIA, or period of impaired blood flow, affecting the part of the brain that processes visual information. Though not a stroke, a TIA is a warning that you are at much higher risk for a stroke. You should immediately consult a neurologist who is expert in diagnosing visual symptoms and prescribing preventive measures.

DIAGNOSIS AND TREATMENT

Along with a physical examination, the most important test for strokes is an MRI scan. It is important that doctors make their diagnosis early because treating many strokes immediately can either eliminate or reduce a permanent loss of vision.

If the cause of stroke is a clot of blood coming from the heart or elsewhere in the body (an embolism), doctors may try to prevent further attacks with anticoagulant medications: Heparin right away, and Coumadin for long-term prevention. People with irregular heart rates due to atrial fibrillation have a 70 percent reduction of stroke risk after they start taking Coumadin. The most modern treatment includes dissolving clots with such medications as TPA (tissue plasminogen activator) if physicians can diagnose an impending stroke within three hours.

The visual symptoms of a stroke do not become more severe as time passes; in fact, if the initial damage was not too severe, a person's vision tends to improve gradually. Loss of vision due to a TIA that is identified quickly and treated effectively is even more likely to improve to normal. As with other visual defects, if you have suffered vision loss from stroke, you must learn to compensate by moving your eyes more frequently and always remaining aware that you cannot see in one area of space.

Hearing Problems

Hearing loss is one of the most common neural impairments. Approximately 1 in 3,000 newborns has a profound hearing loss, and perhaps ten times that number have less than normal hearing. The prevalence of hearing loss increases with age, so that approximately 1 in 3 people over the age of 65 has enough hearing loss to interfere with daily communication. In the United States as many as 28 million individuals have a hearing impairment.

Hearing loss can result from a number of causes: genetic, congenital, infectious, traumatic, toxic, idiopathic (of unknown origin), and immune-mediated. Disorders can occur anywhere along the auditory pathway, so it is useful to examine the anatomy of hearing to better understand the myriad disorders that may affect this sense.

The Ear and Its Common Problems

Your peripheral auditory system includes the external, middle, and inner ear. The external ear consists of the auricle and the external auditory canal, which is separated from the middle ear by the tympanic membrane, or eardrum. The middle ear is an air-filled space connected to the nasal passage by the eustachian tube. It contains three bones, or ossicles—the malleus, incus, and stapes—that move as sound strikes the tympanic membrane. The inner ear includes the cochlea, the auditory nerve, and the vestibular (balance) system.

Sound is a mechanical energy, meaning it depends on something moving—in most cases, the air. That energy is transmitted to your inner ear through the ear canal and middle ear components. In the inner ear there are specialized sensory cells, called hair cells because they have structures that resemble tufts of hair, that transform the mechanical energy of sound into an electrical signal that is then transmitted through the auditory nerve to the central auditory system. The central auditory pathways ascend through the brain stem to the temporal lobes.

The inner ear is organized according to tone, or "tonotopically." Sound energy of high pitch is analyzed and transformed into electrical signals at the base of the cochlea, nearest the middle ear, whereas sound of low pitch is analyzed at the top of the cochlea, furthest away from the middle ear.

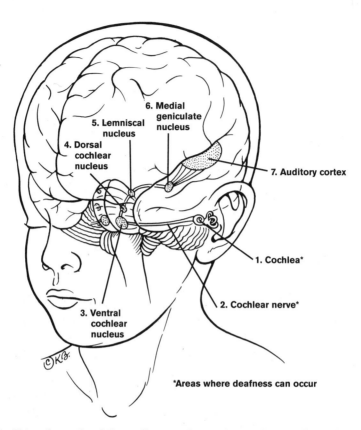

5. Lemniscal nucleus

6. Medial geniculate nucleus

4. Dorsal cochlear nucleus

7. Auditory cortex

1. Cochlea*

2. Cochlear nerve*

3. Ventral cochlear nucleus

*Areas where deafness can occur

This schematic of the auditory pathway shows where auditory signals are processed in the brain. Our sense of hearing starts when the middle ear converts sounds, or vibrations in the air, into signals that travel along the cochlear nerve. On reaching the brain, that information is sent through a series of nuclei in the brain stem to the auditory cortex. Deafness can result from impairments of the cochlea and cochlear nerve. ILLUSTRATION © KATHRYN BORN

There are only 15,000 hair cells to perform this analysis, and they pass the information to the auditory nerve, which contains only 30,000 individual nerves. Unlike other organs, such as the skin and the liver, the inner ear does not have the capacity to regenerate. Thus if your hair cells or neurons are damaged, you may lose hearing permanently.

We can divide hearing loss into two subgroups.

■ Conductive hearing loss: the normal mech-

anisms that transmit sound through the external and middle ears become damaged.

■ Sensorineural hearing loss (also called nerve deafness): the site of damage is in the inner ear, auditory nerve, or central auditory system. The most common causes of hearing loss occur in the inner ear.

A variety of disorders may produce a mechanical or conductive hearing loss. Examples include obstructions of the ear canal, perforations of the eardrum and other injuries, fluid filling the middle ear (serous otitis), chronic infection of the middle ear space, and otosclerosis, a bone disorder that causes the stapes to become fixed. These problems are relatively easy for a doctor to diagnose. In many cases, they can be remedied by cleaning out the ear, giving a person time to heal (while watching any infection carefully to be sure it does not spread to other important areas), or in some cases, performing surgery. If infections have destroyed an ossicle, a surgeon can sometimes create a new one. Conductive hearing loss is not a neurological problem, however, so it is largely beyond the scope of this book. The rest of this section will discuss conditions involving the inner ear, auditory nerve, and central auditory system.

Disorders of the Inner Ear and Auditory Nerve

A number of different diseases may produce either a sudden or progressive deafness in one or both of a person's inner ears. A leading cause of this form of hearing loss is certainly genetic. It is estimated that more than 50 percent of congenital or early-onset sensorineural loss has a genetic basis, and that at least one third of hearing loss that occurs later in life also has a genetic basis. Given that hearing is a complicated process, we should not be surprised that many genes are related to hearing, and thus to possible hearing loss. Researchers have identified a number of these genes, some of which have been linked to problems with the number and efficiency of hair cells.

Many drugs have toxic potential for the inner ear. The best known are generally administered intravenously and include aminoglycoside antibiotics such as gentamicin or kanamycin. However, diuretics, large quantities of aspirin, a variety of antitumor agents, and even such commonly prescribed oral antibiotics as erythromycin may occasionally produce a hearing loss. In most cases, the cause is damage to the hair cells of the inner ear.

Another possible cause of hearing loss is an acoustic neuroma: a benign, noncancerous tumor that generally develops on or near the auditory nerve. Symptoms vary with the size and location of the tumor, but include hearing loss and tinnitus—a ringing or buzzing sensation in the inner ear. Acoustic neuroma is caused by a somatic mutation in the "merlin" gene, located on chromosome 22; it may also be found bilaterally in neurofibromatosis 2 (C7). Acoustic neuromas are relatively uncommon overall, but they are among the most common tumors of the head, affecting approximately 1 out of 100 people. Surgical removal of the tumor is the only treatment that will completely eliminate the acoustic neuroma, though radiation therapy can reduce its size. Early intervention may help people retain most of their hearing.

Immune disorders may result in systemic symptoms, including hearing loss. Examples of these include Cogan's syndrome, syphilis (C38), lupus (C40), polyarteritis nodosa, Wegener's granulomatosis, and giant cell arteritis. Occasionally a disordered immune process may affect the inner ear only, producing a rapid hearing loss in one or, more commonly, both ears. Although some blood tests may indicate an immune disorder, a trial dosage of drugs that suppress the immune system temporarily, such as prednisone, may still be the best method to both identify and treat an inner-ear immune disorder. If an immune disorder of the inner ear is treated early enough, the sensorineural loss may be reversed or further loss prevented.

Circulatory difficulties are a rare cause of hearing loss, although bleeding into the inner ear may accompany blood diseases such as leukemia or may follow certain forms of stroke (**C60**). Transient hearing loss has also been reported in a basilar migraine (**C55**).

A wide variety of other diseases of the inner ear with no specific known causes may produce hearing loss. "Sudden deafness" may occur in one or both ears without any obvious systemic symptoms or any evidence of inflammation of the middle ear. In these cases, doctors often suspect a virus. Ménière's disease is characterized by fluctuating sensorineural hearing loss, vertigo (**C14**), and tinnitus. Although its exact cause is unknown, the disease is thought to stem from a disorder of inner-ear fluids.

One of the most common causes of hearing loss in middle-aged to older people is called presbycusis, or the ordinary hearing loss of aging. This is a progressive, generally symmetrical hearing loss, usually worse in the high frequencies. It occurs with increasing age and probably has several causes: genetic, toxic, and traumatic.

Disorders of the Central Auditory System

Because a relatively small number of cells in the peripheral auditory system are critical for hearing, most cases of hearing loss for which we can name a cause start there. However, the central auditory system can have problems, too. One ex-

SCREENING NEWBORNS FOR HEARING

Hearing loss in children, particularly in newborns, is hard to evaluate. They cannot respond with words to describe what they hear and when, nor can we assume that their physical actions—looking in one direction, for instance—are necessarily responses to what they hear. However, early detection of hearing problems is particularly important because we have increasing evidence that difficulties in hearing speech in infancy may cause irreparable delays in how young children learn to speak themselves (**B14**).

Many states have therefore enacted mandatory screening programs for newborn nurseries. Hearing evaluation at this age uses two techniques. The first, called auditory evoked brain-stem response, extracts auditory neural signals from the brain stem and brain, using electrodes placed on the infant's scalp. The second technique, called otoacoustic emissions, detects sound that is generated within the inner ear and transmitted back to the ear canal when a person has normal hearing. Both of these noninvasive techniques can detect the presence of significant hearing loss in newborns and young children.

If parents learn that their baby has difficulty hearing, they have a range of possible responses. The first option is usually a conventional hearing aid. If the hearing aid does not improve the condition, another option for some families is to ask doctors to insert a cochlear implant when the child is about eighteen to twenty-four months. These implants do not produce normal hearing, however, so parents must still prepare themselves and their child to thrive in a society that expects most people to be able to hear well. With proper support, education, and adjustments for their particular hearing abilities, children can learn to converse through speech, lipreading, sign language, or all three skills.

ample is multiple sclerosis (MS; **C33**). MS produces nerve lesions throughout the central nervous system. Those lesions may affect auditory thresholds (how loud a sound must be before someone can hear it) or more subtle attributes of hearing, such as sound localization and speech understanding. However, since auditory information ascends the brain stem on both sides, only lesions that affect *both* sides of the brain stem will produce a hearing loss.

Brain stem tumors (**C10, C64**) and strokes (**C59, C60**) may also produce hearing loss in the central auditory system.

Diagnosis and Treatment

Many people suspect they or others are losing some of their hearing when it becomes difficult to converse, particularly in a noisy environment. Another indication is when a person must turn up the TV or radio to a level that is uncomfortable for others with normal hearing. Tinnitus, the sensation of ringing or buzzing in the inner ear, is a symptom that commonly accompanies many varieties of hearing loss. And sudden hearing loss is, of course, a cause of concern and should immediately send a person to his or her doctor.

Otolaryngologists (ear, nose, and throat doctors) and audiologists (individuals trained in hearing measurement and rehabilitation) are the medical professionals most likely to evaluate a person for hearing loss. The first step is to examine the ear to rule out such simple causes as cerumen (wax) or foreign bodies in the ear canal, perforations of the drum, or fluid in the middle ear. Then the specialist performs an audiogram, testing hearing at various frequencies, evaluating

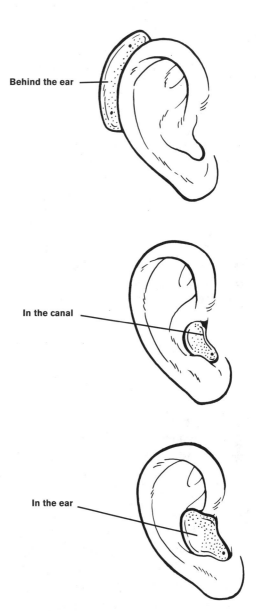

Behind the ear

In the canal

In the ear

The choice of a hearing aid depends on the nature of the hearing loss. Most patients with sensorineural hearing loss do benefit to some degree from hearing aids, and it is important to work with a hearing specialist to decide the most effective device. Anyone with hearing loss should resist the temptation to insist on the most cosmetically pleasing hearing aid: often the most visible behind-the-ear style will provide better hearing. ILLUSTRATION © KATHRYN BORN

COPING WITH HEARING LOSS

It is very important not to become frustrated with a family member's inability to always hear you clearly. There are many resources available for individuals dealing with partial or total hearing loss. This problem can occur as people age, and if you are concerned about a loved one's hearing, it should be checked as soon as possible. Occasionally in an elderly person, it could be as simple a problem as earwax!

- Do not speak loudly, but slowly and clearly, using simple sentences, and try to face the person.

- Maintain eye contact and use hand movements as needed.

- Seek professional help as soon as possible, and if hearing aids are used, be certain they fit and are cleaned correctly and that the batteries are working.

- Try to avoid loud environments and minimize extraneous noises.

Additional sites: www.shhh.org (self-help for the hard of hearing); www.nfab.org (National Family Association for Deaf/Blind); www.deafchildren.org (American Society for Deaf Children); www.nad.com (National Association for the Deaf)

the function of the middle and inner ear, and testing the ability to hear single-syllable words (speech discrimination).

In addition to hearing tests, blood tests and imaging such as computed tomography (CT) or magnetic resonance imaging (MRI) may be useful in diagnosing a specific cause of hearing loss. As discussed earlier, surgery can fix some problems that cause hearing loss. Changing medication may remedy others. Many infections and immune diseases can be slowed, stopped, or even reversed. In other cases, however, a person must learn to live with less hearing and, in some cases, the prospect that the problem will become progressively worse. Most patients with sensorineural hearing loss benefit to some degree from conventional hearing aids, which work by amplifying sounds. Physicians can also provide referrals to services that help the hearing-impaired.

Patients with profound sensorineural loss may regain some measure of hearing by using cochlear implants, which bypass the damaged inner ear. In essence, these tiny devices behave like the inner ear, converting mechanical energy into electrical impulses transmitted to the auditory nerve. They are not yet as sensitive to subtle differences among sounds as the army of 15,000 hair cells— they do not restore a person's hearing. However, they can help some people hear enough to converse in speech without lipreading, and many others to do so while relying on both sound and lipreading.

Since as much as 50 percent of progressive hearing loss may have a genetic basis, we will benefit greatly in the future from better understanding the genetic causes of and predispositions to hearing loss. We will be better able to diagnose individual cases and to predict hearing loss, and even to prevent or reverse loss by correcting genetic errors.

Smelling and Tasting Problems

We rarely think about our sense of smell except when we sniff something particularly pleasant or unpleasant. But in fact our ability to detect and recognize odors does a great deal to shape our mental world. Smells can bring back vivid memories of places and people—and often the emotional states we associate with them. This may relate to the relative uniqueness of some smells, as well as to the brain regions to which the olfactory bulbs connect. Probably the sense of smell was even more important to our evolutionary ancestors. It may no longer be as vital for us as it is for animals that use their noses to hunt (or to avoid being hunted), but being able to smell rotten food, leaking natural gas, and smoke can still be a matter of life and death.

We are more aware of our sense of taste, at least at mealtimes. Our olfactory system works in tandem with our sense of taste to provide us with the flavors of foods and beverages. If people lose their sense of smell, they often feel that they have also lost some of their ability to taste, even though their taste buds are still responding normally.

We call smell and taste the chemical senses because they rely on specialized cells in the nose and mouth that are responsive to the specific molecules they encounter, as opposed to physical changes in air or in light. Together, smell and taste can make eating, a basic animal behavior, into an aesthetic pleasure. It's no coincidence that *gusto*, a word we associate with taking great pleasure in life, is derived from the Latin word for "taste."

Doctors have written about disorders of smell and taste for many years. Indeed, in the third century B.C. the Greek naturalist Theophrastus recognized that a person could suffer anosmia—the loss of smell—due to a head injury or blocked nose. The great nineteenth-century British neurologist John Hughlings Jackson was among the first to note that aberrations in smell and taste often accompany neurological disturbances of the brain's temporal and frontal lobes. He also recorded that strange smells and tastes can precede the paroxysms associated with epilepsy (**C13**).

In recent years research into the sense of smell has benefited from the proliferation of commercial tests of this ability. These have provided scientific standards for measuring many different people's olfactory capacities, opening the door to new discoveries. We now know more about why

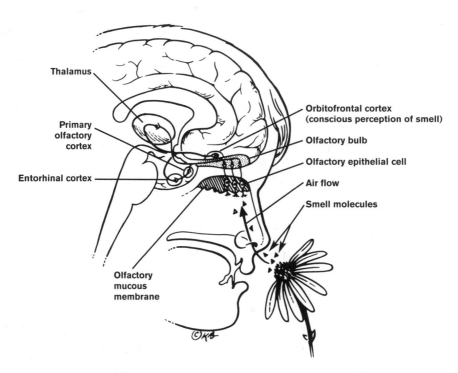

Our sense of smell differs from other senses, in part because olfactory information passes from the receptors, located in the upper recesses of the nose, to cortical regions without relaying through the thalamus. Some of these cortical regions, however, do connect through the thalamus to the orbitofrontal cortex, a region involved in odor identification. Although the sense of smell declines somewhat with aging, actual impairment of smell is likely to be the result of a problem elsewhere, ranging from a cold to the effects of more serious disorders, such as stroke. ILLUSTRATION © KATHRYN BORN

people lose their sense of smell, and how losing that sense can be a clue to a more far-reaching neurological disorder.

Loss of the Sense of Smell

The most common cause of permanent olfactory loss appears to be a severe upper respiratory infection, usually caused by a virus, which damages the layer of nerve cells (neuroepithelium) in the nasal cavity. It is rare for people under 45 to lose their sense of smell this way. People tend to experience such anosmia as they grow older, with men having greater and earlier loss than women. While we estimate that less than 2 percent of Americans under 65 have meaningful olfactory loss, approximately half of the population between the ages of 65 and 80 does. Over the age of 80, three quarters of the population experiences this problem. Age-related olfactory loss explains, in part, why many older people report that their food lacks flavor, and why a disproportionate number of elderly die from accidental gas poisoning.

There are probably a number of mechanisms

PROBLEMS WITH TASTING

If a person perceives less flavor in his or her food while chewing and swallowing, that usually reflects a problem not with taste but with smell. Much of what we "taste" in food is actually odor sensed in the back of our noses. Taste buds pick up only the basic sweet, sour, bitter, and salty sensations, as well as possibly metallic (iron salts), umami (the taste imparted by glutamate), and chalky (calcium salts) sensations. Such beloved flavors as coffee, chocolate, chicken, vanilla, steak sauce, pizza, cheese, and so on are mediated via the first cranial nerve, which is comprised of the olfactory receptor cells.

Many elderly people experience such losses of "taste," but when the function of the taste buds is evaluated, it becomes clear that the nerves there are working fine. It is the olfactory system that is declining.

In addition, older people often experience distortions of their taste perception (dysgeusias), which can be very debilitating and difficult to manage. Such distortions, along with persistent and unpleasant phantom tastes, can arise from various medications (for example, antihypertensive, cholesterol-lowering, and antibacterial agents), poor oral hygiene, radiation therapy, and small blockages of the arteries in the brain stem and thalamus. Fortunately, most of these problems resolve spontaneously over time.

Another source of odd taste sensations is the presence of different metals in a person's dental fillings and appliances. In the wet environment of the mouth, electrons from one device start to flow toward the other, based on which metal holds on to them more strongly. This very small electrical current can cause a peculiar taste in the mouth. If you experience an odd taste shortly after having a new dental device installed, talk to your dentist about the problem.

---

responsible for age-related decreases in the ability to smell. It has been suggested that most loss of smell reflects cumulative damage to the olfactory epithelium from viruses, bacteria, and airborne toxins. When the nerve cells have already suffered damage over time, a sudden but minor problem, such as a bad cold, can produce perceptible and often permanent loss. Some cases of age-related olfactory loss may be caused by hardening of the sievelike bone through which the olfactory nerves pass on their way to the brain.

The second most common cause of olfactory dysfunction is head trauma (61). Between 7 percent and 15 percent of patients suffering such injuries appear to suffer measurable olfactory loss, usually anosmia or severe microsmia (being able to smell much less than normal). In most such cases, the injury has caused the nerves from the nose to be sheared off at the cribriform plate. Bruising particular areas of the brain can also cause olfactory problems; some people may regain their sense of smell over time as the brain swelling or hematomas caused by a head injury clear up.

The third most common cause of prolonged smell loss is a nasal or sinus disease such as polyposis (growths in the mucous membranes) or such inflammatory disorders as allergic rhinitis (hay fever). Usually, this simply means something is physically blocking odorant molecules in the air from moving to a person's olfactory region—in other words, the person has a stuffed-up nose. Fortunately, most people benefit, at least to some degree, from such therapies as surgery to remove polyps or steroidal medication to reduce allergy symptoms. However, chronic inflammation of the nasal regions can result in permanent loss of a person's smelling powers.

Disorders of taste and smell can arise from other sources as well, among them:

- congenital causes
- growths inside the nose and skull, such as olfactory groove meningiomas and frontal lobe gliomas
- radiation therapy for cancer
- nutritional and metabolic deficiencies—cirrhosis of the liver, thiamine deficiency
- endocrine problems—Addison's disease, diabetes, Kallmann's syndrome
- accidental damage to a cranial nerve during tonsillectomy or other surgery
- epilepsy (**C13**)
- kidney disease and hemodialysis

Fortunately, these cases are rare.

Loss of Smell as a Sign of Neurological Disease

Because of our increased ability to test people's smelling abilities in a standard fashion, we now know that decreased olfactory function can be among the first signs of some common neurological and psychiatric disorders.

New research suggests that psychosis may impair a person's ability to identify odors. In schizophrenia (**C25**), odor-identification test scores are the only objective measurement known to correlate with the disease's duration. In other words, schizophrenics who have the most difficulty distinguishing odors also have the longest intense, or fulminant, period of illness. That finding suggests that there is a progressive, perhaps degenerative, component of schizophrenia that we have not yet recognized.

Interestingly, about 90 percent of people with Parkinson's disease (**C41**) from an unknown cause suffer olfactory loss—more people than show the disease's characteristic tremor. The loss of smell does not respond to medical therapy and, unlike the motor symptoms, does not change over time. Therefore, smell testing is useful in differentiating Parkinson's from progressive supranuclear palsy (PSP; **C42**), a similar disorder in which people usually suffer no major olfactory problems.

In the elderly, two other conditions that are often hard to distinguish at first are Alzheimer's disease (**C67**) and depression (**C20**). Many doctors use the Mini-Mental State Examination to unearth clues about which disorder might be affecting an individual. Recent studies have shown that scores on a simple three-item odor-identification test are even more effective. Moreover, an epidemiological study of 1,604 people 65 or older found that individuals' scores on a 12-item odor-identification test were better at predicting who would show a cognitive decline over the next two years than their scores on a global cognitive test. People who were anosmic and who possessed a particular genetic marker had almost five times the risk of cognitive decline than people with ordinary smelling ability and without the gene. The difference was even more apparent for women: those with both anosmia and the genetic marker were almost ten times more likely to show cognitive decline than the other women. Though the individuals with the genetic marker and normal smelling ability were also more likely to suffer cognitive decline than people without the gene, the difference was not as striking as when anosmia was involved.

For most neurological diseases that affect a person's sense of smell, we do not know why that change occurs. An exception is multiple sclerosis (MS; **C33**), where people's loss of smell is strongly correlated with the number of MS-related plaques in their subtemporal and subfrontal lobes—the regions involved in central olfactory processing. Brain plaques outside these two areas show no effect on olfactory test scores. Recent studies of people with MS have shown that over time their sense of smell waxes and wanes in direct association with the number of active plaques in these target regions.

Diagnosis and Treatment

In sum, it is worthwhile telling your physician about any smelling or tasting problems that you experience. It is important, however, that you receive quantitative testing of this sense to be certain you have a true problem. In some cases, loss or reduction of the olfactory sense can be an early sign of a serious neurological disorder, and early detection and treatment might improve your prognosis. In the best outcome, a smelling or tasting problem might be remedied with medication, surgery, or a change in whatever treatment might be causing the side effect. For many people, the loss of smelling ability is simply a problem that comes with age. The bad news is that in most cases physicians can do little to restore the sense of smell (and thus a full sense of the appreciation of food flavors), but the good news is that such anosmia usually does not lead to other problems.

Autonomic Disorders

Our autonomic nervous system is essential for our survival. This system of nerve cells continuously monitors and controls our visceral organs: the heart and blood vessels; the pupils; the glands for tears, saliva, and sweat; the lungs' bronchi; the stomach and intestines; the bladder; and the sexual organs. Control of these organs regulates our bodies' response to exercise, emotion, and environmental challenges. Several areas of the brain are involved in the working of the autonomic nervous system, including the cerebral cortex, amygdala, hypothalamus, brain stem, and spinal cord. Neurons of the brain stem and spinal cord send nerve fibers to the autonomic ganglia, which, in turn, send nerve fibers to all visceral organs.

The autonomic nervous system has two main divisions, sympathetic and parasympathetic. The sympathetic system is activated in response to stress, exercise, exposure to heat or cold, low blood glucose, and other environmental challenges. This system is critical for maintaining blood pressure as we stand up; an autonomic reflex constricts the vessels in our legs and abdomen to keep blood from pooling in these regions and rushing away from our head. The sympathetic system also increases the frequency and strength of heartbeats during exercise, and controls sweating and blood flow to the skin to maintain healthy body temperature. The parasympathetic system is important for digesting and absorbing nutrients, slowing the heart during sleep, emptying the bladder and bowel, and penile erection. In many organs, the effects of the parasympathetic system oppose those of the sympathetic; for example, the sympathetic dilates the pupil and the parasympathetic constricts it.

Problems and Their Causes

Given how many parts of the nervous system control the visceral organs, and the many functions of the autonomic system, it is not surprising that problems with this system can show up in many ways. Any disorder affecting the hypothalamus and brain stem, the spinal cord, the autonomic ganglia, or the sympathetic or parasympathetic nerves may result in autonomic failure or, in rarer cases, excessive autonomic activity. For example, lesions in the hypothalamus, the spinal cord, or the sympathetic ganglia and nerves that connect to the sweat glands can produce an inability to sweat. Diseases of the spinal cord or parasympathetic nerves may make people retain urine and men become impotent. The body's own immune system can be keyed off by an infection to mistakenly attack the autonomic nerves.

One of the most frequent and disabling forms of autonomic failure is chronic light-headedness or fainting when a person gets up from a chair or a bed. This problem can result from lesions in the medulla oblongata, the spinal cord, or the sympathetic ganglia or fibers. That damage blocks the autonomic reflex that normally keeps blood from rushing into our lower limbs as we stand. A person without this reflex instead experiences a drop in blood pressure, called orthostatic hypotension. When the blood pressure falls, so does the blood flow to the brain, and the person feels dizzy or faints. Orthostatic hypotension may also show up as blurred vision, fatigue, and neck and head pain that disappears when the individual sits or lies down. A person with this condition can learn to recognize all these symptoms and can sit down as soon as they appear to avoid fainting.

People with orthostatic hypotension commonly have *high* blood pressure when they are lying flat, and excrete excessive amounts of salt and water during the night. The symptoms of orthostatic hypotension are typically worse early in the morning, after a heavy meal rich in carbohydrates, after exposure to heat, or during heavy exercise or straining. Orthostatic hypotension can prevent people from engaging in normal daily activity. They may be unable to stand for more than a few minutes, or they have to sit down frequently to prevent fainting. Falling down, of course, can

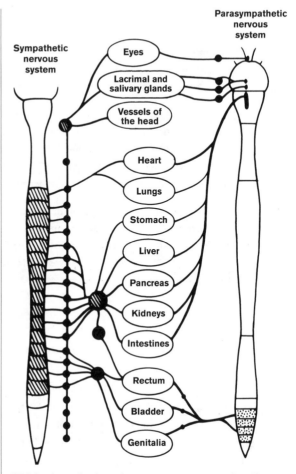

Within the spinal cord, two systems are active: the sympathetic nervous system, responsible for signals that run our bodies' many organs; and the parasympathetic nervous system, which slows down these same organs as needed. Illustration © Kathryn Born

result in head injuries or bone fractures—creating even worse problems.

Most often, autonomic disorders show up as failures of both sympathetic and parasympathetic systems, and can thus cause multiple problems at once, affecting perspiration, appetite, excretion of waste, and sexual arousal. The consequences of these failures can be very harmful to our bodies and our sense of self. Inability to sweat means that

WHEN THE AUTONOMIC SYSTEM GOES TOO FAR

A person's autonomic nervous system can also produce problems if it is *too* active. The most common cause of excessive autonomic activity is anxiety—we're almost all familiar with the proverbial sweaty palms and racing heart that lead up to delivering a speech, for instance.

Excessive autonomic activity can be much more serious than that, however. People with this condition may experience heart palpitations, high blood pressure, excessive sweating and cold skin, excessive salivation, abdominal cramps, diarrhea, or an urgent need to empty the bladder. Left untreated, the cardiac problems and high blood pressure may be life-threatening. Excessive sweating can produce wide fluctuations in body temperature, as well as embarrassment and worry.

Many conditions produce excessive sympathetic activation: seizures and strokes involving the cerebral cortex and the amygdala, intracerebral hemorrhage and head trauma, and some tumors in the hypothalamus or brain stem. On rare occasions, lesions of the brain, spinal cord, or peripheral nerves cause too much autonomic activity. Other important causes are intoxication with cocaine or amphetamines, and withdrawal from alcohol, sedatives, or opiates.

a person cannot exercise in a hot environment and faces the risk of heatstroke. Feeling full after only a small meal, decreased appetite, and nausea may result in malnutrition and weight loss. Severe constipation may lead to fecal impaction. Incomplete voiding causes a person to retain urine in the bladder and poses the risk of recurrent urinary tract infections. Erectile impotence, an early symptom of autonomic failure, has profound psychological impact for men and their partners.

Autonomic failure occurs most commonly as a side effect of drugs a person is taking to treat other problems. These medications interfere with the normal transmission of chemicals from the autonomic nerves. The problem appears most frequently in elderly people because as we age we normally lose some autonomic nerve cells and the system becomes easier to disrupt. As a common example, a person found to have high blood pressure while lying down may adopt a low-salt diet and start taking antihypertensive drugs; under this new regime the person may develop orthostatic hypotension—low blood pressure when standing up. Obviously, such a person's physician should adjust the medication dosage. Another familiar case is an individual who experiences a dry mouth or has difficulty emptying the bladder while using an antidepressant drug.

Several nervous system diseases can produce combined sympathetic and parasympathetic failure. These include some degenerative disorders affecting the brain stem and spinal cord, such as multiple system atrophy (previously referred to as the Shy-Drager syndrome; C42) and Parkinson's disease (C41). In these diseases, autonomic failure occurs alongside symptoms, such as shuffling gait, unsteadiness, stiffness, or tremor. About 5 to 15 people out of 100,000 develop multiple system atrophy—not a large number. Parkinson's disease is more common, but autonomic problems in this disease are less severe and occur much later.

The most common peripheral nerve disease, or neuropathy, that produces autonomic failure is diabetes mellitus. Diabetes affects approximately 1.3 percent of the population, and 5 percent to 7 percent of these people suffer damage to their autonomic nerves.

Some spinal cord disorders predominantly affect a person's bladder, bowel, and sexual function; important examples are multiple sclerosis (**C33**) and injury to the spine.

Diagnosis and Treatment

Doctors diagnose autonomic disorders based on a person's history, a physical examination, tests of the autonomic functions, and laboratory results. During the physical examination, physicians assess blood pressure and pulse while the individual is lying and standing, the pupils' reaction to light, and the color and temperature of the skin. Autonomic tests measure sweat production and changes in the heart rate during breathing. The doctor will also check how the blood pressure responds to straining (the patient closes his or her mouth and nose and tries to blow out, called the Valsalva maneuver), to being switched from a horizontal to a vertical position as the patient lies on a tilt table, and to standing. It is sometimes necessary to check how well a person can urinate and move his or her bowels. Blood glucose and other blood tests are done to exclude diabetes and other conditions that may produce similar symptoms.

People diagnosed with an autonomic disorder should work with a health care team: a neurologist, a dietitian, a physical therapist, and in some cases, a urologist or gastroenterologist. The principles for managing these disorders are:

- Learn about your condition.
- Work with your doctor to correct potentially reversible causes, particularly unnecessary medications.
- Adjust your diet and physical activities as necessary.
- Take drugs specific to the autonomic condition, if prescribed.

As an example, here is the usual program of advice for people with orthostatic hypotension:

- Increase your intake of salt to 8 to 10 grams a day and of water to 2 to 2.5 liters (over half a gallon) a day.
- Sleep with the head of your bed raised 20 to 30 cm (8 to 12 inches) to prevent hypertension and excessive urination at night.
- Eat smaller, more frequent meals with low carbohydrate content, and a high-fiber diet to avoid constipation.
- Learn to use small postural maneuvers as standing with your legs crossed and squatting to prevent fainting.
- Perform regular exercise, but avoid heavy exercise and exposure to heat.
- Some people benefit from the use of support stockings.
- Drug treatment potentially includes fludrocortisone (Florinef), which increases the kidneys' retention of sodium from salt, and midodrine (Proamatine), which constricts the blood vessels.

Other drugs used to treat symptoms of autonomic failure are metoclopramide (Reglan) to improve the working of the stomach and intestine, and sildenafil (Viagra) to treat erectile impotence. Although many elderly people take oxybutynin (Ditropan) or tolterodine (Detrol) to reduce excessive bladder contractions and incontinence, individuals with autonomic failure should *not* take these medicines. People suffering from urinary problems caused by an autonomic disorder need to follow a fluid schedule and may eventually have to learn to empty their bladders with a catheter.

For some people, doctors may recommend surgical procedures, such as a gastrostomy (a feeding tube is inserted into the stomach to bypass swallowing problems) or penile implant. Individuals whose autonomic problems stem from diabetes may be advised to have a pancreas or kidney transplant. These surgeries can't fix the autonomic system itself, but they can either alleviate the underlying problem or counteract the troublesome symptoms.

The prognosis for autonomic disorders varies greatly because of their many causes. In multiple system atrophy, autonomic problems worsen along with the other manifestations of the disease. This illness has a poor prognosis; many patients experience potentially fatal breathing difficulties during sleep and may require a tracheotomy. On the other hand, about two thirds of acute autonomic failures following an infection and an immune attack on the autonomic nerves improve within two to four weeks. The prognosis of autonomic failure in diabetes parallels that of the underlying neuropathy and other manifestations of the disease, and may improve with appropriate control of blood glucose and, in some cases, surgery.

Intensive ongoing research is aimed at understanding the brain mechanisms that control autonomic function, as well as the causes of mechanisms of disorders in this system. These investigations may yield results that help prevent and treat not only the diseases associated with autonomic failure but also conditions such as panic attacks (**C21**), high blood pressure, and sudden cardiac death.

Chronic Fatigue Syndrome

Chronic fatigue syndrome (CFS) often, but not always, begins as a flulike illness. However, unlike such infections normally, the fatigue persists even after the individual has rested or reduced his or her activity. Other CFS symptoms can include headaches, muscle pain, aching joints, swollen lymph nodes, difficulty concentrating, memory loss, "foggy" or slowed thinking, disrupted sleep, and other hard-to-measure complaints. Different people report different combinations of these secondary symptoms. Aches, pains, and other flulike symptoms are often the first signs, in addition to the medically unexplained fatigue. According to one study, 48 percent of people with CFS reported that symptoms appeared suddenly, and 40 percent said they came on gradually over time.

Eventually individuals with CFS notice they can't keep up their previous levels of activity. This fatigue is the condition's hallmark symptom. Family members usually perceive the individual's reduced level of activity and might suspect the individual is suffering from a tenacious but mild flu. Typically, a person with CFS first visits a family doctor, thinking the symptoms are related to a cold or flu. When the symptoms fail to improve, or when individuals become concerned about their increasing impairment, they may seek out a specialist to ask about their fatigue. It's not uncommon for CFS to remain undiagnosed for several years after the initial onset of symptoms.

When pain is more prominent than fatigue, doctors often identify the problem as fibromyalgia; considerable overlap exists among CFS, fibromyalgia, and other unexplained fatigue and pain conditions. Patients with these diagnoses usually feel unable to keep up with the pace of their lives and become exhausted easily. Some become so impaired that they can't maintain their jobs or tend to other important responsibilities. For approximately 45 percent of these individuals, their illness is complicated by a concurrent psychiatric diagnosis such as depression (**C20**) or anxiety (**C21**). For many years, in fact, most doctors believed depression or anxiety was the root cause of the fatigue in CFS. Today these psychological factors are still thought to be involved, but they may be cued or worsened by the physical problems. The different symptoms—physical and psychological—can then exacerbate each other.

Despite the many ways it can appear, the impact of CFS on a person's life is unmistakable. It forces people to become less involved in important activities, interferes with their ability to meet responsibilities, and otherwise depletes their personal stamina and resources. Many people with CFS feel unable to meet the demands of their jobs, family, and other commitments. The condition also brings social consequences. Because there are no easily visible symptoms and because an "official" diagnosis can take so long, employers, coworkers, family members, and health care providers often misunderstand the condition and its severity. Some may assume that the individual is exaggerating or even malingering, trying to avoid responsibilities by feigning illness.

There are many myths about the cause, the best treatment, and the contagiousness of CFS. Many support groups exist and tend to be very active. They can be valuable for mutual support, and they have increased awareness of the condition among the public and medical community. But it's important that people with CFS not let their involvement with these organizations limit or bias their evaluation of available treatments. For the sake of their own health, they must find doctors who are abreast of the latest scientific research and willing to address their specific needs.

Definition by Symptoms

CFS is defined as persistent and disabling fatigue lasting more than six months and not improving with rest or reduced activity. In addition, a person must exhibit four or more of the following symptoms over that period:

- Sore throat
- Tender lymph nodes (in the neck or armpits)
- Muscle pain
- Pain in multiple joints without redness or swelling
- Headaches that are new or different since the onset of the fatigue
- Impaired short-term memory or difficulty concentrating
- Unrefreshing sleep
- Malaise or fatigue after exertion

The symptoms tend to become more severe as time passes, although most individuals report a notable fluctuation in their severity. Earlier definitions of CFS also involved fever and muscle weakness; though they're no longer criteria for the diagnosis, people with CFS often experience them.

The symptoms of CFS commonly occur in other disorders as well, so excluding those other explanations is critical to diagnosing CFS accurately and ensuring an individual receives proper treatment. A doctor must rule out the following alternative explanations:

- Infection
- Heart and kidney disease
- Hypothyroidism
- Multiple sclerosis (C33)
- Cancerous tumors (C64)
- Hepatitis
- Lyme disease (C36)
- Sleep disorders (C11)
- Eating disorders (C27)

- Drug or medication use (**C29, C66**)
- Psychotic disorders

Possible Origins

CFS remains an unexplained illness. Its origins are unclear and may involve many factors. Several medical explanations are being evaluated by researchers, including the following.

Neurological. The most popular explanation of CFS is that an individual's nervous system is altered, presumably by a virus or other pathogen, in a manner that reduces the normal levels of arousal and neural activity. This process would resemble the disruption caused by major depression, in which the brain's cells and certain critical pathways become less responsive to key neurotransmitters. Another neurological explanation focuses on the hypothalamic-pituitary-adrenal (HPA) axis, a collection of structures in the brain and the endocrine system. The HPA axis is known to excite and slow neural activity, and to dictate the levels of essential hormones in the blood; it is also involved in maintaining normal sleep, in arousing the body to respond to a threat or stress, and in regulating other important functions. If this system doesn't work normally, the body's general ability to be aroused would be reduced.

Immunological. Another proposed explanation is that people with CFS possess an abnormally active immune system—hence an alternate term for the condition, chronic fatigue immune dysfunction syndrome (CFIDS). Essentially, the immune systems of some individuals appear to be incessantly active, waging a constant battle against a pathogen we haven't yet identified (or, perhaps, waging that battle even though no pathogen exists). All that activity continuously drains the body's resources. Researchers seeking an agent that might cause this immune response have examined a number of poorly understood infectious pathogens, including human herpes virus (HHV) and mycoplasma bacteria, but little evidence exists to support a specific viral or immunological cause. If people's immune systems are being activated even in the absence of a pathogen, CFS could be related to other autoimmune disorders (**C40**).

Psychological. Several mental disorders are known to produce persistent fatigue, slowed thinking and other cognitive problems, reduced energy and motivation, sleep disturbances, and other CFS symptoms. These include depression (**C20**), acute anxiety (**C21**), bipolar disorder (**C24**), and even some psychotic disorders. It is possible, therefore, that CFS is a mental disorder that primarily affects a person in physical ways. As with many chronic illnesses, individuals who have contracted CFS often alter their daily activities and their interactions with others; inadvertently, these changes can worsen their condition. Furthermore, many people with CFS report that their symptoms improve after they try certain cognitive-behavioral psychotherapies. Whether these biopsychosocial factors play a role in producing CFS, continuing it, or both is not yet known.

Chronobiological. Fatigue and pain are common complaints of people with chronic sleep disturbances. CFS might be the result of a sleep disorder (**C11**) or disruption of the body's mechanisms for inducing and maintaining restorative sleep on a regular cycle. Depression and pain are both known to interfere with sleep cycles. Research into this theory is inconclusive but continues to focus on sleep patterns, sleep quality, and physiological markers of the body's circadian rhythms.

Cardiovascular. Some evidence suggests that CFS is related to the body's inability to maintain optimum blood pressure. Some people with CFS show decreased ability to alter blood pressure in response to challenges as simple as standing up. For these hypotensive individuals, parts of the body may not be getting enough blood and vital nutrients during physical exertion or psychological stress. This might produce fatigue and postexertion malaise.

There is no evidence that CFS is contagious or has a genetic component. There does not seem to be an increase in the prevalence of CFS among family members or among children of those with the disorder.

Diagnosis and Treatment

There are no definitive tests for chronic fatigue syndrome, and treatment is largely supportive. However, some patients may very well have an organic illness that can be identified by testing. For example, some cases of CFS are associated with the Epstein-Barr virus. In addition, many patients with CFS symptoms are suffering from depression or other psychiatric disorders that present these symptoms as well. The lack of biological diagnostic tools for CFS, as a result, requires physicians to make a "diagnosis of exclusion." That is, they cannot diagnose CFS without ruling out the other diseases that may have these symptoms.

Only a qualified physician can make a diagnosis of CFS. The process of eliminating the other possible causes of an individual's symptoms starts with a physical examination and a clinical interview. The physical exam determines the presence of fever or swollen lymph nodes, and the extent of symptoms. The interview is required to assess the severity of the person's fatigue, the degree of impairment, and the presence of any mental disorder. Blood tests are often used to rule out an infection or other fatiguing illness. Neurological and neuropsychological examinations determine the extent of neurological and cognitive dysfunctions and rule out other diagnoses. Even brain imaging is occasionally useful for excluding other neurological diseases.

People diagnosed with CFS should seek physicians experienced with treating the condition and related disorders. There is no specialty dedicated to CFS, but specialists in internal medicine and neurology may have a better understanding of the condition. While an early diagnosis may allow a person to start receiving care sooner and thus reduce the severity of symptoms, it may not influence the final outcome.

Currently, there are no specific treatments and no known cure for CFS. Instead, doctors use treatments known to reduce the symptoms and thus increase a person's ability to function. The clinical goal is improvement in a person's quality of life despite the chronic fatigue. Doctors can recommend various techniques that have been shown to help many people with CFS. By using their personal resources efficiently, these people have returned to a normal level of functioning. Interventions that have proven useful include:

- medication for the symptoms, both physical and psychological
- carefully tailored exercise
- cognitive-behavioral therapies, including stress management and sleep hygiene

Many people with CFS are also clinically depressed to some degree, which can worsen their symptoms or interfere with recovery. Antidepressant medications, exercise, stress management, and better sleep habits may all be useful for this problem.

Whenever individuals with CFS hear about new treatments, especially those not recommended by their primary physician, they should consider the possible adverse consequences. One common danger is becoming overmedicated, dependent on painkilling or psychiatric drugs. Making extreme behavioral and lifestyle changes increases stress, at least in the short run, and may isolate people from their supportive social networks. In some situations, treatment may actually increase fatigue, reduce stamina, and worsen the condition overall.

People with CFS tend to get better. As many as 10 percent report a complete recovery. Most people diagnosed with the condition return to an acceptable level of functioning and ability, though too few return to their workplaces after becoming disabled. Periodically, an individual's CFS symptoms will become less or more difficult; the challenge is to manage a fluctuating but chronic illness. A portion of people with CFS report that their symptoms and impairment persist for ten or more years after the onset of their fatigue. It's not yet clear what differentiates these individuals from the majority, or what influences the progression and remission of their symptoms.

CHAPTER 14

Emotional and Control Disorders

C20   Depression   363

C21   Anxiety and Panic   371

C22   Social Phobia (Social Anxiety Disorder)   376

C23   Obsessive-Compulsive Disorder   379

C24   Bipolar Disorder   385

C25   Schizophrenia   390

C26   Borderline Personality Disorder   394

C27   Eating Disorders   399

C28   Post-Traumatic Stress Disorder   405

C29   Substance Abuse and Addiction   409

C30   Alcoholism   419

C31   Violence and Aggression   426

C32   Suicidal Feelings   429

We value social interactions. When people behave abnormally—acting unnaturally sad or euphoric, voicing unrealistic thoughts, repeating actions compulsively, and so on—such behavior can be quite visible to others, and often distressing. In severe cases, such people may pose a threat to themselves or others. We classify this level of disturbed behavior as mental illness.

Doctors have long known that in some cases such behavior is linked to conditions that leave physical signs on the brain, such as lesions in brain tissue, or plaques of Alzheimer's disease (C67). Conditions that left no recognizable signs were generally classified as "psychiatric" and viewed as purely mental. In the last century, many therapists sought the roots of psychiatric prob- lems in people's childhood experiences. More re- cently, however, advances in neurochemistry and imaging technology have revealed that most of these disorders involve recognizable disruptions in the brain's normal activity. In other words, we now know these illnesses are in large part biolog- ical, and we have a growing number of clues about what might be going wrong in the brains of peo- ple suffering from them.

Modern treatment for diseases of emotion and control therefore usually involves medications to normalize the brain's chemistry (psychopharma- cology) and counseling on how to recognize and manage harmful thoughts (psychotherapy, which can take many forms). We are still a long way from explaining these disorders or curing them, but we are making progress.

Depression

The term *depression* describes a group of conditions characterized by significant and sustained periods of low mood, associated with a syndrome, or group, of accompanying characteristics and symptoms. Although writers have described episodes of depression since antiquity, only recently have we recognized that the depressive disorders are among the most common and disabling medical conditions throughout the world. Approximately 5 percent to 7 percent of the adult population of the United States will suffer from a form of depression during any year, and the lifetime risk may exceed 15 percent.

Depressions are outside the bounds of normal fluctuations of mood; they are not simply extreme periods of sadness. The closest parallel to depression in daily life is the grief experienced after the death of a loved one. In addition to the "blue" or melancholy mood, a depressive episode is defined by disturbances of at least four other psychological and physical processes, such as appetite, sleep, energy, concentration, interest, and the ability to experience pleasure.

Some forms of depression are so severe that the person may become completely incapacitated, hallucinate (for example, "hear voices"), or develop delusions (unshakable but absolutely untrue beliefs, such as the conviction that he or she has cancer or is being punished by God for past sins). People with such severe depressions clearly appear unwell—they may be slow in action and thought, or restless, nervously pacing, and picking at their skin or nails. Their posture is often slumped, and their faces marked by down-turned mouth, lowered gaze, and furrowed brow.

On the other hand, milder forms of depression can involve such subtle changes in appearance and behavior that a suffering individual's loved ones or employer may not be sure anything is wrong. Even so, these milder forms of depression can take a toll on work performance, home life, and overall well-being.

Some depressed people are not even aware of their low mood. Instead, they may complain of "burnout" or stress, feeling perpetually tired, or inexplicably losing their enthusiasm. Such "masked depression" often goes untreated, or a person will receive treatment only for a symptom, such as insomnia (**C11**) or vague pain complaints (**C56, C57**), rather than for the overall disorder.

Pessimism is a hallmark of depression; it can make people seem indecisive, irritable, or less confident in their abilities. The depressed person may appear to be preoccupied with past failures, heartbreaks, or grievances. Underperformance and absenteeism negatively affect the workplace. Performance in social roles as a parent, spouse, and friend similarly suffers. Chores go undone, formerly enjoyable hobbies and social activities diminish, and even attention to grooming may decrease. Recent surveys have shown that depression has an effect on the quality of daily life comparable to heart disease and greater than most other common medical illnesses.

Thoughts of death are common in depression, and most depressed people experience at least passive thoughts of suicide—that is, thinking about it without taking action. Across a lifetime, more than 20 percent of depressed people will make a suicidal attempt, such as cutting their wrists or taking a medication overdose, and about 6 percent ultimately will die by suicide (**C32**). In fact, approximately three fourths of people who commit suicide have a depressive disorder.

Depressions also worsen the outcome of common illnesses such as diabetes, stroke (**C59, C60**), and heart disease. Beyond the increased risk of early death, depression costs U.S. society tens of billions of dollars because of absenteeism from work and prolonged periods of disability.

The Forms of Depression

There are two general forms of depressive disorder, as well as a number of subforms and related conditions. The most common form, called major depressive disorder, is diagnosed when the mood disturbance and symptom profile has per- sisted almost every day for at least two weeks. Usually, a depressive episode is characterized by insomnia and decreased appetite. We use the term *atypical depression* when a person is oversleeping or shows an increased appetite.

Sometimes a person's low mood appears to be related to some recent setback or adversity. If such an individual's mood disturbance or symptoms are mild, fluctuating, or short-lived, we might call the episode an adjustment disorder with de- pressed mood. However, once the person's mood or behavior has been changed for long enough to meet the definition of major depressive disorder, that is the diagnosis no matter what has been hap- pening in his or her life.

About 75 percent of major depressive disor- ders are recurrent, meaning that the person will suffer two or more episodes in his or her lifetime. The average number of episodes, studies say, ranges between four and eight. They may be widely spaced, or, in what is called a seasonal pat- tern, they may occur at the same time each year, almost like clockwork.

At least 10 percent of people with depression will also experience episodes of mania, an abnor- mal state of elation and behavioral excitement. In this case, the person is probably suffering from bipolar disorder (**C24**). It is difficult to tell the dif- ference between depressive episodes associated with bipolar disorder and major depressive disor- der, so the key to diagnosis is recognition of the prior manic (or milder, hypomanic) episodes. Bipolar depressive episodes also tend to last longer, have a greater likelihood of psychotic fea- tures, and convey a greater risk of suicide.

The second basic form of depression is called dysthymia or dysthymic disorder, which repre- sents a longer-lasting but symptomatically milder disorder. Dysthymia, which accounts for about one quarter of depressive disorders, is defined by at least two years of continued mood disturbance, along with at least two associated symptoms. Despite involving fewer symptoms, dysthymia causes as much impairment in quality of life as major depressive disorder. Long-term studies suggest that without treatment, the average episode of dysthymia may last for ten or more years. Frequently beginning in childhood or adolescence, dysthymia may color a person's personality development and negatively affect his or her vocational and interpersonal development for decades. Moreover, people with dysthymia are at great risk of developing superimposed episodes of more severe, major depression (also called double depression).

Factors and Causes

Depression is commonly associated with a number of other psychiatric conditions, including alcoholism (**C30**), nicotine dependence, and other forms of addiction (**C29**); various anxiety disorders (**C21**); and personality disorders. People with schizophrenia (**C25**) often experience significant periods of low mood and suicidal thinking. Depression also frequently accompanies the early stages of Alzheimer's disease (**C67**). Many medical conditions (such as hypothyroidism) and numerous medications (including birth control pills) can cause depressive syndromes. These clinical complexities underscore the importance of receiving a careful diagnostic evaluation before a person assumes that the problem is a major depressive disorder.

Our understanding of the causes of depression has shifted over the centuries. At the broadest level, we now view depression as a state of disturbed brain responses to internal and external signals of stress. Again, we can relate this perspective to how we view grief, as well as to the experimental condition known as learned helplessness (a state of behavioral and neurochemical "exhaustion" observed in animals after exposure to chronic or recurrent, inescapable stress). Studies of important neurochemicals, such as norepinephrine, serotonin, and corticotrophin-releasing hormone, show disturbed brain function in depression, as do alterations in brain wave activity during sleep. More recently, studies using brain imaging techniques have observed changes in cerebral blood flow and metabolism.

The risk of depression is increased by genetic factors. Children of a depressed father or mother will have at least twice the lifetime risk of depression even if they are raised in another home. But heredity is not always a controlling factor, the identical twin of a person with depression has only about a 60 percent to 70 percent lifetime risk. Other factors include a history of abuse or trauma early in life, alcoholism or substance abuse, and (as noted before) many chronic medical illnesses and some medications. People with other psychiatric disorders, particularly the anxiety disorders, are also at greater risk for episodes of depression. Women are at greater risk than men for major depressive disorder and dysthymia.

Most often, the first lifetime episode of depression follows a significant loss, such as a romantic rejection or a failure at work or school. Having strong, supportive personal relationships may help buffer people against the effects of such adversity. Conversely, having loved ones who are harshly critical may have the opposite effect. Psychological factors such as negative attitudes and the tendency to worry or feel overly responsible can also amplify the impact of stress. Psychologi-

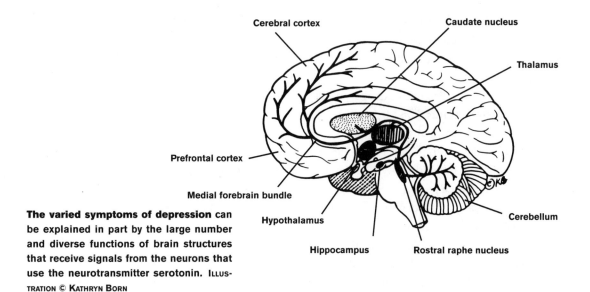

Cerebral cortex

Caudate nucleus

Thalamus

Prefrontal cortex

Medial forebrain bundle

Cerebellum

The varied symptoms of depression can be explained in part by the large number and diverse functions of brain structures that receive signals from the neurons that use the neurotransmitter serotonin. Illustration © Kathryn Born

Hypothalamus

Hippocampus

Rostral raphe nucleus

cal and social risk factors may become less important causal factors in more severe, recurrent, or psychotic depressive episodes, but depression is rarely a strictly medical disease.

Many of the changes in the brain during an episode of depression resemble the effects of severe, prolonged stress. These changes can include a reduction in the activity of brain systems involving serotonin neurons, poor regulation of brain systems involving norepinephrine neurons, and increased amounts of cortisol and related stress-responsive hormones. It is likely that such other brain chemicals as dopamine, acetylcholine, and several neurokinins are also involved. The balance between these chemical systems helps control basic biological processes like sleep, appetite, energy, and sex drive. Together they permit expression of normal moods and emotions.

Low brain serotonin activity in particular has been associated with a greater risk of completed suicide and more violent or impulsive suicide attempts (**C32**). Sustained stress (and, among various animals, a loss of social rank) has been shown

to lower brain serotonin levels. It also appears that some people have reduced serotonin function naturally, perhaps as an inherited characteristic. This may have important therapeutic implications.

Changes in brain wave electrical patterns during sleep have been linked to depression for nearly 40 years. These alterations include a reduction of deep sleep, increased wakefulness, and increased amounts of rapid eye movement (dream) sleep, especially early in the night (**C11**). Other changes in the biology of sleep during depression include a relatively increased body temperature, higher nighttime cortisol levels, and blunted release of growth hormone.

Severe depression has also been associated with shifts in cerebral blood flow and changes in the rate of brain glucose metabolism. Blood flow to the higher cortical areas can be diminished (especially in the prefrontal cortex), whereas we see increased blood flow and metabolism in central brain structures that process more basic emotional and behavioral responses.

There is evidence that trauma early in life may

have persistent, far-reaching effects on brain stress response systems. Further, disturbances in the patterns of sleep brain waves and stress hormones secretion tend to become more marked as people have multiple episodes of depression. Severe, recurrent, and psychotic depressions may actually cause a reduction in the volume of brain tissue in some regions.

Treating Depression

Episodes of major depression range in duration from a few weeks to years. Without treatment, most uncomplicated depressions will remit spontaneously within one year. For the majority of people, therefore, the benefits of effective treatment are reduced time of illness and diminished suffering. Because of the high likelihood of subsequent recurrent episodes and the unpredictability of suicidal behavior, as well as depression's apparent cumulative harm to social and brain functioning, the long-term benefits of prompt and rigorous treatment are extensive. One of the challenges of depression, however, is that it lowers a person's will to change things for the better, and often family members and friends must push a depressed person to find help.

The treatment of choice for depression depends on several factors. When a person has no history of mania and no psychotic symptoms, the initial options usually include counseling or psychotherapy and various forms of antidepressant medications. Bipolar and psychotic forms of depression should *not* be treated with psychotherapy alone. Bipolar depressions usually require treatment with a mood stabilizer (that is, lithium or valproate), either alone or in combination with antidepressant therapy. Psychotic depressions typically warrant treatment with a combination of antidepressant and antipsychotic medications. Electroconvulsive therapy (ECT), sometimes called shock treatment, is usually reserved for more severe depressions that have not responded to medication therapy.

All modern forms of psychotherapy for depression aim to help the person clarify and solve stressful problems, if possible; learn ways to cope more effectively with depressive symptoms; and increase involvement in healthy, nondepressive activities. Modes of therapy differ in how they emphasize the interpersonal, cognitive, or behavioral aspects of depression, but all are intended to help people feel better after a few months of regular sessions. While cognitive therapy might emphasize the decrease in dysfunctional thoughts or distorted information processing, interpersonal therapy might seek to improve social adjustment by dealing with interpersonal disputes or social role traditions. Therapy is usually provided as weekly individual sessions, but forms for couples and groups are also available. Most studies of outpatients with major depressive disorder have found that the newer psychotherapies are as effective as standard antidepressant medications, although the effects of psychotherapy are sometimes slower. If psychotherapy has not resulted in significant improvement within three to four months, other treatments should be considered.

Antidepressant medications are the preferred treatment for more severe depressions or when psychotherapy has not been helpful. Antidepressants are prescribed by both psychiatrists and primary care physicians. There are many different types of antidepressant medication—varying in effects, how safe they are in cases of overdose, and cost. These medications appear to help restore or rebalance the way brain systems involving sero-

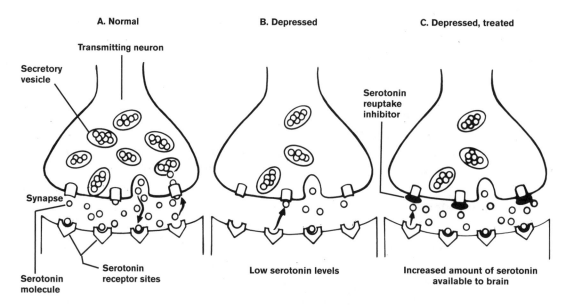

A. Normal **B. Depressed** **C. Depressed, treated**

Transmitting neuron

Secretory vesicle

Serotonin reuptake inhibitor

Synapse

Serotonin receptor sites

Serotonin molecule

Low serotonin levels

Increased amount of serotonin available to brain

Treatment of depression with SSRIs (selective serotonin reuptake inhibitors) **alters the level of the neurotransmitter serotonin in the nerve-cell synapses. Depression appears to involve reduced serotonin, which the antidepressant remedies by blocking "reuptake" of the messenger by the sending neuron.** ILLUSTRATION © KATHRYN BORN

tonin or norepinephrine cells transmit their signals. That effect may in turn cause changes in the genes involved in regulating stress responses and other vital functions.

Antidepressant medications do not dramatically or rapidly lift people's spirits. Rather, they usually work more slowly, typically over four to eight weeks, even though some symptomatic improvement is often noted within seven to ten days. When an antidepressant is effective, a person must usually take it for at least six to nine months to protect against relapse. It is often recommended that people who have suffered repeated episodes of depression remain on antidepressants indefinitely. The major classes of antidepressants are so different from each other that the failure of one type does not mean that another type will not be effective. The medications come in many groupings:

- Selective serotonin reuptake inhibitors (SSRIs): fluoxetine (Prozac), sertraline (Zoloft), paroxetine (Paxil), citalopram (Celexa), and escitalopram (Lexapro). These are the most widely prescribed antidepressants today. As their name implies SSRIs have a much stronger effect on serotonin than on norepinephrine and other brain chemicals.

- Newer antidepressants: venlafaxine XR (Effexor), bupropion (Wellbutrin), nefazodone (Serzone), and mirtazapine (Remeron). With the exception of Effexor, these medications do not have strong effects on serotonin reuptake.

- Tricyclic antidepressants (TCAs): amitriptyline, imipramine, doxepin, and nortriptyline, among others. When compared with the newer medications, TCAs tend to have more side effects and are more dangerous in over-

---

COPING WITH DEPRESSION

How to make life easier:

- Recognize that there may be certain times of the day when you feel better, and use that to your advantage.

- Break large tasks into smaller ones; set priorities and take things one at a time; avoid taking on too much responsibility and setting overly difficult goals.

- Activities such as exercise, attending sports or cultural events, and participating in a religious or social event can help you feel better.

- Avoid alcohol and nonprescribed drugs. Limit caffeine intake as well.

- Seek help immediately if you feel overwhelmed or hopeless.

- Love yourself! Set aside time each day just for you and do something good for yourself. Try to eat right, walk, and try to connect with people you like to be around for emotional support. Do things you really enjoy.

Adapted from www.depression.org (National Foundation for Depressive Illness). Additional helpful sites: www.afsp.org (American Foundation for Suicide Prevention); www.med.jhu.edu/drada (Depression and Related Affective Disorders Association); www.narsad.org (National Alliance for Research on Schizophrenia and Depression); www.ndmda.org (National Depression and Manic-Depressive Association)

---

dose. Nevertheless, they can still be effective if other medications have failed.

- Monoamine oxidase inhibitors (MAOIs): phenelzine (Nardil), tranylcypromine (Parnate). MAOIs have the same comparative drawbacks and potential as TCAs. They require following a diet that is low in the amino acid tyramine (certain cheeses contain this amino acid) in order to prevent sudden high blood pressure reactions.

Antidepressant medications and psychotherapy are commonly used together. For people with more severe, chronic, or recurrent forms of depression, this combination may improve the chances that the problem will respond or remit completely.

Response rates for particular forms of psychotherapy or antidepressant medications usually average about 50 percent to 60 percent within 6 to 12 weeks. Approximately eight out of ten people who begin treatment for depression will respond to the first, second, third, or fourth treatment if applied in sequence. For those still unimproved after multiple courses of psychotherapy or medication, 50 percent to 60 percent response rates are still possible with electroconvulsive therapy.

Newer treatment alternatives include the herb St. John's wort, acupuncture, and "phototherapy" with bright white lights. There is fairly good evidence that the winter form of seasonal depression responds to phototherapy about as well as to conventional treatments, but the treatment can be time-consuming: up to two hours a day in front of a 10,000-lux light box. St. John's wort is a relatively inexpensive (about $15 per month) and usually well tolerated nonprescription remedy that is quite popular in Germany. Despite some evidence of effectiveness, however, its value compared with newer treatments has not been proven. Taking it without a physician's oversight poses some concerns, such as the danger of drug interactions. For example, St. John's wort speeds metabolism of certain medications, including birth control pills and some of the antiviral medications used to treat AIDs, which may lessen their effectiveness. Interest in the potential of acupuncture for depression has only recently surfaced in the West. It is too early to determine whether it is as effective as other treatments.

With all that is now known about depression, well over half of people who suffer from it will experience relief after medical treatment. Research now under way aims to produce both better treatments and better ways of matching people with particular treatments to yield faster and more lasting responses.

Anxiety and Panic

Anxiety is a normal human emotion. We all feel anxious sometimes. The emotion is helpful when it motivates a person to avoid danger or to work hard at difficult or unpleasant tasks that will ultimately bring rewards. At other times, however, anxiety becomes abnormal and harmful, especially in the conditions known as generalized anxiety disorder (GAD) and panic disorder (PD).

Generalized Anxiety Disorder

People with GAD generally experience excessive worry and tension for most of their lives. They may not realize that anything is wrong or unusual with this state because chronic anxiety has become their way of life. But their worry is out of proportion to any real threat. Often people with GAD search their lives for reasons to be so worried, hoping to find an explanation for their feelings. These rationales can be quite convincing. They help explain the usual accompanying symptoms: insomnia, muscle tension, and a variety of aches and pains, including headache and gastrointestinal problems. Those physical problems are products of the tension, but they are also real. They are generally the reason people with GAD first seek medical care. Chronically anxious people rarely seek help for an emotional problem because they do not recognize they may have one.

Left untreated, GAD can cause major, ongoing difficulties. People with this condition are generally unable to remember a moment in their lives when they were calm or relaxed. Their excessive worry makes it difficult for them to complete important tasks. They can transmit high levels of anxiety to their loved ones, often burdening children with excessive fears. The disorder's most dire complication is the onset of major depression (**C20**), which most people with GAD will suffer unless their problem is recognized and treated. Evidence suggests that people with GAD also suffer from higher rates of some medical problems—for example, hypertension and irritable bowel syndrome—but cause-and-effect relationships between these problems have never been established.

Panic Disorder

In contrast to people with GAD, those with panic disorder generally feel well until they experience the first in a series of panic attacks. These are short-lived events (lasting between 10 and 20 minutes), characterized by a crescendo of fear and physical symptoms cued by the autonomic nervous system. Typically, a panic attack includes a suddenly accelerating heart rate, difficulty breathing, shaking, light-headedness, and sweating. People suffering one feel a sense of impending catastrophe. Usually they assume they are in the midst of a grave medical event, like a heart attack, and seek emergency medical attention for that.

If an individual's PD is not identified after the first attack, the condition can become extremely debilitating. Repeated unexplained panic attacks often lead people to become anxious, worrying that another attack will occur, and to develop phobias. The sufferers avoid situations in which they have had attacks in the past, or places where they might have a hard time finding help if one begins. For example, people with PD typically try not to drive in rush hour, travel on subways or planes, sit in crowded theaters, or go to shopping malls. In the worst case, they develop agoraphobia, not leaving the house unless accompanied by a companion they trust to obtain help immediately if an attack occurs. Clearly, the disorder can interfere with an individual's normal social functioning.

People suffering from PD are also at high risk of developing depression (**C20**); when they do, they face an increased risk of suicide attempts (**C32**). PD is also associated with migraine headaches (**C55**), irritable bowel syndrome, asthma and other chronic respiratory diseases, problems with the heart's mitral valve, and increased risk of cardiovascular disease.

Understanding Anxiety Disorders

Because there is no visible, rational cause for the anxiety that people with GAD and PD feel, it is tempting to believe that they can get over their symptoms if they just try hard enough. Sometimes these people are even accused of fabricating their symptoms to get attention. Those notions are clearly false. Though GAD and PD can both be mild, they usually impair a person's life severely. Because of their incessant worry, people suffering from GAD tend to become ineffective and paralyzed when trying to complete important tasks. Those with PD may be unable to do most tasks outside their homes. Both groups frequently resort to alcohol or other abusable substances, and their rates of depression are very high.

Over our lifetimes, about 5 percent of people will suffer from GAD, and 3.5 percent from PD. PD is about twice as common in women as in men. A person is several times more likely to develop PD if a close genetic relative has the disorder. Studies of fraternal and identical twins suggest that inheritance determines about 40 percent of the risk for panic attacks. Data also suggests that a person's risk for PD increases if he or she has suffered significant emotionally traumatic events during childhood, such as the death of a parent, the divorce of parents, or sexual or physical abuse. Both conditions can wax and wane but rarely vanish spontaneously without returning.

A great deal of research in recent years has indicated that both GAD and PD may involve abnormalities in the activity of specific brain circuits, and that these conditions involve both genetic predisposition and exposure to adverse life events. Most scientists now believe that anxiety disorders involve hyperactivity in a channel of the central nervous system called the fear net-

The fear pathway in the brain is vital for our survival. But it can be set off by things that are not really threats, such as the big spider shown in this highly schematic view. Visual information moves from the eyes to the thalamus and then to both the amygdala and the visual cortex. While the visual cortex sorts out the details of the spider, the amygdala, center of emotions, provokes the hypothalamus to initiate such autonomic responses as faster heart rate and sweating. ILLUSTRATION © KATHRYN BORN

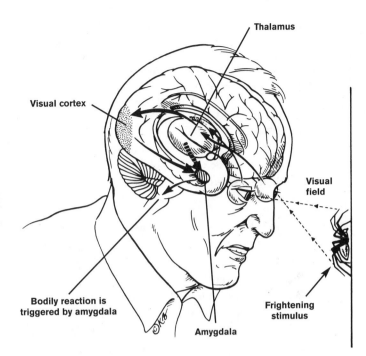

Thalamus

Visual cortex

Visual field

Bodily reaction is triggered by amygdala

Frightening stimulus

Amygdala

work. This involves the central nucleus of the amygdala, its projections to parts of the brain stem involved in autonomic nervous system responses and freezing behavior (that is, sudden immobility due to fear), and its connections to the hippocampus and to the medial prefrontal cortex. Studies have implicated a number of neurotransmitters in the disorders, including excessive activity of noradrenaline in particular areas of the brain and deficient activity of serotonin. We also believe that these anxiety disorders may involve excessive activity of corticotrophin-releasing factor and glutamate, the amino acid most important in exciting the brain.

Another view of anxiety disorders is that the brain has become unable to calm down, to stop being excited. Drugs known as benzodiazepines are effective against anxiety because they bind to a specific receptor in the brain and thereby improve the effects of the brain's major inhibitory neurotransmitter, gamma-aminobutyric acid (GABA). This may indicate that anxiety disorders involve abnormalities in this system as well.

Diagnosis and Treatment

As pointed out above, people with GAD and PD often suspect they are suffering from other problems and can exhibit many physical symptoms. A physician must consider and rule out a wide range of conditions before diagnosing an anxiety disorder. On the other hand, people with anxiety disorders should not be subjected to endless medical evaluations. There is evidence that early treatment of anxiety disorders can prevent many of their complications, such as depression and severe phobic avoidance; delay in treatment worsens a person's prognosis.

In general, a person suspected of having GAD or PD should undergo medical evaluation based on the immediate complaints, his or her medical

THERAPIES COMBINED WITH MEDICATION

In addition to medication to relieve symptoms, treatment for anxiety disorders usually includes either behavioral or cognitive therapy:

- Behavioral therapy focuses on changing specific actions and uses several techniques to decrease or stop unwanted behavior. For example, one technique trains patients in diaphragmatic breathing, a special breathing exercise involving slow, deep breaths to reduce anxiety. This is necessary because people who are anxious often hyperventilate, taking rapid shallow breaths that can trigger rapid heartbeat, light-headedness, and other symptoms. Another technique—exposure therapy—gradually exposes patients to what frightens them and helps them cope with their fears.

- Cognitive behavioral therapy teaches patients to react differently to the situations and bodily sensations that trigger panic attacks and other anxiety symptoms. However, patients also learn to understand how their thinking patterns contribute to their symptoms; they learn how to change their thoughts so that symptoms are less likely to occur. This awareness of thinking patterns is combined with exposure and other behavioral techniques to help people confront their feared situations. For example, someone who becomes light-headed during a panic attack and fears he or she is going to die can be helped by the following approach used in cognitive behavioral therapy. The therapist asks the person to spin in a circle until dizzy. When the person becomes alarmed and starts thinking, "I'm going to die," he or she learns to replace that thought with a more appropriate one, such as "It's just a little dizziness—I can handle it."

history, and routine medical recommendations. Doctors must rule out other psychiatric diagnoses as well, and this can also be challenging. People with anxiety disorders have elevated rates of alcohol and other substance abuse (**C29, C30**), and acute drug or alcohol withdrawal can mimic panic attacks. Other conditions to exclude are somatization disorder, bipolar disorder (**C24**), and anxiety associated with psychotic illnesses.

As described above, anxiety disorders and depression (**C20**) often appear together. Many people with PD and GAD also suffer from specific fears, social phobia (**C22**), obsessive-compulsive disorder (**C23**), and post-traumatic stress disorder (**C28**).

Psychiatrists and some family physicians specialize in treating GAD and PD. There are two forms of treatment that have proven effective for most anxiety disorders: cognitive behavioral therapy (CBT) and medications. CBT generally involves weekly or biweekly sessions with a doctor for about three to four months. These sessions focus on education about one's disorder, training in healthy breathing to stop hyperventilation, learning to think in new ways about one's condition, and gradual exposure to the situations that one associates with the anxiety. It is important that the clinician administering this therapy be specifically trained to provide CBT for anxiety disorders.

Medications for GAD include benzodiazepines, buspirone (BuSpar), and antidepressants. Two antidepressants, venlafaxine XR (Effexor) and paroxetine (Paxil), have been approved by the Food and Drug Administration (FDA) for this purpose.

HELPING SOMEONE SUFFERING FROM ANXIETY

Family and friends can help a great deal in supporting a person dealing with anxiety. Although ultimate responsibility for recovery lies with the patient, family and friends can help by taking part in the treatment program. With the guidance of mental health professionals, they can help ease the person's fear in anxiety-producing situations, offer support and encouragement, and create an environment that promotes healing. Family members can help in the following ways:

- **Recognize and praise small accomplishments.**

- **Modify expectations during stressful periods.**

- **Look for small improvements and expect some setbacks.**

- **Try to be flexible, give needed "space," and try to maintain a normal routine.**

Adapted from www.adaa.org (Anxiety Disorders Association of America)

For PD, the medications include antidepressants and benzodiazepines. Most physicians agree that the first drugs to try are antidepressants of the selective serotonin reuptake inhibitor (SSRI) class: paroxetine (Paxil) and sertraline (Zoloft). The FDA has also approved two benzodiazepines—alprazolam (Xanax) and clonazepam (Klonopin)—for treating panic disorder.

Treatment for anxiety disorders is highly successful at helping a person over immediate problems. Most patients respond well to CBT or medication, and combining the two treatments may be more effective than either alone. Approximately 80 percent of people with GAD and PD respond to a short, intense course of treatment over about 12 weeks. Relapse rates tend to be high, however. Long-term studies suggest that most patients will harbor some residual symptoms, and some will relapse months or years afterward. It is not known whether continuing CBT beyond the initial course improves its long-term effect. Relapse rates after a person with an anxiety disorder stops taking medication are generally high, between 30 and 40 percent, although some data suggest that using effective medication for a year or more may reduce this risk, at least for PD patients. As long as patients remain on medication, relapse is uncommon. Some patients therefore choose to stay on their prescribed drugs for prolonged periods. Fortunately, long-term use of modern antidepressants appears to be safe and relatively well tolerated.

A great deal of research is now going on to identify further risk factors for anxiety disorders in our genes and our early experiences. Ultimately we may be able to prevent the conditions from arising. The concerted effort to study the brain networks and physiology involved in these disorders may result in better treatments. And psychiatrists are doing research to maximize the benefits people can receive from standard courses of cognitive behavioral therapy and medication.

Social Phobia (Social Anxiety Disorder)

Social phobia, or social anxiety disorder, is often mistaken for ordinary shyness. In fact, many people who have this disorder think of themselves as shy, but they are also painfully aware that their shyness is more severe than most people's and that it interferes with their quality of life. Unfortunately, most people with social phobia fail to seek treatment because they do not recognize it as a treatable condition, and perhaps because they are so reticent about calling attention to themselves.

Individuals with social phobia are typically timid, quiet in groups, and uncomfortable being the center of attention. Accordingly, they avoid speaking in public, expressing opinions, or even socializing with peers. Many people with social phobia lack self-esteem, find it difficult to interact with people in authority, and cannot speak or perform in front of even small groups.

People with social phobia fear and avoid social situations because they believe that they will do or say something to embarrass themselves. For example, they may avoid signing checks in the supermarket for fear that their hands will shake and observers will discover that they are anxious. People with social phobia also tend to process neutral social information in ways that reflect negatively on themselves. For example, when talking with a new acquaintance, a social phobia sufferer might think, "Was that a yawn? She thinks I'm boring!" These negative thoughts lead to even more anxiety in social situations, and even to avoiding those situations. When an individual is unable to avoid or easily escape from a frightening social situation, he or she may experience an anxiety attack similar to those that occur in panic disorder (**C21**).

We use the term generalized social anxiety disorder when a person's social phobia interferes with a wide range of social situations. It is this generalized form that is most pervasive and accounts for most cases seen by psychiatric and general medical practitioners, although most people with social anxiety disorder never seek care for this condition. Approximately 5 percent to 10 percent of the general population has some form of social phobia, about a third of which is of the more pervasive, generalized type.

Social anxiety disorder begins early in life and often becomes manifest in childhood. About 50 percent of people with the disorder report that it began before their adolescence, many recalling that they "have always been this way." Others report the onset during or shortly after adolescence. As an early-onset disorder, social anxiety disorder is frequently complicated over time by the occurrence of other conditions, most prominent among them being major depression (**C20**), alcoholism (**C30**), and, more rarely, other substance abuse disorders (**C29**).

Social phobia can result in tremendous disability and impairment in a person's life. It is a disorder of lost opportunities. People with the illness make major life choices in order to accommodate it. For example, an individual with social anxiety disorder may drop out of school early due to fear of speaking in front of groups, or search for jobs that allow workers to avoid interacting with others. People suffering from social phobia often do not date at all, and many become lonely and isolated. If and when they eventually seek treatment, people with generalized social anxiety disorder report tremendous dissatisfaction with their lives.

Searching for a Cause

As with other psychiatric conditions, the causes of social phobia disorder remain obscure. It might seem reasonable to expect that childhood adversities or developmental experiences would confer an increased risk for the disorder, but studies have not yet shown this pattern. The disorder has a hereditary component, particularly in its generalized form; the risk to first-degree relatives (parents, siblings, or offspring) is five to ten times that of the general population. This finding, of course, does not distinguish the family environment in which a person grows up from his or her genetic inheritance of risk, but researchers are trying to isolate those factors.

Researchers are currently testing several biological models of social phobia; one of the most promising is the theory that the disorder involves dysfunction in the brain's systems to regulate dopamine. In support of this possibility, two separate studies using a form of computed tomography (CT) scan called single-photon-emission computed tomography (SPECT) have found that people with generalized social phobia show a significantly lower count of molecules binding to the dopamine transporter, and to the dopamine D2 receptor in their brains, compared with healthy subjects. Additional imaging studies, looking at functioning within neural circuits believed to mediate fear and anxiety (for example, the amygdala and related structures), point to possible alterations in functioning of these neural systems in social phobia.

Diagnosis and Treatment

We now know that social phobia is a treatable disorder, and that several pharmacotherapeutic choices are available to the physician. Treatment with medication for a year or more is usually recommended, but optimal duration of treatment is currently being studied. We also know that many people benefit from cognitive behavioral therapy directed at changing their views about themselves and their expectations for social interactions, in concert with gradual exposure to and practice in the social situations they fear.

Although the efficacy of the monoamine oxidase inhibitors (for example, phenelzine) in the treatment of social phobia has been confirmed, their unfavorable side effects and the need for a special, low-tyramine diet have relegated them to second- or third-line status.

High-potency benzodiazepines (such as clonazepam) are efficacious for social phobia, although their potential for abuse remains of some concern and may limit their use by some practitioners. Beta-adrenergic blockers (such as propranolol and atenolol), although of some use in the treatment of isolated performance anxiety, are probably of no benefit in the treatment of generalized social anxiety disorder. This information still needs to reach some physicians, many of whom equate social phobia with public-speaking anxiety and accordingly prescribe beta-blockers because of their familiarity with this class of drugs. Similarly, buspirone, another medication frequently used to treat anxiety in primary care settings, has been shown to be inefficacious in the treatment of social anxiety disorder.

Recently the effectiveness of selective serotonin reuptake inhibitors (SSRIs) for social phobia has been confirmed in large clinical trials. Currently, newer pharmacotherapies are being tested, and researchers are exploring the possibility of combining pharmacotherapy and cognitive behavioral therapy.

Obsessive-Compulsive Disorder

Recurrent thoughts and rituals can be a part of normal, daily life. Many people wonder when they leave home whether they turned off the coffeepot or locked the door. Some of us might wash our hands every day when we return home from work, or be repelled by the idea of eating from a utensil that has fallen on the floor. It is also quite normal for growing children to go through periods when their playthings, food, bedtime routine, or other aspects of life must be "just so." For some adults and children, however, such obsessions and compulsions can reach a level that causes marked distress, consumes large amounts of time, or significantly interferes with daily life. These people suffer from obsessive-compulsive disorder (OCD).

OCD is an anxiety disorder in which a person has recurrent and persistent thoughts, impulses, or imaginings that are intrusive and inappropriate, and that cause marked anxiety or distress. The individual usually tries to ignore, suppress, or neutralize these obsessions with thoughts and actions. These responses can become compulsive—repetitive behaviors or mental acts that a person may feel driven to perform by an obsession, or to prevent or reduce anxiety or distress.

In general, people with OCD recognize that their anxious thoughts and rituals are unreasonable and excessive, but they feel helpless about stopping them. Thus, while they may have irrational or bizarre thoughts related to their symptoms, they are in touch with reality. OCD is not a psychotic disorder.

The lifetime prevalence of OCD in adults is 2 percent to 3 percent. This level, established by surveys in the 1980s, was considerably higher than expected, indicating the possibility that many people do not have their difficulties diagnosed and treated. One third to one half of adults with OCD report that their illness began in childhood or adolescence. Only about 15 percent of patients with OCD have onset after age 35. "Late onset" OCD (after age 50) is unusual and is most likely to be due to organic causes, such as strokes (**C59, C60**) in the basal ganglia or frontal lobes. In adults, women are more likely to have OCD than men, but before adolescence boys are more likely to have the condition than girls.

Obsessions and Compulsions

A person with OCD may have obsessions, compulsions, or both. Often a person's obsessions and compulsions are characterized by anxiety or fear that something bad might happen. Some people with OCD fear contamination, whether from dirt, germs, certain illnesses (AIDS, rabies), bodily wastes or secretions (urine, feces, saliva), environmental contaminants (asbestos, radiation, toxic wastes), or household items (cleaners, solvents). These people might have the recurring and upsetting thought that someone they passed on the street, or sat beside in a meeting, might have contaminated them. Some individuals go to great lengths to avoid certain places or people, such as not shopping in malls for fear that they might have to use a rest room where they could catch an illness.

Others who suffer from OCD fear that their actions could unwittingly cause harm to themselves or others. A person might worry that leaving an envelope on a table next to a light might cause the paper to catch fire and burn down the house, killing their loved ones. A child might have recurrent thoughts that his or her parents will be kidnapped, whereas a parent might worry that his or her child will be abducted.

Some people with OCD suffer from aggressive or sexualized thoughts or images, fearing that they might harm themselves or their loved ones. For example, a person might have a recurring worry that he or she has caused harm to another person, although no such incident has happened. Other people have recurring fears of doing something embarrassing, such as screaming out in church or temple. Still others are obsessed with doing things perfectly, or being good. Some people are obsessed with the need for reassurance. Occasionally, the obsession can be an image or tune in one's head.

Compulsions (or rituals) are repetitive behaviors or mental acts that a person with OCD might often carry out to "undo" or "neutralize" the obsession. Common compulsions include washing, cleaning, checking, counting, repeating, arranging, touching, and hoarding. Excessive praying is an example of a mental compulsion called scrupulosity. Sometimes the compulsive act has no logical connection to a person's fear: feeling that one must touch particular objects on one's desk before handing in an important report, for instance. At other times, there may be a logical connection between an obsession (cleanliness) and a compulsion (washing), but a person performs the action at an excessive level.

Often compulsive behavior produces clear signs of difficulty. A classic symptom in a person who fears contamination is hands that are red and cracked from excessive washing. Very ritualized showering, grooming, and toothbrushing that is excessive and problematic are also likely to reflect OCD. An individual obsessed with leaving a door locked may feel compelled to check it repeatedly, and may be constantly late to work because of going back home to check. Someone obsessed with cleanliness might do so much laundry that it affects the household bills.

Some people with OCD establish elaborate rituals without knowing why. They may have to do things exactly three, four, or another number of times. Repeating actions—such as turning a light off and on, stepping, touching, or tapping "until it feels right"—might be an OCD symptom. Needing one's possessions to be in the exact right position could be an OCD symptom. Saving sentimental objects is normal, but amassing useless items (used gum wrappers, expired coupons, old newspapers) may be symptomatic of OCD.

Most people with OCD have many different obsessions and compulsions over the course of their illness, and the specific symptoms change in severity. Children with OCD have essentially the same symptoms as adults, although more age appropriate: arranging their toys ritually rather than the items in their offices. It is particularly interesting that individuals from different cultures all over the world have essentially identical obsessions or compulsions, which speaks to the underlying neurobiology of the disorder.

Some activities similar to behaviors associated with OCD, but not actually part of the illness, are grouped under a new term, OC spectrum illnesses. Trichotillomania is the repeated pulling out of one's hair (scalp, eyebrows, eyelashes, body hair). Body dysmorphic disorder is a preoccupation with an imagined defect in one's appearance that causes great distress and impairment; someone who has had multiple unsatisfactory plastic surgeries might have this disorder. Compulsive eating, spending, and gambling are also not considered part of OCD.

What Causes OCD?

Obsessive-compulsive disorder is a heterogeneous disorder, meaning that it may have different risk factors (or causes) in different people. It tends to run in families, so we believe people can inherit a genetic vulnerability. Family studies suggest that OCD and chronic tic disorders, including Tourette's syndrome (C45), may represent alternative expressions of the same gene or genes. In other words, these genes may be expressed as OCD in some people, as tics in others, and occasionally as both.

OCD has both neurological and psychiatric symptoms. One piece of evidence that it is brain based comes from its association with several neurological illnesses: Sydenham's chorea, Huntington's chorea, and illness or trauma that leads to alterations in the basal ganglia. Although these cases of OCD's association with neurological illness are rare, they might provide clues about where the brain is malfunctioning.

Neuroimaging studies of both the brain's structure and function in people with OCD have provided evidence of a change in the normal physiology of connections between the orbitofrontal area and the subcortical areas of the brain (specifically the striatum and thalamus). Some doctors now think that OCD symptoms may arise from an imbalance in the feedback loops in this area of neurocircuitry. Specific neurotransmitter systems—serotonin, probably dopamine, and others—seem to become hyperactive in these circuits. When physicians use cognitive behavioral therapy, medication, or occasionally, surgery to inhibit or interrupt these circuits, OCD symptoms can diminish for many people.

Studies have found that medications that alter the amount of serotonin in the brain's synapses are the most effective way to treat OCD medically. These drugs seem to work by altering the balance in the feedback loops of the neural circuits. Interestingly, cognitive behavioral therapy (CBT) may act on the brain in a similar way. Some brain imaging studies have reported that activity in these circuits changes after successful CBT treatment.

Some researchers also suggest that OCD is a result of "neuroethological" behaviors that we hu-

Obsessive-compulsive behavior seems to be driven by a cycle of abnormal signals in the brain, as in this schematic drawing. This circuit appears to be consistently hypermetabolic when OCD patients are symptomatic. Specific functions associated with the regions making up these brain networks are thought to be involved in obsessive thoughts and impulsive urges. ILLUSTRATION © KATHRYN BORN

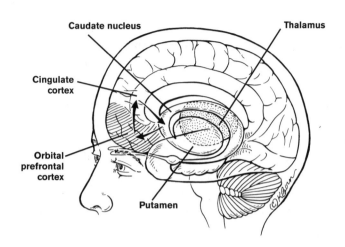

mans developed for survival and retain even though they are no longer necessary. According to this theory, behaviors normally required in the wild—such as perceiving and avoiding danger, protecting the young, and grooming—become magnified and cannot be turned off. Thus, obsessive-compulsive behaviors, such as repeatedly checking on children, excessive washing, or hoarding, may be the unleashing of an innate adaptive behavioral pattern gone awry.

Diagnosis and Treatment

Many people who suffer from OCD are embarrassed by their illness. They may try to hide their symptoms and not seek help. Furthermore, there is no blood test, or brain test, to make the diagnosis clear-cut. Rather, doctors must rely on a clinical interview. They seek to find out if the person spends at least one hour a day in obsessing or carrying out rituals, or if those compulsions significantly interfere with the person's life in other ways. A primary care physician may make an initial diagnosis and refer a person for further treatment, typically to a clinical psychologist with expertise in cognitive behavioral therapy or to a psychiatrist.

Doctors usually do a comprehensive psychiatric evaluation, but unless there is something unusual about a person's case, they won't do a specific medical workup. However, someone who is over 50 and is experiencing the symptoms of OCD for the first time may have another illness, in which case a doctor typically performs a neurological workup.

A psychiatrist or psychologist must distinguish OCD from illnesses that appear similar, such as other anxiety disorders (**C21**), eating disorders (**C27**), depression (**C20**), or a psychosomatic illness. Children may exhibit rigid and ritualized behaviors as symptoms of such developmental disorders as Asperger's syndrome (**C5**) or as a passing stage of normal development. Furthermore, other disorders may coexist with OCD and may obscure the symptoms. It is not uncommon for a person to have other anxiety disorders or a depressive disorder at the same time. A child with OCD has a higher risk of also having a tic disorder or Tourette's syndrome (**C45**), and sometimes a complex motor tic resembles a ritual. Among children with OCD, there is also

IF A CHILD HAS SUDDEN OCD

A small number of preadolescent children develop the symptoms of OCD abruptly and dramatically in response to a streptococcal infection. These children's condition is described by the term PANDAS: pediatric autoimmune neuropsychiatric disorders associated with streptococcal infections. Their immune system responses to the initial infection also seem to disrupt the brain circuits involved in OCD.

Because of that possibility, a child with acute onset or dramatic exacerbation of OCD symptoms, either with or without tics, should be thoroughly assessed for recent medical illnesses. Typically, doctors perform a throat culture and may order blood tests for an antibody to streptococcus.

Once doctors have documented the streptococcal infection and diagnosed PANDAS, they usually prescribe antibiotics to treat the child's infection, helping to fight off the streptococcus bacterium so the immune system can return to normal activity. Research studies are under way to determine if blood plasma exchange or intravenous gamma globulin, which reduce the concentration of the problematic antibodies in the blood, are effective treatments in severe cases. Children with PANDAS are probably a small subgroup of those with either OCD or tics.

a higher than average rate of attention deficit/hyperactivity disorder (**C2**).

We have two effective methods for treating OCD: CBT and drug treatment. There is no clear way to predict which treatment, or what combination, will work best for a particular individual.

A very specific kind of CBT, called exposure with response prevention (ERP), is the psychotherapeutic treatment of choice. It involves progressively exposing the person to the stimulus he or she fears until it no longer brings on the anxious response. Individuals choosing CBT should seek a therapist with experience in delivering this specific form. Some studies estimate that ERP helps people improve their symptoms by 50 percent to 65 percent. More general types of family and individual psychotherapy are sometimes useful for related issues, but not typically for the primary symptoms of OCD.

As we noted above, medications that inhibit serotonin reuptake appear uniquely effective in treating OCD symptoms. These include the serotonin reuptake inhibitor clomipramine (Anafranil) and such selective serotonin reuptake inhibitors (SSRIs) as fluoxetine (Prozac), fluvoxamine (Luvox), paroxetine (Paxil), and sertraline (Zoloft). These drugs are most commonly used to treat depression. Children and adults appear to have similar responses to them.

Many people's OCD symptoms will not respond until after two or even three months of medication, so it is important for the doctor to wait a sufficient time before changing medications, raising doses past target doses, or adding additional medications. It is estimated that one out of three people fails to respond to a given SSRI. Sometimes those who have a partial response to one SSRI are given a second medication as an "augmenting agent." Some doctors believe that drug treatment and CBT are a logical combination and work well together, but studies have not yet

HELPING SOMEONE WHO HAS OBSESSIVE-COMPULSIVE DISORDER

Family members and friends can do many things to help people with obsessive-compulsive disorder. The first and most important thing to do is to learn as much as you can about the disorder, its causes, and its treatment. At the same time, you must be sure the person with OCD has access to information about the disorder. Here are some other suggestions.

- Help the person understand that effective treatments are available.

- Treat people normally once they have recovered, but be alert for telltale signs of relapse.

- When children or adolescents have OCD, it is important for parents to work with schools and teachers to be sure that they understand the disorder.

- Take advantage of the help available from support groups or ask your doctor for the names of individual parents who would be willing to talk with you and offer support.

- Parents of children with OCD should feel comfortable seeking out help for themselves in coping with raising a child with this illness.

Adapted from www.ocfoundation.org (Obsessive-Compulsive Foundation)

been completed to support the superiority of using both treatments together.

For severely incapacitated adults with OCD whose symptoms have not responded to intensive CBT and medication, researchers are studying surgical treatments. The newest investigational procedure is deep brain stimulation (DBS), which involves implanting electrodes into the brain that are connected to an electrical device similar to a heart pacemaker, as in a currently approved treatment for neurological illness such as severe tremor. There is more experience with older operations, such as cingulotomy and capsulotomy. Both of these procedures involve making careful lesions within brain circuits believed to mediate OCD symptoms. In cingulotomy, holes are made in the skull through which a thermal probe is inserted to heat and destroy part of the cingulate gyrus. Capsulotomy, where the target is the anterior internal capsule, was initially done this way as well. A newer capsulotomy procedure allows smaller lesions to be precisely made in the capsule without opening the skull, using a device, a "gamma knife," that focuses many beams of radiation.

Unfortunately, for many individuals OCD is a chronic and debilitating illness. About one third of people get better and stay in remission, one third have continued illness, and one third appear to get worse. Thus, OCD is not a progressive illness in which a person must expect more and more impairment, but those people with a chronic course may never be symptom-free. The development of new drug treatments and specific CBT interventions are believed to improve the long-term prognosis.

Bipolar Disorder

Bipolar disorder, sometimes referred to as manic-depressive illness, is typically defined by alternating episodes of mania and depression—a person may feel unreasonably happy one week, sad and listless the next. It is a recurrent disorder. Individuals who have bipolar disorder usually experience many episodes of both mania and depression over the course of a lifetime. In most cases the illness begins with a depressed episode that appears similar to other forms of depression (C20). In this case, it is not possible to know whether the individual will eventually develop manic-depressive illness or only a pattern of recurrent depressions. However, if a first mood episode is mania, then the individual is diagnosed with bipolar disorder.

The symptoms of depression in bipolar disorder are similar to those of other forms of depression. Individuals experience empty, sad, or irritable mood throughout most of the day. They have no interest in and take no pleasure from all or almost all activities. They often experience loss of appetite or weight loss, although in bipolar depression increased appetite and weight gain are also common. Depressed people tend to report constant fatigue. Their sleep patterns often change; some find it difficult to sleep, while others seem to need to sleep all the time (C11). People suffering from depression cannot concentrate on minor tasks and have difficulty remembering even trivial things. They may also report recurrent thoughts of death or a desire to commit suicide.

A manic episode is defined by a distinctly abnormal and persistently elevated, expansive, or irritable mood. This mood change is accompanied by additional symptoms—extremely high self-esteem or a clearly unrealistically positive view of one's abilities, decreased need for sleep, and pressured speech, flights of ideas, distractibility, high levels of activity, increased sexual interest, and excessive involvement in pleasurable activities, including those with the potential for adverse consequences, such as reckless spending, ill-considered business ventures, and so on. A manic person often has expansive enthusiasm for all kinds of social interaction, including phone calls, e-mails, social gatherings, and others. His or her speech is often rapid and very difficult for others to interrupt. The inflated self-esteem of mania may be so extreme and omnipresent that the manic person starts to suffer delusions about himself or herself. First episodes of mania, especially if they are very severe, may be hard to distinguish from other forms of psychotic illness, such as schizophrenia (**C25**).

Often individuals with mania do not realize that anything is wrong. Only family members, friends, and other people around them recognize that their behavior and level of activity are abnormal. Generally, a person experiencing a mild mania does not look troubled, especially during work; colleagues may just perceive the person as very clever and productive. But if the mania is more severe, it will be obvious to any observer that something is wrong. What the affected person says and does will make no sense and often will be completely inappropriate.

In both manic and depressed episodes, family members and friends often notice changes and encourage the individual to seek help. Frequently a manic person must be taken to the emergency room against his or her will, not believing that anything is wrong. In contrast, a depressed person can sometimes be persuaded to make an appointment with a mental health clinician, although the hopelessness that is a core feature of depression can often make the person feel that he or she is beyond help.

A rare but striking manifestation of bipolar disorder occurs in individuals who show symptoms of both mania and depression at the same time. This is called a mixed state and is tremendously distressing to the sufferer.

Searching for the Cause

Bipolar disorder typically begins in early adolescence; somewhere between 15 percent and 20 percent of adolescents with diagnosed depression go on to develop bipolar disorder. The prevalence of classical manic-depressive illness is generally found to be between 1 percent and 2.5 percent of the population, although some studies suggest that up to 8 percent of people experience the more broadly defined bipolar spectrum disorder, which involves milder forms of depression and what is called hypomania, a milder form of mania.

The rate of bipolar disorder is relatively consistent across cultures. According to projections by the World Health Organization and the World Bank, in the year 2020 bipolar disorder will be one of the world's ten leading medical problems in terms of its cost to society. The risk of suicide (**C32**) among those suffering from bipolar disorder is 10 percent to 15 percent and is as high during mania as it is during depression.

Brain imaging technologies such as positron-emission tomography (PET) and magnetic resonance imaging (MRI) have provided researchers with unprecedented opportunities to study brain function and structure in bipolar disorder. Researchers have identified regions in the brain that function abnormally during the depressed and manic phases of the illness. In addition, the brains of people with bipolar disorder show other abnormalities that persist even after the symptoms have remitted—in the frontal and temporal lobes and in the basal ganglia, which regulate emotional, behavioral, and stress responses.

Autopsies of people who had bipolar disorder, guided by these imaging findings, have revealed regions where the volume of the cortex and the number of glial cells are abnormally low. Very preliminary evidence suggests that ongoing treatment with mood-stabilizing medications, such as lithium, may partly reverse these structural abnormalities.

Studies of families have provided considerable evidence that there is a genetic component to bipolar disorder. For example, studies comparing identical twins (who share 100 percent of their genes) with fraternal twins (who, on average, share 50 percent of their genes) indicate that while about 60 percent of the identical twins of individuals with bipolar disorder will also have the illness, only about 7 percent of fraternal twins of individuals with the disorder will also have it. No specific genes that "cause" bipolar disorder have yet been identified, however.

Diagnosis and Treatment

Bipolar disorder is a chronic, persistent illness that requires long-term treatment. Currently, there is no cure. Repeated episodes of mania and depression over time can bring increasing difficulties in a person's work and family life. On the other hand, adhering to treatment to limit the effects of these episodes can restore many individuals to almost full or even full functioning.

Modern psychopharmacology has transformed bipolar disorder from an essentially untreatable condition to one with the clear possibility of a good outcome. Doctors have prescribed lithium for approximately 40 years as a treatment for mania and as a mood stabilizer to prevent the return of both manic and depressive episodes. The medications used to treat acute episodes have evolved from such neuroleptics as chlorpromazine (Thorazine) and haloperidol (Haldol) to the current atypical antipsychotics (olanzapine), all of which are usually successful.

The treatment of depression in bipolar disorder, however, has not been as satisfactory as the treatment of major depression in individuals with nonbipolar, or unipolar, depression. Lithium alone is sometimes effective for the treatment of bipolar depression, but in many cases an antidepressant medication is required. Most of the traditional antidepressants have demonstrated modest success in the treatment of acute bipolar depression; these include the tricyclic antidepressants, the monoamine oxidase inhibitors (MAOIs), and the current group of selective serotonin reuptake inhibitors (SSRIs). Several studies have indicated that the MAOIs may be the best treatment for bipolar depression, but the dietary restrictions and possible adverse effects of these drugs have minimized their general uses.

New antimanic and mood-stabilizing drugs in-

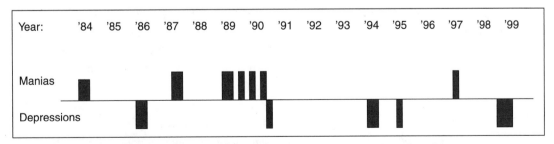

Cycles of mania and depression in bipolar disorder may include long stretches of respite from the disorder, but also clusters of episodes, as this patient's history shows. GRAPH COURTESY OF ELLEN FRANK, PH.D., WESTERN PSYCHIATRIC INSTITUTE, UNIVERSITY OF PITTSBURGH SCHOOL OF MEDICINE

PREVENTING RELAPSE IN BIPOLAR DISORDER

Relapse prevention involves adhering to many guidelines, some of which are discussed below.

■ **Your medications are very important in helping you live with the chemical imbalance in your body. You must take your medication exactly as your doctor ordered. If you have difficulty getting your medication because of transportation problems or paying for your medicine, you should talk to your doctor or counselor. You should also let them know if you think the medication is bothering you in any way.**

■ **Try to decrease the stress in your life as much as possible. Do things you enjoy each day and try to stay away from people or situations that are stressful to you.**

■ **Go to bed at a regular time and have a schedule you keep for exercises and all your other daily routines.**

■ **Talk to friends and family for support. Get involved in activities at work, school, your neighborhood, or church to meet people and to have fun. Try to get help in dealing with any problems you might have in relationships with family, friends, or acquaintances.**

Adapted from www.med.jhu.edu/drada/ (Depression and Related Affective Disorders Association); another helpful link: www.ndmda.org (National Depressive and Manic-Depressive Association)

---

clude divalproex (Depakote), carbamazepine, and other anticonvulsants. Several other compounds (topiramate, lamotrigine, and gabapentin/Neurontin) are currently being tested for both the treatment of acute mania and overall long-term mood stabilization. Several of the new atypical antipsychotics are likely to prove effective for the treatment of acute mania (already, olanzapine/Zyprexa has been approved as such a treatment). Over the next decade, we expect that researchers will identify genetic factors defining vulnerability to bipolar disorder more precisely, and that more specific drugs with fewer side effects will then become available.

Psychotherapy and Severe Bipolar Disorder

The initial success of lithium in helping people with mania and, less effectively, depression led doctors to think of bipolar disorder as a purely biological process that could be treated with drugs alone. Psychotherapy for bipolar disorder came to be considered unnecessary and was largely neglected for many years. Beginning in the 1980s, however, reports suggested that treatment with lithium alone was often not enough. Researchers and clinicians became increasingly aware that the chronic course of bipolar disorder may, in the absence of appropriate psychological help, lead a person to suffer unremitting symptoms and fall into a downward psychosocial spiral.

Recently, therefore, research teams have begun to study ways to use specific forms of psychotherapy in combination with drugs. One group is investigating interpersonal and social rhythm therapy (IPSRT), a one-on-one psychotherapy designed specifically for people with bipolar disorder. IPSRT grew from a theory that such people have a genetic predisposition to body rhythm and sleep-wake cycle abnormalities (**C11**). According to this model, both negative and positive events in people's lives may disrupt their social routines in ways that then perturb their body rhythms and lead to the development of bipolar symptoms. Administered in concert with medications, IPSRT combines the basic principles of interpersonal psychotherapy with behavioral techniques to help patients regularize their daily routines, diminish interpersonal problems, and adhere to their medication schedules.

Another promising avenue of research involves family-focused treatment (FFT). This approach assumes that bipolar individuals who live in supportive family environments are at a lower risk for recurrences of their disorder. Family-focused treatment puts emphasis on educating all family members about the disorder, promoting efficient communication within the family, and enhancing family problem-solving skills to handle illness-related conflicts. It also emphasizes collaboration among relatives to prevent relapses.

Several research groups are studying the possible benefits of cognitive therapy in bipolar disorder. Cognitive therapies emphasize the way in which an individual's thinking can influence his or her mood and seek to help the individual "correct" unrealistically negative (or positive) thinking. Soon a large set of multisite clinical trials sponsored by the National Institute of Mental Health should provide new information about both drug and psychosocial interventions.

Schizophrenia

A popular but erroneous myth about schizophrenia is that it means a "split personality," as in the movie *The Three Faces of Eve*. Instead, schizophrenia is an illness that affects a variety of mental functions as well as a person's ability to think clearly and feel intensely. The word itself stresses how the functions of the mind are fragmented: *schizo* means "fragmented," and *phren* means "mind." Schizophrenic symptoms include changes in the entire gamut of human mental activities.

Symptoms of schizophrenia are typically divided into positive and negative categories. In the case of positive symptoms, a person's mental functions are exaggerated or distorted; in the case of negative symptoms, they are diminished or absent. The table on page 391 summarizes each group and the mental functions that are impaired. For doctors to diagnose schizophrenia, the symptoms must be causing a person significant impairment at work, at school, or in personal relationships.

The natural course of schizophrenia can vary, but it typically starts with a person becoming somewhat more apathetic and withdrawn. During this phase of the illness the patient may be misdiagnosed as suffering from depression or a "personality disorder." At some point clear symptoms of schizophrenia appear, and doctors recognize the condition.

Delusions, hallucinations, and some other symptoms of schizophrenia occur in other illnesses as well, such as mood disorders (**C20, C24**), substance abuse (**C29, C30**), and dementia (**C67, C69**). However, it is rare for young people without schizophrenia to experience a decline in their cognitive abilities; this negative symptom is the characteristic and defining feature of this illness.

After onset, people with schizophrenia usually go through a rather rocky period lasting a few months and up to a few years, during which their positive symptoms remain severe or wax and wane in a series of episodes. The underlying negative symptoms tend to persist throughout. The negative symptoms are the most common signs of schizophrenia, but no single characteristic is present in all forms of the disorder.

Factors and Mechanisms

Psychiatrists who have worked closely with schizophrenia recognize it as a brain disease. Unlike many other brain diseases, however, it does not have a single obvious marker or lesion in the brain. We cannot recognize it in physical features of the brain in the same way that, for example, we know plaques and tangles indicate Alzheimer's disease (C67). Our current understanding of schizophrenia is that it is a neurodevelopmental disorder that arises because crucial functional "nodes" distributed throughout the brain are not connected correctly, so that thought processes lose their coherence and coordination.

Schizophrenia is probably not due to an abnormality in any single specific area of the brain. Both structural and functional imaging studies have indicated that many areas are involved together, including the prefrontal cortex, the temporal lobes, the limbic regions, the thalamus, the basal ganglia, and the cerebellum. It is very likely that the symptoms of schizophrenia arise when these various functional regions are unable to communicate with one another in an efficient and coordinated manner.

Throughout the world, 1 percent of all people suffer from this illness. It usually appears in late adolescence or early adult life, and it tends to affect males more frequently and more severely than females. Many children who later develop schizophrenia do not appear very different from their peers. Some, however, do display some early

POSITIVE SYMPTOMS	IMPAIRED FUNCTION
Hallucinations (usually experienced as "hearing voices")	Perception
Delusions (strongly held erroneous beliefs)	Inferential thinking
Disorganized speech (loosely associated, tangential, or sometimes incoherent speech)	Language and communication
Grossly disorganized (inappropriate, unpredictable, or untriggered) or catatonic (unreactive) behavior	Social and motor regulation
Inappropriate affect	Emotional regulation
NEGATIVE SYMPTOMS	**IMPAIRED FUNCTION**
Affective blunting (diminished range of emotional expressiveness)	Emotional expression
Alogia (decreased ability to speak)	Language and communication
Anhedonia (loss of interest or pleasure)	Emotion
Avolition (lack of goal-oriented behavior)	Decision making and planning
Attention impairment	Attention

indicators. Reasonably well documented markers include physical awkwardness, social awkwardness, shyness, or a preoccupation with unusual interests or beliefs. Parents may also become concerned about their child because of a *change* in behavior during middle to late adolescence. Early signs of schizophrenia include a decline in school performance, a loss of interest in sports and other social activities that the child previously enjoyed, or a tendency to withdraw and become isolated. All of these changes can have other causes, however.

Schizophrenia appears to strike independently of social class, and it occurs at approximately the same rate everywhere in the world. A variety of different risk factors have been identified, including birth during winter months (perhaps reflecting an exposure to an infection, either during fetal development or shortly after birth), exposure to such toxins as illegal drugs (particularly amphetamines), and a family history of the illness.

Schizophrenia thus appears to have a genetic component. For example, if one identical twin develops the condition, the risk that the other will is 40 percent. For fraternal twins the risk is 10 percent, the same as for other first-degree relatives. These statistics indicate, however, that schizophrenia must also have a prominent *non*genetic component. Various studies searching for "schizophrenia genes" suggest that the illness is caused by more than one gene, and that other factors must also have a role.

Schizophrenia in Monozygotic Twins
44-year-old males

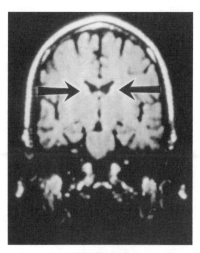 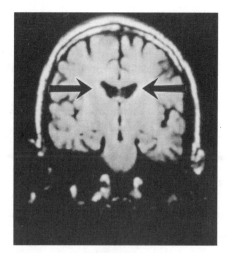

Unaffected   **Affected**

Magnetic resonance imaging shows enlarged ventricles in the brain of an identical twin suffering from schizophrenia. Researchers are trying to learn whether such structural differences are produced by the disease or associated with the causes of it. SCANS COURTESY OF DANIEL WEINBERGER, M.D., NATIONAL INSTITUTE OF MENTAL HEALTH

Diagnosis and Treatment

As there are no specific tests for schizophrenia, doctors make their diagnoses based on the characteristic clinical presentation. Because of the complexity in differentiating between schizophrenia and other conditions (such as depression and substance abuse), a family practitioner will often refer a patient having difficulties to an experienced psychiatric clinician, who then makes the diagnosis. Early recognition and treatment are very important because they may save a person from subsequent psychotic episodes, which have a devastating effect on self-esteem and the ability to perform normally at work or school.

The primary treatment for schizophrenia symptoms consists of neuroleptic medications. Sometimes these drugs are referred to as "antipsychotic" medications, but that implies that the treatment is targeting only a person's psychotic symptoms when, in fact, treating the negative symptoms may be even more important. The brand names of medications commonly used to treat schizophrenia include Risperdal (risperidone), Zyprexa (olanzapine), Seroquel (quetiapine), Zeldox (ziprasidone), Clozaril (clozapine), Haldol (haloperidol), and Thorazine (chlorpromazine). All these examples, except Thorazine and Haldol, which have long been standard treatments, are of the more "atypical" or "second generation" neuroleptics. The positive symptoms of schizophrenia tend to be very responsive to neuroleptic medications, while the negative symptoms are more difficult to treat. The newer atypical medications may be more effective in reducing negative symptoms, however. Most people with schizophrenia need to continue to take medications in order to keep their symptoms under control.

In addition to taking neuroleptic drugs, people with schizophrenia tend to do best if they can strike a balance between returning to the routines of daily life (that is, going back to work or school) and not doing more than their condition permits. Ideally, people should remain as active and engaged in daily life activities as possible. In the era of deinstitutionalization, we are seeing that most people with schizophrenia can live successfully in the community.

When psychiatrists first defined schizophrenia, they thought the prognosis for anyone with the disorder was grim. Recent research indicates, however, that after the initial intense, or fulminant, period of illness, most people stabilize at a level of functioning slightly below their original status. After the initial period of florid psychotic symptoms, many people with schizophrenia have only mild negative symptoms. Therefore, both family members and clinicians can play an important role in maintaining a person's confidence that things will get better, thus reducing relapse rates during the fulminant phase.

Many investigators are studying the causes of schizophrenia. These investigations encompass everything from molecular biology and genetics through the study of the mental systems involved in the illness. It is the long-term goal of researchers to find better treatments and, ultimately, to identify ways to intervene early and prevent the illness from arising.

Borderline Personality Disorder

Borderline personality disorder has two hall-mark features. The first is the emotional in-stability that permeates the lives of people with this condition. People with this disorder are ex-quisitely sensitive to disappointments, frustra-tion, and unmet expectations. Their responses to real or imagined adversity include such emotions as rage, despondency, sadness, or, when their emotional circuits are overloaded, even a bland feeling of numbness.

The second characteristic feature of people with borderline personality disorder is a marked tendency toward impulsive behavior and aggres-sion directed against themselves or others. This can be apparent in angry tirades, verbal abuse, or self-destructive acts such as overdosing, cutting one's wrist or arm, or suicide attempts. Someone with the disorder may also display a variety of other impulsive behaviors, such as reckless driv-ing, alcohol or drug use (**C29, C30**), unsafe sex, binge eating (**C27**), or gambling—though people without the condition do all these things as well. Often such behaviors are ways that people with borderline personality disorder vent their intense emotions and attempt to restore some sense of

well-being. They perceive their actions as survival strategies for the hostile environment they expe-rience.

The personal relationships of individuals with borderline personality disorder are charac-teristically quite stormy, frequently marked by the idealizing of another person in the early stages of the relationship, followed by an inse-cure attachment and fear of abandonment or, in other instances, devaluation. The intense fear of abandonment may result in exaggerated and manipulative behaviors, or cause individuals to cling to abusive relationships. Under periods of high stress, borderlines may become suspicious of others and even feel that people are acting in concert against them.

Because of their tumultuous emotions, people with borderline personality disorder have a hard time sustaining stable relationships and work commitments. They may not perceive how their behavior contributes to their problems, and may find themselves shunned by family members and colleagues. People with the disorder often have difficulties with their sense of identity or such "dissociative symptoms" as feeling unreal or as if

A BORDERLINE PERSONALITY IN THE FAMILY

Family members are often at a loss to know how to deal with the mercurial mood swings and angry tirades that characterize someone with borderline personality disorder. They may urge that relative to seek treatment. On the other hand, they may view the person as simply "impossible" or difficult, not realizing that such problems can result from a treatable brain condition.

Furthermore, borderline personality disorder involves enduring *predispositions* to impulsive or self-destructive acts, emotional shifts, and other behaviors. At any given time, therefore, those behaviors or emotions may not be evident. Indeed, many people with the disorder are able to mask their symptoms at work and in similar contexts. Over the long run, however, these susceptibilities tend to be fairly constant. That means that while a person's symptoms may wax and wane in severity, traits such as impulsivity and emotional instability tend to persist over the long run.

It is especially difficult to definitively diagnose borderline personality disorder in adolescents. Its symptoms may overlap with the more short-lived emotional turmoil and risk taking that often accompanies the transition to adulthood. Nonetheless, the warning signs of self-destructive or self-injurious behaviors, including cutting oneself, affective instability, and impulsivity, are often apparent during the teenage years. If you see such traits in your adolescent child, you should seek a prompt evaluation by a psychiatrist for potential treatment.

the world around them were unreal. They are not frankly psychotic, however.

Individuals with borderline personality disorder often suffer from major depressive illness or bipolar (manic-depressive) disorder as well (**C20, C24**). In fact, at one point this condition was considered a variant of depression, but it is clear now that people with borderline personality disorder may not be depressed most of the time and that not all of them suffer from depression. Nonetheless, the sudden loss of a relationship, often with somebody they initially idealized, often causes them to be overwhelmed with such feelings of despair and abandonment that they seek treatment for depression.

Another disorder that has been associated with borderline personality disorder is post-traumatic stress disorder (PTSD; **C28**). Some researchers have even proposed that borderline is a variant of PTSD. People with borderline personality disorder may indeed have experienced a history of trauma, often sexual abuse, which produces PTSD symptoms, but these seem to be only a minority of cases.

The symptoms of this condition may be very severe, with self-destructive behaviors leading to repeated hospitalizations. Ultimately there is a risk of lethal suicide attempts (**C32**). Thus, borderline personality disorder can be among the most severe of the disorders affecting our brain and nervous system. On the other hand, many people with this condition can function adequately much of the time in work and relationships, even as they also experience a great deal of distress and cause the people close to them similar distress because of their recurring angry, irritable, and manipulative behaviors.

Clues to a Biological Cause

We do not know the exact prevalence of borderline personality disorder, but one study suggests that slightly less than 2 percent of the general population suffers from it. Both men and women have the condition; the prevalence in women may be slightly greater. The symptoms often become apparent during adolescence or young adulthood. There is some suggestion that the prevalence of the disorder may decline or its intensity might decrease with advancing age.

Studies of identical and fraternal twins suggest that genes contribute significantly to the likelihood that a person will have borderline personality disorder, but those genes may be more closely related to impulsivity and emotional instability than to the disorder itself. There are some suggestions that genes related to certain brain chemical systems may contribute to an individual's susceptibility, but definitive studies have yet to be completed. It may turn out that such genetic factors interact with childhood trauma, such as physical or sexual abuse, to contribute to borderline personality disorder. The condition is complex, and the possible explanations are still being explored.

Only a few studies have examined the brain structure and activity of people with borderline personality disorder. That research does suggest, however, that in those who have the disorder parts of the frontal cortex may be less active, while limbic regions may be very easily stimulated. The limbic structures of the brain regulate our emotional responses, and the cortex modulates the limbic region. (Phineas Gage, the railway worker described in chapter 1, sustained damage to his left frontal cortex; he displayed unusually impulsive speech and behavior afterward.) If the limbic system is volatile and the cortex does not act to modulate it, the result might be like driving a runaway train of emotions. That combination might explain the impulsivity and emotional instability that people with borderline personality disorder display.

Serotonin, a brain chemical that regulates our appetite, mood, and temperature and suppresses aggressive behaviors, is an important regulator of frontal brain activity. You can think of serotonin as providing the fluid for our emotional brakes. Many studies have shown an association between the kind of impulsive aggression people with borderline personality disorder display and reduced signs of serotonin activity in the brain. For instance, in most people medications that increase the activity of serotonin activate the area of the frontal cortex directly over the eyes. For people with impulsive, aggressive personality disorders, brain imaging shows these medications to be less efficient. Other imaging studies suggest that the limbic regions of the brain in this disorder are hyperresponsive to drugs that might induce irritability in these brain areas.

These findings have set the stage for the development of medication to specifically treat borderline personality disorder. We suspect that agents that increase serotonin activity might play a role in normalizing frontal function, while agents that reduce limbic irritability, such as mood stabilizers, may dampen people's emotional sensitivity.

Diagnosis and Treatment

Early recognition, diagnosis, and treatment of borderline personality disorder can be quite important. The behaviors characteristic of the disorder can cause serious harm to an individual's occupational and personal development, not to mention his or her physical health and life.

Psychiatrists are the most appropriate physicians to diagnose this disorder; they usually have more experience in recognizing its signs and symptoms, and are in the best position to evaluate people for possible treatment with medication. Clinical psychologists and social workers with specialized training in psychotherapy and personality disorders can evaluate an individual for possible psychotherapeutic treatment.

Physicians and mental health professionals diagnose borderline personality disorder primarily by hearing the history of the person's symptoms and behaviors. It is often helpful for family members and others close to the individual to explain what they have witnessed, because people with the disorder may deny or minimize the extent of their problems. A person's behavior during an evaluation interview or follow-up treatment also offers much useful information. There are no diagnostic tests for borderline personality disorder, but psychological testing can sometimes be helpful in identifying underlying problems.

Treatment for borderline personality disorder almost always makes use of some form of psychotherapy. People with this illness need to change their maladaptive patterns of behavior and develop new ways of coping with stress that involve delay and reflection rather than impulsive actions. There has been considerable research into effective treatments. One that has produced good results in a number of studies is called dialectical behavioral therapy. This is a form of cognitive behavioral therapy that seeks to change behavior and attitudes as well as to develop new skills for emotional regulation and social interaction. It includes a strong focus on reducing self-destructive behaviors. Other forms of cognitive

behavioral therapy that employ anger management have also been successful. In addition to psychotherapy, training in managing interpersonal conflicts and frustration is an important part of treatment for people with borderline personality disorder.

Other types of psychotherapy include supportive psychotherapy, based on helping individuals cope with crises in their lives and become more comfortable with themselves while exploring new ways of handling their emotions. Psychodynamics psychotherapy relies on encouraging conscious decisions and shedding light on more unconscious patterns of behavior, usually in the context of a powerful relationship with the therapist. This provides an opportunity to understand the misconceptions and distortions individuals with the disorder carry with them from their childhood. This technique demands a certain capacity for insight and self-observation that may not be available to many people with the illness, however,

Treatment for borderline personality disorder may also include medications for certain accompanying problems. Antidepressants are usually effective in treating the major depression that an individual may also suffer from. The selective serotonin reuptake inhibitors (SSRIs), one type of antidepressant medication, have also been shown to be effective in treating the impulsive and aggressive behavior typical of the disorder, even in the absence of prominent depressive symptoms. Closely related medications, such as venlafaxine (Effexor) and nefazodone (Serzone), may also be useful in treating the impulsivity. These agents may help correct an underlying problem in the serotonin system. Unfortunately, people with borderline personality disorder can be very sensitive to medications' side effects and often have difficulty taking high doses of the SSRIs or related compounds long enough to experience the beneficial effects.

Mood stabilizers such as lithium and the anticonvulsants valproate (Depakote) and carbamazepine (Tegretol) can be useful in dampening irritability, stabilizing the most rapidly changing emotions, and possibly even reducing the impulsivity. Clinical trials are evaluating these medicines' therapeutic effects more rigorously.

Antipsychotic medications, particularly such newer compounds as Clozaril, Risperdal, and Zyprexa, can be useful in reducing paranoid or psychotic-like symptoms, intense anxiety, and acting out, especially when a person is in acute crisis and needs to check into a hospital. Some-

times administering lower doses of these medications over a longer term can be helpful as well.

Finally, doctors may prescribe antianxiety medications such as buspirone or the benzodiazepines for some of the chronic anxious symptoms of this disorder. The benzodiazepines are potentially addictive, however, and they can have the effect of lowering a person's inhibitions, thus working against the rest of the therapy.

Research into the causes of borderline personality disorder continues, including genetic, brain imaging, and biochemical studies. The more we know about what causes this disorder, the better we will be able to treat it and perhaps one day cure it.

Eating Disorders

The term *eating disorder* usually refers to anorexia nervosa and bulimia nervosa, but applies as well to similar conditions that do not quite meet the exact criteria of these two major eating disorders. The vast majority of people who suffer from eating disorders are women. Approximately 2.5 percent of females in the United States suffer from anorexia nervosa or bulimia nervosa at some time in their lives. Most sufferers are adolescents and young adults ranging in age from 10 to 30. Significantly more women suffer from variants of these disorders. Eating disorders are rare among males.

Because of publicity about eating disorders, you may well be aware of their most common symptoms: eating far less than is healthy, bingeing on food, and vomiting food back up or otherwise purging it from one's body. People with eating disorders often learn to hide such behavior, however. A more visible sign of an eating disorder is therefore an excessive preoccupation with food and body appearance. Other suspicious signs include excessive exercising, refusal to eat foods containing high fat, refusal to eat with family members or friends, gradual weight loss or episodes of weight loss with rapid weight gain, and progressive isolation from friends and family.

Obviously, not digesting enough food is harmful. People with severe eating disorders can suffer damage to the heart, kidneys, liver, immune system, bones, and other organs because their bodies do not receive enough of the nutrients they need. These problems can be fatal. The body also suffers from the unnatural stresses of bingeing and purging.

Even beyond the issues of nutrition and physical health, eating disorders can have a devastating effect on an individual's psychological and social well-being. Afflicted people's isolation from family and friends, difficulty concentrating, irritability, disturbed sleep (C11), and depression (C20) can seriously interfere with their quality of life and their performance at work or school.

Defining Anorexia and Bulimia

Four major criteria define anorexia nervosa:

1. Weight loss and refusal to maintain body weight in the normal range for one's age and height.

2. A morbid fear of becoming fat

3. A disturbance in the way one experiences one's current low body weight: seeing specific parts of the body, such as the abdomen and thighs, as unduly fat even when obviously underweight, and denying the seriousness of one's low body weight.

4. In women, amenorrhea, or the absence of menstruation.

There are two types of anorexia nervosa. The first is the restricting type, in which the person loses

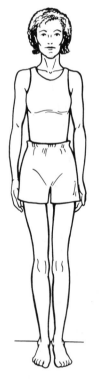 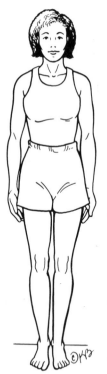

A. Actual size (100 lbs.)

B. Perceived actual size is +20% actual weight (120 lbs.)

A distorted sense of body image is a common feature of anorexia. A young woman with the disorder who weighs only 100 pounds might well resemble the unnaturally thin woman on the left. But she perceives her body to look like the woman on the right, at about 120 pounds. ILLUSTRATION © KATHRYN BORN

weight only by restricting food intake and exercising. The second is the binge-purge type, in which the person regularly engages in binge eating and then purging through self-induced vomiting or the misuse of laxatives, diuretics, and enemas.

Despite their refusal to eat, anorectic people think constantly about food. They may demonstrate this preoccupation by collecting recipes and preparing elaborate meals for others. They may comment incessantly about looking fat and feeling flabby and frequently gaze in the mirror to check their body form. Research on people with anorexia has shown that many have trouble even perceiving their true body size, consistently identifying it as 20 percent larger than it really is.

Bulimia nervosa is defined by five criteria:

1. The person has recurrent episodes of bingeing on food, eating an excessive amount within a discrete period while feeling unable to control the eating or to stop.

2. The person repeatedly uses self-induced vomiting or laxatives, diuretics, enemas, fasting, excessive exercising, or other medications to prevent weight gain.

3. These behaviors occur on average at least twice a week for three months.

4. The person is persistently too concerned with body shape and weight.

5. The person does not meet the criteria of anorexia nervosa. If she or he does, then we call the disorder anorexia nervosa, binge-purge type.

People with bulimia nervosa will often eat huge quantities of food when alone. Family members may return home to find an empty refrigerator or empty cupboards. Bulimic people may also take frequent trips to the bathroom in order to make themselves vomit up food.

There are also people who have most of the core clinical features of anorexia nervosa or bulimia nervosa but do not meet all the criteria stated above. We classify them as having an eating disorder not otherwise specified. Examples are people who vomit after eating small amounts of food but maintain their weight within the normal range and (if they are women) continue to menstruate, or people who binge eat but do not follow these episodes with any efforts at weight reduction. The latter are often referred to as having binge-eating disorder, with the majority of these people being excessively overweight.

There is no single cause of eating disorders. Extensive research indicates that anorexia nervosa and bulimia nervosa begin with simple dieting and that a number of factors—biological, psychological, and societal—propel an individual into developing an eating disorder. The modern West's ideal of a slender body type has been particularly powerful, and individuals who are exposed to this ideal seem to be at risk for developing an eating disorder. There has been a consistent increase in the incidence of anorexia nervosa in industrialized countries during the past three decades. In contrast, the prevalence of bulimia nervosa is remarkably consistent at the rate of 1 percent in adolescent and young adult women.

Searching for Biological Causes

Much of the research into the causes of anorexia and bulimia revolves around neurotransmitters in the brain. Animal studies have shown that eating behavior is strongly influenced by messenger chemicals in the hypothalamus. Serotonin is one such neurotransmitter, helping us to feel satiety or fullness. When researchers inject serotonin into an animal's paraventricular nucleus, part of the hypothalamus, eating behavior is suppressed. Studies have also found that people with anorexia who have been in recovery for a long time have elevated levels of a product left over from metabolizing serotonin. It is therefore possible that having too much serotonin in the brain reinforces a person's urge to abstain from eating.

People who suffer from anorexia nervosa, restricting type, share some personality traits and behaviors also seen in obsessive-compulsive disorder (C23), such as a tendency to be especially rigid, inhibited, ritualistic, and perfectionistic. Researchers have long thought that people with OCD also have serotonin system abnormalities because they respond well to selective serotonin reuptake inhibitors (SSRIs).

We also see an association between low levels of serotonin and impulsive, suicidal, and aggressive behavior (C31, C32). The bingeing and purging behaviors of bulimics suggest they have impulse-control and satiety-regulation problems. Several studies have reported impairment in the system for stimulating serotonin activity in bulimic patients. There seems to be enough evidence of such problems in both anorexia nervosa and bulimia nervosa to consider a vulnerability in the serotonergic neurotransmitter system as a risk factor for eating disorders.

Two other neurotransmitters, norepinephrine and dopamine, also influence how we eat. Studies have indicated that abnormalities in these neurotransmitters may have an effect in precipitating and sustaining eating disorders.

Research in the past two decades has suggested a genetic aspect to eating disorders as well.

Psychological assessments have consistently linked anorexia nervosa to a cluster of moderately heritable personality and temperamental traits, such as obsessionality, perfectionism, and harm avoidance. Studies have found a higher lifetime prevalence of anorexia or other eating disorders in first- degree relatives of people with anorexia, and twin studies have shown that restricting anorexia nervosa was markedly higher for identical twins (66 percent) than for fraternal twins (0 percent). In a twin study on bulimia nervosa, the rate was also significantly higher in identical than in fraternal twin pairs.

Diagnosis and Treatment

People with anorexia nervosa deny the gravity of their illness and are reluctant to obtain medical treatment. Concerned family members usually bring them unwillingly to a doctor after their weight loss or eating habits have become alarming, or after girls have stopped having their menstrual periods. Even then, people with this disorder refuse to acknowledge that the symptoms are serious and are completely uninterested and resistant to treatment.

Many bulimics are ashamed of their bingeing and purging and are thus reluctant to acknowledge that behavior to their physicians. Dentists are often the first to diagnoses bulimia nervosa because they notice the erosion of tooth enamel caused by constant exposure to gastric acid from self-induced vomiting.

For people who make themselves vomit and abuse laxatives, the acute symptoms of fatigue, weakness, and fainting may bring them to a physician or even to an emergency room. People with eating disorders are well aware of what has caused

such symptoms but are often reluctant to describe their behavior or to admit that the problems are serious. Family members may thus worry that the individual has cancer, a chronic infection, or a disturbance of the gastrointestinal tract.

Physicians diagnose eating disorders by obtaining information on a person's weight, menstrual history, and eating behavior, including meals shared with family, dieting, bingeing episodes, self-induced vomiting, or abuse of laxatives and diuretics. Doctors ask questions to determine whether the individual has a preoccupation with and fear of gaining weight. They also inquire about a person's exercise regime and about any depressive symptoms. Weight loss frequently occurs in depressive disorders (**C20, C24**), which have several other features that may appear in anorexia: depressed feelings, crying spells, sleep disturbances (**C11**), obsessive ruminations, and occasional suicidal thoughts (**C32**).

A complete blood count is useful. People with anorexia nervosa often show a low level of white blood cells. Those who make themselves vomit are likely to have a low potassium level and an elevated level of a blood component called serum amylase.

A variety of mental health professionals specialize in the treatment of eating disorders, including psychologists and social workers. Pediatricians who practice adolescent medicine may specialize in both the medical and psychological care of their patients. However, adolescents with severe eating disorders should have psychotherapy from a well-trained psychotherapist in addition to pediatric services. Psychiatrists may also specialize in the treatment of eating disorders. Some psychiatrists who have had special training in internal medicine and pediatrics can treat both the psychological and medical needs of an adolescent with an eating disorder. For the great majority of adolescent and adult sufferers, a psychiatrist's medical training is sufficient. Early diagnosis and intensive early treatment is extremely important for people with eating disorders. Studies have shown that if people with anorexia stay below their normal weight range for longer than six years, their chances of recovery are almost nonexistent. Children treated for eating disorders have a significantly better outcome than patients first treated over the age of 18.

People with anorexia nervosa need treatment that includes medical care, education, and individual therapy. Studies have shown that children and adolescents do better if they have family therapy as well. Nutritional counseling and medication can also be useful, but treatment should never rely on drugs alone.

Chlorpromazine may help a severely ill person who is overwhelmed with constant thoughts of losing weight and has incessant behavioral rituals. The newer atypical antipsychotic medications, such as olanzapine (Zyprexa), are also helpful for such individuals. Cyproheptadine (Periactin) in high doses (up to 28 mg per day) can facilitate weight gain for people with anorexia nervosa, restricting type, and may have a mild antidepressant effect. Fluoxetine (Prozac), an SSRI, has been shown to be useful in preventing relapse into anorexia nervosa and may specifically target the obsessive-compulsive behaviors involving food and weight control.

Almost all antidepressants, including desipramine (Desyrel), imipramine (Tofranil), methylphenidate (Ritalin), amitriptyline (Elavil), and fluoxetine (Prozac), have been shown to be effective in reducing the binge-purge behavior in those with bulimia nervosa by 50 percent to 60 percent. However, the rate of complete abstinence from bingeing and purging in all studies was only about 25 percent.

Cognitive behavioral therapy (CBT) is the first line of treatment for bulimia nervosa. Individuals are encouraged to identify the emotions involved in their binge-purge episodes and perception of body image. CBT interrupts the cycle of bingeing and purging and alters people's dysfunctional thoughts and beliefs about food, weight, body image, and overall self-concept. About 40 percent to 50 percent of bulimic patients stop bingeing and purging at the end of treatment (16–20 weeks). Another 30 percent who do not improve immediately reach full recovery one year after treatment. CBT is also the psychotherapy of choice for anorexia nervosa.

The severity of illness will determine the intensity of treatment for an eating disorder patient. A specialized eating disorder inpatient unit is necessary for those requiring intensive medical management or monitoring for suicidal and impulsive behaviors. Less severely ill people may do well in a partial hospitalization or day program, and those with no serious medical complications and a weight loss of less than 80 percent below the normal range should begin with intensive outpatient treatment.

We expect 25 percent of anorectics to fully recover. About 25 percent will continue to have severe problems with weight control and eating behaviors and will not be able to function adequately at work and in personal relationships. The remaining 50 percent or so will continue to have mild symptoms, such as preoccupation with body weight, that will cause them to practice restrictive eating or controlled exercising but will not interfere with how they function at work or, in most cases, at home. About 40 percent of anorexia nervosa patients will go on to develop normal-weight bulimia nervosa.

CONFRONTING EATING DISORDERS

If you believe that a friend or family member is suffering from an eating disorder, it is important that you express your concern. Your ultimate goal should be to get that person to seek professional help. When you address the problem initially, you need to prepare yourself for all possible reactions. Here are some suggestions:

- Stress the fact that you are bringing up the issue because you care about the person and are genuinely concerned about her or his well-being.

- Be sensitive to the fact that she or he will probably be embarrassed or ashamed.

- Be firm but caring in your approach. Arm yourself with examples of things you have observed that have led you to believe that there is a problem. The more "evidence" you have, the harder it will be for that person to brush off the issue.

- If you think you may have an eating disorder, don't hesitate to get help from your pediatrician or internist. Eating disorders require professional help. Don't forget that you are not alone and that identifying the problem is part of the solution.

Adapted from www.nationaleatingdisorders.org (National Eating Disorders Association)

Mortality rates for people diagnosed with anorexia nervosa are 6.6 percent after ten years, and 18 percent to 20 percent after 30 years. Most follow-up studies show that anorectic patients with an earlier age of onset (under age 18) have a better chance of recovering. Purging behavior, self-induced vomiting, and laxative abuse usually indicate a worse outcome.

For bulimia nervosa, 50 percent of people fully recover. The remaining patients are not symptom-free: 30 percent have a less severe form of the disorder, and 20 percent continue to meet full criteria. Relapse is a serious problem: about one third of recovered bulimics relapse within four years after treatment. Mortality has been estimated to be below 3 percent. There is some suggestion that personality disorders marked by problems with impulse control (B8) suggest a worse prognosis in patients with bulimia nervosa.

Researchers continue to seek clues to the biological basis of these disorders. Imaging studies may identify particular areas of the brain affected by them, as well as impaired receptor functioning for various neurotransmitters. We need more studies to determine new treatment strategies that will help people with eating disorders overcome these difficult and disabling conditions.

Post-Traumatic Stress Disorder

Post-traumatic stress disorder (PTSD) develops in response to a terrifying event or ordeal that a person has experienced, witnessed, or learned about from others. The event is usually life-threatening or capable of producing serious bodily harm, and typically involves interpersonal violence or disaster. Examples include but are not limited to being a victim of or witness to natural or man-made disasters, such as fire, earthquakes, and acts of terrorism or war; suffering or witnessing a rape or physical assault; being kidnapped or tortured; and seeing someone else suffer serious injury or death.

Such a traumatic experience causes the person to feel intense fear, horror, or helplessness. The survivor is unable to get the event out of his or her mind. This disorder can affect many aspects of a person's life, particularly day-to-day functioning, quality of life, and relationships.

Three main symptom clusters characterize PTSD:

- The person will reexperience the event through distressing images, unwanted memories, nightmares, or flashbacks. These reexperiences will cause distress and such physical symptoms as heart palpitations, shortness of breath, and other signs of panic.

- The person will avoid reminders of the event, including people, places, or things associated with the trauma, and become emotionally numb, constricted, or generally detached from or unresponsive to surrounding activities and people.

- The person will experience physical symptoms reflecting a state of anxiety (**C21**) or hyperarousal. These symptoms may include insomnia (**C11**), irritability, impaired concentration (**C2**), hypervigilance, and increased startle responses.

If family members know that an individual has experienced trauma, they will probably notice that their relative is anxious and emotionally withdrawn. However, they may not initially be alarmed by these symptoms because they will likely believe the survivor to be displaying a normal response that will pass with time. Indeed, most trauma survivors themselves wait for several weeks or months before contacting a physician about their symptoms in order to give themselves time to "get over" their reactions on their own. Ultimately, for some people, the post-traumatic symptoms do not spontaneously improve, and sleep disturbance, panic, and depression can cause increasing disability in their everyday lives. That is when these individuals or their families seek professional help.

People also seek medical help for problems that may develop after the trauma that can mask or intensify PTSD symptoms. These include chronic pain (**C57**), fatigue (**C19**), headaches (**C54**), muscle cramps, and self-destructive behavior, including alcohol or drug abuse (**C29, C30**) and suicidal gestures (**C32**). Often, survivors are not aware that their physical symptoms are related to their traumatic experiences. They may even fail to mention those disturbing events to their physicians, which can make PTSD difficult to diagnose accurately.

The Mechanisms of Fear

In 1980 the mental health community established the diagnosis of PTSD and revolutionized the way the field views the effects of stress. This change acknowledged that many of the symptoms people experience after exposure to trauma can be long-lasting, if not permanent. Before that shift, the field tended to view stress-related symptoms as a transient, normal response to an adverse life event, not requiring intensive treatment. Furthermore, before 1980, people who did develop long-term symptoms following trauma were viewed as constitutionally vulnerable; the role of the actual event in precipitating their symptoms was minimized. For a while, in a reversal of previ-

ous thinking, experts expected most trauma survivors to develop PTSD. More recent research has confirmed that only about 25 percent of individuals who are exposed to trauma develop PTSD.

So who is likely to develop PTSD following a traumatic experience, and why? The answer is not yet clear, but it now appears that PTSD represents a failure of the body to extinguish or contain the normal sympathetic nervous system response to stress. This failure is associated with many factors:

- the nature and severity of the traumatic event
- preexisting risk factors related to previous exposure to stress or trauma, particularly in childhood
- the individual's history of psychological and behavioral problems, if any
- the person's level of education, and other cognitive factors
- family history—whether parents or other relatives had anxiety, depression, or PTSD

People who develop PTSD are also more likely to develop other psychiatric disorders involving mood (**C20, C21, C24**), personality, eating (**C27**), and substance dependence (**C29, C30**).

For all of us, being exposed to traumatic stress results in an immediate fear response: the body initiates the natural biological reactions that help us assess the level of danger and organize an appropriate response, the familiar "fight or flight." The limbic system in the brain, which is associated with emotion, motivation, behavior, and various involuntary actions, is part of this response. One part of the limbic system, the amygdala, switches on the neurochemical and neuroanatomical circuitry of fear by activating the startle response, the parasympathetic and sympathetic nervous system response, and the hypothalamic-pituitary-adrenal responses to stress. The hippocampus, another part of the limbic system, is involved in helping to terminate these responses. Eventually the adrenal gland releases cortisol to contain the body's response to stress.

In individuals who develop PTSD, there is only a slight rise in cortisol in the immediate aftermath of the trauma and evidence of greater sympathetic nervous system arousal (that is, increased heart rate). That combination suggests that for these people the fear response is not efficiently contained. In fact, people with relatively low cortisol levels following trauma may be at higher biological risk for developing PTSD.

Some researchers now believe that when an individual's sympathetic nervous system remains

---

STRATEGIES FOR COPING WITH POST-TRAUMATIC STRESS DISORDER

Coping with PTSD symptoms and the problems they cause is usually a continuing challenge for survivors of trauma. Often, it is through receiving treatment for PTSD that many learn to cope more effectively. Positive coping actions are actions that help reduce anxiety, lessen other distressing reactions, and improve the situation in a way that does not harm the survivor further and that improves things not only today, but tomorrow and later. Positive coping methods can include:

- **Learning about trauma and PTSD.** It is useful for trauma survivors to learn more about PTSD and how it affects them.

- **Talking to another person for support.** The survivor of trauma must choose his or her support person(s) carefully, and clearly ask for what he or she needs.

- **Talking to the doctor about trauma and PTSD.** A person's doctor can take care of a PTSD sufferer's physical health better if he or she knows about the PTSD; doctors can often refer a person for more specialized and expert help.

- **Practicing relaxation methods.** These can include muscular relaxation exercises, breathing exercises, meditation, swimming, stretching, yoga, prayer, listening to quiet music, spending time in nature, and so on.

- **Increasing positive distracting activities.** Positive recreational work activities help distract a person from his or her memories and reactions.

- **Calling a counselor for help.** Sometimes PTSD symptoms worsen, and ordinary efforts at coping don't seem to work too well.

- **Taking prescribed medications to tackle PTSD.** One tool that many survivors of trauma with PTSD have found helpful is medication treatment in partnership with their doctor.

Adapted from www.ncptsd.org (National Center for PTSD)

aroused after trauma, that leads to higher levels of the neurochemicals dopamine, norepinephrine, and epinephrine in his or her brain. Normally those three neurochemicals (together called catecholamines) help memories form by maintaining the body at a high level of arousal. If cortisol fails to adequately shut them down, a person's traumatic memories become "overconsolidated," or inappropriately remembered. As a result, "every little thing" has a chance of reminding the person of the traumatic event. The person's increased distress every time he or she recalls the trauma further activates the stress-responsive systems, resulting in anxiety, hyperarousal, and ultimately, PTSD.

Diagnosis and Treatment

Studies of PTSD have demonstrated that this condition is the fourth most common psychiatric disorder, affecting about 8 percent of the population at some time in their lives. Women are twice as likely to develop PTSD as men.

Doctors diagnose PTSD if a person has had symptoms from each of the three clusters described above for one month or more, and if those symptoms cause severe problems or distress at home or work, or in general affect the person's daily life. The reason for the time criterion is to differentiate between the acute response to a troubling event, which for most people is to be expected, and the more chronic response. A psychi-

atrist, psychologist, social worker, or other qualified health care professional who provides counseling related to trauma can help determine if someone has PTSD. Early diagnosis and treatment are critical and can substantially improve long-term outcome.

The symptoms of PTSD do not generally become more severe as time passes, but the failure of those symptoms to diminish often results in a cascade of secondary behavioral, emotional, or personality problems. These problems can increase the individual's disability. Exposure to further stress or trauma increases a person's likelihood of developing a recurrence of the symptoms. PTSD can, however, remit spontaneously or following treatment.

People who receive specialized PTSD treatment have a good chance of recovering. Psychotherapeutic or counseling methods, such as cognitive behavioral therapy, including exposure and anxiety-management treatments have been shown to be effective in treating PTSD. Many trauma survivors are reluctant to talk about their experiences, but most experts believe that confronting the event and all of the upsetting and frightening emotions and memories connected to it is essential for the symptoms to dissipate. Medications such as antidepressants and anticonvulsants have also been shown to be effective. Usually some combination of psychotherapy and medication, along with the support of family and friends, results in the best possible recovery.

Substance Abuse and Addiction

Of the thousands of drugs in nature and the many thousands that people have made in laboratories, only a relative handful are used regularly for their effects on our mood, thinking, or behavior. The most commonly used drugs in the world are caffeine (found in tea, coffee, and certain soft drinks), nicotine (in tobacco), and alcohol (in wine, beer, and a variety of distilled liquors). These drugs are legal in most countries, if not always freely available to everyone. Alcohol, the most frequently used brain depressant in most cultures, and a major cause of illness and death, is discussed in greater detail in section **C30**.

Other categories of drugs, such as the opioids commonly used to treat pain, are either restricted to medical use or prohibited entirely. Attitudes toward prohibited drug use (nonmedical use) vary remarkably across cultures. Penalties for illegal possession can range from modest fines to imprisonment, and sometimes to death.

In the United States we use the term *drug abuse* in two very distinct ways. In a legal and legislative context, it refers to using any drug illegally. Technically, the definition would include not just the use of an illicit drug such as marijuana, but also the consumption of alcohol by anyone under the legal age. In a medical context, however, the use of a drug is not by itself "drug abuse," even if the drug is illegal. However, when drug use begins to cause problems for the user, it becomes a medical concern—even if the drug's use is legal. Doctors can designate such behavior "abuse" of that particular drug and consider such use to be a medical or psychiatric disorder. Admittedly, these definitions of abuse can be confusing. Most other countries use a somewhat different system of categorizing disorders, called the International Classification of Disease. This system does not include a concept of drug abuse but uses instead the notion of *harmful use*, defined as a pattern of psychoactive substance use that causes damage to health. Social problems, such as arrests or marital problems resulting from the drug use, are not part of this definition.

We cannot describe the appearance or characteristics of drug abuse or dependence in a simple way, because the concepts cover a wide array of drugs with distinctly different effects on the brain and behavior. The drugs that people use for their effects are generally categorized into ten

THE SIGNS OF SUBSTANCE ABUSE

Because there is no sharp line separating repeated substance use from substance abuse or dependence, medical scientists have developed a set of criteria to help them determine whether an individual's drug-using behavior should be considered a case of substance abuse. The criteria are applied across all of the families of drugs that typically lead to abuse. The presence of one or more of these criteria within a year is generally accepted as indicating the presence of some degree of abuse:

■ Failing to fulfill major work, school, or home responsibilities.

■ Using the drug in situations in which it can be dangerous, such as while driving a car or operating machinery.

■ Having recurring drug-related legal problems, such as arrests for disorderly conduct while under the influence of the drug.

■ Continuing to use the drug despite having persistent relationship problems that are caused or worsened by its effects.

However, if the person's drug use meets the criteria for substance *dependence* (see "The Signs of Substance Dependence," page 412), that diagnosis supersedes the diagnosis of substance abuse.

groups or families. The World Health Organization uses the following categories: alcohol; opioids (opium and its derivatives, including heroin and morphine); cannabinoids (such as marijuana); sedatives or hypnotics; cocaine; other stimulants, including caffeine; hallucinogens; tobacco (nicotine); volatile solvents (inhalants); and other drugs or use of several drugs together.

Choosing 10 categories is somewhat arbitrary, dictated in part by a coding system that permits only ten categories. Other, more flexible classification systems, such as those used by the American Psychiatric Association, define 12 or more categories, allowing separate categories for amphetamine stimulants, phencyclidine, and mixed substances.

We could create several more groups or families since both classification systems have a mis-

cellaneous category that includes a grab bag of drugs with little in common. Some of these substances are rare in the industrialized world but quite commonly used in less developed areas. For example, betel nut, which contains the drug arecoline, is widely used in Asia and India and is thought to be the fourth most commonly used drug in the world (after caffeine, alcohol, and tobacco). Other agents in the miscellaneous category include anabolic steroids and such nitrite inhalants as amyl and butyl nitrite.

The only property common to all these agents is that they affect the brain and that some people choose to ingest, inhale, or inject them to experience their effects. Of course, we take an even wider array of drugs than are in these 10 to 12 categories, but those other drugs are customarily used to alter some function of the body—for example, to reduce a fever, cure an infection, control diarrhea, and so on. In some instances, drugs that affect the brain may be used for another purpose. Wine can be defined as a food or a sacrament; betel nut freshens the breath; opioids relieve pain as well as alter mood and produce euphoria.

Defining and Discovering Addiction

Despite great advances in knowledge over the past decade, experts do not agree completely on the nature of addiction. What is generally obvious is that drug use, whether the drug is alcohol, nicotine, heroin, or cocaine, begins as a voluntary behavior. The user may be entirely ignorant of the risks or entirely familiar with all of them, including the risk of getting "hooked," or, to use the medical term, becoming dependent. The individual tries the drug nevertheless, either because of peer pressure or because he or she is seeking some expected change (euphoria, tranquility, relaxation) that appears to be worth the risk. Not everyone who tries a drug repeats the experience, even if the effects are satisfying. On the other hand, some who initially have an unpleasant reaction, such as nausea from opiates or from too much nicotine, will persist until they can tolerate these unwanted effects.

In time, some users begin to feel that they need the drug just to function normally; they no longer have the same freedom that they once had to choose whether or not to use it. The degree of severity of this loss of flexibility of choice varies from mild to severe. At its extreme it is sometimes described as a chronic, relapsing disorder characterized by compulsive drug seeking in which use of the drug takes priority over other things the user once valued, such as family, friends, reputation, and even health and life.

How the drug dependence affects a person's life depends in part on the specific substance, the culture, the individual, and the circumstances influencing its availability. For example, dependence on smoked tobacco (cigarettes) may at first have very little impact on an individual's functioning. As the financial cost of daily smoking escalates and employers place limits on smoking in the workplace, the dependence can become a burden. And after many years, daily use of cigarettes may lead to lung cancer, heart disease, or emphysema.

When an adult becomes dependent on illicit drugs, such as cocaine or methamphetamine, his or her family might first notice that money is in short supply. The person may show changes in mood and behavior. For instance, both methamphetamine and cocaine induce talkativeness, a sense of exaggerated optimism, and sometimes irritability. The user may need less sleep and less food. When the drug is unavailable, the opposite effects appear. The user may exhibit a depressed mood, sleepiness, and lethargy. As the syndrome progresses, some of the common toxic effects may become more apparent: repetitive behaviors, suspiciousness, and eventually a toxic psychotic state with auditory hallucinations and paranoid ideas.

Many families have difficulty recognizing substance use, abuse, or dependence in young people because the behaviors vary so much depending on the specific drug, and because in the early stages the symptoms are not very specific. With illicit drugs such as heroin or cocaine, the first clue that there is a problem may be an inordinate need for money or the appearance of new and unusual behaviors aimed at getting money. An unusual decline in school grades is typical, although this can be a sign of a variety of problems unrelated to drugs. Changes in mood or sleep patterns (insomnia or hypersomnia) are also common, although these too may be due to other psychiatric disorders, such as depression or anxiety. Young people are far more likely to use and to become dependent on alcohol and tobacco than the more illicit drugs (though purchasing all of these is illegal for teenagers). Parents often first detect a child's regular use of marijuana from a change in attitude toward school or sometimes by the peculiar sweet smell of marijuna smoke. They can also often detect if their children use alcohol during the day or if alcohol is disappearing from the house. Determining from observation alone whether people have become *dependent* on drugs is more difficult.

There is no medical test to determine whether a person is substance-dependent, but toxicology screens (drug testing) done on blood and urine specimens can reveal the presence of many chemicals and drugs in the body. The accuracy of such tests depends on the substance itself, when it was taken, and the testing method used.

THE SIGNS OF SUBSTANCE DEPENDENCE

We apply seven criteria for drug dependence across all of the families of drugs that typically lead to dependence. The presence of three or more of the following criteria within a year is generally accepted as indicating the presence of some degree of drug dependence:

- **Increasing tolerance of the substance.** Either the person has to take much more to become intoxicated or achieve the effect he or she desires, or the same amount of the substance has much less effect.

- **Withdrawal symptoms when a person stops taking the substance.** There are characteristic physical and psychological symptoms associated with each addictive substance. Alternatively, a person may go back to taking the substance, or one closely related to it, in order to avoid those withdrawal symptoms.

- **The person takes the substance in larger amounts or over a longer time than he or she intended.**

- **The person persistently wants to cut down or control his or her substance use, but can't.**

- **The person spends a great deal of time obtaining the substance** (by, for instance, visiting various doctors), using it (chain-smoking), or recovering from its effects (working off a hangover).

- **The person gives up or cuts back on important social, professional, or recreational activities in order to use the substance.**

- **The person continues to use the substance despite knowing that he or she has a persistent physical or psychological problem associated with it.** For example, a person might feel depressed, know that alcohol is often the cause of depression, and yet keep using it.

If the first two signs appear, the substance abuser is said to have "physiological dependence."

Prevalence and Contributing Factors

When we view the full spectrum of psychoactive drugs, legal and illegal, the probability that an individual will develop a drug-abuse or drug-dependence problem at some point in his or her life is surprisingly high. In the United States, a survey in the early 1990s found that when prescription drugs are included, about 26 percent of people 18 or older at some time meet the criteria for either substance abuse or dependence. For illegal drugs and nonprescribed use of prescription drugs, the lifetime rate was about 8 percent.

Many factors contribute to the likelihood of developing dependence on a drug. Perhaps the most important is use, which depends on access. For example, the likelihood of becoming dependent on heroin for the population as a whole is less than 1 percent, but it is 23 percent for those who have used it. For the population as a whole, the lifetime rate of cocaine dependence is less than 2 percent, but it is 17 percent for those who have used it. Not everyone is equally exposed to illicit drugs; those who live in neighborhoods where they are available are more at risk for trying them. For legally available drugs, the lifetime dependence rates are high. Among people who use alcohol at all, the dependence rates are about 21 percent for men and 9 percent for women. Problems of drug dependence are also higher among doctors, nurses, and pharmacists, who have greater access to a wide range of drugs than other groups with comparable socioeconomic status.

Some people who try drugs seem to be more vulnerable than others to becoming drug-dependent. It is now clear that genetic (hereditary) factors play an important role in an individual's vulnerability to virtually all forms of drug dependence. Also increasing the risk of dependence is the presence of certain other psychiatric disorders. For example, the risk of drug or alcohol dependence is substantially higher among young people with conduct disorder and older people with antisocial personality disorder. The risk of alcohol dependence is sharply higher among those with bipolar (manic-depressive) disorder (C24). In the National Comorbidity Survey, 51 percent of people who were diagnosed with some form of addictive disorder in their lifetimes had at least one additional psychiatric diagnosis.

Drugs, Addiction, and the Brain

Over the past 30 years, science has made great progress in understanding how the drugs involved in addictive disorders work and how they affect the brain. Each of the major categories of drugs affects the brain by acting on a distinct set of receptors located on neurons, alcohol being the possible exception (C30). For example, the opioids act at natural opioid receptors located on neurons in the brain and the gut, and on white blood cells. Similarly, the anxiolytics (anxiety-relieving drugs), such as the benzodiazepines, the cannabinoids (any of various chemical components of marijuana), and phencyclidine, act at their own special receptors on neurons in the brain.

Cocaine acts on specific sites on nerve membranes that are very close to the sites responsible for sopping up newly released neurotransmitters and transporting them back into the neuron for recycling. When cocaine binds at this site, the transporter system doesn't work and neurotransmitters such as dopamine, serotonin, and norepinephrine increase in the space between neurons, allowing these transmitters to produce an exaggerated effect.

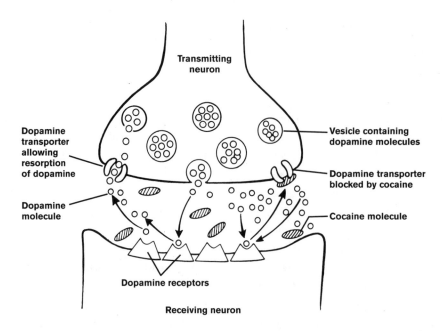

After sending a signal with the neurotransmitter dopamine, the sending neuron removes the chemical from the synapse by reabsorbing it. Cocaine blocks the neuron's transporter, preventing the resorption and prolonging the dopamine signal. This action produces the cocaine "high." ILLUSTRATION © KATHRYN BORN

These neural receptors obviously did not develop just so we could experience the effect of these drugs. They are the sites where our nervous system's signaling chemicals (the neurotransmitters) exert their actions. However, when these receptors are flooded regularly with ingested, injected, or inhaled chemicals that are in higher concentration or that last longer than the body's own neurotransmitters, the brain undergoes changes. Some of these changes probably contribute to the behavioral syndrome that we refer to as "addiction" or "drug dependence."

Some drugs may also lead to either temporary disturbances or long-lasting damage to the brain. These disturbances may lead to a number of abnormal mental disorders other than addiction: psychosis, mood disorders, sleep disorders, and so forth. The table (on page 416) shows the kinds of mental syndromes that may develop with the use of various categories of drugs.

Tolerance and Withdrawal

Recent research has led to a greater understanding of tolerance and physical dependence, the conditions responsible for withdrawal syndromes when people stop taking certain families of drugs after a period of use. Tolerance and physical dependence (physiological dependence) were once considered the essence of drug addiction. Doctors thought that all truly addicting drugs produced obvious withdrawal symptoms. Indeed, when people stop using alcohol or opioids such as heroin, even untrained observers have no trouble seeing the withdrawal symptoms. Opioid withdrawal begins with anxiety, runny nose, yawning, headache, and nausea. If an individual is severely dependent, he or she will also suffer cramps, diarrhea, vomiting, gooseflesh, fever, and kicking movements of the legs (hence the slang "kicking the habit"). These acute symptoms, even when severe, are largely over within a week or two, but it takes much longer—perhaps months—for the person's brain to return to normal functioning. We now believe that subtle, persistent changes in brain function (particularly in those systems that regulate our capacity to experience pleasure from normal activities) may contribute to the high relapse rates for people who try to stop taking addicting drugs.

It is also now clear that withdrawal syndromes need not be dramatic or life-threatening to play a role in perpetuating drug-using behavior and in relapse after drug withdrawal. Until recently, for instance, experts argued that there was no tobacco withdrawal syndrome. It has now become apparent that while no one has ever died from abruptly quitting the use of tobacco, there is a nicotine withdrawal syndrome that consists of irritability or anger, anxiety, dysphoria, difficulty concentrating, insomnia, and weight gain. It is also clear that the syndrome contributes to relapse because treatment with pharmaceutical nicotine (patches or gum) alleviates withdrawal and reduces the rate of relapse. Similarly, withdrawal from cocaine or amphetamines is not particularly dramatic, but the persistent dysphoria and fatigue probably contribute significantly to relapse after a period of abstinence.

Treatment

Since drug dependence results from a complex interplay of many factors, it is possible to intervene in a variety of ways. As a result, a number of distinct treatments have evolved, each emphasizing the importance of changing one or more of the contributory factors. One of the most accessible is the 12-step approach, developed initially by Alcoholics Anonymous, which combines spiritual, psychological, and peer support principles, offering mutual help in a nonprofessional environment. Similar 12-step programs have now evolved to treat opioid and cocaine dependence. For people with alcohol dependence, studies have shown that treatments aimed at encouraging patients to attend AA are comparable in efficacy to cognitive behavioral therapy and to professionally delivered treatments designed to enhance motivation.

For many years, researchers have tried to develop useful medications for treating dependence. Many medicines are effective in controlling acute withdrawal syndromes, but relatively few are useful afterward to help avoid relapse. For tobacco (nicotine) dependence, nicotine patches and gum can increase the likelihood of initial abstinence and decrease the chances of relapse. Bupropion (Zyban), a drug developed for depression, is also effective in decreasing relapse rates. For alcohol dependence, opioid antagonists can reduce the likelihood of relapse to heavy drinking, but they do not increase the likelihood of continuous abstinence; the next section discusses specific medications for alcohol. There are as yet no useful medications for cocaine, amphetamine, anxiolytic, or cannabis dependence.

Two distinct types of medications have been approved for the treatment of opioid dependence. Opioid antagonists, such as naltrexone and nalmefene, have been used to help addicts avoid relapse. Antagonists act by displacing the opioids from their action sites on receptors.

MENTAL SYNDROMES CAUSED BY DIFFERENT KINDS OF DRUGS

	ALCOHOL	AMPHETAMINES	CAFFEINE	CANNABIS	COCAINE
Dependence	yes	yes		yes	yes
Abuse	yes	yes		yes	yes
Intoxication	yes	yes	yes	yes	yes
Withdrawal	yes	yes			yes
Dementia	persistent				
Memory disorder	persistent				
Delirium during . . .	intoxication, withdrawal	intoxication		intoxication	intoxication
Psychotic disorders during . . .	intoxication, withdrawal	intoxication		intoxication	intoxication
Mood disorders during . . .	intoxication, withdrawal	intoxication, withdrawal			intoxication, withdrawal
Anxiety disorders during . . .	intoxication, withdrawal	intoxication	intoxication	intoxication	intoxication, withdrawal
Sexual dysfunctions during . . .	intoxication	intoxication			intoxication
Sleep disorders during . . .	intoxication, withdrawal	intoxication, withdrawal	intoxication		intoxication, withdrawal

Adapted from *Diagnostic and Statistical Manual of Mental Disorders*, 4th edition

Therefore, they cannot be given until a person is completely withdrawn from opioids; otherwise, they would cause severe withdrawal. By occupying the opioid receptors, antagonists prevent opioids from producing their typical effects. When people can be persuaded to take these medications, they have a better chance of avoiding rapid relapse.

Opioid agonists are the second type of approved medication: methadone, LAAM, buprenorphine. These drugs are now used throughout the world to treat people with opioid (usually heroin) dependence. When used in adequate doses, these drugs reduce or prevent the euphoric effects of other opioids and reduce people's craving. Users can function normally once they develop tolerance to these opioid agonists. Since the drugs are themselves opioids, users are physically dependent on them and will experience opioid withdrawal if they stop taking them. But such treatment reduces the use of illicit opioids and thereby reduces the likelihood of adverse consequences associated with such use, such as crime, HIV infection, and overdose deaths.

Prognosis

For many people with typical drug-dependence problems, the toxic effects of the drugs themselves or the conditions under which they are used substantially increase the chances for se-

HALLUCINOGENS	INHALANTS	NICOTINE	OPIOIDS	PHENCYCLIDINE	SEDATIVES, HYPNOTICS, ANXIOLYTICS
yes	yes	yes	yes	yes	yes
yes	yes		yes	yes	yes
yes	yes		yes	yes	yes
		yes	yes		yes
	persistent				persistent
					persistent
intoxication	intoxication		intoxication	intoxication	intoxication, withdrawal
intoxication, plus flashbacks	intoxication		intoxication	intoxication	intoxication, withdrawal
intoxication	intoxication		intoxication	intoxication	intoxication, withdrawal
intoxication	intoxication			intoxication	withdrawal
			intoxication		intoxication
			intoxication, withdrawal		intoxication, withdrawal

rious illness, disability, and death. Even people dependent on legally available tobacco and alcohol will have their lives shortened if their dependence persists for long periods. Cigarette smoking can cause lung and other cancers, heart disease, and noncancerous lung disease. High levels of alcohol consumption can cause liver disease, damage to the nervous system, and higher risk of certain kinds of cancers, auto accidents, and injuries. The use of illicit drugs such as cocaine and heroin is associated with even higher risks of premature death, most commonly from accidental overdoses but also from the effects of infections with the AIDS virus (HIV) or hepatitis viruses that result from sharing needles or engaging in unprotected sex.

Many factors influence the likelihood of successful recovery from drug dependence. Much depends on the drugs involved and the circumstances and characteristics of the individual. Sometimes stopping for a while may require little in the way of formal treatment, as when a long-term cigarette smoker finally decides to quit after an illness. Many people with alcohol dependence have found support through such self-help groups as Alcoholics Anonymous. Some people who quit in this way are able to stay free of drugs for very long periods. More typically there are slips and relapses.

Many experts believe that a person who has been severely dependent on a drug, whether alcohol, opiates, tobacco, or cocaine, cannot ever again use that drug, even occasionally, without a high risk of rapidly becoming dependent on it. The basis for the persistent vulnerability of people who were formerly drug-dependent is not clear. It may be that the same genetic or psychiatric factors that contributed to a person's initial vulnerability still influence his or her behavior, or it may be due to long-lasting changes in neurons during the earlier period of active drug use.

For many people, however, the chances of long-term success go up with repeated efforts to end dependence. After several years of continuous abstinence from a drug, the likelihood of relapse becomes relatively low. Although once a person stops taking a drug, many of the toxic effects of drug dependence are largely reversible, some, such as severe liver damage from alcohol use or lung damage from smoking, may persist indefinitely.

Alcoholism

A lcoholism is a disease that is defined by the compulsive use of alcohol to the point that it interferes with work or personal life or impairs health. A popular myth holds that alcoholics drink on a daily basis and are usually unemployed and unsuccessful. In truth, most alcoholics are successful, intelligent, educated citizens who are able to function normally but become incapacitated gradually due to excessive use of alcohol. Many alcoholics may not even drink every day.

Alcoholism is a substance disorder, and the official definition of alcoholism includes the criteria for substance dependency outlined in section **C29**. Specific to alcohol, these symptoms include the following:

- The person shows increasing tolerance to alcohol. Either the person has to drink much more to become as intoxicated as he or she desires, or the same amount of alcohol has a much less potent effect.

- Withdrawal symptoms (sweating or high pulse rate, hand tremors, insomnia, nausea or vomiting, shakiness, hallucinations, anxiety, and seizures) appear several hours or days after the person has stopped using alcohol following a period of heavy drinking.

- The person drinks larger amounts or over a longer time than he or she intended.

- The person persistently wants to cut down or control his or her drinking, but can't.

- The person spends a great deal of time buying alcohol, drinking, and recovering from hangovers.

- The person gives up or cuts back on important social, professional, or recreational activities in order to drink.

- The person continues to drink despite evidence of alcohol's adverse effects, such as depression, blackouts, or liver disease.

Most, if not all, alcoholics report that they crave alcohol, and that they spend a great amount of time thinking about it. Other symptoms of alcoholism specific to the brain include personality changes, forgetfulness, moodiness with gradual progression to carelessness, and depression. Long-term alcoholics may suffer a gradual onset

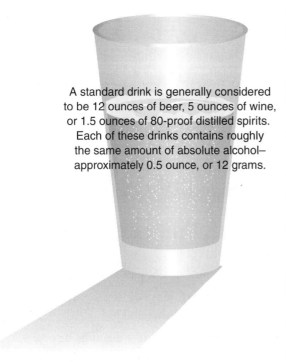

A standard drink is generally considered to be 12 ounces of beer, 5 ounces of wine, or 1.5 ounces of 80-proof distilled spirits. Each of these drinks contains roughly the same amount of absolute alcohol—approximately 0.5 ounce, or 12 grams.

ILLUSTRATION © LEIGH CORIALE

of forgetfulness that can be misdiagnosed as Alzheimer's disease (**C67**). Indeed, alcohol always impairs memory during intoxication, and some people's memories are very sensitive to its long-term effects.

In the most severe cases, drinking alcohol damages multiple nerves in both the central and peripheral nervous systems. In affecting the brain, it impairs memory and such cognitive skills as problem solving and learning. The most distinguishing symptom of this syndrome, known as Wernicke-Korsakof syndrome, is that sufferers will make up detailed, believable stories about their experiences or situations to cover the gaps in their memories. Alcoholic neuropathy is another disorder that can be caused by the toxic effect of alcohol on nerve tissue. It can affect the autonomic nerves that regulate internal body functions as

well as the nerves that control movement and sensation. Damage is usually permanent, and may become progressively worse if the person does not stop using alcohol. Symptoms vary from mild discomfort to severe disability.

Alcoholism is a form of substance dependence, which differs from more general substance abuse (see **C29** for details of this distinction). Alcohol *abuse* thus does not include a craving for alcohol, tolerance, or withdrawal, but does involve other problems. Alcohol abuse is defined as a pattern of drinking in which within 12 months a person fails to fulfill major work, school, or home responsibilities; drinks in dangerous situations; has recurrent legal problems related to alcohol, such as being arrested for driving drunk; or continues drinking despite any persistent relationship problems it exacerbates.

There is also a separate, unofficial category called binge drinking, which applies to the consumption of five or more drinks on a single occasion for a male, and four or more drinks for a female. Very often adolescents and college students are binge drinkers, some of whom go on to develop full-blown alcoholism.

Who Becomes an Alcoholic?

More than 90 percent of adult Americans have consumed alcohol at some time in their lives. About 70 percent continue using it during adulthood. Most adults can drink moderate amounts of alcohol—up to two drinks a day for men, and one drink a day for women—and avoid alcohol-related problems. However, of those exposed to alcohol, 10 percent to 15 percent develop alcohol abuse or dependence, making this a very common disorder.

Nonalcoholic man (36 years old)

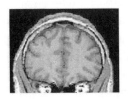 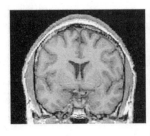 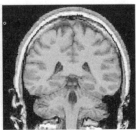

Alcoholic man (39 years old)

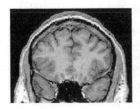 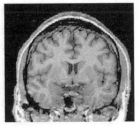 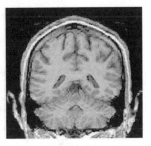

Brain scans of a nonalcoholic man compared with those of an alcoholic man suggest brain tissue shrinkage, although it is not clear whether all the differences seen are the result of damage from alcohol. Scans courtesy of Daniel Hommer, M.D., National Institute of Alcohol Abuse and Alcoholism

We do not know what causes alcoholism, but there is strong evidence from adoption studies that it can be inherited. People whose biological parents are alcoholic have a greatly increased risk of alcoholism even when they are adopted and raised by nonalcoholics. Conversely, people whose biological parents are nonalcoholics do not have an increased risk of alcoholism in adulthood, even when raised in homes where there is at least one alcoholic.

There is also an increased risk of alcoholism for people born with a high tolerance for alcohol. Some people report little effect from relatively large amounts of alcohol when they are quite young, even on their first exposure to alcohol. In a study involving young men tested for sensitivity to alcohol, those with a family history of alcoholism tended to have a higher tolerance compared with those with a similar drinking history but no family history of alcoholism. At follow-up, the men who were very tolerant at age 20 had a much higher incidence of alcoholism by age 30. Thus, it appears that some people may inherit tolerance to alcohol and that this tolerance increases the risk for developing alcoholism.

Beyond biological factors for alcoholism, some psychological and social factors may play a role. These may include anxiety, stress, or low self-esteem; the widespread availability of alcohol and acceptance of its use; and peer pressure, especially among teenagers.

Alcohol and the Brain

Alcohol is a complex, water-soluble drug that distributes itself throughout the body. It affects the central nervous system as a depressant, which in most people results in an initial "high" of stimulation and euphoria and in a decrease of anxiety, tension, and inhibitions. Larger amounts of alcohol result in sedation, unconsciousness, and, in toxic quantities, death. Beyond those basic facts, however, there is much that scientists do not know. Research is under way to move us from educated guesses to solid knowledge.

In one promising avenue of research, scientists are taking a closer look at some of the receptors in the brain—the sites where neurons receive their chemical messages. At one time alcohol was thought to have only a general effect on nerve cells, but research now suggests that alcohol may fit into specific places in many different receptors. This action would differ from that of other addictive drugs, such as heroin, which fit into a few particular receptors. It may explain why alcohol addiction is so complex. (For more information on how drug use alters the brain, see section **C29**.)

Alcohol seems to affect the specific brain pathways for gamma-aminobutyric acid (GABA), the brain's major inhibitory neurotransmitter, or "off" signal. Some studies suggest that alcohol intensifies the effects of this chemical by acting on one type of GABA receptor. Such sedatives as Valium also work on these receptors, which may explain alcohol's ability to lessen anxiety. Individuals who are tolerant to large doses of alcohol also have high GABA inhibition. If these individuals suddenly stop drinking, they lose this inhibition all at once and experience withdrawal seizures.

Alcohol also affects the general central nervous system through the receptors for *N*-methyl-D-aspartate (NMDA), which is an important excitatory neurotransmitter (or "on" signal). NMDA is also thought to be involved in some forms of learning and memory, as well as motor control. When alcohol inhibits this receptor, nerve cells may fire less rapidly, which may explain alcohol's sedative action on the central nervous system.

Another major effect of alcohol is to enhance dopamine activity in the reward pathways of the brain, the same effect that cocaine, nicotine, and opioids have. Alcohol appears to increase this neurotransmitter by releasing endogenous opioids (naturally occurring hormones with sedative effects), which results in more dopamine being released in important brain reward areas. If the opioid receptors are blocked, alcohol does not increase dopamine and the reward from alcohol is significantly less. This mechanism appears to be an important factor in the success of opioid-antagonist medication in treating alcoholism.

Serotonin, which is involved in regulating moods, is yet another neurotransmitter affected by alcohol. Alcohol releases serotonin, decreasing the long-term storage of this chemical in the body. A lack of serotonin may contribute to anxiety and depression. Researchers are now studying whether alcohol also intensifies a serotonin receptor, thereby increasing the reward response in the brain that reinforces the tendency to drink. It is also interesting to note that while most antidepressant drugs enhance serotonin function, they are not consistently helpful in the depression associated with alcoholism.

Diagnosis and Treatment

Alcohol affects a person's life by gradually eroding normal relationships and functions. A typical alcoholic may cope with the impairment produced by alcohol for years before finally succumbing to its behavioral toxicity. As a result, an alcoholic may not come to medical attention until the disease is far advanced. However, early treatment is much more effective than later treatment, after so much social and medical damage has been done.

Typically, a person's alcoholism comes to the attention of a physician because of some precipitating event, such as a car accident, a violent episode, a suicide attempt, divorce, or loss of a job. In other cases, the first evidence of the disease is a medical problem, such as gastrointestinal bleeding, liver failure, memory loss, heart disease, or high blood pressure. Alcoholism may also be noted incidentally when a person has a routine physical or is being evaluated for another problem. Usually, even an early alcoholic will have some abnormal blood test involving blood cells or liver enzymes.

Unfortunately, there are no definitive biological tests for alcoholism since abnormalities in blood tests could be due to other causes. Some medical professionals use the CAGE test, which is a series of questions developed by Dr. John Ewing:

- Have you ever felt you should **C**ut down on your drinking?
- Have people **A**nnoyed you by criticizing your drinking?
- Have you ever felt bad or **G**uilty about your drinking?
- Have you ever had a drink first thing in the morning to steady your nerves or to get rid of a hangover (**E**ye opener)?

One "yes" answer suggests a possible alcohol problem. More than one "yes" answer means it is highly likely that a problem exists.

Determining whether a person is intoxicated is somewhat more straightforward than determining if he or she is an alcoholic. Since alcohol is distributed throughout the body, the level in blood is a good measure of the level in the brain. The amount of alcohol in expired air (measured in a Breathalyzer test) can also give a reliable measure of blood alcohol. In most states, the legal definition of intoxication is 100 mg of alcohol per 100 ml of blood. It is important to note, however, that alcohol begins to produce measurable impairment in brain function at about a third of that level. Thus, even lower alcohol levels greatly increase the risk of car accidents. Most European countries set the limit much lower than the United States. In France the legal limit is 50 mg per 100 ml of blood—about the level achieved after two glasses of wine drunk within an hour.

Impairment of judgment is a critical factor in measuring the effects of alcohol. People who show great tolerance, usually by inheriting some and acquiring more through experience with high doses of alcohol, may be able to show fairly normal motor function at alcohol levels that could kill an average person (200–400 mg per 100 ml of blood). However, these individuals' judgment is still likely to be severely impaired, which can lead them to take dangerous risks.

For many years the medical profession neglected to treat alcoholism. Then, in the 1930s, a physician and a salesman started a self-help movement that became known as Alcoholics Anonymous (AA). This movement has grown into one of the greatest American inventions of all time. AA has spread to virtually every country in the world and has been a great solace to many, many alcoholics.

Today the medical community has come to see the AA movement and other self-help programs as partners in helping alcoholics and other addicts. AA does not consider itself to be a treatment program, however; it defines itself simply as a "worldwide fellowship of men and women who help each other to stay sober." Not everyone responds to AA's style and message, and many alcoholics either refuse to go to meetings or drop out after one or two. Even those who are helped by AA usually find that it works best in combination with other treatment, including counseling and medical care.

The standard medical treatment program for alcoholism consists of an abstinence-oriented residential or inpatient stay of 28 days, followed by aftercare that may consist simply of encouraging a person to attend AA meetings. Throughout the United States the standard goal of treatment is complete abstinence from alcohol, since long-term follow-up studies show that total abstinence is the most stable state and that those who try to take alcohol in moderation more often relapse to uncontrolled drinking. However, some research-oriented physicians have advocated a more flexible approach. Alcoholics are not all alike, and requiring everyone to accept the same treatment and goal does not seem reasonable. In European countries, there is more acceptance of the goal of controlled, nonexcessive drinking. Many alcoholics refuse to join a treatment program that requires total abstinence until their condition has progressed and both social and medical damage have occurred. If, on the other hand, they work to control their drinking, they are limiting the damage. If they continue to relapse, they can switch to total abstinence. Often individuals must make several tries before they stop drinking to excess.

Medical treatment can be important in the acute phase of detoxification, when the sudden abstinence from alcohol may cause seizures and cardiovascular collapse. In severe cases, medication can be essential for preventing death, although in mild cases it may not be necessary. Benzodiazepines have been used for the past 30 years to help people through alcohol withdrawal. The most commonly used of these is oxazepam, which does not require liver metabolism; that is important because alcoholics' livers are often impaired. Oxazepam also has a low abuse potential. Anticonvulsant medications, such as carbamazepine, can also be useful during detoxification.

Even after a person has achieved detoxification and stopped drinking to excess, he or she is still considered an alcoholic. Alcoholism is a chronic disorder that is rarely cured. Those who try to return to controlled drinking after successful treatment usually relapse. The most stable condition is total abstinence, and even then people can slip, sometimes after years of total abstinence.

Recently it has been found that the incidence of relapse can be reduced if doctors prescribe a medication that blocks the reward from alcohol. Naltrexone is one such drug. After being detoxified, approximately 50 percent of alcoholics show some degree of relapse within three to six months. With naltrexone, that relapse rate has been reduced by about half. The major weakness of naltrexone is that it is necessary to take it regularly; researchers are working at developing a monthly injection. Furthermore, there is no indication that naltrexone permanently changes behavior, so people still have a tendency to relapse when their medication is stopped. This is why behavioral rehabilitation is essential, and naltrexone is often used very effectively in combination with AA meetings.

Another medication, called acamprosate, has been approved for use in Europe and is currently in clinical trials in the United States, on its own and combined with naltrexone. Acamprosate works on a different brain mechanism from naltrexone, so the combination may have an added benefit. It appears that acamprosate acts on the GABA system to reduce the hyperarousal often seen during alcohol withdrawal and for months afterward.

The long-term prognosis for alcoholism depends on the stage at which it is treated, the long-term treatments and supports that are available, and the characteristics of each person. For example, alcoholics with more eduction, better job prospects, better family supports, fewer medical problems, and fewer psychiatric problems have a better prognosis than those with severe problems in these areas.

Research continues into the relationship between alcohol and the brain, with the hope that with better understanding we will find more effective treatments. Perhaps once we know why some people become alcoholics, we will be able to eliminate the disease and its destructive effects on alcoholics and those close to them.

Violence and Aggression

The prevalence of violence in our society has motivated both sociologists and biological scientists to search for the predictors and causes of this destructive human behavior. Scientists are specifically searching for biological factors that might predispose an individual to this aberrant form of behavior. The propensity for impulsive aggression appears to be associated with a lack of self-control over certain negative emotional responses and with a lack of fear or understanding of the negative consequences of behaving aggressively.

Psychological research has examined the relation between aggression and emotion. Numerous studies show that negative affect (a term that describes a mixture of emotions and moods including anger, distress, and agitation) can cause or intensify aggressive behavior. The forms of aggression that are relatively unplanned and spontaneous, termed *impulsive aggression*, are different from premeditated aggression. Although most neurobiological studies of aggression and violence typically do not differentiate between premeditated and impulsive aggression, the distinction is probably relevant in understanding

their genetic, neurochemical, and functional neuroanatomical bases. In other words, a person who commits a violent act in the heat of passion may possibly display different neurological and chemical brain symptoms than someone who plans and commits a violent act.

Defects in the normal dispersal of serotonin in the brain have been linked to aggression and violence by a variety of methods. Researchers have found evidence that serotonin exerts inhibitory control over impulsive aggression. Measurements of the levels of a chemical known as 5-hydroxy-indoleacetic acid (5-HIAA) in cerebrospinal fluid (CSF) are believed to reflect serotonin activity in the brain. For example, reduced CSF 5-HIAA has been found in aggressive psychiatric patients; impulsive, violent men; and victims of suicide by violent means. Furthermore, low levels of 5-HIAA concentration have been found to predict aggression two to three years in the future in boys with conduct disorders and repeat criminal offenders. Finally, lower CSF 5-HIAA levels have been reported in impulsive violent offenders and impulsive fire setters.

Scientific findings suggest that genetic abnormalities may contribute to serotonin function as well as to individual differences in aggressive behavior. In a study of 251 community volunteers, researchers examined the association between a specific genetic abnormality in the serotonin system and measures of aggression and anger-related personality traits. Subjects having the mutation scored significantly higher on several measures of aggression, including the tendency to experience unprovoked anger, than individuals with the other form of the gene. The prefrontal cortex (PFC) is known to be a crucial brain area in emotion regulation and has been implicated in aggressive and violent behavior. Scientists have discovered abnormalities in serotonin activity in the prefrontal cortices of persons with impulsive aggression.

Imaging studies with positron-emission tomography have revealed prefrontal abnormalities in glucose metabolism in individuals prone to impulsive aggression. A study of 41 murderers found lower levels of glucose metabolism in areas of the prefrontal cortex and increased metabolic activity in the right amygdala compared with age- and sex-matched controls. An increased metabolic rate was also observed in the hippocampus, amygdala, thalamus, and midbrain in the right hemisphere in impulsive murderers, compared with both the control group and those murderers who had planned their crimes in advance.

Brain lesions in the orbital frontal cortex (OFC) and adjacent PFC regions have been shown to produce syndromes characterized by impulsivity and aggression. Researchers reported in a 1999 medical study that a 56-year-old man who sustained bilateral damage to the OFC and some damage to the left amygdala showed unpredictable, impulsive aggression and violence. The patient was described by a relative as "a quiet,

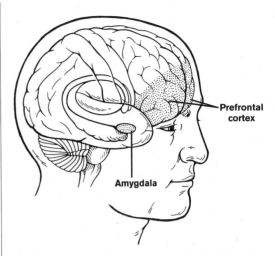

The prefrontal cortex acts as mediator, taking impulses from the amygdala and deciding whether or not to act on them. Studies have shown that persons with damage to the frontal lobes are more likely to engage in impulsive acts of aggression. ILLUSTRATION © KATHRYN BORN

rather withdrawn person who was never aggressive" before the brain damage.

Emotion Regulation, Aggression, and Violence: Common Neurological Connections?

Impulsive aggression may be the product of a failure of emotion regulation. Normal individuals are able to control negative feelings voluntarily and can also profit from restraint-producing cues in their environment, such as facial and vocal signs of anger or fear, that also serve a regulatory role. Some studies suggest that individuals predisposed to aggression and violence have an abnormality in the central circuitry responsible for these adaptive behavioral strategies—a defect in the brain regions that control emotional regulation. The evidence suggests that abnormalities in serotonin function in regions of the prefrontal cortex may be especially important. Other neurotransmitters, neuromodulators, and hormones are probably also involved.

The evidence indicates that the OFC and the structures with which it is interconnected (including other prefrontal territories, the anterior cingulate cortex, or ACC, and the amygdala) constitute the core elements of a circuit that underlies emotion regulation. The OFC, through its connections with other zones of the PFC and with the amygdala, plays a crucial role in restraining impulsive outbursts, and the ACC recruits other neural systems, including the PFC, in response to conflict. In normal individuals, activations in these brain regions that occur during anger arousal and other negative emotions restrain the impulsive expression of emotional behavior. Deficits in this circuit are believed to increase a person's vulnerability to impulsive aggression.

Many factors influence the structure and function of this circuitry. Genetic factors clearly play a role, as revealed by the association of one particular genetic difference associated with traits of anger and aggression. However, these factors undoubtedly interact with early environmental influences. The very circuitry identified here as playing a crucial role in emotion regulation is dramatically shaped by early social influences. Biological factors alone do not determine whether a person will be aggressive. Environmental factors such as upbringing and social interactions surely also contribute to one's propensity for aggressive or violent behavior. Novel behavioral training procedures based on experimental research that investigates how people suppress negative emotion need to be developed and then rigorously evaluated to determine whether they can be used to benefit those with a propensity for aggression. Drugs that affect the serotonin system may also be useful in counteracting aggressive tendencies. Nevertheless, the first important step is to recognize that impulsive aggression and violence, irrespective of the distal cause, reflect abnormalities in the emotion-regulation circuitry of the brain. Parents who notice such tendencies in their children should see a child psychiatrist who can evaluate the causes of such problems and suggest an appropriate treatment. More research is needed to develop better and earlier treatments for those potentially devastating conditions.

Suicidal Feelings

Suicidal feelings are not uncommon. Many people experience transient thoughts of death during a crisis. People under great stress or threat may fleetingly wish they were dead; we call these "passive" suicidal thoughts or feelings.

Suicidal feelings become a cause for more concern if a person experiences them often or starts to consider specific details about ending his or her life. Prolonged or recurring thoughts of suicide are frequently a serious indication of psychiatric illness. And, of course, taking any *action* to commit suicide is a sign that a person needs mental health treatment. Most suicide attempts are not lethal, but they are much more than an emotional "cry for help."

Because we often associate suicidal thoughts or behavior with life stresses, we may not realize that the vast majority of suicide victims have an actual psychiatric illness. That condition renders them incapable of coping with stress or loss in healthy ways. Suicidal thoughts are relatively common as a manifestation of clinical depression (**C20**). A person suffering from severe depression may experience persistent strong impulses to end his or her life, making specific plans to use highly lethal methods.

Suicidal feelings are not tied to one psychiatric disorder alone, however, but occur most commonly in a range of disorders, including bipolar disorder (**C24**), alcoholism (**C30**), schizophrenia (**C25**), and severe forms of borderline personality disorder (**C26**). Suicidal people frequently display depressive symptoms, no matter what primary diagnosis their doctors make. Often physicians find that patients meet the criteria for more than one diagnosis at the same time, a condition called comorbidity. People at risk for suicide also often have a history of impulsive behavior or agitation (physical hyperactivity often associated with anger or anxiety). This may be associated with a history of substance abuse (**C29**).

Though symptoms of depression are a common thread, there is no one type of person at risk for suicide. Different individuals experience or express their feelings in different ways. Some examples are:

- Severe hopelessness coupled with anguish experienced as "psychic pain"; in this condition, a person may suffer in silence, without complaint.

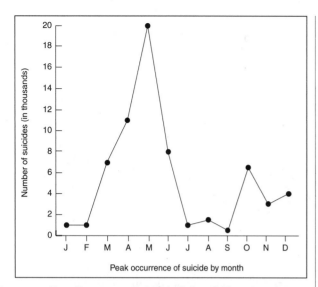

Peak occurrence of suicide by month

Despite conventional belief, suicide rates are not highest during the Christmas holiday season, when persons may become more depressed and thus vulnerable to suicidal feelings. The month of May is actually the highest month for suicides statistically. GRAPH ADAPTED BY LEIGH CORIALE FROM *MANIC-DEPRESSIVE ILLNESS,* BY FREDERICK GOODWIN AND KAY R. JAMISON, 1990, OXFORD UNIVERSITY PRESS, BY PERMISSION

- Increasing anxiety over physical symptoms, either those of a diagnosable medical illness or those that doctors cannot pinpoint, along with symptoms of depression.

- A history of substance abuse, followed by the loss of an important relationship because of that behavior.

- Severe personality disorder, which makes people impulsive and very demanding, quick to feel that others do not support them, and unable to soothe their anger over feelings of rejection. If they face a discharge from a hospital, a therapist's vacation, or the loss of a relationship, they may make repeated suicide attempts, usually by hanging or asphyxiation, escalating the danger each time.

In the United States, suicide is the eighth most common cause of death among adults, with the rate of suicide increasing dramatically in men after age 65. The suicide rate for females is about one fourth the rate in males, but females have a much higher rate of suicide attempts. Women, however, choose methods that are less often lethal.

Recognizing Suicidal Feelings

How do the conditions that can lead to suicide or suicide attempts first appear to others? Depressive illness can begin at any age, but people most commonly show its signs first in young adulthood or adolescence. Often their first symptoms are social withdrawal and a loss of interest in activities that they previously enjoyed. They may experience persistent insomnia or inability to sleep (**C11**) and sometimes a loss of appetite coupled with weight loss (**C27**). About half the time clinical depression begins after a major life stress or setback, such as the loss of a relationship or physical illness. In a depressed state, people commonly feel increased fatigue, have trouble concentrating, and express hopelessness about life ever improving. While this condition commonly leads to suicidal feelings, not every depressed person is suicidal, and only a small percentage ever complete a suicide. However, an untreated clinical depression can worsen in severity and lead to such problems as lost jobs, financial stresses, and fractured relationships. It is a serious disorder, and people of all ages can get help—see section **C20**.

How can we tell the difference between depressed patients who are at an immediate risk of suicide and the majority who may not be at risk? This judgment is difficult even for professionals.

SUICIDE AMONG TEENAGERS

Adolescents are not the most likely people to commit suicide (in fact, the elderly are), but they have the second highest rate of suicide. Also, consider the absolute numbers: while suicide rates are higher in the elderly, the number of deaths by suicide in adolescents is much greater. Plus, suicide is the second or third leading cause of death in the young. That increased risk, together with the feeling that teenagers have so much potential ahead of them, makes suicide by teenagers a great concern for parents, educators, and counselors.

The 1997 Youth Risk Behavior Survey found that an average of 20 percent of youths in grades nine through twelve reported that they had "seriously considered attempting suicide." The same survey noted that 7.7 percent of these high school students reported a suicide attempt (with the rate among females double the rate of males), and 2.6 percent reported that the suicide attempt "required medical attention." Though the national death rate from suicide for all individuals ages 15 to 19 in 1997 was about .01 percent, or about 1,800 teens, suicide constituted the third most frequent cause of death in this age group.

As with adults, suicide attempts in adolescence are frequently linked with diagnosable psychiatric disorders. Sixty percent of adolescent patients who committed suicide were found to have suffered from mood disorders. Furthermore, 54 percent had shown disruptive or antisocial behavior, 42 percent substance abuse, and 27 percent an anxiety disorder. (That these percentages total more than 100 percent shows how most suicides are associated with more than one condition.) Over half of these adolescents' parents knew about these conditions (except for the anxiety disorder) at the time of their child's suicide.

Other surveys have found that teenagers who feel attracted to people of their own sex are far more likely to attempt suicide than other teenagers, as are those using addictive drugs, Native American youths, and those with a history of agitation, impulsiveness, or violence.

Certainly expressing a suicidal idea or feelings of hopelessness is an important sign. Other behaviors that indicate a person faces an increased danger of attempting suicide are:

- Abusing alcohol or other drugs.
- Impulsive behavior, such as tantrums, violent outbursts, or episodes of agitation.
- A history of rapid mood swings between hyperactivity and depression.
- Recurrent severe anxiety, often in the form of incessant worry and rumination.
- Recurrent panic attacks in addition to symptoms of depression.

Again, not every depressed person who shows one of these signs will commit suicide, but it is cause for extra concern.

It is not uncommon for people who have suicidal feelings to mention them to loved ones or friends. A classic study of suicide in adults reported that over 90 percent of individuals who committed suicide had a diagnosable psychiatric illness at the time of their death, and over 60 percent of those had communicated their suicidal feelings to others—

A CASE STUDY IN SUICIDAL FEELINGS

A man in his early 30s, with a history of depression, asked a woman to marry him and was turned down. He became severely depressed, agitated, hopeless, and nearly delirious, to the point that he expressed the feeling that life was too painful to continue. The man's friends stayed with him around the clock and removed all dangerous weapons from his presence. They watched him like this for a week. Later, one of them took the young man into his home, paying his living expenses as well as his law school tuition. After many more disappointments and failures, the man became our sixteenth president. What would our nation's history have been like if Abraham Lincoln had acted on his suicidal feelings and taken his own life?

three people, on average—in the year before they died. On the other hand, the same study found that only 18 percent of this group conveyed their suicidal thoughts to a helping professional, such as a physician or mental health counselor. This shows the importance of taking a friend's suicidal feelings seriously and reporting them to the person's doctor or therapist. You cannot assume that the doctor or counselor will have heard about them.

Mechanisms

While individuals who commit suicide have a range and often a combination of diagnoses, there is some evidence that the vulnerability to kill oneself may run in families independent of any one diagnosis. Studies have similarly shown that such traits as impulsivity and anxious depression also run in families. It is therefore possible that impulsivity, severe anxiety or panic symptoms, or even the degree of hopelessness a person feels while depressed may have a genetic component that confers increased risk of suicide to people in certain families.

Studies of serotonin function that measure receptors in the brains of suicide victims have shown evidence of up-regulated—that is, hyperactive—receptors, suggesting that serotonin was functioning less than normally in their brains. We do not know if these findings apply to nonsuicidal patients with depression.

Other researchers have found increased corticotrophin-releasing hormone (CRH) in the brains of suicide victims. That is important because CRH stimulates the release of adrenocorticotrophic hormone (ACTH) from the pituitary, which in turn stimulates adrenal enlargement and hyperfunction of the adrenal gland, which has been shown to be associated with suicide. Also, CRH may stimulate cells in the brain stem to release norepinephrine, which is associated with emotional arousal. This would fit with doctors' observation of severe anxiety and agitation in many people talking about or attempting suicide.

There are also studies that show a correlation between low cholesterol levels and suicidal behavior, as well as deaths from suicide, accidents, and violence. It is not clear what those findings mean. There could be some interaction between our cholesterol metabolism and neural membranes, resulting in altered brain function relating to depression and perhaps an increase in impulsive behavior.

Diagnosis and Treatment

If a friend or relative shows signs of being suicidal, do not leave that person alone until he or she has been assessed by a mental health profes-sional. Remove any dangerous implements from the person's access, including guns, knives, car keys, and toxic substances. This support can be life-saving. The person may seem to change his or her mind and deny such thinking. Emphasize that it is still important to seek psychiatric help. It is not unusual for individuals who have expressed suicidal feelings to deny such thoughts to loved ones and doctors or counselors shortly before they actually attempt suicide. If necessary, walk the person to an emergency room or call 911.

Doctors and counselors will try to identify what conditions are causing a person to consider suicide, while at the same time taking steps to pre-vent that act and relieve the acute suicidal feel-ings. There are several levels of treatment and ap-proaches to avert suicide. Sometimes, a severely depressed and acutely suicidal individual must be hospitalized for protection and treatment. The successful treatment of depression or other major underlying illness can reduce the risk of suicide, but it may rise again if the person relapses. Treat-ing severe anxiety symptoms, panic attacks, or ag-itation in depressed individuals can reduce acute suicide risk.

For people with recurrent episodes, such as patients with bipolar disorder or recurrent depres-sion, there is evidence that taking lithium reduces suicide by seven to nine times. Further research should lead to further advances in detecting acute suicide risk and preventing needless loss of life.

CHAPTER 15

Infectious and Autoimmune Disorders

C33 **Multiple Sclerosis** 435

C34 **Shingles/Herpes Zoster** 444

C35 **Neurological Complications of AIDS** 448

C36 **Lyme Disease** 453

C37 **Meningitis** 458

C38 **Viral Encephalitis** 462

C39 **Creutzfeldt-Jakob Disease** 468

C40 **Systemic Lupus Erythematosus** 471

Like other systems of the body, our nervous system is vulnerable to infections by bacteria, viruses, and other pathogens. Some of these diseases have limited effects, but others can be debilitating or even fatal. It is useful to recognize what can be done against different threats. For bacterial infections, doctors can prescribe antibiotic medicines like penicillin. As long as the disease has not caused too much damage to a person's vital organs, he or she usually recovers well. However, we have no such medications for viruses. The best physicians can offer is treatment for symptoms, such as pain. The body's own immune system must fight off that sort of invader. In the case of Creutzfeldt-Jakob disease, the damage is caused by a prion, a normal brain protein that has taken on an abnormal shape; as yet we have no treatment for prion diseases.

Our immune systems can also go out of control, perceiving some of the body's own cells as foreign and attacking them. In recent years we have recognized many more of these autoimmune disorders. They include not only multiple sclerosis and systemic lupus erythematosus, found in this chapter, but also Guillain-Barré syndrome (**C49**), myasthenia gravis (**C52**), and paraneoplastic syndromes (**C63**).

Multiple Sclerosis

Multiple sclerosis, often referred to as MS, gets its name from the multiple areas of scarring (sclerosis or gliosis) that it causes in the nervous system. MS is a major cause of disability in Western societies because of its frequency, tendency to begin in young adulthood, and chronic course. However, manifestations of MS can range from relatively minor symptoms to major incapacity.

Most often the first symptoms of MS appear gradually over hours or days, but they may also begin suddenly. MS symptoms that begin rapidly are referred to as an attack or, if they have happened before, a relapse. The most common initial symptoms of MS are:

- Weakness. This may cause fatigue, difficulty walking, or trouble using fingers for fine movements or handling objects. Facial weakness may produce a drooping mouth, mimicking a stroke (**C59, C60**) or Bell's palsy (**C50**). Stiffness, which may be one-sided, and spasms often accompany the weakness.

- Imbalance. MS damage in the cerebellum and its connections can render individuals unable to walk in a straight line (heel to toe) or stand with both feet together without falling. These troubles worsen when the individuals close their eyes. The imbalance can be accompanied by dizziness (**C14**), sometimes enough to cause vomiting. In severe cases, a person's speech can become slurred, or "scanned," as he or she loses some capacity to articulate and coordinate the flow of words.

- Vision problems of two sorts (**C15**). Optic neuritis manifests itself as a sudden difficulty reading, blurred vision in one eye, dimness, or inability to see red and other colors clearly. Many people feel pain around the affected eye. In this condition, MS has affected an optic nerve and the pathway that transmits images from the retina to the brain; in extreme cases, optic neuritis can produce blindness. The other type of visual disturbance is double vision, indicating damage to the nerve fibers in the brain stem that coordinate eye movements; the eyes cannot move together to focus on one image. The double vision disappears when the person with MS covers either eye.

▦ Sensory problems. Tingling, pins and needles (paresthesias), pain, or numbness can appear on the limbs, torso, or face. People with MS often describe abnormal sensations of swelling, squeezing, "water running on the skin," burning or cold, or "being wrapped." Some suffer trigeminal neuralgia, a recurrent shocklike pain in the temples and cheeks (**C58**). Lhermitte's sign is another sensation like an electric shock that runs down the spine when one bends the neck forward; it can occur with several disorders of the spinal cord.

The signs and symptoms of MS, especially the fatigue, tend to be exacerbated by heat, usually during periods of hot weather or after a hot bath or shower. Weakness or other symptoms may appear only during exercise.

When a person first suffers an MS attack, he or she might think the problem is a stroke (**C59, C60**). Other conditions that can mimic an attack include carpal tunnel syndrome (pain or tingling and numbness of hands), a herniated disk or compression of the spine (numbness or weakness of one side or in a limb; **C56**), and the aura of a migraine attack (**C55**). Trigeminal neuralgia may be misinterpreted as dental or eye pain (**C58**). In addition to the most common symptoms, people with MS may experience problems with their bladder and, less often, bowel functions. Some people of both sexes experience impotence. Memory loss, impaired attention, and changes in mood may accompany MS, and more than half the people with the disorder develop depression (**C20**).

Following the first attack, MS can follow several clinical patterns, each of which can be mild, moderate, or severe. In more than 80 percent of cases, MS begins with attacks coming and going, often without leaving any permanent deficit between them. This pattern is termed relapsing-remitting MS. Some people experience very few such attacks over their lifetime. Others suffer increasing numbers, leading to a degree of permanent disability. On average, a person with relapsing-remitting MS experiences one new clinical attack every 6 to 12 months; magnetic resonance imaging (MRI) studies have suggested that unnoticed attacks occur much more often. Approximately half of people with relapsing-remitting MS shift to a chronic progressive course by 15 years after onset. This form of disease is termed secondary progressive MS. Another 10 percent to 15 percent of people experience what we call primary progressive MS, in which the disease advances steadily from its onset, without remission.

The initial symptoms of a group of diseases termed acute disseminated encephalomyelitis (ADEM) can resemble an MS attack but may be much more explosive. These frequently start after a viral infection or vaccination. ADEM's symptoms are similar to those of MS, but it is rare for further attacks to occur.

Mechanisms and Factors

Current evidence indicates that MS results from an abnormal response of the body's own immune system against parts of the brain. We thus classify MS as an autoimmune disease, along with systemic lupus erythematosus (SLE; **C40**), myasthenia gravis (**C52**), rheumatoid arthritis, insulin-dependent diabetes mellitus, and others.

MS is a disease of the central nervous system: it involves the structures in the brain and spinal cord responsible for sending commands to the

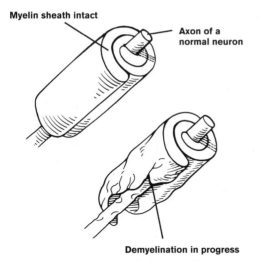

Myelin sheath intact

Axon of a normal neuron

Demyelination in progress

An immune system attack in multiple sclerosis targets the insulating myelin sheath around nerve fibers. Myelin helps speed nerve cell communication, and its loss from MS damage results in the weakness and other nerve signal impairments characteristic of the disease. ILLUSTRATION © KATHRYN BORN

body and receiving and processing information from sensory organs. This pattern distinguishes MS from peripheral nervous system diseases, in which nerve fibers outside the brain and spinal cord are damaged, such as myasthenia gravis. However, both groups of diseases can cause similar weakness, numbness, and pain.

The symptoms of MS result primarily from damage to myelin, the fatty whitish substance that insulates nerve fibers. The myelin sheath narrows at regular intervals along the fibers; such narrowings are termed nodes of Ranvier. When the myelin sheaths are in normal condition, information travels to and from the brain and spine at very high speeds: electrical impulses "jump" from one node of Ranvier to the next. When MS has destroyed those myelin sheaths, these impulses may be blocked, just as a wire that has lost its insulation may no longer conduct properly.

Failure of conduction is responsible for most of the symptoms of MS. The brain can no longer communicate efficiently with the peripheral nerves, muscles, and other organs. The particular nerves that are involved determine a person's symptoms. Also, demyelinated nerves may conduct impulses under normal conditions but fail under such stresses as repeated use or elevated temperature. That "conduction block" seems to explain why people with MS find their symptoms become worse with exercise or fever.

Recent research has shown that the immune attack in MS may damage not only myelin, but also nerve fibers and neurons. We do not know whether this is a consequence of the destruction of the myelin sheath or due to actual attacks on the nerves.

In temperate climates, MS affects approximately 1 in 1,000 individuals. In both the northern and southern hemispheres, it becomes increasingly common as one moves from the equator to the poles. Thus, MS is common in Scandinavia and northern Europe but rare in Japan and other countries in Asia.

MS affects women about twice as often as men. In both sexes, the incidence rises from adolescence to age 31, then declines gradually. It is unusual but not unknown for MS to begin as early as age 2, or as late as the eighth decade of life.

MS appears to develop in people who inherit genes that make their immune system likely to respond to certain environmental exposures—possibly viruses—by attacking the myelin insulation of nerve fibers. MS is not a genetic condition in a strict sense, but heredity influences how susceptible people are to the condition. Although most people with MS have no relative who is also affected, some families are particularly prone to MS. The lifetime risk for MS is approximately 5 percent for a brother or sister of an affected individual, 5 percent for a fraternal twin, and 30 percent for an identical twin. Spouses of people with MS and children adopted into MS-prone families show no increase in risk, strongly suggesting that the aggregation of MS in some families is due to genetic and not environmental factors.

It is likely that MS susceptibility is the effect of several genes together. To date, the most important is a gene labeled human leukocyte antigen [(HLA)-DR2], which seems to be responsible for 10 percent to 50 percent of genetic susceptibility. We believe that DR2 binds strongly to a fragment of a myelin substance termed myelin basic protein, triggering an immune response.

Most likely, the immune system misinterprets components of myelin as foreign and therefore seeks to destroy them. It has two basic ways to destroy these invaders: white blood cells called T cells, and antibodies, which are vital mechanisms to fight infections, tumors, and other diseases. In MS both T cells and antibodies may be involved; T cells may initiate the process of inflammation, whereas antibodies appear to act in concert to destroy the myelin. This "joint attack" from the immune system may result from a phenomenon called mimicry. When certain components contained in common microbes look like brain components, the T cells or antibodies mistakenly attack the brain and myelin, and may keep doing so even though the microbes are long gone. This theory could explain the global distribution of MS, which could correspond to the location of certain microbes. However, despite numerous claims, no specific infectious agent has been convincingly linked to MS.

Diagnosis

Currently, no test can identify MS, and since its symptoms can occur in other diseases, one of the first steps in diagnosing it is to rule out several alternate possibilities. These include other autoimmune disorders, such as ADEM, systemic lupus erythematosus, and Sjogren's syndrome (**C40**); sarcoidosis; Lyme disease (**C36**); vitamin B_{12} deficiency (**C65**); infections such as HIV (**C35**), HTLV-1, and syphilis (**C38**); spinal cord compression (**C56**); and tumors, especially when the symptoms have worsened steadily (**C64**).

Then, to make a diagnosis of definite MS, doctors must find evidence that scarring has occurred

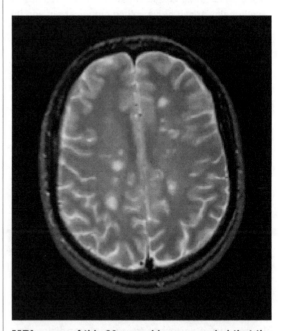

MRI scans of this 30-year-old man revealed that the cause of the numbness and tingling he reported experiencing in his legs was multiple sclerosis. The white circular or oval areas on this image indicate the "plaques" of MS. Scan courtesy of Keith Johnson, *The Whole Brain Atlas*, www.med.harvard.edu/AANLIB/home.html

in two or more areas of brain white matter in ways that alter a person's neurological functions. There must also be two or more attacks at least one month apart, each time with symptoms lasting more than 24 hours.

MRI is the method most often used to detect scarring; 98 percent of people with MS have MRI abnormalities of the brain or spinal cord. MRI typically reveals many more lesions than doctors can detect from a clinical examination alone. Doctors can inject the heavy metal gadolinium to make the lesions appear even more clearly. However, the abnormalities an MRI detects are not absolutely specific for MS. On the other hand, if someone with symptoms has a normal MRI of the brain and spinal cord, physicians should focus first on other possibilities.

Other tests include the evoked response test, which records the changes in electrical activity of the brain following stimulation of a nerve pathway, as recorded by electrodes applied to the scalp. Responses are measured after stimulation with light, sound, or electrical current. If the time between the stimulation and the brain recording is unusually long, the electrical impulses must be blocked. These tests are sensitive to lesions in both the brain and spinal cord.

Cerebrospinal fluid, sampled by spinal tap, can show increased concentrations of antibodies in people with MS. In a minority of individuals, there is also a small increase in the number of inflammatory cells.

Treatment

We do not have therapies to prevent or cure MS, but we have treatments that partially alter its course, and a number of effective treatments for MS-related symptoms, which are listed in the table on page 440. MS attacks that are moderate or severe are treated with high doses of glucocorticoid (steroid) medication, given by intravenous infusion (methylprednisolone) or by mouth (prednisone). These medications can be administered to people who experience attacks despite disease-modifying therapy, and they are usually offered on an outpatient basis. Side effects of glucocorticoids include fluid retention, high blood pressure, excitability and insomnia, and stomach ulcers.

Rehabilitation and related therapies are important complementary treatments that help people with MS maximize their capacities. Occupational counseling and other support services may assist these people and their families in coping with the effects of the disease. Stress reduction, eating a balanced diet, getting adequate rest, and other generally healthy behaviors are very useful. We recommend that people with MS keep vaccinations to a minimum because of the possibility that they may stimulate the immune system and trigger an attack. However, it is reassuring that recent controlled studies of hepatitis B, influenza, and tetanus vaccinations have shown no MS-related adverse effects.

Disease-Modifying Therapies for Relapsing-Remitting MS

In the United States, four therapies are approved for people with relapsing-remitting MS: interferon beta-1b (Betaseron), interferon beta-1a (Avonex and Rebif), and glatiramer acetate (Copaxone). Currently Avonex is the most commonly prescribed. We do not know how these drugs act with certainty, but they appear to suppress the

TREATMENTS FOR MS SYMPTOMS

SYMPTOM	MEDICATIONS AND OTHER TREATMENTS	SIDE EFFECTS
Spasticity (stiffness)	Lioresal Tizanidine Diazepam (Valium) Cyclobenzaprine HCl Clonazepam (Klonopin)	Limited effect Worsening of weakness Dry mouth Drowsiness
Pain	Carbamazepine (Tegretol) Gabapentin (Neurontin) Acetazolamide (Dazamide, Diamox)	Stomach and liver toxicity Drowsiness
Tremor	Clonazepam (Klonopin) Primidone Ondansetron Isoniazid (Laniazid) Propranolol (Inderal LA) Stereotaxic surgery (thalamotomy)	Limited effect Drowsiness
Bladder incontinence	Oxybutynin (Ditropan) Tolterodine (Detrol) Propantheline (Pro-Banthine)	Fluid retention
Bladder retention	Bethanechol (Urecholine) Terazosin HCl Self-catheterization	Incontinence
Bowel dysfunction	Laxatives Enemas Low-fiber diet (for incontinence)	
Impotence	Male: Sildenafil citrate (Viagra), penile prosthesis Female: antispasmodics, lubricants, counseling	
Fatigue	Amantadine (Symmetrel, Symadine) Fluoxetine HCl Modafinil (Provigil) Pemoline (Cylert) Change of work hours	
Mood swings	Amitriptyline (Elavil) Fluoxetine (Prozac)	Dry mouth Drowsiness
Depression	Psychiatric appointment if needed Antidepressants Psychotherapy	

myelin-reactive T cells, prevent them from entering the brain, and/or counteract the harmful substances that they make.

Clinical trials show that people receiving these drugs on average experience 30 percent fewer attacks and fewer new lesions in MRI scans. The interferons also significantly delay the development of new disability. However, these medications are only partially effective and may not be useful for all people with MS.

Betaseron is given by subcutaneous injection every other day, Avonex by intramuscular injection once weekly, Rebif by subcutaneous injection three times weekly, and Copaxone by subcutaneous injection daily. For all medications, the main side effects include local allergic reactions to the shots. Both interferons produce flulike symptoms that tend to disappear after two or three months of treatment and can usually be managed by over-the-counter medications. For some individuals, Betaseron, Rebif, and, less commonly, Avonex may also give rise to neutralizing antibodies, which impair their efficacy. In 15 percent of people Copaxone produces allergic reactions that may be severe but usually do not recur. Betaseron has been associated with depression.

Disease-Modifying Therapies for Secondary Progressive MS

In 2000 the FDA approved mitoxantrone (Novantrone) for treating secondary progressive MS. The drug is administered every three months by intravenous infusion, which is generally well tolerated. Mitoxantrone reduces the attack rate and MS activity, and delays the onset of new disability. Its use is of concern because of dose-related toxicity to the heart and a potential long-term risk of malignancies. Most physicians do not treat individuals with advanced forms of

secondary progressive MS who can no longer walk. Individuals with secondary progressive MS who also have ongoing attacks are candidates for therapy with one of the interferons.

Disease-Modifying Therapies for Primary Progressive MS

There are no effective disease-modifying treatments for primary progressive MS. However, clinical trials with a variety of agents, including interferon, glatiramer acetate, and mitoxantrone, are currently under way.

Other Treatment Options

Some medical centers use a variety of treatments that are not FDA-approved for various forms of MS. The "general immunosuppressive therapies" include azathioprine every day orally; methotrexate every week orally; cyclophosphamide, by monthly infusion; methylprednisolone, by monthly infusion. Recent trials of intravenous immunoglobulin infusions suggest that this treatment may also be useful. Finally, plasma exchange has been shown to be helpful for severe MS attacks that have not responded to glucocorticoid therapy.

Unfortunately, there are also many claims for therapies of uncertain value. The National Multiple Sclerosis Society is an excellent source of information on the most effective therapeutic options for MS.

Prognosis

Most people with MS eventually experience progressive disability, although some can remain stable for a very long time. In studies that preceded the current disease-modifying thera-

OPTIC NEURITIS

It has been estimated that about 55 percent of people with MS will have an episode of optic neuritis. Frequently, it is the first symptom of MS.

Optic neuritis is generally experienced as an acute blurring, graying, or loss of vision, almost always in one eye. It is rare that both eyes are affected at the same time. There may or may not be pain in the affected eye. Loss of vision usually reaches its maximum extent within a few days and generally improves within 4 to 12 weeks.

Recent studies suggest that a short course of methylprednisolone administered intravenously, followed by a tapered course of oral steroids, may be useful in helping to reverse the inflammation and restore vision. There is, however, no definitive evidence that treatment with steroids produces a more complete recovery than would have occurred without treatment.

Adapted from www.nationalmssociety.org (National Multiple Sclerosis Society). Other informative sites: www.msaa.com (Multiple Sclerosis Association of America); www.msfacts.org (Multiple Sclerosis Foundation)

pies, more than 80 percent of people with MS were found to have some functional limitation 15 years after diagnosis. Half required help to walk, 70 percent were limited or unable to perform daily living activities, and 75 percent were unemployed.

These traits are signs that a person with MS might have a more favorable prognosis than the average:

- optic neuritis as the only initial symptom
- complete recovery from the first attack
- onset before age 40
- being female
- having fewer than two relapses within the first year

The degree of impairment five years after the first attack and the number of MS lesions detected on a brain MRI after the first attack also appear to predict disability 10 to 15 years later.

Pregnancy may affect the course of MS. Although there is no proven effect of pregnancy on the overall course of disability, pregnant patients tend to have fewer attacks during gestation but more in the first three months after delivery. This is probably related to hormonal effects that influence the activity of the immune system. Because pregnant mothers should not undertake disease-modifying and immunosuppressive therapies, women with MS should carefully review their health, goals, and family support before deciding to bear a child.

The MS research community has clarified the underlying biology of the disease and shown great promise for developing improved therapy for it. Areas of research that hold promise in the near future include:

- Developing drugs that block the movement of myelin-attacking T cells from the bloodstream into the brain.

REDUCING COMPLICATIONS OF MULTIPLE SCLEROSIS

There are many means available to minimize or prevent complications of severe, advanced MS. This is a brief overview.

- Bladder dysfunction may lead to incontinence or repeated urinary tract infections. Bladder control can often be achieved with drugs, or by intermittent or continual catheterization, which involves inserting a thin tube into the bladder to remove urine. Patients can be taught how to do this themselves.

- Bowel problems can be managed through the judicious use of stool softeners with bulk-forming laxatives, or, in more difficult cases, with suppositories and enemas.

- Depression may be caused by the stresses of life or be the result of MS damage in brain areas involved in the regulation of emotions. Depressed people tend to withdraw. The resulting lack of activity and stimulation makes matters worse. Although social activities will not replace lost myelin, they can have a positive effect on a person's outlook on life. But often depression does not respond to commonsense remedies. Professional help is then needed.

- Mobility problems are common among those with advanced MS. Assistive devices, such as canes, walkers, and motorized scooters, can be useful to those who maintain some ability to walk. Patients who can no longer walk or lift themselves up can be moved or repositioned with mechanical lifts, electric beds, and special recliners and wheelchairs that raise a person to a standing position. These measures may help prevent skin breakdown and osteoporosis. Before a person uses these types of assistive devices, trained professionals should be consulted to make sure the devices fit the patient and meet his or her needs, and that the patient and caregivers know how to use them.

- Spasticity, an increase in muscle tone that can cause stiffness, pain, and awkward and unwanted movements, can be managed with a combination of exercise, medication, and possibly surgical intervention.

- Swallowing difficulties are very common. An evaluation by a speech/language pathologist may be recommended. Management strategies may include changing types of food and their consistencies.

Adapted from www.nationalmssociety.org

- Engineering drugs that specifically inhibit the damaging T cells or antibodies.

- Finding approaches that promote remyelination (myelin repair), which may allow individuals to regain function.

- Studies of MRI, immune, and genetic variables that improve our ability to predict the disease course and tailor or engineer therapy to individuals with MS.

Shingles/Herpes Zoster

Shingles, or (to use the medical term) herpes zoster, is characterized by pain and a localized rash. The rash usually covers a few inches of skin encompassing one to three dermatomes, each dermatome being the area supplied by a single nerve root. The rash of shingles is characterized by many small blisters superimposed on an angry red, inflamed base. Shingles always occurs on only one side of the body at a time.

The pain of shingles is severe; most patients describe it as burning. The area usually becomes exquisitely sensitive to touch (the medical term for this is allodynia). At the same time, the inflamed skin may be *less* sensitive to a painful stimulus, such as a pinprick (this is called hypalgesia). Because of allodynia, people with shingles often wear loose-fitting clothes. They may be reluctant to rub the affected skin when washing or showering.

The rash and pain usually develop within a few days of each other, although the pain can come first by many days or even weeks, making the diagnosis difficult. Sometimes people ascribe their rash to exposure to toxic materials, allergies, or animal bites.

Chicken Pox in Childhood

The same virus that produces chicken pox (varicella) causes shingles. Typically, when children develop chicken pox they have a rash over most of the body rather than a small portion. This is be-

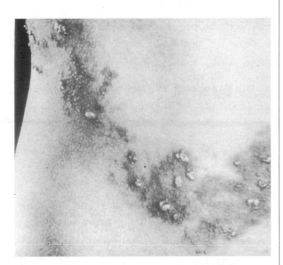

The painful rash of shingles appears in a characteristic pattern on just one side of the body. PHOTO COURTESY OF DONALD H. GILDEN, M.D., DEPARTMENT OF NEUROLOGY, UNIVERSITY OF COLORADO HEALTH SCIENCE CENTER

THE CHICKEN POX VACCINE

Millions of American children are now being administered an effective chicken pox vaccine every year. No one yet knows if this will also help against the development of shingles 40 to 60 years from now. The vaccine contains a live, attenuated (weakened) virus that becomes latent in ganglia with a potential to reactivate. Thus, this vaccine may not eradicate shingles.

The possibility of shingles in the future is no reason to prevent your child from being vaccinated against chicken pox today. As this section notes, it is almost impossible for a child to avoid being infected with VZV sometime, so he or she is best off contracting the weakest form. Furthermore, while most children survive chicken pox handily, the disease can be fatal or lead to such debilitating conditions as Reye's syndrome.

Researchers are evaluating the effect of giving the chicken pox vaccine to people around the age of 50. We know that vaccination in midlife can boost immunity to the virus, so this might prevent elderly individuals from developing shingles.

cause individuals encountering the varicella-zoster virus (VZV) for the first time have no immunity to it. Children almost always survive chicken pox, developing strong resistance to VZV. However, there are two important residual effects. First, the virus does not disappear—it becomes hidden, or latent, in collections of nerve cells in ganglia. Second, as we age, our immunity to VZV declines naturally. Thus the latent virus can reemerge from ganglia decades after chicken pox. Fortunately, most people still have some immunity to VZV that limits its reactivation to one area of the skin.

VZV is ubiquitous. Nearly everyone in the world develops chicken pox; each year, more than 3 million American children have it. Even some adults who have never had chicken pox have been found to have VZV antibodies, meaning their original infection was subclinical (no history of chicken pox). Thus, nearly everyone has the virus latent in their ganglia, with the potential to reactivate.

People can develop shingles at any age, even less than ten years after chicken pox. However, it does not usually appear until after age 50. The longer a person lives, the more likely he or she is to develop shingles. As our population grows older on average, we will have more cases. Even now, over half a million Americans develop shingles every year. Men and women are equally affected, as are all ethnic groups.

Shingles and the Immune System

Any medical condition that impairs an individual's immune system also predisposes that person to shingles. Years ago, people with cancer, lymphoma, or leukemia were the most likely to develop shingles. Such people usually have poor resistance to infections and are frequently treated with drugs and X rays that further impair their immune response. Many organ-transplant recipients also develop shingles as they take immunosuppressive drugs to prevent rejection of their newly received tissue.

Today the condition most commonly associated with shingles is AIDS, which also weakens a person's immune response (**C35**). Shingles can occur any time during the course of AIDS, and sometimes it is the first sign that a person has encountered the human immunodeficiency virus (HIV) that causes AIDS.

For a healthy person to develop shingles before age 50 does not mean the individual has cancer or AIDS. Although the disorder is most common in older people, it can even affect a teenager. Its appearance is usually not significant. However, if the individual is at high risk for HIV infection because of drug abuse or sexual practices, doctors will usually recommend an HIV test.

Diagnosis and Treatment

Most doctors can readily diagnose shingles from hearing about the severe pain and seeing the characteristic rash over a few inches of a person's skin. Fortunately, for most people the immune system is already at work driving the virus back to the latent state, and we have treatments to help.

There is also a rare condition called zoster sine herpete (shingles without the rash), which is harder to diagnose. This is characterized by chronic pain, usually in the same three- to five-inch distribution in which a rash usually occurs, but a rash never develops. Blood and cerebrospinal fluid tests can sometimes show that the VZV virus is causing this pain. Although these cases are rare, patients can be treated effectively.

VZV is one of eight known human herpesviruses, the only family of viruses for which we have effective antiviral therapy. The three main drugs we use today are acyclovir (Zovirax), valacyclovir (Valtrex), and famciclovir (Famvir). Acyclovir has been used the longest; people with shingles need to take it five times a day for seven to ten days. In contrast, famciclovir only needs to be taken three times a day, so many physicians prefer it.

For people over age 50, most physicians prescribe one of the oral antiviral agents (usually famciclovir or valacyclovir) for a period of seven to ten days. For people who have normal immune systems and are under 50, however, many doctors prescribe pain-relieving medicines only. Antiviral agents are not required. Other physicians give antiviral drugs even to young people because they are safe.

When immunocompromised patients develop shingles, doctors usually prescribe intravenous acyclovir, administered in a hospital or by a visiting nurse at the patient's home, for seven to ten days. This treatment is designed to prevent the virus from spreading. When the virus spreads beyond the usual two or three dermatomes to all areas of the skin, and to the liver, lungs, and other organs, the condition is called disseminated zoster. It can be fatal if not treated early.

Along with antiviral agents, physicians will prescribe medication for pain. Usually aspirin and anti-inflammatory agents are not enough. Often treatment requires acetaminophin with codeine (Myapap with codeine). Other medications prescribed are carbamazepine (Tegretol) and gabapentin (Neurontin), two medicines usually used to prevent seizures (**C13**) that can also reduce pain in some people with shingles.

In individuals under 50, the rash begins to resolve within a week and pain disappears within a month. In individuals over 50, and particularly over 60, however, the rash disappears but pain may persist for months or years. This condition is called postherpetic neuralgia (PHN). Forty to fifty percent of individuals over 60 develop it. This is a difficult problem because it requires continued doses of strong medications. All the drugs we have to treat shingles have side effects, such as confusion, unsteadiness, lethargy, and impaired balance. Furthermore, oxycodone is addictive. Elderly people are particularly sensitive to these medications. Other long-term treatments include anesthetics applied to the skin, such as lidocaine patches (which require a prescription) or Aspercreme or Flexall 454 (which can be purchased over the counter). Physicians frequently combine topical agents with the systemic drugs described above.

Healthy individuals with no known condition impairing their immune response have less than a 5 percent recurrence rate of shingles. In contrast, in immunosuppressed patients, shingles may recur. The VZV may even spread to other parts of the body and produce new neurological conditions. These may include the following:

■ In the spinal cord, myelitis—pain, tingling, and weakness in the legs, along with bladder and bowel incontinence.

■ In arteries outside the brain, granulomatous arteritis—shingles on the face followed a few weeks later by a stroke (**C59**) that produces paralysis of the opposite side of the body.

■ In arteries around and inside the brain, encephalitis—headache, fever, weakness of one or both sides of the body, and trouble with speech and balance.

Both brain conditions are serious and require intravenous treatment with acyclovir for seven to ten days. Many doctors also give steroids for their anti-inflammatory effect.

In addition to research on new drugs and the chicken pox vaccine, many investigators are studying the physical state of VZV in latently infected ganglia, often from people who have recently died of unrelated causes. Understanding the latent virus's DNA, RNA, and proteins may lead to drugs that prevent it from reactivating, thus eradicating shingles and its attendant serious neurologic complications.

Neurological Complications of AIDS

Acquired immune deficiency syndrome, or AIDS, was first recognized 20 years ago when a cluster of unusual infections were detected in homosexual men. Within two years of this recognition, its viral cause—now called human immunodeficiency virus type 1, or HIV—was identified, and within four years the FDA licensed a test that detects infection by this virus. Through a massive research effort, we now know a great deal about how this virus is transmitted, how it persists, and how it eventually causes fatal disease. Fortunately, treatments that are effective in suppressing HIV, and in preventing or delaying the development of AIDS, have also resulted from this research.

The primary target of this virus is the immune system, and particularly one of its components, the CD4 T lymphocyte, which is critical in orchestrating defenses against certain types of infections. The gradual loss of this system leads to vulnerability to these infections, which are rare in those with intact immunity and so are called *opportunistic* infections. However, infection also results in damage to different tissues by other mechanisms. As a result of both opportunistic in-

fections and these other effects of HIV, the nervous system is frequently altered by the virus, particularly in its more advanced stage, and the resultant neurological diseases are a cause of considerable disability and suffering.

Treatment of HIV Infection

Because the disease complications of HIV ultimately relate to active HIV infection, the major approach to treatment of those who have this virus is to suppress the infection. This is now accomplished by the use of combinations of antiviral drugs, usually three or more different drugs taken several times a day. The reason several different drugs are needed is that the AIDS virus replicates very rapidly and undergoes extensive mutation, which allows the selection of strains of virus that are resistant to drugs. Current drugs target enzymes that are "coded" by the viral nucleic acid and are essential to the reproduction of new virus particles. One of these enzymes is called reverse transcriptase (RT). RT allows the nucleic acid in the virus particle, which is RNA, to produce a DNA copy that is then inserted into the target cell's DNA (a component of the human genome), where it can serve as a template for production of new RNA to be inserted into the new virus particles. The production of DNA from RNA reverses the process normally used by the cell in its own reproduction. The first effective anti-HIV drugs were RT inhibitors. There are now two classes of these drugs and within each class there are several different drugs. The other major class of drugs inhibit a second viral enzyme, the HIV protease, which is essential for production of "mature" virus particles capable of infecting other cells. There are now also several different protease inhibitors.

Several drugs are used together to decrease the rate of virus reproduction and to make it more difficult for viable mutations to develop. Because these drugs target different enzymes or different parts of these enzymes, they are said to have synergistic, rather than simple additive, effects. When taken faithfully, these drug combinations are often remarkably effective in suppressing the virus and preventing immune dysfunction or even restoring immunity in those already damaged. However, there are also a number of problems. Because of HIV's capacity to mutate and develop resistance and because such resistance is fostered by exposure to low levels of the antiviral drugs, patients must be very careful in adhering to medication schedules. With multiple drugs available, patients can switch to a new combination when resistance develops, but with time the various options may be exhausted. These drugs are also expensive and may have undesirable side effects in some patients. Because the DNA copy of the HIV genome discussed earlier can remain in certain long-lived lymphocytes, treatment does not eradicate infection but only suppresses viral replication. There is no cure, only the prevention or delay of progression.

Despite these difficulties, the development of combination anti-HIV therapy has restored many patients to normal or near-normal activity and well-being, and has clearly reduced the death rate. Monitoring infection and treatment now involves sophisticated tools to track the infection (by measuring the number of viral particles in the blood), its effect on the immune system (by counting the number of CD4 T lymphocytes in the blood), and even the development of drug resistance. This has all brought great hope to those infected by HIV within the developed world. Unfortunately, this cannot be said of the poorer regions of the world, such as Africa and Asia, where the great majority of the world's infected population lives without benefit of these advances of modern biotechnology.

In the developed world, the major approach to preventing neurological complications in those infected by HIV involves suppressing HIV replication with these drugs. This has clearly reduced the incidence of these disorders. However, treatment is not successful in all, and some individuals develop neurological problems without previous awareness that they harbor HIV infection. Thus these problems have not been eliminated even in the United States.

Central Nervous System Infections

The central nervous system (CNS) includes the brain and spinal cord. While HIV renders these structures susceptible to several infections late in its course, three stand out as the most common.

- Progressive multifocal leukoencephalopathy (PML) is probably now the most common of these three central nervous system infections. PML is caused by another virus, known as JC (its name is taken from the initials of the person in whom this virus was first identified). This is a virus that infects the majority of the population but is seemingly harmless, causing no clinical disease in those with normal immunity. However, in some immunosuppressed people, including those with AIDS, it can spread to the brain and destroy the cells that manufacture myelin, the layered substance surrounding axons. This demyelination causes loss of neurological function, with particular difficulties depending on what part of the brain is infected. There is currently no specific treatment for PML, but in about one half of patients the condition may stop progressing when they are started on anti-HIV medications, which are thought to help by reversing the immunosuppression and restoring the person's ability to fight this virus.

- Primary central nervous system lymphoma is a malignant tumor that grows and compresses the surrounding brain and may be lethal. This lymphoma also has "opportunistic" characteristics and is related to infection with Epstein-Barr virus (the virus that causes infectious mononucleosis). It is treated with radiation and formerly was usually fatal within a few months; antiviral treatment of AIDS has both reduced the frequency of this tumor and prolonged the survival of those affected.

- Cerebral toxoplasmosis involves the development of brain abscesses caused by a parasite that otherwise causes serious disease almost exclusively in newborns. While it was formerly the most common brain infection in AIDS, its incidence was reduced when sulfa drugs began to be used widely to prevent a common type of lung infection. Its incidence has been further reduced by combination anti-HIV therapy. Unlike the other two common brain disorders, cerebral toxoplasmosis can be effectively treated by antibiotics.

Diagnosis

A weakness on one side of the body, difficulty with speech, or some other neurological anomaly may serve as a first indicator of one or another of these CNS infections. An important first step in diagnosis is usually some type of imaging of the brain, frequently magnetic resonance imaging (MRI). MRI can often reveal features that are characteristic of each of these infections (or other, less common, diseases). For instance, in PML infections, MRI can help detect any loss of myelin in white matter. In both toxoplasmosis and lymphoma, it can spot mass lesions in the brain's cerebral cortex and deep nuclei, such as the basal ganglia.

For more certainty about the diagnosis, doctors may call for other tests. To better pin down PML, for instance, they might extract spinal fluid with a lumbar puncture (spinal tap) to test for JC virus DNA. When they suspect lymphoma, doctors usually do a biopsy to confirm the nature of the brain tumor. In the case of toxoplasmosis, the standard practice is to start a person on antibiotic therapy right away, assuming that he or she has the disorder. If the lesions get smaller, then the diagnosis was correct.

AIDS Dementia Complex

AIDS dementia complex (ADC) differs from the opportunistic infections in relating in a more fundamental way to HIV itself and to brain infection by this virus. While there remain some fundamental questions about how the brain is injured, most feel that HIV infection of macrophages in the brain causes the release of toxic chemicals that secondarily damage the essential functional elements of the brain—the neurons and other supporting cells. Thus, HIV causes a characteristic neurodegenerative disorder by triggering release of these toxins, some of which are produced as part of the host's defenses but, in excess amounts in the brain, lead to disease. Affected patients lose their capacity to concentrate and think quickly, and, in severe cases, to remember and reason. Motor function can also be affected, so that movements are also slow and walking becomes unsteady. In the early years of the AIDS epidemic, this was a common and dreaded complication of the late stage of HIV infection. However, with the widespread use of combination anti-HIV therapy it is far less common, although it still affects some patients. The diagnosis depends on careful assessment of the patient's abnormalities on examination and of tests that may affirm the diagnosis or suggest alternatives. These tests usually include an MRI scan and often a spinal tap.

ADC is treated with anti-HIV drugs, usually given as an 'aggressive' combination. Some patients, particularly those with a shorter period of dysfunction, do very well with reversal of their neurological abnormalities and return to or near their previous level of function. Others with more longstanding disease and more severe impairment may obtain more modest improvement. A variety of strategies to improve the outcome of treatment, including some aimed at interfering with the toxic processes just discussed, are under active study.

Neuropathies

HIV can also lead to abnormalities of the peripheral nervous system (**C48**), with several types of neuropathy. Indeed, one type of neuropathy is quite common in people with HIV infection and AIDS. It is referred to as a *distal* (because it causes symptoms in territories of the longest nerves, particularly in the feet and lower legs and sometimes in the fingers) *sensory* (it alters sensations, causing tingling and, sometimes, pain and loss of feeling, while largely sparing muscles so that strength remains normal) *poly-* (many nerves are involved so that it develops symmetrically, involving the right and left equally) *neuropathy*. Although the condition is not fatal, in some people it can be extremely painful and interfere with their mobility and normal life.

It has been estimated that 20 percent to 40 percent of people with HIV infection experience some degree of neuropathy, though this too may be decreasing with widespread use of antiviral therapy. Although the cause of this neuropathy remains uncertain, the leading theory is that it is an indirect consequence of the HIV infection, with mechanisms similar to those causing ADC. In other words, the virus does not injure nerve fibers directly but causes the secretion of toxins that do.

Diagnosis and Treatment

In most cases the combination of HIV infection and the characteristic complaints of the patient and findings on examination by the physician are sufficient to establish a diagnosis of distal sensory polyneuropathy. One exception is when the patient is taking certain of the anti-HIV drugs that themselves can cause a very similar neuropathy. In this case the drugs should be stopped and another drug substituted that does not cause neuropathy. If there is question about the diagnosis, or certain features are not typical, special electrodiagnostic studies that assess the function of the nerves may be helpful.

Other than management of the patient's HIV infection, treatments aim principally at reducing pain when it is part of the neuropathy. Most effective are certain anticonvulsants (including gabapentin) or tricyclic-type antidepressants, but some patients may require opiate analgesics or other measures. While these treatments do not change the course of the neuropathy itself, they can very much help patients live with this problem. Other approaches that might be of more direct benefit in restoring the altered nerves are under study.

Research

While major problems remain, particularly in the application of tools available in the developed world to more impoverished societies, the remarkable progress made by the intense research effort devoted to HIV and AIDS provides a stunning example of the power of modern science to understand and treat disease. Work on AIDS has set many examples that are influencing other areas of medical research and treatment, including examples applicable to neurological disease. These include the integration of the newest and most sophisticated molecular diagnostics into daily clinical care, the rational design and rapid development of new drugs, and some fundamental concepts of brain degeneration. AIDS research also provides examples of the usefulness of well-informed patients and the power of advocacy groups.

Lyme Disease

Although Lyme disease has taken on almost mythical proportions in the public mind, it is in fact a simple bacterial infection. Caused by a spirochete (a corkscrew-shaped bacterium) known as *Borrelia burgdorferi*, this infection is transmitted almost exclusively by bites from hard-shelled *Ixodes* ticks. The bacteria live in a unique ecosystem—their survival requires a reservoir of infected animals, usually a combination of field mice and larger mammals such as deer, bear, and sheep. Ticks transmit the bacterium from one animal to another. When humans live or play in areas where these infected ticks reside, such as rural and suburban areas, they can become infected too.

When an infected tick attaches to a host, it ingests some blood, which triggers the spirochetes to proliferate. The multiplying bacteria ultimately spread to the tick's salivary glands and can then be injected into the host. This sequence typically requires at least 24 to 48 hours; if a tick is attached for a shorter time, therefore, it is highly unlikely to transmit an infection. In fact, experts have estimated that only about 2 percent of bites by infected ticks result in human infection. Since the incidence of side effects from the antibiotic treat-

ment is at least that high, doctors do not recommend routine antibiotic treatment for all tick bites.

Symptoms of Lyme Disease

If a person becomes infected with *B. burgdorferi*, the most common first sign is a unique rash

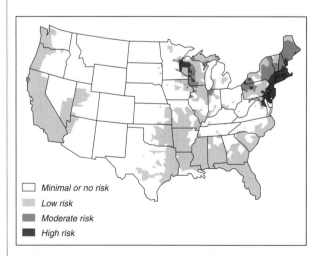

□ Minimal or no risk
▒ Low risk
▓ Moderate risk
■ High risk

Areas of risk for Lyme disease in the United States.
MAP COURTESY OF THE CENTERS FOR DISEASE CONTROL, ATLANTA, GA; ADAPTED BY LEIGH CORIALE

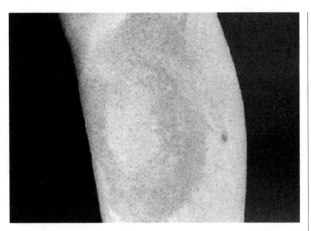

Infection from the bite of a tick carrying the Lyme disease bacterium causes a unique rash, although not every case of the disease will begin with this sign. Photo courtesy of the Centers for Disease Control, Atlanta, GA

called erythema migrans. This consists of a slowly enlarging circular or oval red rash, which surrounds the site of the initial bite. Typically the rash is not particularly painful or itchy, but if left untreated, it can grow to become many inches in diameter over the course of days to weeks. Diagnosis of this rash does not require laboratory testing since it is virtually unique to Lyme disease. Physicians usually give an infected person antibiotics immediately, which almost without exception results in a cure.

If the bacteria spread from the initial site through a person's body, he or she may develop a fever, diffuse achiness, and a generally run-down feeling, just as with any disseminated infection. Several specific problems may arise from this early bacterial spread. Some people may develop the erythema migrans rash in several spots. About 5 percent develop irregular heartbeats or a slow pulse. Occasionally patients develop joint pains or, rarely at this stage in the illness, arthritis, with painful, red swelling of individual joints.

About 15 percent of people with the spreading infection will experience problems with their nervous systems. The most common manifestation is meningitis: an infection within the central nervous system that inflames the lining of the brain (**C37**). Symptoms typically include headaches, sensitivity to light, and fever and may be mild or severe; individuals usually recover regardless of treatment, but, as with all neurologic forms of infection, antibiotics speed recovery and limit the possibility of persistent infection.

Some people suffer damage to the nerves that exit from the central nervous system. Involvement of the cranial nerves can lead to different problems, depending on the nerve affected. The most common is Bell's palsy (**C50**), a paralysis of one side of the face; on occasion this palsy can be bilateral. Involvement of other cranial nerves can result in double vision (**C15**), facial numbness or pain, vertigo (**C14**), hearing loss (**C16**), or in rare cases, difficulty swallowing or vocalizing. When the nerves exiting the spinal cord are involved, individuals can develop symptoms mimicking those of pinched nerves—severe burning or shooting pain in a limb or on the trunk, often associated with some weakness of nearby muscles or loss of sensation in the region of the affected nerve.

Other neurologic manifestations can be somewhat subtler, coming about because *B. burgdorferi* grows unusually slowly and does not provoke a very vigorous or effective response from our immune systems. As a result, some people may develop syndromes that evolve slowly—again with a loss of neurological function. Most common is neuropathy with damage to peripheral nerves either singly, in groups, or in widespread fashion (**C48**). This leads to loss of sensation, muscle strength, or reflexes. Infected people may experience symptoms of nerve damage—burning, tingling, or other abnormal sensations. However, these symptoms must accompany other evidence of nerve damage to indicate a serious problem; when they occur in isolation, they are generally not considered evidence of a serious disease.

Similarly, *B. burgdorferi* infection can involve the central nervous system. In rare cases, this can be severe, with damage to the brain or spinal cord resulting in weakness or paralysis; difficulty with sensation, coordination, or sphincter function; and even alteration of consciousness. This is encephalitis (**C38**). Fortunately, it can be treated, and it occurs in less than 0.1 percent of people not originally treated for Lyme disease. Like anything that damages the brain, it may cause some long-term effects. If these problems are treated early, however, they tend to be manageable.

Some patients develop alterations of memory and reasoning. In some, this is a manifestation of a mild form of encephalitis. These people's brains often display abnormal areas on magnetic resonance imaging (MRI) scans, and their cerebrospinal fluid (CSF) is virtually always abnormal. More often, this syndrome appears in people who do not have encephalitis but rather a chronic inflammatory arthritis or other form of systemic disease. For these individuals, the problem is analogous to that seen in other non–nervous system infections—when people have a disseminated infection, they usually do not function at their intellectual best. Unfortunately, this has created a great deal of confusion and concern among individuals who perceive a decline in memory and intellectual functioning, but who lack any other evidence of Lyme disease. In such a setting, invoking a diagnosis of Lyme disease is illogical and can lead to unnecessary treatment, with significant attendant cost and potential for complications. Finally, Lyme disease does not cause psychiatric problems any more than any other comparable chronic illness.

Diagnosis and Treatment

Diagnosis of a disseminated *B. burgdorferi* infection usually relies on testing for antibodies created by the individual's immune response against the offending organism. An ELISA test measures the level of antibodies in a person's blood. A more sophisticated test, known as a Western blot, demonstrates the specific constituent proteins of the bacterium against which the antibodies are directed and is used in combination with the ELISA. The Western blot tends to eliminate much of the confusion created when antibodies are actually responding to other bacteria. However it is not as sensitive as the ELISA and is not invariably positive in all patients with Lyme disease. Interpretation requires thoughtful consideration of the two tests and the individual's symptoms.

If a person's central nervous system (CNS) may be infected, examining the CSF can be invaluable. This requires a spinal tap (lumbar puncture). As in all other CNS infections, a local inflammatory reaction to *B. burgdorferi* is almost always evident, with increased numbers of white blood cells and increased concentration of protein. Specific testing to find local production of antibodies directed against *B. burgdorferi* can be highly informative. Moreover, reexamining CSF after treatment can be helpful in showing a decrease in the intensity of the inflammatory reaction (decreased white count, protein), although antibody production may remain elevated for years.

Two common misconceptions about antibody

"A TICK BY ANY OTHER NAME . . ."

Lyme disease is transmitted by *Ixodes* ticks, but that name encompasses a large variety of ticks:

■ **In the northeast United States, *Ixodes scapularis* is commonly known as the deer tick.**

■ **In the midwest United States, the same tick is known as the bear tick.**

■ **In California, Lyme disease is spread by *Ixodes pacificus*, which is partial to lizards.**

■ **In Europe, *Ixodes ricinus* spreads the infection and is commonly known as the sheep tick.**

■ **In Asia, the main culprit is *Ixodes persulcatus*.**

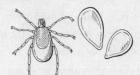

To scale: adult deer tick and sesame seeds

testing can lead to confusion. First, it takes time for the body to generate a measurable level of antibodies. Hence, at the time of the rash, very early in infection, a test may not find any Lyme disease antibody. This does not negate the diagnosis. If the rash looks like erythema migrans, a person should receive antibiotic treatment regardless of the test result. Second, our immune systems are designed to remember past infections in order to prevent reinfection, so antibody measures typically remain elevated for years, or even permanently. Therefore, a positive test may reflect prior exposure but have nothing to do with current symptoms or how well a treatment has succeeded.

Treatment for Lyme disease is highly effective. Early in the disease, a course of oral antibiotics for three to four weeks results in a cure for about 95 percent of infected people. Doxycycline/ Vibramycin (which should not be taken by pregnant women or children under age eight) or amoxicillin is highly effective. There is good evidence that these regimens also work against more advanced forms of the disease, such as arthritis or even meningitis. For those individuals with more

severe disease (typically central nervous system disease, arthritis, or other manifestations that have not responded to oral medications), doctors usually prescribe intravenous drugs—usually ceftriaxone, cefotaxime, or a very high dose of penicillin. Carefully performed studies have indicated that treatment with these medications for two weeks cures the vast majority of infections. There has been a tendency for doctors to expand this treatment to four weeks because some patients have relapsed after two. However, there are no data to indicate that routine treatment for any period longer than four weeks is either necessary or reasonable.

A partially effective vaccine against Lyme disease has been developed, but incomplete efficacy and concerns about possible adverse effects resulted in limited acceptance and withdrawal from the market. Individuals at risk of tick exposure because of where they live and work will still need to exercise caution.

In sum, Lyme disease is a somewhat unusual infection that can affect the nervous system in a variety of ways. Diagnosis and treatment are usu-

AVOIDING LYME DISEASE

In tick-infested areas, the best precaution against Lyme disease (LD) is to avoid contact with soil, leaf litter, and vegetation as much as possible. However, if you garden, hike, camp, hunt, work outdoors, or otherwise spend time in woods, brush, or overgrown fields, you should use a combination of precautions to dramatically reduce your chances of getting Lyme disease.

When spending time outdoors, make these easy precautions part of your routine:

- Wear close-toed shoes and light-colored clothing with a tight weave to enable you to spot ticks easily.

- Scan clothes and any exposed skin frequently for ticks while outdoors.

- Stay on cleared, well-traveled trails.

- Use insect repellent containing DEET (diethyl-meta-toluamide) on skin and clothes if you intend to go off trail or into overgrown areas.

- Avoid sitting directly on the ground or on stone walls (havens for ticks and their hosts).

- Keep long hair tied back, especially when gardening.

- Do a final, full-body tick check at the end of the day (also check children and pets).

When taking the above precautions, consider these important facts:

- If you tuck long pants into socks, and shirts into pants, be aware that ticks that contact your clothes will climb upward in search of exposed skin. This means they may climb to hidden areas of the head and neck if not intercepted first; spot-check clothes frequently.

- Clothes can be sprayed with either DEET or Permethrin. Only DEET can be used on exposed skin, but never in high concentrations; follow the manufacturer's directions.

- Upon returning home, clothes can be spun in the dryer for 20 minutes to kill any unseen ticks.

- A shower and shampoo may help dislodge crawling ticks but are only somewhat effective. Inspect yourself and your children carefully after a shower. Keep in mind that nymphal deer ticks are the size of poppy seeds; adult deer ticks are the size of sesame seeds.

Adapted from www.aldf.com (American Lyme Disease Foundation)

ally quite straightforward, although some controversies remain to be resolved. The best treatment is prevention—avoiding tick bites in the first place, or removing ticks carefully and rapidly after they have attached. But even if infection occurs, we are fortunate to have readily available and safe antibiotics that do an excellent job eliminating the bacteria.

Meningitis

Meningitis is an infection or inflammation of the lining over the brain and spinal cord (the meninges) and in the fluid produced by that lining (cerebrospinal fluid, or CSF). Often people fear meningitis because some forms can be contagious and rapidly fatal. Fortunately, other kinds are much less harmful, and the disorder remains relatively uncommon in the United States. Each year there are only about 2 cases in every 100,000 people.

Different types of microorganisms can cause meningitis. The infections produced by bacteria

are often the most acute and severe and can be fatal. Viral meningitis is much more common and much less severe; it usually does not require treatment and leaves no lasting effects. Unusual types of meningitis, such as that caused by fungal infections, occur primarily in people whose immune systems are weakened. All these microorganisms can infect other parts of our bodies as well; it is just by chance that in some cases they infect the meninges and CSF.

Symptoms of meningitis appear rapidly, over

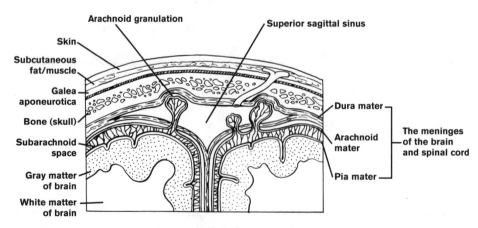

The meninges of the brain and spinal cord envelop both and include the dura, a tough protective layer. Bacterial and viral infection may attack the meninges. Illustration © Kathryn Born

hours or a few days. They usually include fever and headache; over 90 percent of people diagnosed with the disease report these symptoms. People with meningitis will often complain that light hurts their eyes (photophobia) and may complain of a stiff neck (meningismus). Some may vomit. Over time, the sufferer may become restless and irritable and might develop seizures (**C13**) and experience neurological problems such as weakness, hearing loss (**C16**), or visual changes (**C15**). Over 80 percent of people experience some sort of neurological symptom. In severe cases, a person with meningitis may lapse into a coma (**C61**).

In the very young and the very old, meningitis symptoms may be much subtler, making diagnosis more difficult. In newborns, elevated CSF pressure may cause a bulge in the fontanels (the gaps between the developing bones of the skull) or hydrocephalus (**C8**).

Bacterial Meningitis

The danger of bacterial meningitis, and the ease with which it spreads, varies greatly depending on the bacterium involved.

Meningococcus

Only one form of meningitis is truly contagious—an infection by the bacterium *Neisseria meningitidis,* also called meningococcus. This form of bacterial meningitis accounts for about 25 percent of cases in the United States, most occurring in children and young adults. Of all the people who contract meningitis from *N. meningitidis,* only 3 percent die. Because the disease is potentially contagious, people who come into close contact with someone infected with meningococ-

cus, such as members of the same household, are often given prophylactic antibiotics such as rifampin to halt its spread and prevent disease.

Meningococcal meningitis outbreaks have occurred in crowded settings, such as day-care centers, army barracks, and dormitories, because it is airborne (caught and spread through coughing). The disease also occurs in epidemics in some areas of the world, such as sub-Saharan Africa.

A meningococcal vaccine is available for four types of *N. meningitidis* infections—A, C, Y, and W135. Physicians give this vaccine when one of these four types might cause an outbreak in susceptible people, such as military recruits, college students in the United States and abroad, and travelers spending long periods in crowded conditions in high-risk areas of the world. It is not recommended as a routine vaccination in the United States because many of the sporadic cases here involve *N. meningitidis* type B, which is not prevented by the current vaccine.

Hib

Until 1985, most cases of bacterial meningitis occurred in children under 5 years old (up to 60 cases per 100,000 children each year). The overwhelming majority of these infections, about 10,000 cases a year, were caused by *Haemophilus influenzae* type b (Hib). This kind of meningitis has a 6 percent mortality rate. Since 1985, when the first Hib vaccine became available to all children starting at two months of age, the incidence of Hib meningitis has declined by 90 percent. The vaccine has been improved recently to be even more effective. In parts of the world where the vaccine is not available, Hib meningitis remains a devastating disease of childhood and is mildly contagious among very close contacts, particularly other children.

Pneumococcus

Streptococcus pneumoniae (pneumococcus) is the most common cause of meningitis in adults, although it can also affect children and the elderly. This bacterium can cause a more severe disease than others, with the highest overall mortality—21 percent. Like the other organisms, it usually reaches the meninges through a person's breathing, or it follows an infection in the blood. Pneumococcal meningitis, too, can be prevented and reduced through a vaccine, which is recommended for high-risk individuals over the age of 2. These individuals include the elderly and people with underlying disease such as cancer, diabetes, kidney disease, AIDS, and lung and heart disease. A new formulation pneumococcal vaccine has recently become available to protect high-risk children under 2; it may become a routine vaccination in all children, similar to the improved Hib vaccine.

Other Forms

Specific groups of people may contract less common forms of bacterial meningitis. Newborns can get meningitis from Group B streptococcus picked up while passing through the birth canal of an infected mother. Newborns can also get meningitis from gut flora such as *Escherichia coli* and *Klebsiella.* These bacteria, as well as *Staphylococcus aureus,* can also cause meningitis in individuals who have had severe head trauma (**C61**) or neurosurgical procedures. *Listeria monocytogenes* is a less common bacterium that can cause meningitis in people whose immune systems are compromised, as well as in the elderly. It is usually acquired by eating contaminated foods such as cheese and other dairy products. Other bacterial diseases that in rare cases cause meningitis include syphilis (*Treponema pallidum;* **C38**), Lyme disease (*Borrelia burgdorferi;*

C36), pneumonia (*Mycoplasma pneumoniae*), Rocky Mountain spotted fever (*Rickettsia rickettsii*), brucellosis, nocardiosis, and tuberculosis (*Mycobacterium tuberculosis*).

Viral and Other Types of Meningitis

Viruses account for over half of all cases of meningitis, generally causing a much less severe form of the disease than bacteria. Viral meningitis usually lasts 7 to 14 days and is associated with headache, a stiff neck, and fever. Most cases occur in late summer and early fall and are caused by one of the many enteroviruses belonging to the Coxsackie or ECHO families. However, many other viruses, including mumps, herpes simplex II, and even HIV (**C35**), can produce viral meningitis. Each virus spreads in its normal, characteristic way.

Various fungi and parasites can cause meningitis if they infect the spinal column. These cases of meningitis are uncommon and are more likely to occur in people whose immune systems are compromised because of other diseases. Each type has its own specific treatment, and physicians must also bear in mind the infected person's other possible health problems.

Diagnosis and Treatment

Doctors diagnose meningitis by examining the individual and by testing his or her cerebrospinal fluid. They obtain the CSF through a procedure called a lumbar puncture, or spinal tap. The person usually lies on his or her side, often curled in a fetal position. The doctor or nurse cleans the lower spine well and applies a local anesthetic to numb the area. The physician then inserts a needle between the patient's L3 and L4 vertebrae and draws out a sample of CSF. The fluid is sent to a laboratory for testing.

Typically, meningitis produces an inflammation that causes a higher than usual CSF pressure, white blood cell count, and protein level. In viral meningitis, testing the spinal fluid reveals a mild elevation of white blood cells, primarily in mononuclear cells. In bacterial meningitis, there is also likely to be an increased number of neutrophils (a specific type of white blood cell) and a somewhat lower sugar level.

Doctors can have a person's CSF cultured to check for bacteria, including tuberculosis; viruses; or fungi. The fluid may also be tested to identify less common causes of meningitis, such as syphilis and cryptococcus. Recent advances have made it possible for doctors to diagnose some specific types of meningitis within hours of testing.

The quicker a person receives treatment for bacterial meningitis, the better. In fact, if doctors even suspect bacterial meningitis, they usually perform a spinal tap immediately and start therapy *before* receiving the test results. If they cannot do the spinal tap for some reason, they give antibiotics immediately anyway. Bacterial meningitis is truly a case of "Better safe than sorry."

Treating Bacterial Meningitis

Treating bacterial meningitis consists of giving high-dose intravenous antibiotics that penetrate the meninges and spread in high levels through the CSF and brain tissue. Only certain antibiotics get through the meninges adequately. It is therefore very important that doctors use the appropriate antibiotics. Initially doctors use a combination of antibiotics to cover all possible causes, but once they have identified the exact cause of the meningitis they can use specific ther-

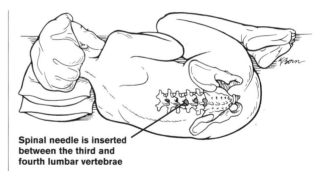

Spinal needle is inserted between the third and fourth lumbar vertebrae

A spinal tap is used to diagnose meningitis. Cerebrospinal fluid is drawn from the subdural space surrounding the spinal cord for testing. ILLUSTRATION © KATHRYN BORN

apy against it. In children who have Hib meningitis, the use of steroids in conjunction with antibiotics has been shown to reduce the risk of hearing loss.

Meningitis can be fatal because it can cause severe neurological damage that, in some cases, cannot be reversed by treatment. For people who survive the infection, bacterial meningitis may leave lasting effects. Newborns and young children may have mild to severe learning disabilities, as well as significant hearing loss, seizures, blindness, or other neurological deficits.

Treating Viral Meningitis

While physicians have treatments for bacterial and fungal meningitis, we cannot yet treat the viral form directly. (This is equally true for many other viral diseases, starting with the common cold.) Instead, doctors focus on alleviating a person's symptoms and reducing discomfort. This treatment includes pain relief and fever control. The rate of death or disability associated with viral meningitis is minimal, and the condition usually leaves no lasting effects. New antiviral agents to treat viral meningitis, such as pleconaril, are being tested but are not yet available.

Viral Encephalitis

Encephalitis means simply "inflammation of the brain," and encephalomyelitis translates as "inflammation of the brain and spinal cord." The two terms are often used interchangeably. Inflammation can result from infections or from immune (allergic) reactions. Infectious encephalitis is most commonly caused by viruses, and more than 100 different viruses have been related to acute encephalitis; acute disseminated encephalomyelitis, or postinfectious encephalomyelitis, is an autoimmune disease that follows infections or, occasionally, immunizations with vaccines containing brain tissue.

The varied viruses that can cause encephalitis can be spread by people (some through saliva or respiratory droplets, and others through breast milk, fecal contamination, sexual contact, blood transfusion, or organ transplantation), by domestic or wild animals (through bites or urine), or by female mosquitoes and ticks when they inject saliva while taking blood meals from humans. Many viruses that can cause encephalitis are common infections that only rarely affect the brain; encephalitis is therefore usually a rare complication of a common systemic infection.

Fever, headache, stiffness of the neck, and depression of consciousness are the hallmarks of encephalitis. Paralysis, changes in sensation or vision, and seizures may also occur. To make a positive diagnosis, a doctor will examine the spinal fluid for inflammatory cells, a leakage of serum proteins, and sometimes an increase in pressure, which can indicate inflammation and swelling of the brain. Modern imaging studies (computed tomography, or CT, and magnetic resonance imaging, or MRI) may also be helpful.

To discuss the varied features of encephalitis, we focus on three diseases: herpes simplex virus encephalitis, the most common form of fatal nonepidemic viral encephalitis; arthropod-borne virus encephalitis, the most common form of fatal epidemic encephalitis; and postmeasles encephalitis, a major cause of serious autoimmune encephalomyelitis before the worldwide immunization program. Neurosyphilis, a fourth disease, will then be discussed as an example of chronic brain infection and inflammation and as an example of infection by a bacterium rather than a virus.

Herpes Simplex Virus Encephalitis

This is the most common fatal, nonepidemic form of encephalitis worldwide. Herpes simplex virus is ubiquitous: half of all people show evidence of a prior infection by adolescence, and 90 percent of adults have antibodies. Infection is spread by saliva and respiratory droplets, commonly by family contacts. The primary infection is either asymptomatic or a mild respiratory disease. The virus is then moved along peripheral nerves from the mucous membranes of the mouth and throat to sensory nerve cells in ganglia near the base of the brain, and it is in these nerve cells that the virus remains latent for life. Periodically the virus is activated, spreads down the nerves, and may, in some individuals, cause cold sores (herpes labialis). In other individuals the virus is shed in the throat without symptoms; this happens particularly at times of stress. We are all commonly infected with this virus, and most are unaware of it except for the 25 percent who are inconvenienced or embarrassed by cold sores. On very rare occasions, however, with new infections, the virus may spread from the mucous membranes of the nose into the brain along the neurons related to smell, or, with activation, the virus may spread to the underside of the brain rather than to the lip. In either case this life-threatening brain infection localizes in the lateral lower, or so-called temporal, part of the brain, and it is thought that infection remains localized because the individual's immune status prevents generalized spread of the virus.

Because of the localization of the infection, in addition to signs of headache, fever, stiff neck, and depression of consciousness, there are often signs of temporal lobe abnormalities, such as bizarre behavior, hallucinations, strange smells, a feeling of unfamiliarity—signs that have also been recognized with temporal lobe tumors and other abnormalities. The disease may run an acute course over a few days or a rather protracted course over several weeks. It may be localized to one temporal lobe or involve both lobes. The infected person progresses from confusion, to stupor, to deep coma, and to death in the majority of untreated patients.

Diagnosis and Treatment

The diagnosis of herpes simplex encephalitis is suspected because of the localization of signs and symptoms; this localization is often confirmed by an electroencephalogram that shows characteristic patterns over one or both temporal lobes, or by imaging with computed tomography or magnetic resonance that shows evidence of tissue destruction and inflammation in one or both temporal lobes. In the past, definite diagnosis required a

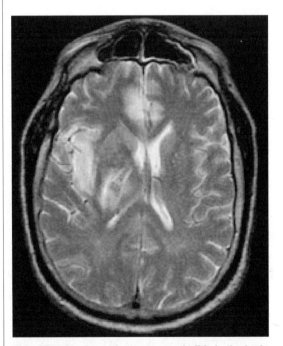

This CT scan shows herpes encephalitis in the brain of a 65-year-old man. Scan courtesy of Keith Johnson, *The Whole Brain Atlas,* www.med.harvard.edu/AANLIB/home.html

biopsy of the brain to isolate the virus or identify the viral proteins. In recent years, however, a highly sensitive and specific method has become available that uses polymerase chain reactions to detect tiny fragments of the viral DNA in spinal fluid.

Before the advent of modern antiviral drugs, the fatality rate of herpes simplex virus encephalitis was approximately 70 percent. With antiherpes drugs such as acyclovir, given intravenously for 10 to 14 days, this mortality rate has been reduced to 20 percent. Many patients now survive with few if any long-term effects, although one of the most distressing is an inability to form new memories because of the involvement of the more central parts of the temporal lobe on both sides.

Two factors strongly influence the outcome of treatment. First, younger patients survive at a higher rate with fewer problems than older patients. Second, treatment early in the course of the disease, when the patient is still alert and oriented, results in a far better outcome than if treatment is delayed until the patient is in a coma. Thus, in patients thought to have viral encephalitis the two most important factors the physician must deal with are 1) whether this may be herpes simplex virus encephalitis requiring specific treatment, and 2) whether it is something other than a virus for which other treatments are available.

Arthropod-Borne Viruses

Unlike herpes simplex virus encephalitis, which is a worldwide disease with no seasonal variation, the arthropod-borne viruses, or arboviruses, are localized geographically and occur only in seasons when the arthropods (usually mosquitoes or ticks) are feeding. These viruses undergo a biological cycle in the arthropods; thus these viruses are not transferred like an enteric virus that may contaminate the feet or mouthparts of flies or cockroaches and then be passively spread to our food. Arboviruses go through an incubation period in the mosquito or tick and eventually infect the creature's salivary glands, from which they can be injected into a warm-blooded host. The viruses cause little if any disease in the arthropod, and the arthropod may remain active and infected for life—in some cases the viruses are passed on to their offspring by infection of the eggs. The warm-blooded hosts are usually birds or small mammals that may or may not become ill but do circulate virus in their blood, so that further arthropods can be infected and complete the cycle.

There are over 400 different arboviruses. Some cause hepatitis, such as yellow fever virus. Others cause tropical fevers, such as dengue. More than 20 are known to cause human encephalitis, and 8 of these occur in various regions of the United States. Eastern equine encephalitis virus occurs mainly along the Atlantic Coast. Western encephalitis occurs west of the Mississippi. The LaCrosse strain of California virus occurs in the midwestern United States, Venezuelan virus in Florida and along the Texas border. A tick-borne virus exists along the Canadian border, and in 1999 an African virus, West Nile virus, was transported to New York City. St. Louis virus causes the largest epidemics, with several thousand cases in the summer of 1975, and it has the widest distribution, from coast to coast. The LaCrosse strain of California virus is the most consistent from year to year, causing several hundred cases of childhood encephalitis each year. These epidemics are often preceded by warnings—for example, increasing mosquito populations in particular areas due to rainfall and temperature. Some outbreaks are heralded by the death of other animals, such as the sudden death of horses on the East Coast prior to a human case of Eastern equine encephalitis, or the death of crows and exotic birds in some zoos before the human cases of West Nile virus.

Most infections with arboviruses are either asymptomatic or cause general muscle aches or rash. Only on rare occasions do they enter the central nervous system from the blood and cause severe encephalitis. Worldwide, the most important of these viruses is Japanese encephalitis, which causes from 30,000 to 50,000 cases of encephalitis each year over a very large area of Asia and is spread by mosquitoes that breed in rice fields.

Encephalitis due to arboviruses is usually characterized, like other forms of encephalitis, by headache, fever, stiff neck, confusion, or coma and often seizures. These tend to lack the localizing signs of herpes simplex virus encephalitis. The severity of the encephalitis varies with each particular virus. Less than 1 percent of LaCrosse virus encephalitis cases are fatal, and very few of the children infected with this virus sustain permanent damage. At the other extreme, about 50 percent of persons, adults or children, with encephalitis due to Eastern equine encephalitis virus die, and many survivors are left with permanent disabilities. Japanese encephalitis virus, which accounts for the majority of arbovirus encephalitis, causes about 20 percent to 30 percent fatality, and about 30 percent of survivors are left with permanent brain damage.

Diagnosis, Prevention, and Treatment

The diagnosis of an arbovirus infection is suspected because of the season, an increase in mosquitoes, and, usually, public health warnings.

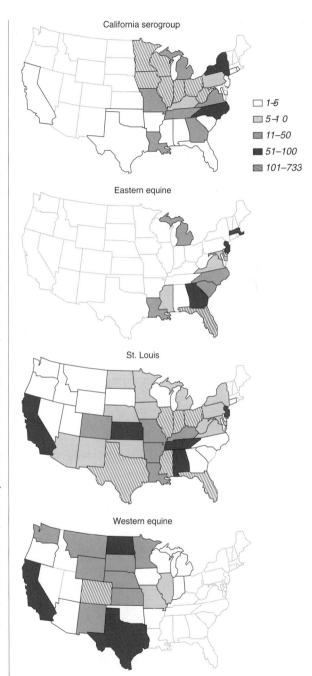

The diagrams show the incidence rates of different encephalitis arboviruses (spread by mosquitoes or ticks) across the United States. Illustration © Leigh Coriale, courtesy of the Centers for Disease Control

Arboviruses must also be suspected in people who have traveled in areas where other arboviruses are spread, such as travelers in Asia during the summer months, or to the woodlands in southern Germany or Austria, where tick-borne viruses cause encephalitis in the spring and summer.

There is no specific antiviral drug that is effective against arboviruses. Once encephalitis has developed, treatment is limited to supportive intensive care. Some of the more severe infections can be prevented by vaccines. These are available for Japanese encephalitis virus in Asia and for tick-borne encephalitis virus in Europe. Some of these vaccines, however, are made in mouse brain, and on rare occasions they can cause an autoimmune encephalomyelitis resembling postinfectious encephalomyelitis.

Postmeasles Encephalomyelitis

The measles virus is a highly infectious virus with no known host other than humans. Before there were immunization programs, measles was usually acquired when children first gathered for schooling. Although measles is often thought of as a mild childhood rash, it has been one of the three most common infectious causes of death in the world, second only to malaria and dysentery. Indeed, 3 million children used to die every year from measles, and in areas where immunization has not been universal, over a million children still die every year from pneumonia, gastroenteritis, and secondary bacterial infections related to measles. Acute encephalomyelitis occurs in 1 in 1,000 cases of measles and is not associated with infection of the brain but is a complication of the systemic infection, which disrupts normal immune responses. In the course of the immuno-

suppression and deregulation that accompanies measles virus infection, an autoimmune disease against brain myelin can occur. It occurs most commonly in children over age 2 and adults, and, unlike pneumonia and gastroenteritis, it is unrelated to malnutrition.

Encephalitis usually follows uncomplicated measles and occurs five to eight days after the rash, when the child has gone back to school or is resuming normal activities. There is suddenly a recurrence of fever, depression of consciousness, and a variety of neurological abnormalities, such as paralyses, unsteadiness, abnormal movements, and loss of sensation. This may proceed to coma and death in about 25 percent of those who develop this complication.

Diagnosis, Prevention, and Treatment

The diagnosis is not difficult, because measles is a readily diagnosed disease and this autoimmune form of encephalitis follows directly thereafter. A similar encephalitis can follow chicken pox or rubella, where again, the diagnosis of the antecedent disease is straightforward. When an autoimmune encephalomyelitis occurs after nonspecific upper respiratory or gastrointestinal infections, it is very difficult to differentiate from cases of direct infectious encephalitis. Often the spinal fluid shows less of an inflammatory response than is seen in acute viral encephalitis. Imaging studies, either computed tomography or magnetic resonance imaging, may show multiple areas of inflammation specifically in the white matter of the brain.

Although steroids are commonly given to patients with this disease, there is no evidence that they alter the course or outcome. Fortunately, the disease is almost totally preventable with immunization, and postmeasles encephalomyelitis has essentially disappeared in the western hemisphere, where persistence of the virus in the population has been eliminated by vaccine programs.

Neurosyphilis

In contrast to the acute diseases of the brain caused by viruses described earlier, syphilis is caused by a spiral mobile bacterium (*Treponema pallidum*), which causes a chronic inflammation of the brain that can remain symptomatic or cause a variety of diseases years after the primary infection. After the introduction of penicillin in the mid-1940s the frequency of neurosyphilis fell more than tenfold, but in recent years there has been a modest increase in the frequency of this disease.

Syphilis is spread through sexual contact, blood transfusions, or across the placenta to the fetus. After sexual spread, a painless genital sore called a chancre usually develops. Several weeks later the bacteria spread via the blood, when a rash is often seen and other organs are seeded. In approximately a quarter of persons the brain and spinal cord are involved, and this involvement usually occurs within 3 to 18 months after the primary infection. Some patients at the time of bacterial spread suffer a mild meningitis, with headache, fever, and stiff neck, but this clears within a few days. The infection, however, remains in the nervous system, with a chronic mild inflammatory response. Years later some patients may develop vasculitis with strokes, chronic involvement of the gray matter of the brain resulting in dementia, or inflammation and thickening of the thin covering of the brain, causing sensory loss and pain in the legs or blindness.

Meningovascular neurosyphilis is primarily an involvement in and around blood vessels, with a marked inflammatory response and strokes. This commonly occurs within 5 to 10 years after the primary infection. Paretic neurosyphilis is a syndrome of slowly progressive dementia and typically occurs 10 to 15 years after the primary infection. Tabetic neurosyphilis, or tabes dorsalis, is an indolent fibrosis (slow growth of the fibrous tissue) of the meninges (delicate coverings of the brain) around the nerve roots coming into the spinal cord, and leads to a loss of sensation and reflex in the legs, often accompanied by pain referred to as lightning pains. This usually occurs 15 to 20 years after the initial infection.

Diagnosis and Treatment

The diagnosis of neurosyphilis may be suspected when a positive reaction to syphilis is found in blood tests, but the critical factor in diagnosis is examination of the cerebrospinal fluid, which during asymptomatic neurosyphilis will show a positive reaction to the spirochete. But during the active phases of meningovascular syphilis, paresis, or tabes dorsalis, the spinal fluid also shows an increase in cells and an elevation of spinal fluid protein.

The treatment is penicillin, but there has long been a controversy as to how much penicillin should be given and for how long. Because of the difficulty with which penicillin enters the cerebrospinal fluid in the absence of marked inflammation, it is probably better to use daily large intravenous doses of penicillin for a period of 14 days. Subsequently, the patient's spinal fluid should be reexamined at six-month intervals to ensure that the spinal fluid abnormality has reversed, with a disappearance of cells, a reduction of protein, and a decrease in the amount of reactivity to the organism.

Creutzfeldt-Jakob Disease

Creutzfeldt-Jakob disease (CJD) is a very rare but fatal brain condition. It causes dementia that rapidly worsens from week to week. The disease may begin with subtle psychiatric signs, such as anxiety (**C21**), depression (**C20**), or insomnia (**C11**). This phase of the illness is followed within a few weeks or months by more obvious abnormalities—most commonly forgetfulness, confusion, and disorientation. Sometimes people experience visual disturbances (**C15**). Poor balance and loss of coordination (**C46**) also occur in many cases of CJD and may be among the earliest clear signs of the disorder. Of course, all of these symptoms can result from other, far more common conditions.

In CJD, a person's symptoms usually worsen rapidly and eventually involve all parts and functions of the brain. It is not unusual for an individual to decline from the first subtle symptoms to a state of complete unresponsiveness in a few months. A characteristic feature of the disease is irregular jerking of the extremities, known as myoclonus. The disease progresses relentlessly, and any major fluctuation in severity—in which the symptoms plateau or improve—suggests that the person is actually suffering from another condition. As of now, people with CJD usually die within a year of diagnosis, usually from infectious complications of the disease.

There are also a number of rare, variant forms of CJD. These forms may mimic Alzheimer's disease (**C67**) or cerebellar degeneration. Severe insomnia is the first major symptom of a variant called fatal insomnia. The variant CJD seen in Great Britain begins with difficulty balancing, pain in the limbs, and psychiatric disturbances.

What Causes CJD?

CJD is the most common form of prion disease. All prion diseases stem from the misshaping of a particular protein called PrP. Proteins are complex molecules that sometimes do not fold up properly after our bodies make them; they therefore cannot function in the brain as they were genetically designed to do. It is not clear how the brain rids itself of misfolded proteins, but most seem to be broken down by enzymes before they cause much damage. Some researchers suspect misfolded proteins to be factors in many brain diseases, including Alzheimer's (**C67**), Parkinson's (**C41**), and Huntington's (**C47**) diseases.

A prion refers to misfolded PrP. Prion disease

is unusual because the misshapen protein causes normal PrP molecules to misfold as well. In other words, the abnormality can be passed from a few affected molecules to much of the brain's supply of PrP. Because of this property, prion disease can in extraordinary situations be transmitted from one person to another, and in even more unusual cases, from one species to another.

Apparently, any region of the brain can be affected by CJD. The dysfunctions we can see probably result from the accumulation of large amounts of abnormally folded PrP in nerve cells, but we do not know exactly how this occurs. Under a microscope, the brain is seen to be full of little blobs or holes, making it look like a sponge (hence the description "spongiform"). Nerve cells elsewhere in the body are not usually affected.

Fortunately, CJD is a rare disease. There is only about one case per million people each year, and it has been estimated that in our lifetime about 1 person in 10,000 will eventually develop any form of prion disease. For 85 percent of CJD cases, the only known risk factors are age (most victims are between 55 and 70 years old) and a weak genetic predisposition based on a common variation, or "polymorphism," in the PrP gene. Most cases of prion disease are thus sporadic, meaning there is no factor we can identify that causes the PrP misfolding to begin. Fifteen percent of prion disease is inherited. In these cases, a mutation in the gene for PrP causes it to produce an abnormal form of the protein. This abnormal form seems more likely to spontaneously misfold into the form that causes CJD.

In unusual cases, people develop prion disease because they have been exposed to prion-infected brain tissue or have eaten prion-infected food. In the United States, most of those cases have occurred in people who received growth hormone

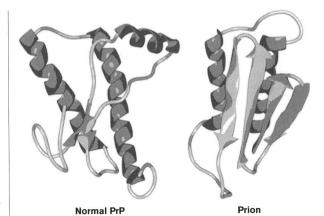

Normal PrP   Prion

Proteins fold in a characteristic way, but in a prion disease such as Creutzfeldt-Jakob disease, a protein called PrP is misfolded, becoming a "prion." A prion is considered infectious because it is able, in ways still not understood, to cause normal PrP molecules to misfold. ILLUSTRATION BY FRED E. COHEN, M.D., D.PHIL., UNIVERSITY OF CALIFORNIA AT SAN FRANCISCO

derived from the human pituitary gland, which is located at the base of the brain. Worldwide, there have been about 100 such cases. Physicians now use a growth hormone that is not extracted from human brains and does *not* transmit CJD. In Japan, a number of people contracted CJD after they received contaminated grafts of dura mater, a connective tissue derived from the human brain; neurosurgeons are now aware of this danger and take steps to avoid it.

More than 125 people in Great Britain, France, and Ireland, many of them young, have been diagnosed with a variant form of CJD. Since CJD rarely appears in young people with no family history of it, these cases produced great concern. It appears that these people contracted CJD from eating the meat of cattle infected with another form of prion disease—bovine spongiform encephalopathy. This condition received its popular name, "mad cow disease," from the way cattle behave after contracting it; just as CJD causes dementia and balance problems in humans, farmers observed their cows staggering around. Cattle and human brains both make PrP, but in slightly different forms; the prions in the two species are not exactly the same, but they are similar enough for people to become infected. Bovine spongiform encephalopathy occurs mainly in Great Britain, but newly developed ways to test for the disease have uncovered small numbers of cases in several other European countries, as well as in Israel and Japan. The European Union and the United States have instituted strict measures to quarantine and destroy affected herds.

Other forms of prion disease affect different animals. Scrapie affects sheep and goats in many areas of the world, including Europe and the Americas. Most evidence indicates that scrapie is *not* transmitted to humans who eat sheep or goat meat. Chronic wasting disease (CWD) is a prion disease of deer, found only in North America. We do not know whether CWD can affect humans who eat venison.

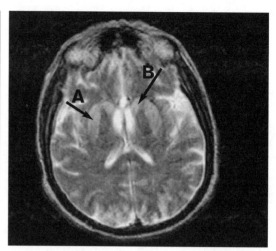

Creutzfeldt-Jakob disease is a "spongiform" disease, so called because the disease produces areas of abnormal tissue that under a microscope are seen to be full of little holes, with a texture reminiscent of a sponge. On an MRI scan, these areas may be seen as abnormally bright. The structures in the MRI above, known as the putamen (A) and caudate (B), are affected. SCAN COURTESY OF KEITH JOHNSON, *THE WHOLE BRAIN ATLAS*, WWW.MED.HARVARD.EDU/AANLIB/HOME.HTML

Diagnosis and Treatment

Neurologists must diagnose CJD by recognizing its characteristic symptoms and excluding a number of other illnesses that might mimic the condition. Chief among these are certain drug intoxications (especially with lithium or bismuth), an inflammation of the blood vessels of the brain (vasculitis), certain brain infections, and a rare condition known as Hashimoto's encephalopathy. Useful diagnostic tests include a magnetic resonance imaging (MRI) scan of the brain, a lumbar puncture (spinal tap), an electroencephalogram (EEG), and a test for antithyroid antibodies. Genetic testing can confirm the diagnosis of the familial forms of the disease, but not the sporadic or infectiously ac-

quired forms. The only test that can conclusively diagnose CJD is a biopsy of brain tissue. Pathologists can see the microscopic changes typically produced by prions in the biopsied tissue, and test directly for misfolded PrP.

Unfortunately, there are no treatments that can cure or slow the progression of prion disease. Currently, it is always fatal. However, despite the rarity of CJD, we know its basic biology better than we understand most other neurodegenerative diseases. Excellent animal models of prion disease exist, allowing us to test treatments effectively. A number of compounds are currently under investigation in laboratories throughout the world. These treatments seek either to block the conversion of the normal form of PrP to a misfolded form or to allow the brain to rid itself of the misfolded proteins.

Systemic Lupus Erythematosus

Systemic lupus erythematosus (SLE, or "lupus" for short) is a chronic autoimmune disease that can inflame any and all organs of the body—hence the term *systemic*. Lupus can produce a wide range of symptoms, the most common of which include arthritis, rashes (particularly on the cheeks), fever, a low number of white blood cells, or platelets, and kidney and brain disease. Few people with lupus have all the possible symptoms, but up to half have neurological symptoms or complications, which this section will concentrate on. Please refer to Appendix C, "Resource Groups," at the back of this book for contacts that can provide you with information on the disease in its full range of manifestations.

We do not know why, but lupus and related diseases spontaneously wax and wane ("flare" and "remit"), so their symptoms vary considerably over time. Lupus can be very mild, or it can be lethal. Because its symptoms are so varied, we are really not sure how many people suffer from it. Its onset is difficult to pin down, and we do not know its cause. We do know that lupus mostly affects young women, particularly those who are non-

Caucasian. It has been estimated that up to 1 in 250 black women between 15 and 45 develop the disease, compared with 1 in 800 white women of the same age. The fact that lupus tends to run in families suggests that there is a genetic component to the disease, but no specific gene has been identified.

Lupus is an autoimmune disorder, which means that the immune system, which normally controls a person's defenses against infection, turns against the body and produces antibodies against its own cells. This leads to direct damage and to inflammation, which often blocks small blood vessels (a condition called vasculitis). Because many lupus symptoms reflect loss of blood flow to a specific part of the body, those symptoms can be as varied as our organs and tissues are.

Neurological Symptoms

It is common for people with lupus to develop some neurological symptoms, but rare for these to be the first symptoms to show up. Most often people are diagnosed with the disease because of

OTHER AUTOIMMUNE DISEASES

Lupus, myasthenia gravis (**C52**), and rheumatoid arthritis are the best known of the diseases we classify as autoimmune disorders because our bodies' immune systems are at the root of the problems. Several other rare diseases seem to belong to this category as well, and can produce neurological problems.

- **POLYARTERITIS** refers to inflammation of many arteries at once. If the vessels involved supply a person's brain or spinal cord with blood, the result can be serious neurological difficulties.

- **SCLERODERMA** causes patches of skin, muscle, or blood vessels to become hard. In causing problems with arteries, it can affect blood flow to the brain or nerves.

- **BEHÇET'S DISEASE** causes the inflammation of small blood vessels anywhere in the body, a condition called vasculitis. This can lead to strokes (**C59**, **C60**); central nervous system damage, producing difficulties in speaking, moving, or memory; and peripheral neuropathy (**C48**).

- **WEGENER'S GRANULOMATOSIS** usually affects the upper respiratory tract, lungs, and kidneys; when it involves the peripheral nerves, it can lead to numbness, tingling, shooting pains, and sometimes weakness in a foot, hand, or limb (**C48**).

- In **SJÖGREN'S SYNDROME**, the immune system attacks the moisture-producing glands; again, it can also affect the central nervous system.

symptoms affecting other parts of the body. Neurological symptoms can be caused by lupus antibodies, which directly inflame the brain; by blocked blood vessels; and by such lupus complications as high blood pressure, spontaneous hemorrhage, and kidney failure. Furthermore, many of the drugs used to combat the disease can also cause brain symptoms.

Symptoms Due to Lupus Antibodies

Some individuals with lupus make antibodies to various brain, spine, and nerve cells. We do not know precisely how these antibodies injure the brain, but when they do the injury is widespread. Often people with lupus antibodies to their brain cells complain that it is difficult to focus their thoughts or to remember things. Some show bizarre behavior (lupus psychosis). Sometimes a magnetic resonance imaging (MRI) or computed tomography (CT) scan will show that parts of the brain have atrophied, but usually they show nothing. In rare cases, people with severe brain disease will develop seizures (**C13**) or coma (**C61**).

When antibodies attack the spinal cord, the result is either a disease like multiple sclerosis (**C33**) or meningitis (**C37**) or a localized inflammation of the cord, called transverse myelitis, that causes paralysis from the site of the injury downward. A few individuals will develop antibodies against their peripheral nerves, which can cause numbness and weakness in the feet and hands (polyneuropathy).

Lupus antibodies can also block the chemical message passed between a nerve and a muscle, causing quick fatigue and weakness. This is similar to the disease process found in myasthenia gravis (**C52**). Still other people develop muscle inflammation (myositis), usually in the muscles nearest the torso, which weakens their shoulders and thighs but leaves their hands and feet strong. Lupus can also produce depression (**C20**) and hallucinations, usually paranoia; these episodes almost always remit completely.

Fortunately, in most cases brain cells recover from the injury they suffer from lupus antibodies, so the neurological impairment is not permanent. Most people return to their usual lives.

Symptoms Due to Blood Vessel Blockage

About one third of people with lupus have an unusual antibody, called antiphospholipid antibody, that can cause clotting and blockage in blood vessels. Lupus can also inflame those blood vessels (vasculitis). Both blockage and inflammation can cause brain, spinal cord, or peripheral nerve symptoms. When the affected vessels are large, a person can suffer strokes in any part of the brain (**C59**). Generalized obstruction of the small blood vessels results in thinking disorders and dementia (**C69**).

If only the small blood vessels in the parts of the brain that control motion are affected, a person may suffer from involuntary flailing or twisting motions (chorea) and sometimes loss of balance (ataxia; **C46**). In people with these symptoms, MRIs and CT scans often show evidence of injury to the related part of the brain.

When lupus causes blood flow to the spinal cord to be cut off, a person becomes paralyzed (transverse myelitis). Loss of blood flow to a peripheral nerve can result in a sudden loss of power or sensation in the corresponding part of the body (mononeuritis multiplex). Unfortunately, brain or nerve injury due to blood vessel blockage is usually permanent.

Symptoms Due to Lupus Complications

Lupus can damage parts of the body that, in turn, produce problems for the brain. The most common of these complications include kidney damage, which results in uncontrolled blood pressure and causes seizures or stroke (**C13, C60**); kidney failure, which causes twitching, seizures, and coma (**C45, C13, C61**); and low blood platelets, which can cause spontaneous hemorrhage into the brain (**C60**). Some people with lupus develop premature hardening of the arteries and heart disease, which can lead to cholesterol blockage of their blood vessels and eventually to ischemic stroke (**C59**).

Symptoms Due to Treatment and Its Complications

Many of the medications used to treat lupus can cause neurological symptoms as side effects. The drug most commonly used for lupus is prednisone, a corticosteroid, which can cause psychosis. The psychosis is dose-related and disappears when the person stops taking the medication. The same class of drugs (steroids) can cause muscle weakness that closely resembles the weakness we see in lupus-induced muscle inflammation, so identifying the effect of the dosage can be tricky. Steroids can also bring on diabetes, which can lead to diabetic coma, and they markedly suppress our immune systems, making a person vulnerable to brain abscess and other infections. Immunosuppressants, which are used in severe cases of lupus, can also make the person vulnerable to infection.

In addition, lupus sufferers are very sensitive to other drugs. Even low doses of the simple medications used to control nausea can cause people with lupus to suffer uncontrolled facial movements. Because of all these possible complications, people with lupus and their doctors become very mindful of drugs' potential side effects.

Evaluation and Treatment

Most people with lupus develop only a few of the total number of possible symptoms. This diversity of clinical symptoms and possible mechanisms of brain injury makes it difficult for doctors to evaluate people with new neurological symptoms and immediately diagnose lupus as the cause. Furthermore, other autoimmune and rheumatic diseases may affect the nervous system in a similar way: dermatomyositis, scleroderma, vasculitis, rheumatoid arthritis, and others.

No single test can determine whether a person has lupus. Doctors faced with neurological symptoms commonly run blood tests, brain wave and other electrical tests, MRI and X-ray tests, and cerebrospinal fluid analysis, but these tests do not provide any specific indication of lupus. They may show evidence of a hemorrhage, vessel blockage, inflammation, or infection that led to an individual's disorder, but not what caused that problem. Often these tests are normal, even though a person may be suffering from lupus.

Due to the absence of a single diagnostic test, doctors must identify lupus by recognizing its constellation of symptoms, and then attempt to confirm the diagnosis by testing for the specific antibodies that the body makes against its own tissues (called autoantibodies). We use the antinuclear antibody to screen people for lupus, and the antibody to DNA to diagnose the disease. Un-

fortunately, some drugs, infections, and other diseases can also produce positive results on these tests, and some people who have lupus might nonetheless test negative.

To further complicate the diagnosis of lupus-related neurological disease, only a few of the many lupus autoantibodies can affect the brain, and even the little information we have on those autoantibodies is controversial. Antineuronal antibodies are more common in people with brain disease than in those without, but we do not know whether they actually cause the brain disease. Antibodies to the microsomal P antigen may sometimes identify people whose mood disorders (C20) are due to lupus. Antiphospholipid antibody and lupus anticoagulant are clues to spontaneous clot formation. The only way to make the final diagnosis is careful clinical assessment using all available diagnostic tools. The autoantibodies can only serve as clues.

Treating lupus is often a team effort involving the affected person, the family, and several types of health care providers. Each person's treatment depends on the specific symptoms. Once lupus has been diagnosed, a treatment plan is tailored to the individual's needs, and it often changes over time. Neurologists are most likely to work with individuals suffering from symptoms involving the brain or nervous system.

People with lupus and their doctors must be extremely vigilant for *any* possible neurological symptoms. The initial signs may be quite subtle. Early and aggressive treatment of these complications can prevent severe brain injury. Our current treatment cannot repair damaged brain tissue, but it can reduce inflammation, thus improving a confused person's thinking or awakening someone in a coma. Treatment can also prevent problems from recurring.

ROUTINES THAT HELP IN LUPUS TREATMENT

For the vast majority of people with lupus, effective treatment can minimize symptoms, reduce inflammation, and maintain normal bodily functions. Preventive measures can reduce the risk of flares.

- For photosensitive patients, avoidance of (excessive) sun exposure and the regular application of sunscreen will usually prevent rashes.

- Regular exercise helps prevent muscle weakness and fatigue.

- Immunization protects against specific infections.

- Support groups, counseling, and talking to family members, friends, and physicians can help alleviate the effects of stress.

- Negative habits are hazardous to people with lupus. These include smoking, excessive consumption of alcohol, too much or too little of prescribed medication, or postponing regular medical checkups.

- Regular monitoring of the disease by laboratory tests can be valuable because noticeable symptoms may occur only after the disease has significantly flared. Early treatment may decrease the chance of permanent tissue or organ damage and reduce the time one must remain on high doses of drugs.

Adapted from www.lupus.org

Several types of drugs are used to treat lupus. When the disease is active, blood vessels are inflamed, or a person is suffering from acute brain symptoms (seizures, coma, confusion), doctors prescribe high doses of corticosteroid hormones (such as prednisone) and immunosuppressive drugs (such as cyclophosphamide). If the problem is blood clots, the treatment is anticoagulant drugs (aspirin, warfarin/Coumadin, heparin/Calciparene). People may also take antihypertensives and anticonvulsants for the relevant conditions. Many of these drugs can cause severe side effects, and doctors aim to use the lowest possible dose for the shortest possible time to achieve the highest possible benefit. Some people seek alternative approaches, including special diets and homeop-

athy, but no research has proven these methods to be successful.

Even with the symptoms of lupus and the potential side effects of treatment, many people with the condition maintain a high quality of life. Perhaps as many as half of those affected have only mild illness, and others develop strategies to prevent or minimize their flares. Around 76 percent of people diagnosed with lupus survive for at least ten years, and around 69 percent for at least twenty. Symptoms involving the central nervous system make a person's prognosis worse, but lupus is most deadly when it affects the kidneys. Much research is under way to determine what causes lupus, what new drugs can treat it, and what someday may cure it.

CHAPTER 16

Disorders of Movement and Muscles

C41   Parkinson's Disease   477

C42   Parkinsonism Plus   484

C43   Tremors   490

C44   Dystonia, Spasms, and Cramps   494

C45   Tourette's Syndrome and Tics   497

C46   Ataxia   501

C47   Huntington's Disease   505

C48   Peripheral Neuropathy   511

C49   Guillain-Barré Syndrome   516

C50   Bell's Palsy   520

C51   Myopathies   523

C52   Myasthenia Gravis   530

C53   Amyotrophic Lateral Sclerosis   535

For you to move a muscle, a signal from your brain must travel across a long chain of connections to that muscle tissue. That chain starts with the brain's system for initiating and regulating movement, centered on the motor cortex. The cerebellum must coordinate all the body's movements and maintain balance. A few of the neurons involved require the neurotransmitter dopamine, while most use glutamate to carry the signal. After entering the spinal cord, the message to move must travel safely down to the nerves that connect to the appropriate muscle. The connecting nerves from spine to muscle use the neurotransmitter acetylcholine. Finally, the muscle itself must have the power to contract.

Disruptions along this chain of connections produce the movement disorders discussed in this chapter. Some of these disorders, such as tremors and tics, can be minor embarrassments. Others cause more or less severe handicaps. In the most serious of these conditions, a person's lack of ability to work his or her muscles produces slow movements, clumsiness, and paralysis. If a movement disorder affects the involuntary muscles as well, it damages the body's ability to keep itself alive.

Parkinson's Disease

Parkinson's disease (PD) is a progressive neurological disorder that most commonly develops between the ages of 55 and 65. First described in England in 1817 by James Parkinson, PD today afflicts around 1 million individuals in the United States and approximately 1 percent of those over 55. The disorder's cardinal features are difficulty in initiating movement (akinesia), slowness of movement (bradykinesia), muscular stiffness (rigidity), and tremors at a rate of four to five per second. As the disease progresses and these symptoms become more pronounced, people who suffer from it may have difficulty walking, talking, and writing.

The onset of PD, which is typically subtle and gradual, is most often unilateral, with tremors the most common symptom. In its earliest stages, doctors may miss the diagnosis if a person does not have the characteristic resting hand tremor. Some of the other common earliest symptoms are decreased eye blinking, reduced facial expression, and shrinking handwriting (micrographia). This early period might last one to two years before more pronounced symptoms appear. Tremor, slowness of movement, and stiffness usually cause a person to seek medical help.

Doctors describe the tremor as "pill rolling," meaning the motion one makes in rolling a pill across the tips of the fingers with one's thumb; it is present *at rest* and is frequently a source of embarrassment. The tremor typically disappears with movement; driving is not affected early on. Other difficulties are slowness, clumsiness, and increasing fatigue in carrying out normal activities, as well as stiffness, or increased muscle tone (rigidity). A person with Parkinson's disease typically develops a flexed posture, bending forward at the waist, with the arm on the affected side slightly flexed.

In addition to motor problems, people with PD commonly suffer from depression and anxiety. Depression (**C20**) affects as many as half of the patients. It may occur at any stage of the illness but is often missed because the decreased blinking and reduced facial expressions that are characteristic of the disease can mask depression. Or it may go untreated because of the inappropriate expectation by both patients and physicians that patients with Parkinson's should be depressed because of their condition.

Up to 30 percent of people with PD suffer

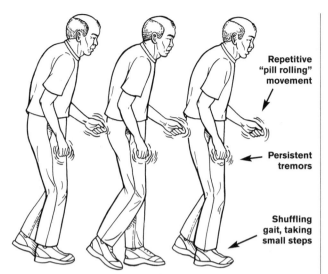

Repetitive "pill rolling" movement

Persistent tremors

Shuffling gait, taking small steps

Parkinson's disease produces typical signs in gait and movement. Two of the most frequent effects are a shuffling gait and the "pill rolling" tremor. ILLUSTRATION © KATHRYN BORN

some degree of cognitive impairment—memory loss, impaired judgment, poor planning—usually with advanced illness, and sometimes proceeding to dementia. But people with PD can develop similar problems from other causes: depression (**C20**), drug side effects (**C66**), and unrelated conditions, such as Alzheimer's disease (**C67**). Doctors must therefore rule out those other causes before assuming that a person's difficulties in thinking are related to PD.

Sleep disturbances (**C11**) are common in PD at any stage, with many people getting fewer hours of sleep or sleeping poorly. These individuals are often significantly less alert during the day, compounding their other challenges. Many factors may play a role in these sleep disturbances, including side effects of drugs, difficulty turning in bed, restless legs, vivid dreaming, and sleep apnea (the repeated obstruction of breathing). Correct diagnosis and treatment of sleep dis-

turbances can greatly improve daytime functioning.

Other symptoms of PD include sexual, urinary, and bowel dysfunction. These, too, often respond to appropriate drug therapy. Speech becomes low-pitched and indistinct; the skin may develop seborrhea.

The course of PD varies considerably. Those who have tremor as their major symptom, may do exceedingly well for a decade, while others may progress rapidly to more disability over several years. Most people respond excellently to drug treatment for the first three to five years, but thereafter enjoy less benefit because of drug-related

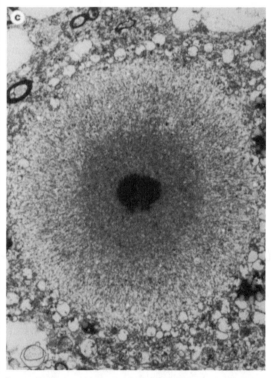

Lewy bodies, a characteristic of Parkinson's disease, consist of a dense, granular core surrounded by a halo of radiating filaments. Lewy bodies form in the neurons of the cerebral cortex in Parkinson's patients. IMAGE © *NATURE,* MAY 2001

complications, especially "wearing off" of drug effects and involuntary movements (dyskinesias).

As the disease progresses, patients have increasingly frequent and severe difficulties with gait and balance. One hallmark of PD is the episodic "freezing" of gait: a patient will be walking and will suddenly be unable to take another step. Postural instability is one of the most disabling and difficult-to-treat features of PD, as well as a major factor contributing to falls, injuries, and dependence.

What Causes Parkinson's Disease?

PD is one of the best-understood neurodegenerative disorders. The pathological hallmarks of this disorder include the degeneration of a small group of dopamine-containing neurons in a part of the brain stem, in a structure called the substantia nigra. Dopamine is a chemical messenger that is released in portions of the basal ganglia involved in the control of movement. Loss of dopamine causes nerve cells to fire abnormally and excessively, which disrupts the functioning of other portions of the motor system that are directly responsible for movement.

Loss of dopamine neurons in the substantia nigra occurs gradually over many years, and PD symptoms develop only when 50 percent to 80 percent of those cells have been lost and compensatory mechanisms fail. Many researchers are intensely studying the causes of cell loss. It is generally believed that the vast majority of PD cases result from an interaction between genetic and environmental factors, but the relative roles of

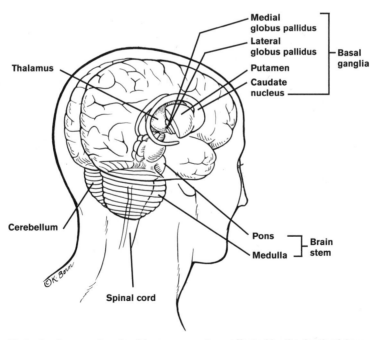

These brain areas involved in movement are affected by the death of dopamine cells in Parkinson's disease. ILLUSTRATION © KATHRYN BORN

heredity and environment are still uncertain. PD strikes men and women in almost equal numbers across social, economic, and geographic boundaries. Studies have shown that the disease risk is higher among those who live in rural areas, drink well water, or are exposed to pesticides. Recent research has uncovered specific genetic mutations in a small number of familial forms of PD. While this provides new insight into the disease's causes, it does not in itself explain the vast majority of cases—approximately 95 percent—that appear "spontaneously," without obvious genetic triggers.

How the loss of dopamine in the brain leads to the symptoms of slowness, stiffness, tremor, and the other features of PD has received considerable study. This research has led to new medical and surgical treatments for the disease's symptoms.

Diagnosing Parkinson's Disease

Parkinson's disease is a clinical diagnosis; that is, there are no specific medical tests for the illness. Neuroimaging with positron-emission tomography (PET) or single-photon-emission computed tomography (SPECT) may help rule out other conditions that clinically resemble PD. These syndromes are often difficult to distinguish from "atypical forms" of parkinsonism or "parkinsonism plus" (C42). These conditions share some of the four primary symptoms described at the beginning of this section, but not all are the result of losing dopamine-producing brain cells. It is important to distinguish PD from other types of parkinsonism because treatment and prognosis differ significantly. Here are some indications that a person's symptoms are *not* due to PD:

- The presence of clinical findings indicating other disorders.

- Gait and balance difficulties appear early rather than later.

- The symptoms do not respond satisfactorily to antiparkinson medications (levodopa or dopamine agonists).

- Imaging studies (magnetic resonance imaging, PET) show that structures other than the basal ganglia are involved in a person's difficulties.

Treating Parkinson's Disease

Although there is no cure for Parkinson's, people can be treated effectively for many years with medication, physical exercise, and conditioning. Surgical approaches provide new hope for patients for whom drugs no longer control symptoms adequately. The goal of these treatments is to maintain active functioning and quality of life.

Advancing the medical treatment of PD is one of the major accomplishments of modern medicine. Until the mid-sixties, the drug treatment of PD consisted mainly of anticholinergic drugs. These medications are still occasionally used to treat tremors, but they cause considerable side effects: memory impairment, visual blurring, and urinary difficulties. The discovery that people with PD have less dopamine in their brains led to the use of the dopamine precursor, levodopa. On entering the brain, this substance is chemically transformed into dopamine, which acts on the dopamine receptors in the basal ganglia. Levodopa therapy has become a mainstay of treatment. It vastly improves the quality of life of

TRANSPLANTATION

Another surgical approach to treating PD is to replace the missing dopamine neurons with new cells derived from fetal or other tissue. This approach remains experimental. One of the more promising recent avenues of research for Parkinson's disease, and for other neurodegenerative disorders, involves what are called stem cells. These cells can develop into the different sorts of cells that make up our bodies. Stem cells can be either embryonic or adult. Embryonic stem cells are derived from the earliest stage of development and have the greatest potential because they can lead to any tissue or cell type in the body. Adult stem cells are found in many tissues of the body—for example, blood, skin, and even brain. These cells can generate all of the cell types of their respective tissues. Blood stem cells, for instance, can become red cells, white cells, or platelets. Adult stem cells appear to have some capacity to cross tissue lines, but less than that of embryonic stem cells.

Stem cells hold potential for medicine in several ways. First, by observing and testing how they behave, we can learn more about how we normally develop and how cellular growth can go wrong, as in cancer. We might also be able to use these cells to create tissues on which we can test new drugs without endangering human (or animal) lives. But most of the public excitement over stem cell research involves the potential of growing cells to replace those the body lacks. Researchers have begun to manipulate human stem cells to produce new dopamine-producing neurons; people with PD, who are missing those crucial cells, could have a new supply inserted into their brains.

There are many challenges to overcome before we achieve such therapies, however. One difficulty is learning exactly how stem cells are guided to become one type of cell or another. Another is figuring out how to graft the new cells in place so that the body does not reject them and so that they work as the brain and body need them to.

---

people with PD and has led to a nearly normal life span.

Soon after its introduction, however, it became evident that levodopa does not arrest progression of the disease. Even more problematic, it can lead to drug-induced motor impairment (dyskinesias) and cognitive complications. The introduction of alternative drugs has helped lessen and delay these complications. Levodopa is now given together with a drug called carbidopa, which prevents the metabolism of levodopa in the body. This reduces the side effects of nausea and vomiting and maximizes the amount of levodopa that enters the brain. Newer drugs that directly activate the brain's dopamine receptors (called dopamine agonists) are now prescribed before levodopa because they appear to delay and mitigate drug-related complications. Amantadine is quite effective at reducing the severity of drug-induced dyskinesias.

Attempts are under way to find so-called neuroprotective treatments that will delay or arrest the progression of PD. Approaches that use substances known as growth factors and antioxidants are in this group. Studies using experimental models of PD have shown that destroying the

HEALTH STRATEGIES WITH PARKINSON'S DISEASE

Treating Parkinson's disease is not exclusively the doctor's job; the patient can do a lot to stay as well as possible for as long as possible. Here are three things patients can do for themselves.

■ **Exercise:** For people with Parkinson's, regular exercise and physical therapy are essential for maintaining and improving mobility, flexibility, balance, and a range of motion and for warding off many of the secondary symptoms that can occur with the disease. Exercise is as important as medication for the management of PD.

■ **Support groups:** These groups play an important role in the emotional well-being of patients and families. They provide a caring environment for asking questions about Parkinson's, for laughing and crying and sharing stories and getting advice from other sufferers, and for forging friendships with people who understand each other's problems.

■ **Staying active:** PD seems to advance more slowly in people who remain involved in their pre-Parkinson's activities, or who find new activities to amuse them and engage their interests. In a word, getting joy out of life has proved to be good for health.

Adapted from www.pdf.org (Parkinson's Disease Foundation)

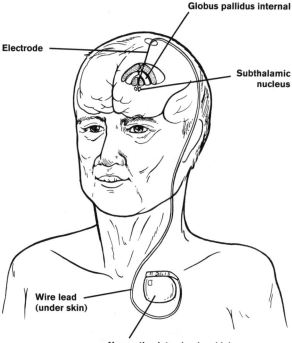

Globus pallidus internal

Electrode

Subthalamic nucleus

Wire lead (under skin)

Neurostimulator (under skin)

A new alternative to surgery for Parkinson's disease that no longer responds to medication is deep brain stimulation. For many years, a surgical procedure called pallidotomy has been performed, in which a lesion is made in the globus pallidus, one of the areas affected by the loss of dopamine signals in PD, to quiet tremors. A deep-brain-stimulator implant works in the same area and interferes with the faulty signal, thereby reducing tremors. The advantage to the implant is that the signal can be adjusted or turned off as needed. ILLUSTRATION © KATHRYN BORN

part of the basal ganglia called the subthalamic nucleus can immediately reduce stiffness and tremor and improve mobility in the limbs on the opposite side of the body. This discovery renewed interest in surgical approaches to treating PD. To control tremor and rigidity, doctors can also perform a thalamotomy, in which a small section of the thalamus, a part of the brain that relays signals coordinating movement, is destroyed. Another surgical procedure, pallidotomy, targets the globus pallidus, a part of the basal ganglia whose output leads directly to the symptoms of PD. All these surgeries carry some risk of damage to adjacent brain structures, but they can be highly effective. It is as yet unknown how long the beneficial effects will persist.

Another procedure, which mimics the effect of lesions without actually destroying brain tissue, is deep brain stimulation (DBS). DBS uses a device similar to a cardiac pacemaker. The surgeon, with imaging and physiological guidance, inserts an electrode into the subthalamic nucleus and the globus pallidus internal (GPi) that is connected to a small pulse generator placed under the skin. The pulse generator can be adjusted so that the optimal benefit is achieved by varying the voltage, frequency, and pulse duration. The advantages of this method over surgery include the ability to adjust the generator or stop using it.

People with PD should consider having surgery before the disease takes too great a toll on their independence, employment, and self-confidence. Younger people with unilateral symptoms and intractable drug-induced dyskinesias are the best candidates for surgery, but there is no true age limit or lack of substantial benefit for older individuals. Patients who have developed dementia or have atypical parkinsonism are not suitable candidates. Before they consider surgery, or if they experience complications related to treatment, patients should consult a movement disorders specialist. The Parkinson's support groups listed in the back of this book can help in finding one.

Parkinsonism Plus

A number of other diseases can cause the symptoms we most often see in Parkinson's disease (**C41**): slowness, clumsiness, and increasing fatigue in performing various voluntary activities (referred to as akinesia or bradykinesia) and stiffness or increased muscle tone (rigidity). We therefore use the terms *parkinsonism* and *akinetic-rigid syndrome* to describe this group of symptoms.

Sometimes, especially early in the course of a disease, doctors have no way to determine which disorder is causing these symptoms. As a person's condition progresses, important differentiating features usually (but not always) develop. The term *parkinsonism plus* indicates these additional abnormalities. Even though most physicians are aware of the potential for diagnostic error, up to 25 percent of people classified as having Parkinson's disease are found after death to have had one of these other conditions. This highlights the need for more effective methods of diagnosing parkinsonian disorders.

Symptoms of Parkinsonism

A number of complaints are common to all causes of parkinsonism. People with parkinsonism typically experience a general slowing of their movements. They note increasing clumsiness and less dexterity in their hands, which often interferes with such activities as brushing their teeth, doing up buttons, getting arms into sleeves, and writing. Walking commonly slows, and they feel less stable on their feet. Eventually, poor balance may make them need help with walking, and even a wheelchair. Although this problem generally occurs later in the course of the illness, poor stability on the feet and even spontaneous falls can sometimes develop early. Speech frequently becomes softer and hard to understand, and an individual may develop other unusual speech and language difficulties. Chewing and swallowing may become difficult, particularly later in the course of these disorders, and can impair a person's ability to take in adequate nutrition and also result in such complications as pneumonia.

In contrast to Parkinson's disease, tremors evident when the limbs are at rest (for example, arms in one's lap or by one's sides while walking) are relatively uncommon in other parkinsonian disorders. If a person has any tremor, it most often occurs only during activity, as in bringing a cup to the mouth or writing.

Another important feature distinguishing Parkinson's from other neurodegenerative causes of parkinsonism is evident in the disorder's response to the drug levodopa and other dopamine-replacement treatment. Parkinson's disease, which is a disorder primarily of the cells that manufacture and release dopamine, typically responds very well to these treatments. Most other neurodegenerative causes of parkinsonism damage both this region of the brain and others. The additional brain dysfunction generally means dopamine-replacement therapy is inadequate. Although some individuals obtain modest benefit from these treatments early on, the response is usually incomplete and is largely lost over the course of the illness.

Causes of Parkinsonism

There is a long list of causes of parkinsonism. Some of these are exceedingly rare or occur only in certain age groups; causes of the infrequent instances of parkinsonism in children and young adults are very different from those late in life.

In rare cases, strokes cause parkinsonism (**C59, C60**). This problem can usually be recognized because the onset of symptoms is abrupt, and people rarely get worse unless they have further strokes or other complications.

Early in the twentieth century parkinsonism was often the result of what we presume was a viral infection of the brain known as encephalitis lethargica. This form of parkinsonism is extremely rare nowadays.

Most of the major Parkinson's symptoms (rigidity, slowness, tremor) result from the deficiency of the critical neurotransmitter dopamine. Therefore, neuroleptics or other drugs that block the effects of dopamine in the brain may produce parkinsonism. Doctors generally assume that anyone who displays the syndrome while taking one of these agents has drug-induced parkinsonism (**C66**).

For most people who develop parkinsonism in middle or late life, however, the cause of the symptoms is neurodegenerative, meaning a gradual loss of some functioning in the brain. This section will focus on the most common of this type of disorder. Neurodegenerations typically appear insidiously, with a slow, progressive increase in neurological disability over months or years. Parkinson's disease (**C41**) is the most common neurodegenerative cause of parkinsonism, accounting for about 80 percent of the cases. Among these disorders, it is also one of the slower to develop.

Because of the symptoms' faster progression and the poorer response to dopamine-replacement therapy, the prognosis for other neurodegenerative causes of parkinsonism is generally worse than for typical Parkinson's disease. This serious state of affairs has encouraged considerable research into these disorders, directed both at the possible underlying causes and at new treatments that might alter their natural history. In addition, speech, occupational, and physical therapy may provide people with some useful benefits even when drug therapy fails.

The more common neurodegenerative causes

of parkinsonism include progressive supranuclear palsy (PSP), multiple system atrophy, and corticobasal degeneration. Although we say these are the "more common" causes, they are still relatively rare disorders, especially in comparison to Parkinson's disease. Together they account for perhaps 10 percent of all people with parkinsonian symptoms. Other common neurodegenerative causes of parkinsonism, discussed elsewhere in this book, include Alzheimer's disease (**C67**) and Lewy body dementia. A number of other neurodegenerative causes of dementia (**C69**) often show some parkinsonian features, especially later in their course.

Progressive Supranuclear Palsy

The name of this disorder highlights one of its most prominent clinical features and most important clues for physicians. "Supranuclear palsy" refers to a disturbance of eye movement that removes a person's ability to look down. Slowing of up-and-down eye motion precedes this complete loss of downward gaze. These eye-movement disturbances may cause people to look wide-eyed and vacant. Some people with early PSP have few or no visual complaints, while others notice that they have trouble seeing the food on their plate or other practical problems. While many people have the walking and balance difficulties that appear in other forms of parkinsonism, people with PSP may have spontaneous falls early in the course of the disease, or they may trip or fall simply because of the difficulty of looking down, which means they cannot see where they are walking. As the disease progresses, they may also notice disturbances of their hand and arm function, such as clumsiness

and impaired fine coordination of the hand in writing, as well as the major symptoms of parkinsonism.

As with other neurodegenerative forms of parkinsonism, we do not know the cause of PSP. The degenerative process is relatively widespread in the brain but especially affects the midbrain (which accounts for the eye-movement abnormalities) and other regions of the brain stem, and the basal ganglia (accounting for the parkinsonism). In recent years the involvement of the cerebral cortex has been more widely recognized. The combination of problems in the basal ganglia and cerebral cortex can result in cognitive and behavioral disturbances. Doctors have used the term *subcortical dementia* to refer to the slowness of mental processes, apathy, and other so-called frontal lobe disturbances they often see in people with these types of problems in PSP.

We estimate that PSP occurs in approximately 6 in 100,000 individuals in the general population. To date, we know of no risk factors for it. PSP generally begins in middle to late life, affects both sexes equally, and is not linked to specific ethnic groups. Rare examples of "familial PSP" have been reported, suggesting that there might be a genetic factor. A number of recent reports have confirmed a type of genetic predisposition involving the gene for the protein tau. But many normal individuals have the same variant gene, so other factors are obviously critical to the development of the disorder. Indeed, recent reports of PSP-like features in residents of the Caribbean islands of Guadeloupe who ate or drank certain fruits or herbal teas suggest that an environmental toxin might be a factor (**C66**).

As with most other neurodegenerations, there are no specific tests that allow an accurate or early diagnosis of PSP. Magnetic resonance imaging

(MRI) scanning may be helpful in showing shrinkage (atrophy) in the regions most affected, especially in the midbrain. MRI will also exclude disorders that can mimic PSP, including multiple strokes and rare examples of brain hydrocephalus (**C8**).

As with most other parkinsonism-plus disorders, treatment of PSP is relatively ineffective. Although doctors regularly use the standard anti-Parkinson drugs, good responses are uncommon and most people can eventually stop taking these drugs without obvious deterioration. None of the surgical techniques currently available for Parkinson's disease have shown any benefit in PSP.

Unfortunately, the prognosis for PSP is poor. People die (usually of pneumonia or infections) generally within five to ten years after diagnosis, and current treatments have little or no impact on this course. The most promising paths of research relate to the mechanisms of cell death. We expect that advances in understanding the biology of the tau protein will boost the treatment of PSP as well as a number of other conditions that also involve abnormalities of this critical component of brain cells.

Multiple System Atrophy

Multiple system atrophy (MSA) is another important cause of parkinsonism plus. It is marked by a combination of symptoms—affecting movement, blood pressure, and other body functions—that were originally thought to be several different disorders: Shy-Drager syndrome, striatonigral degeneration, and some forms of olivopontocerebellar atrophy. In Shy-Drager syndrome, the most prominent symptoms involve the autonomic nervous system. Striatonigral degeneration causes parkinsonian symptoms, while olivopontocerebellar atrophy principally affects balance, coordination, and speech. It is now recognized that these conditions are different manifestations of a single disorder.

Most people with MSA have typical parkinsonian symptoms. A smaller proportion will first experience a predominant cerebellar syndrome, usually gait imbalance (ataxia). Eventually, most people with MSA show some features of both.

Parkinsonian MSA is probably the most difficult neurodegenerative cause of parkinsonism to distinguish from Parkinson's disease. Important clues include a lack of the typical resting tremor of Parkinson's disease, poor response to levodopa and other dopaminergic drugs, a relative lack of common motor complications of levodopa seen in Parkinson's disease (the motor fluctuations and dyskinesias described in **C41**), and more rapid progression of the condition. Other clues relate to the more widespread distribution of the pathological changes in the brain and spinal cord. However, these features may be lacking, and the patient may demonstrate a picture completely indistinguishable from Parkinson's disease.

For a clinical diagnosis of MSA, physicians must see signs of degeneration in the autonomic nervous system, which controls, among other things, blood pressure and sexual and bladder and bowel function. People with MSA commonly experience a fall in blood pressure when they move to a more upright position (for example, from sitting to standing, or from lying to sitting), with consequent light-headedness, "dizziness," and even fainting. This symptom may be aggravated by the drugs used to treat the parkinsonism (and may first appear when these drugs are started). In men, sexual dysfunction may be the first symptom of the disorder, and difficulty in gaining an erection and eventual impotence may predate the development of other neurological complaints by months or even years. Bladder disturbances include increased frequency of urination during the day and night, and particularly, difficulty controlling the urge to urinate, which sometimes results in loss of bladder control (incontinence). Constipation is very common, but this is also a frequent complaint in other parkinsonian disorders.

MSA involves a variety of brain areas: the basal ganglia, several locations in the brain stem, and the cerebellum. It also affects the spinal cord, particularly those regions that serve the autonomic nervous system. Dysfunction of these regions accounts for the disorder's broad range of symptoms. The cerebral cortex is relatively spared, so significant cognitive decline and behavioral changes are uncommon, in contrast to many other neurodegenerative causes of parkinsonism. This is probably why psychiatric side effects, such as hallucinations, from anti-Parkinson drugs are less common in MSA than in Parkinson's disease.

It has been recently estimated that MSA occurs in 4 of 100,000 people in the general population. It affects a wide age range, usually from middle to late life and typically not before the age of 40. Men and women are affected equally. The cause of MSA is completely unknown, and there are no recognized risk factors that increase the likelihood of developing this disorder. Examples of more than one individual in a single family having MSA are extremely rare, so it is not believed to be genetic.

As with other neurodegenerative causes of parkinsonism, the diagnosis of MSA is largely clinical. MRI brain scans show abnormalities characteristic of the disease (typically involving the basal ganglia, brain stem, and cerebellum) in some people, making a definitive diagnosis possible. However, other people with typical clinical features may not exhibit these changes in their brains.

More than most other forms of parkinsonism, MSA may respond to some degree to levodopa and other dopaminergic drugs. Occasionally people receive a quite pronounced benefit. Usually the response diminishes gradually with time, although many individuals continue to feel some effect. Some people will experience motor complications, with fluctuations and dyskinesias similar to those seen in Parkinson's disease, but these are generally less obvious. Other drug therapies are generally ineffective, as are currently available neurosurgical interventions.

MSA is an inexorably progressive disease, with pronounced disability developing within two to three years, and death from pneumonia or infection generally within five to ten years. Neurotransplantation is a treatment approach that is currently being explored in animals, with the hope that we will be able to use it one day in humans.

Corticobasal Degeneration

Corticobasal degeneration (CBD) is an even rarer cause of parkinsonism than PSP and MSA. This is another condition involving abnormalities of the tau protein. Some people with pathological changes of CBD in the brain develop a syndrome dominated by features of parkinsonism, while others primarily experience predominant behavioral and cognitive disturbances (that is, dementia) with little or no parkinsonism until very late in the illness. Doctors once believed that the parkinsonian form predominated, but they have increasingly recognized that the dementia may in fact be the more common of the two forms. Given this complex state of affairs, it is impossible to know how common this disorder really is.

In addition to possible parkinsonism and mental changes, other features of CBD include:

- abnormal postures of the limbs (most often the hand and arm), termed *dystonia*
- jerky movements of the limbs, particularly when trying to move or in response to a light touch or other stimulation, called stimulus-sensitive myoclonus
- abnormalities of complex movements we have learned to use in everyday life, as if the person has forgotten how to perform tasks (apraxia; **C71**)
- "pins and needles" or numbness in the hand
- disturbances of language functions (aphasia), most often causing difficulties with finding words
- peculiar wandering, or seemingly purposeful but involuntary, movements of a limb (called alien limb phenomenon)

The nature of the disability varies greatly from one individual to the next, and the prominence of each of these symptoms varies over the course of the disease.

CBD seems to affect both sexes equally, beginning generally in later adult life. Although most people with the disease lack a family history of it, genetic factors are increasingly recognized as important. Both pathological and genetic overlap exist between CBD and PSP, and investigators are discussing potential links between the two disorders.

Once again, the diagnosis of this form of neurodegenerative parkinsonism is largely clinical. MRI, single-photon-emission computed tomography (SPECT), or positron-emission tomography (PET) scanning of the brain may reveal characteristic changes. For example, it is relatively common for people with CBD to have one side of the body much more affected than the other, and in these situations brain imaging may show that one side of the brain is more shrunken or atrophied. However, no abnormalities are completely specific for the diagnosis.

As is the case in many other types of parkinsonism, people's response to anti-Parkinson medication is generally very poor. Occasionally some symptoms will show modest improvement after drug therapy (for example, myoclonic jerking may respond to clonazepam, and painful dystonia may be lessened by injections of botulinum toxin into the most affected muscles). However, no treatments have an impact on the course of the disease, which is progressive over a period of five to ten years. As with other neurodegenerative parkinsonism-plus diseases, patients become bedridden and typically die of infections.

Once again, we hope that better understanding of the cause(s) of cell death and the possible genetic predisposition to CBD will alter this dismal prognosis over the next few years.

Tremors

Although people may think of tremors, spasms (**C44**), and tics (**C45**) as similar, in that all can involve unusual movements, the three conditions have different medical definitions and different origins within the nervous system. Tremors are rhythmic, involuntary, oscillatory movements of muscles around a joint. These movements result from alternating contractions of opposing muscle groups, or from simultaneous contractions of muscles working against each other.

Tremors can appear when

- hands are at rest (for example, parkinsonian tremor)

- hands are outstretched (postural tremors, most commonly essential tremor)

- hands are in motion (action tremors, such as kinetic or writing tremors)

- fingers reach a target (intention tremors, caused by cerebellar disorders)

These variations help physicians diagnose what type of tremor a person has. In addition, different sorts of tremors usually have characteristic fre-quencies, as measured in hertz (repetitions per second), but there is a large overlap of frequencies among tremor disorders.

Essential Tremor

Essential tremor (ET) is the most common type; indeed, it's the most common movement disorder. It is characterized by rhythmic oscillations of the arms or hands when a person holds them in a sustained position (postural tremor) or moves them (kinetic tremor). The tremor usually has a frequency of 4 to 12 Hz. To diagnose ET, doctors must rule out such causes of tremors as toxins or drugs, which can create similar shaking, and such neurological conditions as multiple sclerosis (**C33**) and Parkinson's disease (**C41**). ET is not a symptom of another condition but a disorder in its own right, with the tremor its primary characteristic.

About 5 percent of people aged 40 and older have ET, and for elderly individuals in institutions that rate rises to 10 percent. ET usually starts as a postural tremor of the hands or arms, sometimes more on one side than the other. It may progress to affect a person's head, voice, and, less frequently, trunk and legs. Such tremors usually appear in adulthood, and initially may be more prominent when a person is under emotional stress. ET is most apparent when people hold their arms outstretched. It increases when an individual starts to move (kinetic tremor), and (unlike parkinsonian tremor) rarely shows up when a person is at rest.

ET may be static for many years, but usually progresses slowly in severity. Eventually it can interfere with the activities of daily life, to the point of disabling a person. One of its most obvious manifestations is a rhythmic bobbing of the head, either vertically or horizontally. Despite its progressive nature, however, ET is not associated with increased mortality.

Most patients with ET have postural and kinetic tremors to varying degrees. Other types of tremor disorders appear to be related to the condition. These include:

- combined resting-postural tremor resembling the tremor of Parkinson's disease

- primary writing tremor—that is, tremor primarily occurs when writing

- isolated chin tremor; "isolated" means the only symptom is chin tremor

- isolated voice tremor

- isolated tongue tremor

- orthostatic truncal tremor—that is, a tremor of the trunk when standing

- kinetic-predominant hand tremor—which appears mostly when people move their hands, with little or no tremor when they are trying to keep still

Often people with these conditions have a family history of ET, and, as with that condition, their tremors frequently improve when they drink alcohol.

Other Types of Tremors

Parkinsonian tremor appears in a limb at rest (resting tremor), is usually asymmetrical, and has a frequency of 4 to 6 Hz. The amplitude of parkinsonian tremor declines during voluntary movements. It typically involves the hands—fingers opening and closing, or fingertips rubbing together continuously (pill-rolling tremor). This tremor is characteristic of Parkinson's disease (**C41**).

Cerebellar tremor, so called because it arises from the cerebellum, is a tremor with a frequency of 2 to 8 Hz that occurs when a person performs fine voluntary movements. It appears clearly, for instance, when individuals touch their noses with one finger, or touch one shin with the opposite heel. This tremor is accompanied by other cerebellar features, such as titubation—back-and-forth oscillation of the trunk and head, as if one is losing one's balance. One cause of cerebellar damage that commonly produces such tremors is multiple sclerosis (**C33**).

Physiological tremor occurs as a postural tremor and results from peripheral mechanical properties of the musculoskeletal system. The frequency of physiological tremor is between 5 and 15 Hz.

Neuropathic tremor occurs in the context of peripheral neuropathies (**C48**) and arises from problems in how the body's nerves signal each other. Around 10 percent of people with hereditary motor and sensory neuropathy display a tremor when they move as well. There is no correlation between the tremor and the severity of the neuropathy, however. Some of the clinical features of this tremor—age at onset, response to alcohol, and family history—overlap with those of ET, which suggests an association between the two conditions.

Factors

Medications can cause tremors or, more often, intensify a physiological tremor that already exists. Physostigmine or other anticholinesterases can augment or enhance parkinsonian tremor. Other drugs capable of causing tremor include intraventricular baclofen (used to treat cerebral palsy; C4), valproate (for seizures; C13), lithium (for bipolar and other mood disorders; C24), and trimethoprim-sulfamethoxazole (for AIDS; C35).

ET may be sporadic or familial, but it tends to run in families. Studies have found that between 17 percent and 70 percent of people with such a tremor have a relative with the same condition. Swedish geneticists conducted a comprehensive study of people in the geographically and ethnically restricted north of their country, tracing 210 cases of ET to nine ancestral families. The inheritance pattern of ET was found to be autosomal dominant, meaning that only one parent needs the unusual gene for children to inherit the condition. Other studies have identified specific chromosomes linked to forms of ET and related conditions.

We do not know where in the brain or nervous system the possible neural generators of ET reside. The condition may result from the activity of an abnormal oscillator, a sort of "tremor pacemaker," within the central nervous system.

Diagnosis and Treatment

Usually a person with a tremor is aware of the condition when he or she goes to a doctor for advice. Sometimes the shaking is simply mysterious and embarrassing, and sometimes it is interfering with the person's daily life. The physician's first task is to determine the nature of the tremor, which will indicate the most appropriate treatment and the long-term prognosis.

If doctors diagnose a serious disease underlying a person's tremor, the treatment they recommend will be focused primarily on that disease. In many cases, however, ET or a related tremor appears on its own. In this case, a thorough neurological examination will eliminate other possible diagnoses. Doctors should evaluate all people with tremors for an overactive thyroid gland (thyrotoxicosis) and, if necessary, screen their urine for toxins. In cases of neuropathic tremor, they should also perform nerve-conduction studies.

ET may be misdiagnosed as parkinsonian tremor, especially in elderly people. But the lack of such other parkinsonian features as resting tremor, rigidity, bradykinesia, and loss of postural reflexes should help neurologists differentiate these two diseases (C41). Other neurological diseases that may be associated with tremor include multiple sclerosis (C33), Wilson's disease, Huntington's disease (C47), and cerebellar degenerative diseases. In addition, physicians must exclude the possibility that the tremors are induced by drugs, toxins, and systemic illness (C29, C30, C65, C66). Occasionally, ET may be misdiagnosed as anxiety disorder (C21).

Some people with ET do not require treatment, just reassurance that the problem is not more serious, and advice about how to deal with it. One useful step is to minimize caffeine consumption. Drinking small quantities of alcohol may lessen the tremor, though of course such a drinking habit can affect us in other ways (C30). ET disappears during sleep. A person's tremor may also vary, not only over the course of years but even over the course of a single day.

The main pharmacological options include primidone and beta-blockers. Some people respond only to high doses of primidone, but physicians must start with a small initial dose (25 mg) to avoid its possible side effects: nausea, vertigo, weakness, and ataxia (C46). If an individual shows no sign of those problems, the physician can then gradually increase the dose to the usual range, 100 to 250 mg at bedtime. If the tremor remains, the doctor may add or switch to another medication, such as propranolol.

Propranolol, which blocks peripheral receptors of adrenaline, can suppress tremors. The medication may be administered as a short-acting formulation, as a person needs it (for example, 10 to 20 mg half an hour before a public event) or a few times daily. However, propranolol has possible adverse effects, including depression (C20), weight gain, orthostatic hypotension (low blood pressure), sedation, and impotence. People with asthma, chronic obstructive pulmonary disease, and congestive heart failure should not take propranolol. Benzodiazepines may reduce anxiety but do not have a direct effect on ET.

Botulinum toxin type A is effective for a variety of movement disorders, including dystonia and hemifacial spasms (C44). It works by relaxing the muscles involved in these disorders. The drug appears to have some good effect on ET of the head and voice, but less for hand tremors. Research continues into new therapeutic agents for people whose tremors do not respond to the currently used medications.

For people with severe ET that interferes with their daily activities and is resistant to medications, doctors may recommend surgical options. These operations all involve manipulating areas of the brain involved in the tremors and therefore carry risks of severe complications. The target for some of the surgeries is the ventralis intermedius nucleus of the thalamus. In one procedure, a thalamotomy, surgeons use magnetic resonance imaging (MRI) to guide them in placing a probe at that site that destroys a small area of brain tissue through radiation or freezing. This can stop the errant signals that produce tremors. However, side effects may include temporary intellectual deficits and transitory paralysis on the corresponding side of the body, though a lasting weakness is unusual. Other rare adverse outcomes include seizures (C13), involuntary movements, and cerebellar dysfunction.

Bilateral thalamotomy—performing the same operation on both sides of the brain—is associated with much more serious complications. In particular, people can experience a severe, persistent difficulty articulating words (dysarthria) and permanent mental changes. Therefore, people should undergo bilateral operations only with the utmost caution.

A more modern surgical intervention consists of implanting a permanent electrode in the appropriate part of the brain that is connected to an electronic stimulator placed under the skin (deep brain stimulation, or DBS). The configuration of the electrode and the intensity of its stimulation can be adjusted to best suppress an individual's tremors. DBS of the thalamus is highly effective in reducing ET and appears to produce fewer adverse reactions than thalamotomy. This procedure can be done on one or both sides of the brain. See section C41 for more information.

Dystonia, Spasms, and Cramps

What dystonia, spasms, and cramps have in common are unwanted, involuntary, excessive muscle contractions. These symptoms may be manifestations of a larger problem, especially if they are persistent and widespread, or they may occur on their own.

Spasms and Cramps

The term *spasms* is perhaps the least specific of the three. Spasms are typically brief contractions that can appear in any muscle in the body, with or without pain. They can be due to many causes, including a reaction to pain, such as when a muscle contracts to avoid pain. This is common when a person has a pinched nerve that causes pain when he or she moves; by contracting, the muscle prevents movement and thus prevents the pain. An example would be a painful herniated disk, which results in involuntary contraction of a back muscle to guard against the pain.

Spasms can be the result of irritated nerves; a common example is facial spasms when a blood vessel is pressing against a facial nerve. This con-

dition has been given the name hemifacial spasm. A change in a person's blood electrolytes, particularly a reduction of calcium, can produce muscle spasms. Because the term *spasm* is rather general, people sometimes apply it to various twitches, tics, and other jerks they might encounter, although neurologists prefer to label these other muscle contractions by their distinctive names (**C45**).

Muscle cramps are painful spasms. The most common occur in the middle of the night, waking a person from sleep. They usually involve the foot or big toe, and the pain is due to excessive shortening of a muscle. These are relaxed by stretching the muscle. Some of these foot cramps are due to decreased sodium in the blood, often from sweating in hot weather without taking in enough salt to make up for the loss. Intestinal cramps are also common. These result when the muscles of the intestines contract excessively.

Dystonia

Dystonia is a neurological disorder in which a person experiences sustained muscle con-

CONSIDERATIONS IN DYSTONIA TREATMENT

There are many techniques to help ease the symptoms of dystonia, including relaxation therapy, medication, and physician attention.

■ Techniques that result in a lessening of stressful feelings may help ease dystonia in a stressful situation. Getting rid of all stress in life is not possible. Relaxation techniques can therefore be of considerable help.

■ Over-the-counter pain medications should be tried first to deal with pain. Pain is difficult to treat if symptoms don't respond to oral medications or botulinum toxin injections—often by relieving dystonia contractions and spasms, you can relieve the pain caused by these symptoms.

■ When it comes to joint pain, it may be that a joint has developed arthritis from all of the actions of the dystonia working on that joint. This needs to be checked by a physician. If the pain is due to arthritis, the arthritis should be treated.

■ Depression can aggravate dystonias and make them worse. If a person is affected by both depression and dystonia, treating the depression often results in an improvement in the dystonia.

Adapted from www.dystonia-foundation.org (Dystonia Medical Research Foundation)

tractions, usually causing twisting movements and even abnormal posture. The involuntary movements can be slow or fast; when fast, they can resemble repetitive muscles spasms.

Dystonia can affect any of the voluntary muscles of the body. Most commonly the condition is confined to a specific body part, producing what is called focal dystonia. Focal dystonias are so common that many have been given their own names, including:

■ torticollis (wry neck, or cervical dystonia)

■ blepharospasm (blinking and closure of the eyelids)

■ dysphonia (dystonia of the vocal cords)

■ writer's cramp and musician's cramp (dystonia of the hand and arm)

■ oromandibular dystonia (sustained jaw clenching or jaw opening)

But dystonia can also spread from one site to adjacent areas, or even the whole body (generalized dystonia). It is usually not painful, except when the neck muscles are involved.

Dystonia is due to a variety of diseases involving the central nervous system, particularly the deep nuclei in the brain. When this condition appears without a known cause or is due to a genetic abnormality, it is called primary dystonia. Several genetic types have been identified. Primary dystonias are not associated with loss of nerve cells—in other words, they are not degenerative disorders. They are more likely due to abnormal physiology in the person's nerve cells.

Secondary dystonias are the result of an injury

to the brain, such as from trauma (**C61**), encephalitis (**C38**), strokes (**C59, C60**), birth injuries (**C4**), and various toxins and drugs (**C66, C29**). Some degenerative diseases of the brain can cause dystonia when they damage neurons in the deep nuclei. These include Huntington's disease (**C47**), Parkinson's disease (**C41**), Hallervorden-Spatz syndrome, and Wilson's disease.

A neurologist must determine the cause of a patient's dystonia. The presence of other neurological features on examination would suggest a secondary or degenerative dystonia, because primary dystonia is not associated with other neurological features besides the presence of dystonia and sometimes tremor. Gene testing for one of the primary dystonias is available. For many of the secondary dystonias, the diagnosis can be made on the basis of a detailed history of an insult to the brain or exposure to drugs or toxins. Imaging of the brain, such as a magnetic resonance imaging (MRI) scan, is very helpful. The MRI scan is often abnormal in secondary dystonia and in dystonia due to various neurodegenerative disorders, whereas it is normal in primary dystonia.

Treatment varies, depending on what is appropriate for the condition, and may consist of oral medications, injections of medications into the contracting muscles to weaken them, or surgery involving the deep nuclei in the brain. When a person's dystonia is severe and disabling and medications have failed to provide sufficient relief, doctors may employ a new technique: implanting electrodes that stimulate the deep nuclei artificially (hence the name deep brain stimulation; **C41**). This treatment provides relief by neuronal depolarization—that is, blocking conduction of the signals causing the muscle contraction.

Tourette's Syndrome and Tics

Tourette's syndrome (TS) is a neurological disorder manifested by motor and vocal tics, usually starting in childhood. It is often accompanied by obsessive-compulsive disorder (OCD; **C23**), attention deficit/hyperactivity disorder (ADHD; **C2**), poor impulse control, and other behavioral problems. Once considered a rare psychiatric curiosity, TS is now recognized as a relatively common and complex neurobehavioral disorder affecting up to 3 percent of the general population. Many notable historical figures, including Samuel Johnson and possibly Mozart, are thought to have been afflicted with TS, like some accomplished individuals today.

The French neurologist Georges Gilles de la Tourette first described the disorder in 1885. He had noticed nine patients who shared one feature: they all exhibited brief involuntary movements he called tics. In addition, six made noises, five shouted obscenities (coprolalia), five repeated other people's words (echolalia), and two mimicked others' gestures (echopraxia). Although Tourette considered the disorder hereditary, for nearly a century afterward, most physicians felt the behavior had psychological causes. The perception of TS began to change in the 1960s, when doctors recognized that people with the symptoms benefited from drugs that block dopamine receptors in their brains.

The cause of TS is still unknown, but most people with the disorder appear to have inherited it. Many studies have found that people often inherit a genetic susceptibility from both parents. How the genetic defect surfaces in behavior varies from one person to another, even within families. In addition, individuals' symptoms often fluctuate.

Tics

The tics that characterize TS are of two sorts: motor and vocal. Motor tics are abrupt, brief, rapid, repetitive movements. They may fluctuate in distribution and severity, and a person can often suppress them for a while. Common motor tics include eye blinking, eye deviation, facial grimacing, neck popping or stretching, and shoulder shrugging.

Tics that produce sound from air moving through the nose or mouth are called vocal or phonic. The most common include sniffing, coughing, grunting, screaming, and squealing.

We also classify tics as either simple or complex. Simple motor tics involve the repetitive movement of one muscle group, such as shoulder shrugging, eye blinking, or neck popping. Complex motor tics involve the integration of learned, sequenced movements, such as touching someone or something, tapping, jumping, or socially inappropriate gestures.

The most overemphasized TS symptom is a complex vocal tic: coprolalia, the shouting of obscenities or profanities. Only about a third of all people with the disorder ever actually have this problem. Other complex vocal tics include palilalia (repeating the last syllable, word, or phrase in a sentence) and echolalia (repeating someone else's words or phrases).

Motor and vocal tics may persist during all stages of sleep (C11). They are usually exacerbated by stress and by suggestion. People with TS, especially children, often exert energy to suppress their tics in order to avoid embarrassment or social ridicule. This can reduce the attention students can give to their schoolwork, and cause their symptoms at school to appear different from their symptoms when alone with family members.

People with TS often feel premonitory sensations before tics; they describe these as increased tension or discomfort, a need to stretch the muscle, or an urge to tic until it "feels just right." The "just right" desire may also relate to the compulsive behaviors of OCD. Frequently, TS patients engage in these activities until things look "just right" or their bodies feel "just right."

Behavioral Symptoms

ADHD and OCD commonly accompany tics in TS, as do such other behavioral problems as poor impulse control, anxiety (C21), mood and conduct disorders (C24), and self-injurious behavior (C26). These behavioral symptoms may contribute to poor academic, social, and work performance. For many people, they are more troubling and debilitating than the motor tics.

About half of all people with TS have symptoms of ADHD (C2) sometime during the course of the disease. Although attention deficit is certainly one of the most common and disabling symptoms of TS, for many individuals the inability to pay attention is due not only to a coexistent ADHD but also to poor motivation, unwanted intrusive thoughts, the mental concentration needed to suppress tics, sedation from anti-TS medications, and associated migraine headaches (C55).

Some people with TS cannot pay attention because of a compulsive fixation of gaze. While they are sitting in a classroom or a theater, for instance, their gaze can become fixed on a particular object. Despite concentrated effort, they are unable to break the fixation. As a result, they might miss a teacher's lesson or a particular action in a play. This can also happen during conversations, leading others to think they are choosing not to listen.

That OCD is a part of the spectrum of neurobehavioral manifestations in TS is now well accepted. Most people with OCD have been found to have a lifetime history of tics, suggesting a link to TS.

Diagnosis and Treatment

The Tourette Syndrome Association, scientific programs, and the media have increased professional and public awareness of TS. As a result, more people with tics have consulted with their doctors about these symptoms, and doctors are correctly diagnosing TS earlier than in the past. Many individuals, however, still wrongly attribute their symptoms to such things as habits, allergies, asthma, dermatitis, hyperactivity, and nervousness.

Diagnosing TS depends on a careful evaluation of a person's symptoms and signs by an experienced clinician. Tics do not automatically point to TS, though that is their most likely cause. Tics appear in other neurological disorders, and there are other symptoms of TS to look for.

Once a doctor has confirmed that a person has TS, the next task is for the doctor and patient to discuss what sort of treatment seems most useful. The goal should not be to completely eliminate all symptoms. Often the side effects of the drugs or other therapies needed to achieve that goal outweigh the benefits. Rather, treatment should be aimed at suppressing tics and other symptoms so that each individual can function at his or her best. Doctors must also consider which component of TS is causing the most difficulty. For instance, a person might have an obsession that triggers a tic; treatment might target the obsession, the tic, or both. Similarly, when an individual with TS has an attention deficit, the doctor cannot assume the problem is due to ADHD but must consider other possible causes before selecting the best therapeutic approach.

TS is a chronic condition that people must learn to manage. It does not have to be debilitating. Even people with severe TS tics, such as touching the faces of people with whom they speak—normally a social taboo—have been able to adapt and enjoy happy, successful lives. Especially for children with TS, the best treatment requires the integrated experience of educators, physicians, psychologists, and social workers.

Treating Tics

Most physicians believe that the treatment of choice for reducing the frequency and severity of tics involves medications that act by blocking dopamine receptors or by depleting dopamine. The neuroleptic (dopamine receptor–blocking) drugs include fluphenazine (Prolixin), haloperidol (Haldol), risperidone (Risperdal), and pimozide (Orap). While they have proved effective in reducing tics, they can also bring a variety of side effects: gastrointestinal upset, sedation, restlessness, and weight gain. Face and neck spasms, lockjaw, or involuntary eye deviation may occur with all these drugs, but these side effects can be reversed with anticholinergic medications such as benztropine (Cogentin) or diphenhydramine (Benadryl). People taking pimozide are advised to have regular electrocardiogram (ECG) tests. In rare cases, dopamine-blocking agents may cause involuntary repetitive movements that usually involve the lower face and mouth, called tardive dyskinesia.

Another antidopaminergic drug, tetrabenazine, may be effective in treating tics without the risk of tardive dyskinesia, but this drug has not yet been approved by the Food and Drug Administration. Other drugs occasionally found useful in the treatment of tics include clonidine, guanfacine, and clonazepam.

Yet another alternative for treating tics is the use of botulinum toxin injections in the area of the most problematic tic. The botulinum temporarily paralyzes or weakens the muscles. Such injections are safe and effective in reducing the severity and frequency of the tic, as well as the premonitory sensation or tic urge, without the side effects of systemic medications. Depending on the site of injection, the most common side effects include drooping eyelids, weak neck, and low vocal volume (hypophonia).

When TS and ADHD are both present, behavioral modification, school and classroom adjustments, and stress management may provide important emotional support for the person with TS and family members, helping to improve self-esteem and motivation. But while these behavior strategies may be useful in ADHD, for most people they are rarely fully effective by themselves. Pharmacological therapy is usually required as well. The central nervous system (CNS) stimulants used to treat ADHD, such as methylphenidate (Ritalin), controlled-release methylphenidate (Concerta), dextroamphetamine (Dexedrine), mixture of amphetamine salts (Adderall), and pemoline (Cylert), can exacerbate or precipitate tics in up to 25 percent of people with TS. If the symptoms of ADHD are the most troublesome for an individual, however, it is reasonable to use these stimulants while keeping the dosage at the lowest effective level. Further-more, many people report that their tics return to baseline levels several days or weeks after they start taking a stimulant medication. Alpha-2 agonists and tricyclic antidepressants are also useful in treating ADHD, particularly if people cannot tolerate CNS stimulants. Clonidine (Catapres) improves symptoms of ADHD and of impulse-control problems but only occasionally has been found to be effective against tics.

The most effective drugs for OCD are the selective serotonin reuptake inhibitors (SSRIs). These drugs usually do not relieve typical motor or phonic tics, but they may be beneficial in controlling the premonitory urges and compulsions (that is, "compulsive tics"). It may take two or three months for people's symptoms to respond, and about a third of all people show no response to one or another SSRI. For more on the treatment of OCD, see section **C23.**

Ataxia

The word *ataxia* is derived from Greek roots that mean "without order." In a medical sense, it refers to lack of coordination. The first sign of the condition is usually walking with poor balance and a slow and unsteady gait. That is often followed by impaired hand coordination, including deteriorating handwriting and difficulty with complex hand motions. Later a person may have slurred and inarticulate speech. Ataxia can also be associated with shaking or tremors, especially when a person tries to use his or her hands. It occasionally shows up as altered eye movements, producing distorted vision and impaired perception of movement.

To outsiders, a person suffering from ataxia may seem drunk: reeling unsteadily, slurring his or her speech, and making uncoordinated hand gestures. But people with the condition, their family, and their friends know that alcohol is not the cause. Usually the person's obvious difficulty in walking causes the family to seek medical attention quickly. They are often concerned that the symptoms are due to a stroke, brain tumor, multiple sclerosis, or other serious neurological disorders, and indeed ataxia might be the first sign of those problems. Diagnosing ataxia and its cause as rapidly as possible is important to prevent further losses of coordination and to obtain the best chance for full recovery.

Ataxia can indicate a serious medical emergency, especially when the problem is associated with any of these additional symptoms:

- headache (**C54**)
- nausea or vomiting
- decreased alertness
- impaired coordination on only one side of the body

It is therefore important to note how the problem begins and how quickly it grows. If the ataxia is one-sided and develops suddenly, it may be due to a large stroke (**C59**) or hemorrhage (**C60**) affecting the part of the brain that controls coordination and balance. The presence of other serious symptoms—headache, nausea, vomiting, and decreased alertness—might indicate that an abscess or tumor (**C64**) is putting pressure on that part of the brain. This increased pressure may also compress the brain stem underneath, causing more neurological symptoms: altered breathing; dizziness and paralysis of muscles in the face, arm, or leg; impaired swallowing; and impaired comprehension of language and speech. Once again, a person should see a neurologist as quickly as possible when ataxia appears.

The Many Possible Causes

Like hearing loss or dizziness, ataxia is a symptom that can be produced by many conditions. Something is interfering with the brain's elaborate system to regulate and coordinate the movement of muscles. The main component of this motor regulatory system is the cerebellum, located in the back of the brain near the junction of the head and neck. The cerebellum lies over the brain stem and is neuroanatomically connected

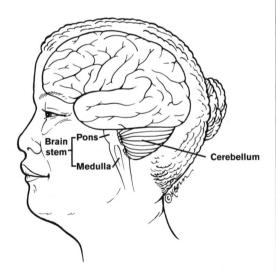

In ataxias, or movement disorders, the cerebellum and brain stem may be affected. Ataxias most often result from stroke involving one of these areas. ILLUSTRATION © KATHRYN BORN

to it. When the brain issues a command to move a set of muscles for a specific activity, the brain's motor neurons send electrical messages through the brain stem to the spinal cord motor neurons, which in turn activate the appropriate set of muscles. At the same time, electrical messages go to the cerebellum, telling it exactly in what direction, how fast, and how forceful the intended motor activity should be. The job of the cerebellum is to modulate the motor neurons so that the motion occurs in the precise direction, at the correct speed, and with the proscribed amount of force. If the cerebellum or its connections to the brain stem are impaired, it can't send these corrective electrical signals. That results in the poorly coordinated motor functions that define ataxia.

Ataxia is a rather common neurological condition, occurring most often after a stroke or hemorrhage in the brain. As noted above, ataxia on only one side of the body is frequently the first sign of these underlying conditions. The treatment for stroke and hemorrhages is discussed in detail in sections **C59** and **C60**. Here we will emphasize the best ways to prevent these problems, and thus to prevent this form of ataxia. People with high blood pressure, elevated serum cholesterol and lipids, or diabetes mellitus are at particular risk for stroke or brain hemorrhage. Individuals with these medical conditions therefore need to seek medical attention as soon as possible to correct them. People over 60 years old are also more at risk for these disorders and should have a medical evaluation at least once a year.

There are several other possible causes of ataxia as well, especially when it's not accompanied by the additional symptoms listed above. In determining the cause of the problem, a physician will have to consider all of these:

- A tumor, abscess, or other growth within the brain (**C64**).

- Medication that reaches a toxic level in the blood (**C66**). The drugs that most commonly cause problems include lithium, diphenylhydantoin (Dilantin for epilepsy), and barbiturates.

- Exposure to mercury, solvents, gasoline, and glue, among other poisons (**C66**). Doctors will test for traces of these substances if the person's history indicates they might be the cause.

- A recent infection, such as pneumonia.

- Deficiencies of specific vitamins, such as B_1 and B_{12} (**C65**).

- Hypothyroidism—an underactive thyroid gland.

- The human immunodeficiency virus (HIV; **C35**). AIDS-related disorders can result in a severe form of ataxia, and a test for HIV is necessary.

- Tumors outside the brain that have caused the body to form antibodies that react with the cerebellar tissue in the brain, producing a paraneoplastic syndrome with ataxia (**C63**). If a person is at high risk for a systemic cancer—for instance, a tocacco smoker facing the increased likelihood of lung cancer—doctors will look into this possibility carefully.

Finally, ataxia may also be due to a genetic disorder. If one person in a family develops ataxia without a clear cause from the list above, then a child or sibling of that person should seek genetic counseling and have a neurological examination. A careful family history should be obtained to determine if an inheritance pattern can be found. This pattern will be important to decide the percent of risk to develop ataxia for a child of an affected parent.

Diagnosis and Treatment

Diagnosing the problem underlying ataxia starts with taking a careful history of the onset and development of the symptom, and doing a detailed neurological examination to determine the pattern of the neurological abnormalities. Measuring a person's blood pressure and heart function is useful, as are blood tests for drugs, vitamin levels, thyroid function, toxins and metals, HIV and other infections, and paraneoplastic antibodies when a person's history suggests any of these might be the cause of the problem. A brain scan is often helpful for spotting growths or other problems within the skull. If the ataxia suggests the problem may be multiple sclerosis or infection, a spinal tap to obtain cerebrospinal fluid may be necessary.

The history of the condition, the neurological examination, and the laboratory tests combine with a high level of accuracy to determine the cause of the ataxia. Strokes, hemorrhages, or tumors are quickly identified. Tests for toxic substances, infections, and systemic cancers help zero in on these potential causes or rule them out. Genetic tests, especially the new DNA tests, are also highly specific; because neurologists are trained to diagnose the cause of ataxia in general, however, consulting a neurogeneticist may be necessary for the rarer genetic diseases.

Treatments will, of course, depend on the cause of the ataxia and the amount of damage a person has already suffered. Doctors will pay careful attention to the person's airway, and if increasing brain pressure starts to affect his or her natural respiration, a breathing tube and respirator may need to be used for a short time. Large lesions inside the cerebellum may be harming the brain stem, requiring urgent surgery to relieve this pressure. Antibiotics are required if there is a bacterial or fungal infection in the cerebellum and the membranes lining the brain, causing meningitis (**C37**). High-dose steroids are indicated if the cause is acute multiple sclerosis (**C33**).

Sometimes the ataxia is the result of a series of problems, all of which need to be treated. If a stroke or hemorrhage has occurred in the person's cerebellum, doctors will focus on correcting any remaining high blood pressure; this is essential and can be life-saving. Such a stroke may have been caused by a blood clot traveling from the heart to the brain; in this case, carefully thinning the blood with anticoagulants may be necessary to prevent further clots from developing. And such a blood clot may have been the result of an underlying heart attack, which itself demands intensive care.

Ataxia can be a mild neurological condition, or it can rapidly develop into a serious problem. Recovery depends on how much the brain tissue has been compromised and how rapidly the condition is corrected, either spontaneously or due to therapy. Most people with ataxia arising from common causes, such as stroke, recover nicely. Long-term improvement is common and helped along by careful medical reevaluations and physical rehabilitation. Some ataxias with less common origins do not allow as good a chance at recovery. Many excellent laboratories are studying how to regenerate brain tissue using stem cells, which could be one way to counteract the problem. Other researchers are seeking ways to correct or compensate for the genetic mutation that can cause ataxia.

Huntington's Disease

Huntington's disease (HD), previously referred to as Huntington's chorea, is a hereditary neurological disorder. Typically, individuals who have inherited the responsible mutant gene see the first signs of illness in adulthood. The average age at HD onset is about 40, with an average duration of illness of about 20 years. Therefore, the "typical" individual who has inherited the HD gene spends the first two thirds of life healthy and the last one third with emerging and progressive features of HD. It should be noted, however, that the onset of HD may vary from as early as childhood to as late as the eighth decade of life.

The first signs of illness develop gradually over months or years. They consist of changes in movement and dexterity, alterations in personality and mood, and occasionally disordered thought and impaired judgment. The motor symptoms are perhaps the most conspicuous and uniform features of the disease. An individual who has previously been healthy, agile, and adroit gradually develops the symptoms of fidgeting, incoordination, impaired dexterity, and involuntary movement. Over time, dancelike movements referred to as chorea (from the same root as *cho-*

reography) may appear in the person's fingers, toes, face, head, neck, or torso. In some individuals, the movements may be very slow and take the form of posturing or dystonia (sustained muscle contractions; **C44**). General movements often become slow (bradykinetic), leading to impaired coordination and dexterity.

As HD progresses, the person's movements may become more intense or widespread, altering gait and balance. The involuntary movements frequently affect the muscle groups responsible for speaking and swallowing, resulting in slurred speech and difficulty eating and drinking. Eventually people with HD can no longer balance easily or take care of themselves because of the progressive worsening of their motor functions.

Changes in intellect, another cardinal feature of HD, may precede or follow motor symptoms by months or even years. The first signs of intellectual damage typically include an impaired ability to carry out a fluid sequence of tasks such as preparing a recipe, maintaining a changing work schedule, or overseeing family finances. Eventually a person's memory, recall, and learning are affected. Many other intellectual operations, such as language and spatial and recognition processing, as well as the general fund of knowledge, may remain relatively well preserved. With time, however, a person's progressive intellectual decline may affect his or her judgment, analytic skills, and capacity for self-care.

A variety of psychiatric disorders may develop in HD patients, some even preceding the motor symptoms. About 40 percent of HD patients develop features of depression, characterized by apathy, low mood, and poor self-esteem (**C20**). At times, agitation and irritability may accompany the mood disorders. On occasion, the features of depression are cyclical, with periods of depressed mood alternating with intervals of unrealistic expectations and falsely elevated mood (**C24**). About 10 percent of HD patients develop psychotic features—thought disorders, loss of one's sense of reality, and paranoid thinking—virtually indistinguishable from schizophrenia (**C25**).

Individuals and families who are aware of their risk for inheriting the HD gene may engage in "symptom searching." They may interpret such common mishaps as dropping objects as a harbinger of illness, but we all fumble things sometimes. In contrast, people who are not aware of the HD gene in their family legacy may not recognize the symptoms for many months or years.

The Genetics of Huntington's

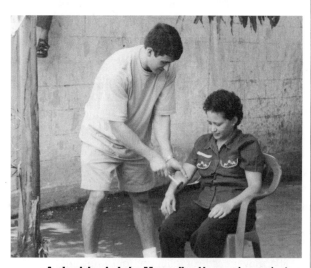

A physician in Lake Maracaibo, Venezuela, conducts a reflex test on a local woman, one of many residents there who are at high risk for Huntington's disease, a fairly rare genetic disease characterized by lesions in the basal ganglia in the brain. Lesions of this kind result in malfunctions in the normal reflex actions of the arms and legs. PHOTO COURTESY OF JULIE PORTER/HEREDITARY DISEASE FOUNDATION

George Huntington, an American physician, first described the clinical features of HD and its hereditary nature in 1872. More recently, the disorder has been definitively tied to a mutant gene. The origin of the HD mutation remains unknown, but it is likely that it arose in Europe several hundred years ago. With increasing migration, the HD gene has been distributed worldwide, but there are areas of high occurrence, such as the Lake Maracaibo region of Venezuela. In the United States, HD affects about 5 to 10 people in every 100,000, and about 30,000 individuals have the clinical features of HD. In addition, approximately 150,000 healthy individuals are at risk of having inherited the HD gene.

Huntington's disease develops only in individuals who have inherited the gene responsible for this disorder from their mother or father. The HD gene is autosomal, meaning that men and women have equal risk of inheriting HD from an affected parent. The HD gene is also dominant, meaning that each offspring of an HD parent has a 50 percent risk of having inherited the gene.

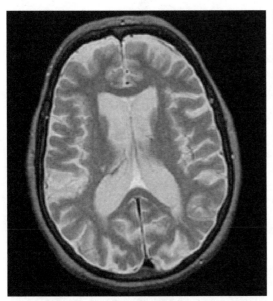

Huntington's disease is a neurodegenerative disease. This MRI scan shows the massive loss of brain tissue resulting from H.D. Scan courtesy of Keith Johnson, *The Whole Brain Atlas*, www.med.harvard.edu/AANLIB/home.html

Most important, the HD gene is highly penetrant, meaning that individuals who have inherited it carry a 100 percent lifetime risk of developing the illness.

Over the past century researchers recognized that HD results from the mutated gene's delayed but gradual adverse impact on particular regions of the brain responsible for the automatic (unconscious) operations controlling movement and intellect. Within the past two decades, the gene responsible for HD has been located in a region of DNA on the short arm of chromosome 4. This discovery has allowed healthy adults who are at risk for inheriting the HD gene to learn whether or not they carry it. Because there are no treatments to prevent, postpone, or slow the disorder, however, there are few practical rewards to knowing that one has the gene. Therefore, only a small propor-

tion of individuals at risk for HD have decided to undergo DNA testing.

How the HD gene is triggered to cause selective brain neurons to die prematurely remains unclear. The gene is present in all tissues, but only certain regions of the brain are vulnerable. The basal ganglia and particularly the striatum (consisting of the caudate and putamen nuclei) are the regions most susceptible to the gene's deleterious effects. Specific groups of cells in the striatum lose normal function and vitality, and eventually degenerate and are replaced by brain scar tissue (composed of glia, which fill in the space where the neurons they were supporting have died). The resulting shrunken basal ganglia can be seen through such neuroimaging techniques as computed tomography (CT) and magnetic resonance imaging (MRI). The selective degeneration of brain cells is progressive and parallels the onset and progression of illness and disability.

Diagnosis and Treatment

Although we can detect the presence or absence of the HD gene, a skilled and experienced neurologist or psychiatrist must still conduct a clinical evaluation of an individual to diagnose HD itself. A key to recognizing and confirming the disorder is a detailed and accurate family history that goes back for as many generations as possible. If an individual has a family history of HD, the presence of a movement disorder that cannot be explained otherwise, by medications or illness, confirms the diagnosis.

Although disorders of intellect and mood commonly occur in HD, and sometimes precede the characteristic difficulties with movement, they

WHAT DOES THE HD GENE MEAN?

The HD gene was one of the first to be connected to a major neurological disorder, and it provides one of the clearest examples of such a link. It is therefore a useful example of how our genetic makeup can lead to specific disorders.

Our genetic legacy consists of the 46 chromosomes we inherit from our parents, half from each parent. Copies of those chromosomes are present in the nucleus of every cell in our bodies (except sperm and egg cells, each of which contains 23 chromosomes to pass on to another generation). Every chromosome is a long, twisting molecule of deoxyribonucleic acid (DNA).

DNA is not a specific chemical compound, like water (H_2O) or salt (NaCl), but a family of molecules that share the same basic makeup and structure. Every DNA molecule contains two long strands made up of chemical building blocks that are called bases. Each base on one strand is linked to a corresponding base on the other strand, creating a sort of twisting ladder. There are only four types of bases, each paired with one other: adenine (A) with thymine (T), cytosine (C) with guanine (G). Thus, if one sequence of bases is GTATCGATCA, the corresponding segment on the other strand is CATAGCTAGT. A sequence of bases can "spell out" a gene or be meaningless, just as letters can combine to produce words or nonsense. It takes an average of 3,000 bases in proper sequence to make one gene.

The HD gene consists of a mutated form of the IT-15 gene, found on the short arm of chromosome 4. Normally, individuals have between 17 and 30 repetitions of the sequence CAG in the working part of that gene. In the mutant gene that causes HD, the CAG sequence is repeated 37 or more times. That change must affect how the gene functions in brain cells, though its exact effects are still unclear.

In addition, DNA analysis of blood samples from thousands of affected individuals shows a strong relationship between the number of CAG repeats in the HD gene and the age at which a person starts to show signs of the disease. The more repetitions, the earlier the clinical onset. People who inherit an HD gene with many CAG repeats, say 50 or more, may see the first symptoms in adolescence or even childhood. People who inherit an HD gene with closer to 37 repeats tend to develop illness in their fourth, fifth, or sixth decade of life.

Despite this general trend of CAG repeats, there is enough variation among individuals that we cannot predict when a person with the HD gene will develop the disorder. We can come no closer than a range of several years or even decades. Other genetic factors, not yet defined, and a host of environmental factors seem to be as influential as the CAG pattern in determining the disease's timing. Once a person has developed clinical features of HD, the progression of the illness does not seem to be related to the number of CAG repeats in his or her gene.

NUTRITION AND HUNTINGTON'S DISEASE

More and more people are coming to realize the importance of good nutrition in maintaining health and preventing disease. Advice has been issued by many organizations about diet as it relates to the major killer diseases: heart attacks, strokes, and cancer. This advice focuses on:

- reduction of fat and cholesterol

- increased consumption of fruits, vegetables, and grains

- maintaining a body weight slightly above desirable weight

People with Huntington's disease may have higher calorie needs than the average person, possibly due to chorea (frequent brief, rapid, jerky movements), metabolic changes (increased energy requirements of the body), or a combination of both.

People with increased caloric needs must often be encouraged to eat even when they are not hungry in order to meet their nutritional requirements. This is usually not true of people with HD. They often have excellent appetites and sometimes eat very quickly. Frustration at being unable to get sufficient food down quickly enough without choking on it can exacerbate the psychological problems associated with food and eating in Huntington's disease. One approach to this problem is to provide six to eight smaller meals per day instead of the usual three.

Adapted from www.hdsa.org (The Huntington's Disease Society of America)

are not as specific or uniform in their appearance as the movement disorder. Furthermore, mood disorders like depression are common in the general population. Therefore, we do not use the isolated appearance of such disorders to confirm the diagnosis of HD.

Individuals who have features resembling HD but do not have (or cannot provide evidence for) a family history of the illness must undergo a rather deliberate and extensive evaluation. Neuroimaging tests such as CT and MRI may show evidence of loss of tissue (atrophy) in the area of the basal ganglia and striatum. With the necessary consent and counseling, these individuals may also be tested for the HD gene. The results of that testing will usually clarify whether the person's symptoms are indeed due to HD.

We do not have medications to halt or slow the progression of HD. There are pharmacological treatments, including antipsychotic (dopamine-blocking) drugs, to help suppress involuntary movements. The benefits of these medications are often transient, however, and they can have such adverse effects as excessively slowed movements, apathy, and problems with swallowing and speaking.

There are also drugs to treat some of the psychiatric disorders that accompany HD. People can manage depression effectively for many years using a variety of antidepressant medications;

the new selective serotonin reuptake inhibitors (SSRIs) seem to be well-tolerated and effective antidepressants for HD. For individuals who develop psychotic features, a range of antipsychotic medications may help improve thinking, behavior, and functioning.

There are other, nonpharmacological interventions to help people with HD and their families, including genetic counseling; group and individual psychotherapy; and physical, speech, and occupational therapy. Effective care depends on counseling, a supportive environment, and help for the family as well as the individual. One concern for HD families is confidentiality, particularly for healthy individuals who are coping with the ramifications of their genetic risk and considering such aspects of life as having children, working, and buying insurance.

There remains no effective treatment to stem the degeneration of brain cells from HD and the progressive impairment and disability that result. However, we can see promise for the future in the remarkable revolution in our understanding of the HD gene over the last two decades. That advance gives us hope for developing a treatment to postpone or prevent the onset of HD. Researchers are also examining a variety of pharmacological and neurosurgical treatments. The outlook for substantive therapeutic gains within the next decade is good.

Peripheral Neuropathy

The term *peripheral neuropathy* refers to disorders of the peripheral nerves, the wiring that connects the body to the brain and spinal cord. Older terms for the same disorders are *neuritis* and *peripheral neuritis*. The term actually covers more than 100 medically distinguishable conditions. Their symptoms are highly variable and depend on how many nerves are affected, why, and at what rate. In general, the most common symptoms are weakness, usually of the limbs (that is, motor symptoms), and numbness, frequently accompanied by unpleasant and painful sensations (sensory symptoms). The sites affected may range from the size of half of one finger or toe to almost the entire body. The rate at which a peripheral neuropathy evolves can be as rapid as a few hours, as in Guillain-Barré syndrome (**C49**), or as slow as 60 or 70 years, as in some hereditary neuropathies. If this sounds confusing, it is, because the only common thread among these disorders is that some part or all of the peripheral nervous system is involved.

It is easiest to think of the peripheral nervous system as an enormously complex network that connects your brain and spinal cord (the central nervous system) to every bit of the rest of the body, which means every millimeter of your skin surface, your internal organs, your muscles, tendons, bones, ligaments, arteries, and every other organ. The system includes the nerves for your eyes and ears; the olfactory patches in your nose; the taste buds on your tongue; the lining of your sinuses, mouth, throat, esophagus, stomach, intestines, bladder, lungs, heart, liver, spleen, and pancreas; and even the sheaths of the nerve trunks themselves.

The peripheral nervous system never sleeps. There is a constant flow of nerve impulses from all the organs, particularly the skin, to the spinal cord and brain. There is also a continuous flow of nerve impulses from the central nervous system through the motor nerves to the muscles and the complicated apparatus that monitors and modifies how the muscles contract to make you move. Most of this activity is processed subconsciously to regulate bodily functions, balance, orientation in space, and the like. Certain specialized cranial nerves connect directly to the brain to convey special senses, including sight, sound, smell, taste, and feeling on the face, scalp, and tongue. All of these functions

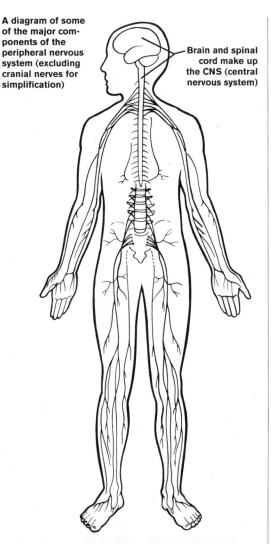

A diagram of some of the major components of the peripheral nervous system (excluding cranial nerves for simplification)

Brain and spinal cord make up the CNS (central nervous system)

Peripheral neuropathy most often strikes nerves in the extremities, but the term actually covers more than 100 medically recognized conditions. The most common symptoms are weakness, usually of the limbs, and numbness, frequently accompanied by unpleasant and painful sensations. ILLUSTRATION © KATHRYN BORN

are usually coordinated seamlessly and unnoticeably—unless something goes wrong. When this connecting network between our bodies and our central nervous system does fail, we use the general term *peripheral neuropathy* to describe it.

Single-Nerve Neuropathies

In sorting out the various forms of peripheral neuropathy, one helpful distinction is between problems that involve a single nerve and those that are more general.

Carpal Tunnel Syndrome

Carpal tunnel syndrome is the most common peripheral neuropathy. The affected nerve, called the median nerve, carries the sensory fibers to the thumb, index finger, middle finger, and the adjacent side of the ring finger, plus motor connections to the muscle at the base of the thumb. The median nerve courses through the forearm and enters the hand at the wrist underneath a broad, tough band of tissue called the carpal ligament. The median nerve has to share the space beneath the carpal ligament with nine tendons. In almost all instances, carpal tunnel syndrome comes about by mechanical compression of the median nerve beneath the carpal ligament.

Repetitive hand and wrist movements may cause the median nerve to become compressed or inflamed. When this happens, symptoms appear, particularly at night. Often individuals wake up because of intense tingling and discomfort in their thumb and first two fingers and have to get up and shake the hand vigorously to soothe the symptoms a bit. Numbness in the thumb and index and middle fingers, especially in the tips, can occur, and a person may lose a strong pinch grip because of weakness of one of the muscles at the base of the thumb. A typical case is an avid gardener who overdoes it with a trowel or in repotting plants and that evening first notices the tingling, painful sensations and numbness.

Often carpal tunnel symptoms will subside

with the simple use of a splint, but if they persist, particularly with numbness in the fingers and thumb, surgery on the wrist is necessary. An electrodiagnostic examination (usually referred to as an electromyogram, or EMG) of the median nerve is helpful in establishing the diagnosis and how much of the nerve is involved.

Ulnar Neuropathy

The ulnar nerve is the second most frequently affected nerve trunk. This nerve provides sensation to that part of the hand that the median nerve does not. Like the median nerve in carpal tunnel syndrome, the ulnar nerve is usually damaged mechanically, either by a blow or by chronic compression at the elbow or just an inch below the elbow, in the upper forearm. Both motor and sensory symptoms appear. The little finger and occasionally the side of the palm adjacent to it become tingly and numb. A person may feel weakness in trying to spread the fingers on that hand and sometimes in straightening the ring finger and little finger. Usually, symptoms appear slowly over weeks or several months, although a sharp blow to the elbow ("hitting the funny bone") may cause immediate ulnar neuropathy symptoms. The first symptoms are the tingling sensations in the ring finger and little finger, but any unusual numbness or weakness in the fingers should send you to the doctor. As with carpal tunnel syndrome, the physician will probably do an EMG to determine the severity of the nerve damage. As for treatment, surgery can either decompress the ulnar nerve at or near the elbow or, if symptoms progress or persist, actually reroute it to a safer, damage-free channel. In less severe cases, simply using an elbow guard to protect against further injury is the conservative management.

Other Single-Nerve Injuries

There are three major nerve trunks in each leg and each arm. A major nerve or branch may be injured at any one of a number of sites. This will result in motor symptoms (weakness), sensory symptoms (tingling and numbness), or both, in a distinctive pattern for each nerve trunk or branch.

Generalized Neuropathies

Generalized peripheral neuropathies are those that affect more than a single nerve. These neuropathies, which are much less frequent than carpal tunnel syndrome or ulnar neuropathy, come in two kinds:

- a patchy affliction of several individual nerve trunks, resulting in the equivalent of many single neuropathies

- a more even, symmetrical pattern, in which individual nerve fibers are affected according to their diameter, length, function (motor or sensory), or all three—the result is tingling numbness, sometimes painful, and weakness in the feet and hands; the problem is worse in the toes, soles, and fingertips

To evaluate these neuropathies, physicians determine the type and distribution of symptoms, how they began and how quickly they developed, and the degree of dysfunction. They ask about such background events as family history, toxic exposures, systemic illnesses, heavy alcohol use (**C30**), as well as such factors as diabetes and medications, the latter being particularly important (**C66**). Combined with these data, an EMG can distinguish most peripheral neuropathies. Doctors can then decide on more specialized tests, usually blood tests or imaging procedures, to pinpoint an exact basis for the neuropathy, if possible.

Here are brief descriptions of common generalized neuropathies, also referred to as polyneuropathies.

Sensory Peripheral Neuropathy

Sensory peripheral neuropathy is a quite common disorder characterized by tingling, aching, burning, searing discomfort beginning in the toes and spreading to the soles of the feet and then to the tops of the feet, the ankles, and on occasion, the knees. The symptoms are symmetrical and even in distribution, and seem to depend on nerve length. Numbness of the feet, which is usually also painful, frequently occurs. The nerves most affected are the small-diameter fibers that carry sensations from the skin. A person's motor strength, balance, and (usually) reflexes remain intact. Generally the problems do not rise above the knees, though some people's fingertips and hands may also be affected. Outwardly, individuals with sensory peripheral neuropathy appear normal, and friends, relatives, and colleagues may not realize the discomfort they feel.

An electrodiagnostic study of this condition yields relatively ordinary results because it is difficult to measure abnormalities in the small-diameter sensory nerve fibers. All test results for a systemic disorder usually come back normal as well. A specialized skin biopsy may pinpoint the problem but not the cause; this type of test is done only at certain academic medical centers. There is no known cause for this disorder.

HEREDITARY NEUROPATHIES

Hereditary neuropathies are relatively widespread, occurring in as many as 1 person in 2,000. By far the most common of these are the dominantly inherited neuropathies, which are often called Charcot-Marie-Tooth neuropathy. This condition is passed down for multiple generations. Usually family members know of others' problems, but not always.

Dominantly inherited neuropathies can be relatively mild. Some individuals, affected only with high arches in their feet and few symptoms, may not know anything is wrong. Others may sense symptoms as early as their teens and for many years feel them progress very slowly, sometimes almost seeming to stop. People with this inherited disorder tend to have few sensory symptoms, so the main problems are foot drop, slapping gait, some unsteadiness, and wasting of the calves and other lower leg muscles. The hands may become affected, and wasting of the hand muscles is particularly apparent. In a majority of families, affected individuals have very abnormal results on electrodiagnostic testing (EMG), with marked slowing of the speed at which their nerve trunks conduct electrical signals. This is true even for mildly affected persons. Genetic testing using blood samples will usually identify such persons as having Type I dominantly inherited neuropathy. No effective therapy has been developed.

Other families have so-called Type II dominant hereditary neuropathy. On electrodiagnostic testing (EMG), they show little or no slowing of nerve conduction velocity. The affected genes are only now being discovered, and some blood tests are now becoming available.

The usual medications for treating sensory peripheral neuropathy are antiepileptic medications, particularly gabapentin, and tricyclic antidepressants, mainly nortriptyline and desipramine. All have selective effects on pain. Such treatment is not a cure, simply a way to reduce symptoms. In fact, there is no known cure for this common and frustrating disorder.

Diabetic Peripheral Neuropathy

The symptoms of diabetic peripheral neuropathy also begin with tingling and burning pain and then numbness in the toes and feet. In this case, however, we can link those symptoms to diabetes. Peripheral neuropathy is common in people with long-standing diabetes, usually of ten to twenty years' duration or more. Prolonged elevation of blood sugar appears to be the important factor, but exactly how this produces nerve damage is still controversial. The only known way to stabilize and sometimes improve diabetic peripheral neuropathy is through strict control of a person's blood sugar levels.

Peripheral Neuropathies That Develop over Months or Years

Many other chronic peripheral neuropathies also begin in the feet and spread gradually over months or years but involve motor nerve fibers. This causes weakness of the feet and ankles. A person ends up slapping his or her feet on the ground while walking. Eventually, the wasting of leg muscles may make walking or rising from a chair difficult. The person may still feel tingling, numbness, and perhaps pain alongside this weakness because of involvement of the sensory fibers. The sensory symptoms may slowly ascend from the feet to the legs and then appear in the hands and forearms if the condition continues to progress.

There are many possible causes for this motor-sensory type of peripheral neuropathy. The condition can be brought on, for instance, by prolonged exposure to such toxins as lead and arsenic (**C66**). In particular, certain medications can produce this side effect: these include some of the cancer chemotherapy drugs, strong immunosuppressants used after organ transplants, amiodarone (Cordarone) for heart irregularity, and statin medications for high cholesterol. The problem can arise from excessive doses of vitamin B_6 (pyridoxine), as advocated by some "nutrition experts," and heavy alcohol use (**C30**). These are all best managed by avoiding that toxin, if it can be identified.

Guillain-Barré Syndrome

Guillain-Barré syndrome (GBS) is an auto-immune disease of the peripheral nerves that causes weakness in the limbs and other body parts. It can be triggered by something as common and inescapable as a cold virus. Now that polio has been eradicated in developed countries, GBS has become the most common cause of general paralysis. Fortunately, the condition improves on its own or with treatment in most cases.

The illness usually begins with a feeling of pins and needles (paresthesias) in the feet and hands and with weakness of the legs. Both of these signs worsen over several days. Some people also suffer weakness of the facial muscles, similar to Bell's palsy (**C50**). GBS symptoms, both sensory and motor, characteristically affect both sides of the body more or less equally, which is quite different from the paralysis and sensory loss of a stroke (**C59**). As the illness worsens, weakness can become quite severe; most people who contract GBS are unable to walk within a week or so. About one in four will eventually have weakness of the muscles of breathing, which of course is very serious.

There are many variations on this pattern, and some people experience other symptoms of GBS:

double vision (diplopia; **C15**), severe clumsiness of walking and limb movement (ataxia; **C46**), severe weakness without changes in sensation, trouble swallowing, and so on. One particular constellation of problems is double vision and clumsiness, called Miller Fisher syndrome. Some people suffer rapid worsening over one or two days instead of several. GBS does not affect the mind, however; only the nerves in the arms, legs, and facial areas are involved.

In most instances the weakness worsens for several days, or up to two or three weeks, until the person's condition levels off. The severity of the weakness at this point is highly variable. A fraction of people with GBS—fewer than 10 percent—are still able to walk. Most are bed-bound at the disease's worst point. Some are almost completely paralyzed and need a respirator to keep breathing. The last group must be cared for in a hospital's intensive care unit. Being on a respirator means a patient must have a tube inserted in his or her trachea, which prevents speaking and eating, so the hospital must supply other means of communication and feeding. Many other problems occur in people severely affected by GBS because of their weakness and immobilization; pneumonia, urinary infections, and blood clots in the legs and lungs are the most frequent. A few people have an unusual problem with their autonomic nervous system that causes their blood pressure and pulse to fluctuate greatly (**C18**); this, too, requires special treatment.

What Causes Guillain-Barré Syndrome?

Throughout the world GBS occurs in about 2 people per 100,000 each year. Among these patients there is a very slight predominance of women, but the disease has no age, ethnic, regional, or seasonal predilection. Inheritance is not thought to be a factor; the cases in which different family members have contracted the illness have been very infrequent. There are no known ways to prevent GBS, but fortunately there are no signs that it is contagious.

More than one third of GBS cases begin some days after an infection with fever. The triggering infection is most commonly a cold or flulike illness, but it can also show up as diarrhea or other problems. Because people are often still getting over the fatigue and overall poor feeling of these illnesses, they sometimes attribute the GBS symptoms in their fingers and toes to the infections. Of the many people who suffer a particular infection in any given period, however, only a few—or none—will develop GBS. And in one-third of GBS cases, the individual and his or her doctors can identify no triggering infection.

In rare cases, GBS follows vaccinations of various sorts. Because of that slightly increased incidence, some have questioned the safety of administering vaccinations to people who have developed the condition before. After much dis-

cussion in the field, most doctors have decided in favor of giving vaccinations to those individuals who may be at risk of contracting the flu because the chances of serious complications from influenza are still far greater than the chance of contracting GBS from the immunization.

From these and other indications, we have come to recognize GBS as a temporary autoimmune disease. An infection or other challenge to a person's immune system leads his or her white blood cells to produce an immune protein that attaches to and damages the nerves. For instance, there is strong evidence that the body produces antibodies to fight off the diarrhea-causing bacterium *Campylobacter;* the antibodies then also react to the person's nerves. Other infections that often precede GBS are mononucleosis from the Epstein-Barr virus, pneumonia from mycoplasma bacteria, HIV infection, and hepatitis due to cytomegalovirus. In many cases an individual may not notice the infection, even as a low-grade fever, but his or her immune system still reacts. The misdirected immune attack usually strikes the cylinder of fatty material, myelin, that surrounds nerve fibers—a process called demyelination. In about 10 percent of cases the nerve fiber itself (the axon) is the site of the main damage. And many people with GBS have a combination of these two types.

Treating GBS

GBS is fairly easy for doctors to identify from a person's description of his or her symptoms and a neurological examination. They can establish the diagnosis with more certainty through electrical testing of the nerves (electromyogram) and sampling the spinal fluid to see if it shows an

CHRONIC INFLAMMATORY DEMYELINATING POLYNEUROPATHY

A small number of people with GBS, perhaps 5 percent, will get progressively worse over weeks and months instead of reaching a plateau after a few weeks and then gradually improving. Most of these have a chronic form of nerve disease termed chronic inflammatory demyelinating polyneuropathy (CIDP), which is similar to GBS except for its long duration and lack of reversal. Most cases of CIDP begin more slowly than GBS. In diagnosing the condition, doctors must differentiate it from a large group of other chronic neuropathies, such as those caused by diabetes (C48). CIDP may be treated similarly to GBS, but it also responds to corticosteroid drugs such as prednisone. Most people with this illness can retain their basic body functions with tolerable symptoms; however, only a few patients become nearly normal over time, and cure is infrequent. As with GBS, we now know no way to prevent CIDP.

increase in the amount of protein. Cases with unusual features may be more difficult to diagnose.

Neurologists usually direct the care of people with GBS. If major medical problems arise, or if respiratory failure requires the use of a ventilator, a specialist in intensive care, pulmonary medicine, or anesthesia usually becomes involved as well.

Several treatments seem to shorten the course of GBS, but they are not cures and they do not seem to influence the disease's course in all individuals. The first therapy shown to be effective was plasma exchange. This process starts with removing some of the patient's blood and spinning it in a centrifuge machine in order to separate the plasma from the blood cells. Only the cells are returned to the patient's body, with the missing

plasma replaced by an artificial fluid. In this procedure, a tube must be placed in one of the large veins of the chest or neck to bring enough blood to the centrifuge machine. Several treatments are performed over a week or two, each taking about two hours. The main risks have to do with injury to the lung from the tube. Most patients tolerate the treatment well, but some experience low blood pressure, fatigue, and tingling from time to time.

A newer and easier alternative is administering intravenous immunoglobulin (IVIG), several bottles daily for four or five days. The IVIG is obtained from the blood donations of many individuals, screened for viruses; the risk of contracting an illness from this procedure is extremely low. As with plasma exchange, improvement is usually not apparent immediately after treatment. Nevertheless, most studies have shown that these therapies cut in half the time it takes for a person to walk again. Certain patients are less likely to improve—for example, those with severe damage to the nerve fibers (axonal GBS).

A person with GBS is typically hospitalized for one to several weeks, during which he or she experiences slow improvement. The person then goes to a rehabilitation hospital or is discharged home with physical therapy visits. More severe cases—people who have been on a ventilator or have been virtually paralyzed—require months in the hospital and various types of rehabilitation afterward. Almost no people who develop GBS stay on a ventilator for the rest of their lives, but about 5 percent remain so weak that they need canes and braces or a wheelchair for years or indefinitely.

Improvement may continue in the most severely affected people for about two years. After that time it is still possible to make gains, but they are largely the result of overtraining of muscles with physical therapy and assistive devices. That is, improvement is not due to recovery from the neuropathy but to increased physical stamina and strength as a result of the exercise. Older people, particularly over 70, and those with severe damage to the axons are more at risk for having a long and probably incomplete recovery, but some patients in these categories have done well. Although medical teams have used many forms of rehabilitative therapy, no one program has proven superior overall; treatments must be tailored to the individual's pattern of weakness. Vitamins, health-food supplements, acupuncture, electrical stimulation, and other alternative treatments have not proven to be of any benefit.

Bell's Palsy

Bell's palsy involves a paralysis of the seventh cranial nerve. The condition is named after Sir Charles Bell (1774–1842), a surgeon and neurologist who described this nerve in detail and wrote the first clear descriptions of the disorder.

The cardinal symptom of Bell's palsy is a painful weakness of one side of the face. This weakness may develop within just hours, raising concern about a stroke (**C59, C60**), but it usually appears progressively over several days. The affected side of the face becomes smooth and wrinkle-free because the underlying muscles lose their tone. Weakness around one eye may interfere with a person's ability to blink and close that eye; on the lower face, the one-sided weakness can make it impossible to whistle, result in the face being pulled toward the side with normal muscle tone, and cause food to collect on the weak side of the mouth during eating.

Pain behind the ear often precedes the facial weakness by a day or two. Such pain associated with Bell's palsy is frequent but transient and not debilitating.

As for other symptoms, people may describe the heavy feeling caused by the facial muscles' paralysis as "numbness," but they do not really lose sensation there. Some astute observers may notice a loss of taste on half of the tongue. Sounds often appear louder on the side of the palsy. Because a person may blink less on one side, which is sometimes combined with a decrease in tear production, the affected eye can become dry and irritated from exposure to the air.

The muscle weakness bottoms out within a week, usually in two or three days. Then, after remaining unchanged for several weeks to several months, a person's face begins to improve. Satisfactory results, with problems limited to mild residual weakness and some difficulty coordinating the facial muscles, occur in more than 90 percent of Bell's palsy cases.

Diagnosis and Treatment

It is common for people suffering from Bell's palsy to worry about a stroke, and indeed paralysis or other neurological symptoms on one side of the body can be the first sign of that emergency. Some other neurological conditions begin with facial

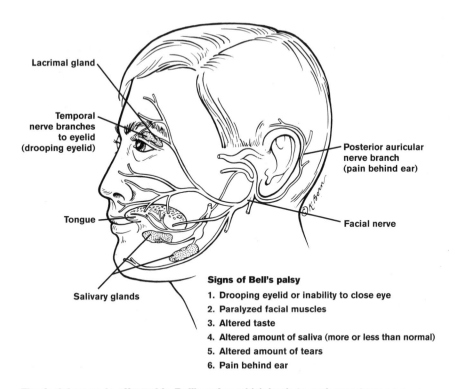

Lacrimal gland

Temporal nerve branches to eyelid (drooping eyelid)

Posterior auricular nerve branch (pain behind ear)

Tongue

Facial nerve

Salivary glands

Signs of Bell's palsy
1. Drooping eyelid or inability to close eye
2. Paralyzed facial muscles
3. Altered taste
4. Altered amount of saliva (more or less than normal)
5. Altered amount of tears
6. Pain behind ear

The facial nerve is affected in Bell's palsy, which leads to such symptoms as a drooping eyelid and paralyzed facial muscles. ILLUSTRATION © KATHRYN BORN

weakness as well, including sarcoidosis, multiple sclerosis (rarely), occasionally Guillain-Barré, and sometimes tumors. It is very important, therefore, to see a physician promptly when facial weakness or paralysis appears. Even if the problem turns out to be nothing more than Bell's palsy, prompt treatment has been shown to improve the already good chance of an excellent recovery.

While strokes affect the brain. Bell's palsy involves a nerve outside it. The seventh cranial nerve, which connects the brain stem to the facial muscles, is prone to attack by viruses. Several different viruses are implicated in the disorder, but herpes simplex appears to be the most frequent cause. Bell's palsy is a common affliction, annually affecting about 25 people out of every 100,000.

If doctors confirm the diagnosis of Bell's palsy within a week after symptoms start (and if there are no contraindications), they usually prescribe a seven-to-ten-day course of steroids (prednisone) and antiviral therapy (acyclovir).

Doctors will also offer therapy for the most damaging symptoms of the condition, which most often involves minimizing damage to an individual's eye from exposure. When a person cannot close one eyelid—his or her blinking is limited and the eye opens during sleep—the cornea of that eye is at risk. Measures to protect it may include:

- taping the eye partially shut using paper tape along the upper eyelid

- taping the eye completely shut using paper tape stretched from the upper lid to the cheek

- applying a neutral eye ointment underneath the taped lid at bedtime

- wearing glasses or sunglasses in waking hours to somewhat reduce exposure to the air

Artificial tears (methylcellulose eyedrops) may offer some relief, but they tend to wash out of an open eye rapidly. If you see the eye becoming red, you should quickly return to the doctor.

Stimulating the facial muscles by massage, acupuncture, or electrical stimulation offers no proven benefit. They usually recover on their own. In the rare event of severe residual weakness, a plastic surgeon can tighten the affected side of the face to "reanimate" it and improve a person's appearance.

Myopathies

Myopathies are disorders of the skeletal muscles, involving changes in either the structure or the function of those muscles. Their major symptoms include muscle weakness, pain, and fatigue. In their early stages, they can resemble diseases of the nerves that control the muscles, such as peripheral neuropathy (**C48**), myasthenia gravis (**C52**), and amyotrophic lateral sclerosis (**C53**). Therefore, even though myopathies do not necessarily involve the nervous system, physicians must consider them alongside nervous system disorders when trying to diagnose the cause of a person's weakness or fatigue.

Many myopathies arise from problems in the muscle tissue itself, either through a genetic defect (as in the various forms of muscular dystrophy) or as an acquired condition (most commonly in what are called inflammatory myopathies). This book cannot cover all the myopathies in detail but will focus instead on how doctors distinguish them from neuromuscular disorders and how they can be linked to other neurological problems.

Symptoms of Myopathies

Muscle weakness. Most muscle disorders cause persistent weakness, with the muscles closest to the trunk (the proximal muscles) weaker than those farther away (the distal muscles). Some diseases affect the muscles of the eyes, causing eyelid drooping (ptosis) and double vision (diplopia), as in myasthenia gravis (**C52**).

In certain disorders, the muscle weakness is intermittent. Symptoms may fluctuate drastically between severe weakness at one time to complete recovery at others. This is particularly characteristic of disorders in which the sources of energy for a muscle (fats and carbohydrates) are deficient and unable to support vigorous activity. Overworking the muscle causes its tissue to break down, accompanied by the release of a chemical called myoglobin into the bloodstream, which turns a person's urine dark brown. Intermittent symptoms are also typical of myasthenia gravis, especially of the eye muscles late in the day; swallowing and limb muscle strength also varies during the day and from day to day.

A doctor's examination may reveal a pattern of

weakness that helps in diagnosing a specific myopathy. Gowers' sign is particularly useful in revealing proximal weakness; individuals "climb their own limbs" as they get up from the floor.

When people's trunk and hip muscles are weak, their gait reveals an arching of the back and a tendency to walk on the toes. These same individuals demonstrate a "waddling gait" caused by their muscles' inability to hold the hips in a horizontal position; thus the hip drops or dips with each step.

Thigh muscle weakness causes a characteristic gait with a tendency for the knee to lock and curve backward (hyperextend) with each step.

If ankle muscles are weak, individuals tend to exhibit what is called foot drop—with each step, they have a hard time raising their moving foot. This predisposes an individual to tripping and falling (and perhaps breaking a bone).

Fatigue. Any disorder that causes muscle weakness can also bring on fatigue, which in this context means an inability to maintain a force. With weak muscles, individuals cannot sustain physical activities for very long; they become excessively tired. After all, they are attempting to perform the same movements with fewer or damaged muscle fibers. Such fatigue occurs in a variety of conditions: myasthenia gravis (**C52**), disorders altering the energy production of the muscles, such as mitochondrial myopathies, and many of the myopathies that cause a significant loss of muscle (such as muscular dystrophy).

The fatigue from myopathies is different from the excess tiredness or lack of energy that many individuals experience, although people may confuse these conditions. Tiredness usually also involves feeling sleepy and having difficulty concentrating.

Muscle pain. Symptoms of muscle pain, also called myalgia, may or may not be accompanied by weakness or swelling. Certain drugs, particularly those taken to lower cholesterol, cause true myalgia ("true" meaning that the pain is in the muscle, not merely felt there). Two important painful muscle conditions are not associated with muscle weakness:

- Fibromyalgia is a common but poorly understood pain syndrome. People with this condition complain of severe muscle pain and tenderness with specific trigger points, disturbed sleep (**C11**), and easy fatigability.

- Polymyalgia rheumatica occurs in people over age 50 and is characterized by stiffness and pain in the shoulders, lower back, hips, and thighs. A blood test called the erythrocyte sedimentation rate (ESR) shows values that are well above normal. Blood vessels to the scalp (temporal arteries) and eyes may be inflamed, with a risk of blindness and strokes. It is important to recognize polymyalgia rheumatica because doctors can relieve the discomfort and risk of blindness and strokes with corticosteroids, medication that reduces the inflammation of the blood vessels.

Muscle cramps. These are painful, involuntary, localized muscle contractions with a visible hardening of the muscle. They are usually abrupt in onset and short in duration, but the muscle may remain sore for an extended period. Cramps often occur when a muscle is irritated from overwork, or if there is a pinched or damaged nerve. They can also accompany Duchenne and related forms of muscular dystrophy.

Myotonia is a distinct form of cramp consisting of a prolonged muscle contraction followed by slow muscle relaxation. Myotonia always follows muscle activation, usually voluntary, but a doctor can elicit myotonia by striking the muscle with a reflex hammer. Myotonia makes it difficult for a person to release an object after grasping it firmly. Usually it becomes worse in cold temperatures and eases with continued activity. Myotonic muscular dystrophy is named for its symptoms of muscle weakness and myotonia.

Muscle enlargement or atrophy. In most myopathies, fat and scar tissue replace lost muscle tissue, so the size of the muscle is usually not affected. However, in Duchenne muscular dystrophy a person's calf muscles typically grow, due to increased fibrous tissue and fat replacement. A muscle can also appear enlarged when a tendon has ruptured, especially the biceps brachii tendon in the upper arm.

In contrast, *atrophy* refers to a decrease in the size of the muscle. It occurs slowly over time in long-standing myopathies. Muscle atrophy also occurs when there is nerve damage, as in polio, because the size of the muscle depends on nerve input.

Testing and Diagnosis

Doctors can diagnose any suspected myopathy with a limited battery of tests. Nearly all individuals require electrodiagnostic studies and blood tests. For some conditions, a muscle biopsy or DNA analysis may be very useful.

Electrodiagnostic studies. A very important test that measures the electrical activity of a person's muscle is often called an EMG. In actual practice, however, the term EMG applies only to an elec-

tromyogram, a needle examination of muscle. An EMG can determine whether weakness is due to an inflamed muscle, or which muscle is appropriate to sample for biopsy, and is also especially helpful in detecting myotonia.

Nerve conduction studies are almost always done as part of the electrodiagnostic examination. By electrically stimulating a nerve, doctors can measure how fast that nerve conducts the impulse. This may indicate that weakness is due to nerve damage rather than muscle damage. In combination, the EMG and the nerve conduction studies provide enough information to differentiate myopathies from other conditions causing weakness.

Another component of the electrodiagnostic examination, called repetitive nerve stimulation, detects the type of fatigue in a muscle that is characteristic of myasthenia gravis. This requires that the nerve be stimulated at very high frequencies and can be uncomfortable.

Enzymes. Another standard part of testing for myopathies is to take a blood sample and look for certain enzymes. The most important is creatine kinase (CK), which leaks into the blood after damage to muscles.

DNA analysis. Molecular biology now allows us to precisely identify certain myopathies caused by genetic mutations and the resulting defective proteins. After a doctor takes a blood sample, laboratory technicians extract DNA from the person's white blood cells and look for particular genetic markers. In some cases, a DNA test leads to a diagnosis without the need for other tests.

Muscle biopsies. Muscle biopsy analysis is an important step in establishing the final diagnosis of a suspected myopathy. This procedure requires removing a small sample of muscle for laboratory examination. The muscle selected depends on a variety of factors, including the degree of weakness and how the surgical procedure may affect the individual. Choosing a very weak muscle may show only scar tissue, so doctors try to avoid that.

A biopsy involves evaluating the muscle sample on a microscopic, cellular scale, using a combination of techniques.

- Histochemistry, or chemical tests on the cells: this can identify certain disorders leading to energy failure or pain in the muscle.

- Immune staining: a standard battery of antibodies can be applied to the sample to identify missing components of the muscle, thus helping to diagnose specific types of muscular dystrophies.

- electron microscopy: viewing the cells at great magnification to spot structural changes.

A muscle biopsy is of particular value in diagnosing the inflammatory myopathies.

Muscular Dystrophy

Muscular dystrophy is an umbrella term for a group of hereditary progressive diseases affecting the muscles. All are neuromuscular disorders.

Duchenne Muscular Dystrophy

This inherited disorder affects only boys: about 30 out of every 100,000 male babies. It is usually recognized when a boy of about age 3 or 4 falls frequently and has difficulty keeping up with his friends when playing. The problem is progressive, and by age 12, most boys who suffer from Duchenne use wheelchairs. By age 16 to 18, young men are predisposed to serious, sometimes fatal pulmonary infections. Boys with Duchenne dystrophy commonly also have some intellectual impairment, more so than children with comparably disabling disorders. This usually affects verbal ability most but, unlike the muscular problems, does not get worse over time (**C3**).

To diagnose Duchenne muscular dystrophy, doctors must perform a muscle biopsy or DNA blood test, looking for an abnormality in the protein dystrophin or the gene that creates it. If a mother has the defective gene, there is a 50 percent chance that it will be passed to a son or daughter. A son would develop the disease; a daughter would become a carrier. The DNA mutation can be identified in a fetus before birth through amniocentesis or chorionic villus sampling (CVS; see chapter 5).

Becker Muscular Dystrophy

Becker dystrophy results from defects of the same gene as in Duchenne dystrophy but is about ten times less frequent; it also strikes only boys. The defect is not as severe: though this condition also involves muscle wasting, it progresses much more slowly. Most people with Becker first experience difficulties between the ages of 5 and 15. By definition, those with Becker walk beyond age 15, while Duchenne boys are typically in a wheelchair by age 12. People with Becker dystrophy have a reduced life expectancy, but most survive into their fourth or fifth decade. The disorder affects the heart and in some cases leads to heart failure. Mental retardation (**C3**) in Becker dystrophy is not as common as in Duchenne.

Limb-Girdle Muscular Dystrophy

Limb-girdle muscular dystrophy (LGMD) actually represents more than one disorder, now distinguished by genetics:

■ LGMD1 refers to cases that are dominantly inherited, with a child having a 50 percent chance of inheriting the disease if one parent is affected. Five forms have been identified.

■ LGMD2 indicates autosomal recessive transmission, meaning that *both* parents must carry the affected gene for a child to inherit it. It is rare for either parent to have the condition. Ten forms of LGMD2 have now been identified, with more added every few months.

Muscle weakness in LGMD of any type affects both males and females, with onset ranging from the first to the fourth decade. Most cases are progressive and affect the pelvic and shoulder girdle muscles. A person's diaphragm may become so weak that he or she needs help to breathe. In some individuals the disorder weakens the heart muscle. The pattern of weakness and the rate of progression vary from person to person. Most people maintain normal intellectual function.

Myotonic Muscular Dystrophy

This disorder has an incidence of 13.5 per 100,000 live births, affecting males and females equally. It is the most common adult muscular dystrophy. Diagnosing the condition does not require a muscle biopsy. An EMG will show the myotonia, and a DNA test will easily reveal the genetic defect that causes it.

The symptom of myotonia usually appears by age 5, making it difficult for people to release objects after a firm grasp. The condition also produces weak neck muscles, wrists, hands, and fingers. Ankle weakness may cause foot drop. People's proximal muscles remain stronger throughout the course of the disease, in contrast to most types of muscular dystrophy, although many individuals develop weakness and selective atrophy of the quadriceps (thigh) muscles.

It is common for people with myotonic dystrophy to develop a nasal voice and swallowing problems. Some suffer weakness in their diaphragm and chest muscles, which results in breathing problems. Affected adults typically have a narrow-faced appearance due to atrophy of muscles of the face and jaw. Men are usually bald, and woman may have thin hair; how these latter signs relate to the muscle weakness or the genetic defect is unknown.

Most people with myotonic dystrophy suffer disturbances in their heartbeat, and some require pacemakers. Other features associated with myotonic dystrophy include mild intellectual impairment, sleep apnea and excessive daytime sleepiness (**C11**), and cataracts.

A very severe form of myotonic dystrophy occurs in about 25 percent of infants with affected mothers (not fathers). It is present at the time of birth and often causes swallowing and breathing problems. This congenital form of myotonic dystrophy is usually associated with mental retardation (**C3**).

Facioscapulohumeral Muscular Dystrophy

This form of muscular dystrophy affects approximately 1 in 20,000 people. It is inherited as an autosomal dominant disorder affecting males and females. The condition typically comes on in a person's teenage years or young adulthood. In most cases the first symptoms appear subtly in facial muscles: an inability to smile, whistle, or fully close the eyes. Later, individuals develop weakness of the shoulder girdles, making it hard to raise their arms. That weakness usually cues a young person to seek medical attention.

For most individuals, the weakness remains restricted to facial, upper extremity, and distal lower extremity muscles. In about 25 percent of cases, weakness progresses to involve the proximal lower extremities, producing great difficulty walking and perhaps necessitating the use of a wheelchair. Characteristically, people with facio-scapulohumeral dystrophy do not have heart involvement. A few individuals develop nerve deafness or loss of vision from retinal detachment; why this disease affects these senses is unknown.

Researchers have located the gene for facio-scapulohumeral dystrophy on chromosome 4 but have not detected the specific missing protein. Nevertheless, a very accurate diagnosis can be established by a DNA test.

Treating Muscular Dystrophies

The current treatment for muscular dystrophies is mostly supportive, aimed at improving people's quality of life. Individuals need help tailored for their physical needs—for example, braces, canes, scooters, and wheelchairs to get around.

Prednisone, a powerful anti-inflammatory drug in the corticosteroid family, has been shown to delay the progression of Duchenne muscular dystrophy. It must be administered cautiously, however, because of potentially severe side effects. It has not been shown to be helpful for other types of muscular dystrophy, with the exception of rare individuals with LGMD.

Experimenters continue to seek a definitive way to replace the proteins that are missing or abnormal because of these genetic diseases. Attempts to replace the protein directly have not

been successful; usually the protein breaks down before it reaches the muscle. Most researchers have turned their attention to gene replacement, trying to deliver to defective muscles a normal gene that will make the missing protein. Such treatment is not yet available for patients, but encouraging results in experimental animals with muscular dystrophy demonstrate that gene therapy looks promising for the future.

Inflammatory Myopathies

There are many forms of myopathies that are acquired during life rather than inherited. The three most prevalent all cause muscles to become inflamed and are grouped under the label "inflammatory myopathies." They all tend to come on slowly and insidiously, with weakness developing over weeks or months. They usually affect the proximal muscles and cause difficulty swallowing, among other symptoms. Despite overlap in symptoms, the disorders are distinct.

Dermatomyositis

This disorder can begin at any age from childhood to late life. The slowly progressive weakness affects the proximal muscles more than the distal, but both are involved. The weakness is commonly accompanied by fatigue and muscle aching. Many myopathies can produce these symptoms, but dermatomyositis is distinguished from all other conditions by a skin rash. Its name in fact comes from the root words for "skin" (*dermato-*) and "muscle inflammation" (*myositis*). The rash may precede the muscle symptoms and involve the fingers, the backs of the hands, the elbows, and the skin around the eyes. Many people develop a purplish discoloration of the eyelids, with swelling around the eyes and the rash extending onto the cheeks and forehead. Some people develop small calcium deposits over pressure points on their buttocks, knees, and elbows. The inflammation can affect other organs, causing heart failure, fibrosis (scarring) of the lungs, and swelling of the joints.

People with dermatomyositis have an increased risk for cancer, especially in the lung, breast, and colon. Dermatomyositis patients should be tested for cancer and be especially careful to avoid known cancer risk factors, such as smoking.

The diagnosis requires blood tests showing an elevated CK level, an EMG demonstrating irritability of the muscles from inflammation, and a muscle biopsy showing characteristic changes. The findings on biopsy distinguish dermatomyositis from other inflammatory myopathies.

Treatment can be very effective. A new approach is to use intravenous immunoglobulin (IVIG) as the first treatment—an infusion of antibodies straight into the blood system, usually repeated over several weeks or even months. In many cases this treatment must be combined with prednisone or other anti-inflammatory drugs. Individuals must work closely with their physicians to be sure that side effects are kept to a minimum.

Polymyositis

This disorder mainly affects adults; it is relatively rare in children. As with dermatomyositis, the symptoms may include slowly progressing weakness of the proximal muscles and swallowing difficulties, but there is no skin rash. Polymyositis can cause heart failure, fibrosis of the lungs, and joint swelling accompanied by aching. The risk for cancer is not as high as with dermatomyositis, but individuals do need to be screened for underlying tumors. The diagnosis is established by a CK blood test, EMG, and muscle biopsy. Polymyositis responds to prednisone and other anti-inflammatory drugs, but not to IVIG.

Inclusion Body Myositis

The third major type of inflammatory myopathy is a disease of older adults: most people with the disorder develop symptoms over age 50. The weakness in inclusion body myositis (IBM) has some unique features. In addition to causing proximal muscle weakness and swallowing problems, it typically affects the distal muscles. Individuals have notable hand weakness and may exhibit foot drop. CK in the blood is usually not as elevated as in the other inflammatory disorders and may even be normal. An EMG reveals the inflammatory process. The final diagnosis of this disorder depends on a muscle biopsy; the microscopic features permit an unequivocal diagnosis distinct from other inflammatory myopathies.

Unfortunately, treatment for IBM has minimal benefits. Prednisone or other anti-inflammatory drugs may help to a small degree but not significantly for any length of time. IVIG does not help people with IBM any more than drugs. This lack of effective treatment is frustrating both for individuals and for their doctors. Many researchers are now studying IBM to find a way to help people with this disorder.

Myasthenia Gravis

Myasthenia gravis means "serious muscle weakness," which indicates this condition's essential symptoms: weakness of the voluntary muscles and muscular fatigue. In this case, fatigue does not mean a feeling of tiredness but rather that a person's muscles become progressively weaker during activity. Often this weakness appears in characteristic patterns. The most common pattern affects the muscles of the eyelids and eyes. One or both lids may droop, or the person may experience double vision or blurriness with both eyes open. Early on, these symptoms may come and go at variable levels, but later they may become constant and more severe.

In about 80 percent of people with myasthenia, the initial eye symptoms become more severe and spread to additional muscle groups. These individuals may also develop difficulty in swallowing, trouble chewing (especially tough foods),

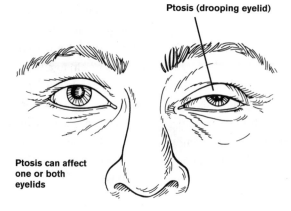

Ptosis (drooping eyelid)

Ptosis can affect one or both eyelids

A drooping eyelid, or ptosis, is the most frequent early sign of myasthenia gravis, a disease that produces extensive muscle weakness. ILLUSTRATION © KATHRYN BORN

slurred (dysarthric) speech, difficulty keeping their head erect, and weakness in their limbs.

An important characteristic of myasthenia is the variability of its symptoms from time to time. Characteristically, people suffering from the condition are somewhat better after waking up in the morning or after rest, and worse later in the day or after physical exertion.

Usually the visual symptoms and weakness cause a person with myasthenia to seek medical care. Because the early symptoms are so often variable, however, they can be easily confused with psychiatric disorders. Also, because many of the early symptoms affect the eyes, physicians often suspect some intrinsic eye problem. Double vision, for example, can also result from disorders of the eyes or orbits, aneurysms or tumors affecting the nerves to the eye muscles, and occasionally thyroid disorders (C15). The symptom of weakness is also common to a wide variety of problems affecting the brain, spinal cord, peripheral nerves, and muscles. The most important step in diagnosing myasthenia gravis may therefore be to suspect it in the first place. Since it is relatively uncommon, many physicians have either never seen a case or do not think of it. There is often a long period between the onset of symptoms and the diagnosis.

The Mechanism Behind Myasthenia

Myasthenia gravis is an autoimmune disease, meaning that it develops from within the body's own defense system. In fact, due to remarkable advances over the past 25 years, it is the best understood of all the autoimmune diseases. In this type of condition, a person's immune system, which normally fights germs and other invaders, produces antibodies that attack his or her own cells. Myasthenia gravis results when the body's defenses mistakenly produce antibodies that attack the acetylcholine receptors on skeletal (voluntary) muscles.

To understand how myasthenia causes problems, we must start with how nerves and muscles interact. To move any muscle—to breathe, swallow, speak, smile, or look in any direction—your nerves must transmit a signal to that muscle. An electrical impulse traveling down the motor nerve releases the neurotransmitter acetylcholine. The muscle receives this chemical signal in a specialized area, below the nerve, that is tightly packed with acetylcholine receptors. When the acetylcholine released from the nerve combines with the receptor on the muscle, a new electrical impulse is initiated within the muscle, which causes the muscle to contract.

If something interferes with the signal's transmission from nerve to muscle, the result is weakness and fatigue. In myasthenia, the problem is that antibodies attack the acetylcholine receptors, leaving too few of them available to receive the signal. The brain itself is not involved in myasthenia gravis, and the body's mechanisms for initiating movement at the level of the brain and spinal cord are intact. Even the peripheral nerves remain healthy. Only the acetylcholine receptors on the skeletal muscles are abnormal.

As we have learned more about myasthenia gravis, we have come to recognize it in more people. About 1 in every 7,000 individuals has the condition, and the rate may even be three times that. Females often develop it in their teens and twenties, while in men it usually appears in the fifth to eighth decades. However, myasthenia can occur at any age.

Why some people's immune systems erroneously attack their acetylcholine receptors is not clear. The answer in many cases seems to be re-

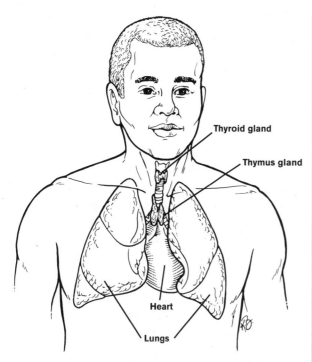

Thyroid gland

Thymus gland

Heart

Lungs

Although myasthenia gravis does not originate in the brain or nerves, it is an immune system attack on the receptors for acetylcholine, the neurotransmitter that commands muscles to move. About three quarters of all people with myasthenia have abnormalities of the thymus gland, which is suspected of being the source of the immune system's error. ILLUSTRATION © KATHRYN BORN

lated to the thymus gland, a lymph gland located under the breastbone that serves its main function during early development. About three quarters of all people with myasthenia have abnormalities of the thymus gland. Eighty-five percent of these show evidence of overactivity (hyperplasia) of the gland, and the other 15 percent have tumors there. We therefore suspect that the immune system's error may originate in the thymus gland.

Myasthenia may also occur in association with other autoimmune diseases, such as thyroiditis, lupus, and certain blood diseases. This suggests a more generalized error by the immune system in distinguishing between "self," which should not be attacked, and "nonself," which could represent a threat.

It is rare for myasthenia to be inherited. However, similar disorders of nerve-to-muscle transmission do have a genetic component. These are termed congenital myasthenic syndromes, and they are extremely rare.

Diagnosis and Treatment

Early diagnosis and treatment of myasthenia gravis are helpful because recovery is generally quicker the earlier a person begins treatment. The condition is diagnosed by the following methods:

1. Typical clinical features, such as the symptoms described earlier.
2. A blood test measuring antibodies to acetylcholine receptors; 80 percent to 90 percent of myasthenic people show these antibodies in their blood. (Surprisingly, only about half of people with weakness limited to the eye muscles seem to have positive results for this antibody test.)
3. Electrical tests with nerve stimulation and recording from muscles, to check how strongly signals are getting through.
4. Injection of edrophonium, which temporarily increases acetylcholine in the body by blocking the enzyme that usually breaks it down. If the body's response to this drug is better neuromuscular transmission for a short time, that is a useful clue to the problem.

It is also important to exclude other possible diagnoses.

One of the common myths about myasthenia is that it is severe, chronic, disabling, and untreatable. In fact, well over 90 percent of people who develop the condition can return to fully productive lives with proper treatment. Neurologists who specialize in neuromuscular disorders or immunological disorders have the most experience in treating myasthenia gravis successfully. Treatments fall into several categories.

Thymectomy. This is the surgical removal of the thymus gland; it provides long-term benefit for most patients. About 30 percent eventually achieve remission or resolution of their symptoms. About another 50 percent benefit partially. The surgery does not have an immediate benefit, however; improvement takes months to many years. As mentioned above, about 10 percent of people with myasthenia have tumors of the thymus gland. These tumors must be removed because they may spread locally and damage the important structures in the chest. Thymectomy should never be done as an urgent or emergency procedure, however. A person's overall condition, particularly his or her breathing, should be optimized before the surgery in order to assure a smooth and safe recovery. A thymectomy should only be done at a hospital where surgeons commonly perform the operation for myasthenia.

Anticholinesterase medications. The neurotransmitter acetylcholine acts very quickly on its receptor and is then rapidly broken down by an enzyme, as mentioned above. That enzyme is acetylcholinesterase. Drugs that cut back on the acetylcholinesterase in a person's body allow the existing acetylcholine to interact repeatedly with the receptors. In other words, the muscle receives multiple signals from a single neurotransmitter molecule. This partially improves muscle strength and function but is only a temporary measure.

Immunotherapy. The goal of immunotherapy is to modify the body's autoimmune attack against the acetylcholine receptors. Some treatments act more quickly or last longer than others. For relatively fast, short-term improvement, usually to get a person over a difficult period or to prepare him or her for surgery, doctors may carry out one of two procedures. *Plasmapheresis* uses a machine that separates the liquid portion of blood, which contains the troublesome antibodies, from the blood cells, and then returns only the cells to the person's veins. For most people this produces improvement within a week or so, but the effect is only temporary since their immune cells continue to produce antibodies. On average, the benefit lasts four to nine weeks. Infusing large amounts of immunoglobulin into a person's blood also produces benefits in a short time, benefits that last for weeks or a month or two. The immunoglobulin is available commercially, prepared from the blood serum of many individuals. Like plasmapheresis, this treatment is used to get a person with myasthenia over a difficult period.

There are several drugs that help suppress the immune system, thereby decreasing the autoimmune disease process. Adrenal corticosteroids (such as prednisone) and cyclosporin A are the most common. These drugs have many side effects, so they must be used with care. Working with skilled and experienced doctors, a person can usually avoid the medications' problems. Both types of drug work in a time frame of one to three months and often provide excellent benefit. Often these drugs are used in conjunction with other medications that work over the long term.

CONSERVING ENERGY IN MYASTHENIA GRAVIS

Many things can exacerbate myasthenic weakness temporarily, including infections (such as a cold, pneumonia, or even a tooth abscess), fever, excessive heat or cold, overexertion, and emotional stress. Here are some everyday tips on how to conserve energy.

■ Don't stand when you can sit.

■ Plan all activities and eliminate extra steps; assemble all the necessary equipment before beginning. Don't be embarrassed to ask for help.

■ Use a cart, wagon, or basket to carry several things from one part of the house to another, eliminating unnecessary trips back and forth.

■ To ease difficulty getting up from a sitting position, try leg extenders to elevate chairs.

■ Try a shoulder pad or intercom phone to completely free your hands when talking on the phone.

■ Avoid hot and cold weather extremes; they exaggerate weakness.

■ Try an electric toothbrush and toothpaste pump to conserve hand strength.

Adapted from www.myasthenia.org

This allows a person to take moderate doses of each drug, thereby minimizing the side effects while optimizing the therapeutic benefit. Two drugs that are prescribed for long-term benefit are azathioprine and mycophenolate. It is worth emphasizing that physicians with experience in managing myasthenia and prescribing these drugs should be in charge.

People with myasthenia gravis should learn as much as possible about their condition, any warning signs that it might get worse, and the side effects of their drugs. It is particularly important for people with myasthenia gravis to seek prompt attention in the event of an infection. Infection can make myasthenia worse because it prompts the body's immune system to work harder. At the same time, the immunosuppressive medications useful in treating myasthenia may increase a person's susceptibility to infections.

The goal of research is to devise new methods that will cure myasthenia gravis specifically. Current treatments require some suppression of the immune system as a whole, and, of course, a working defense system is important for a healthy body. An ideal treatment would suppress only the *abnormal* immune response affecting acetylcholine receptors. Research is now under way to target and eliminate the specific cells of the immune system that are responsible for the disorder. In the meantime, new immunosuppressive agents with fewer side effects are greatly improving the treatments available to people with myasthenia.

As noted above, most people with myasthenia can already expect to live virtually normal lives if they are properly treated. Their life expectancy and the variety of activities they can enjoy should be well within the ordinary range. Without treatment, however, the prognosis for myasthenia is serious. That makes early diagnosis all the more important.

Amyotrophic Lateral Sclerosis

In the United States, amyotrophic lateral sclerosis (ALS) is often called Lou Gehrig's disease, after the renowned baseball player who died of the condition in 1936. In France, ALS is called Charcot disease for the physician who first described it. "Motor neuron disease" is yet another name for the condition, because it affects the nerve cells that control movement, as opposed to those involved in sensation.

Whatever its name, the hallmarks of ALS are the degeneration and disappearance of the motor neurons. People affected by the disease gradually lose the ability to control voluntary movements. Almost all the symptoms of ALS are due to the resulting weakness. There are no sensory aberrations: no pain, numbness, or feelings of "pins and needles." The problems may start with clumsiness of the hands or, if the legs become weak, difficulty walking. Sometimes the muscles used in speech and swallowing are affected, so slurred speech may be another early manifestation. Other common symptoms are twitching muscles or cramps. Involuntary movements are not affected, so there are no problems with the stomach, intestines, or bladder. Sometimes people who are developing

ALS, or their family members, fear that they have had a stroke (**C59, C60**). More often, they are mystified by the symptoms.

Once ALS symptoms start, they become gradually worse and spread from one part of the body to another. The course is progressive, with no evident plateaus or periods of improvement. The disease produces increasingly severe disability. The average life expectancy with ALS after onset of symptoms is three to five years; about 20 percent of patients live more than five years. Progress in research has accelerated in the last decade, improving our hope for developing a cure, but we do not have one yet.

How ALS Works

ALS always affects the lower motor neurons, which send out the nerves that control the skeletal (voluntary) muscles. Motor neurons in the lower part of the brain control the tongue, speech, and swallowing. Lower motor neurons in the spinal cord are also affected, leading to weakness, wasting, and twitching, or "fasciculation," of muscles in the limbs. The normal function of

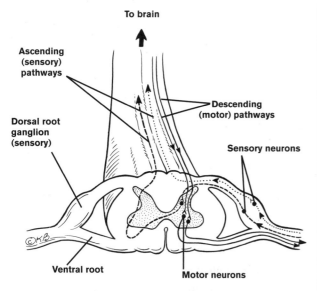

To brain

Ascending
(sensory)
pathways

Descending
(motor) pathways

Dorsal root
ganglion
(sensory)

Sensory neurons

Ventral root

Motor neurons

The lower motor neurons send out the nerves that control the skeletal (voluntary) muscles. Motor neurons in the spinal cord control muscles in the limbs, and those in the lower part of the brain control the tongue, speech, and swallowing. These neurons degenerate in ALS. When ALS affects upper motor neurons (located in the motor cortex and sending fibers down to the lower motor neurons), the result is stiff, clumsy arm and leg movements. ILLUSTRATION © KATHRYN BORN

muscle is dependent on receiving connections from lower motor neurons, and in their absence muscle degenerates.

Additionally, ALS affects neurons in other parts of the brain that control movement. One set lies in the motor cortex: the upper motor neurons, which send fibers down to the lower motor neurons. If these are malfunctioning, a person suffers stiffness and clumsiness of the arms and legs, with overactive tendon jerks. Among the signs that clearly indicate difficulties in the upper motor neurons, doctors find two especially helpful:

■ Babinski sign: normally when a doctor strokes the sole of a person's foot, the big toe moves

down. If the big toe goes *up* instead, that is a sign of malfunctioning upper motor neurons.

■ Hoffmann sign: when the doctor flicks the tip of a person's finger, the muscles normally do not react. If the person's upper motor neurons are not working properly, that finger quickly flexes.

The clinical diagnosis of ALS is accurate in about 95 percent of all patients. Physicians take a history and do a neurological examination, supplementing that information with findings in the electromyogram (EMG) that confirm the lower motor neuron disorder. Nerve conduction tests exclude diseases of the peripheral nerves that can simulate ALS (**C48**). Other procedures used include magnetic resonance imaging (MRI), lumbar puncture for examination of the cerebrospinal fluid, tests for antibodies that might attack nerves, and DNA tests if there is a family history of the condition. To diagnose the disease, a doctor must see signs of problems in the lower motor neurons; the diagnosis becomes more certain if, as in most cases, there are also upper motor neuron signs.

All these tests yield clues to ALS, but the diagnosis can be *proven* only by autopsy. This postmortem procedure can be done so that it does not alter the appearance of the body. It is of vital importance in confirming the diagnosis and also providing tissues crucial for research into what causes the disease and thus what may be effective treatment.

The nerve cells of people who die from ALS show abnormal structures called Bunina bodies. In addition, their muscle cells show accumulations of ubiquitin, a protein that seems to mark each cell for destruction through a process called apoptosis. The more we learn about these structures, the more likely it is that we will be able to intervene and spare the cells from premature death.

We do not know the cause of the nerve cell degeneration in ALS, but several possible abnormalities may lead to the death of motor neurons. Most researchers now favor an explanation called excitotoxicity, whereby accumulations of the amino acid glutamate overstimulate the cells. Other theories blame the formation of free radicals or the excessive accumulation of normal neuronal structures called neurofilaments, which may block the transport of essential nutrients within the nerve cell. Researchers are investigating all of these theories in hopes of finding a way to prevent or treat and reverse ALS.

Patterns of ALS

About 25,000 people have ALS in the United States on any day. This contrasts with 500,000 to 1 million people with Parkinson's disease, and 4 million with Alzheimer's disease. But life expectancy is the shortest with ALS.

Most people with ALS suffer no loss of intellectual functions. About 5 percent to 10 percent suffer a particular kind of cognitive loss called frontotemporal dementia; this affects memory and other brain functions needed for normal daily life (**C69**).

About 95 percent of all cases of ALS are sporadic, meaning that no relatives of the affected person have had the disease. The cause of sporadic ALS is not known. The only clear risk factor is advancing age. There are almost no cases before age 20; 10 percent to 20 percent of people with ALS develop it before 40; and after that age, the frequency increases with each decade. Men are slightly more likely to be affected than women.

Some studies have found evidence that occupation, trauma, and rural life are factors in ALS, but this evidence is inconsistent. A form of the disease may be associated with cancers, and viral infections have also been suspected without consistent proof.

The remaining 10 percent of all cases of ALS are familial, usually in the pattern called autosomal dominant. Every child of a person with this type of ALS has a 50 percent chance of developing the disease. In 1993 one form of familial ALS was found to be associated with mutations in the gene for an enzyme called superoxide dismutase. This discovery opened the gates for a flood of research pointing to different mechanisms that could cause ALS in both sporadic and familial forms. We should learn even more about the overall disease when we isolate the causes of other forms of familial and nonfamilial ALS.

Treatment and Care

As ALS advances, the person requires more and more help with daily tasks: walking, sitting up, eating, going to the bathroom. The final stages of the disease are characterized by paralysis of limb muscles, inability to speak or swallow, and finally inability to breathe. The challenge to the ALS care team is to keep the patient comfortable by treating these symptoms as necessary. There are effective ways to help patients who have difficulty communicating, swallowing, or breathing. Throughout the country ALS centers have been formed, bringing together the skills of neurologists, nurse clinicians, physical therapists, respiratory specialists, psychiatrists, clergy, and hospice workers. In most of these centers, a neurologist leads the team. These facilities are the best resource for families facing the multiple challenges of ALS.

Such a grave disease brings nonmedical problems as well. Both patients and their families face the emotional challenges of dealing with the disability and looking ahead to further deterioration. Financial problems arise because a person with ALS cannot work and needs a full-time caregiver, either another member of the family, who must forgo earning money, or a paid professional. Legal questions may complicate the picture. No aspect of family life is spared. The guiding principle of managing the disease is patient autonomy, and medical teams must provide people with ALS and their families with the information they need to make choices. Ultimately the choice is between living as long as possible while depending on a mechanical ventilator, or using a hospice service to be as comfortable as possible without prolonging life.

The Food and Drug Administration has approved only one drug for the treatment of ALS: riluzole (Rilutek). It works against glutamate, the natural amino acid that plays a normal role in the excitatory functions of motor neurons and is thought to accumulate in ALS. Riluzole is believed to extend the life of a person with ALS by an average of three to six months, but there is no visible effect—there is no improvement either in symptoms or quality of life. Frustrated by this limited benefit, researchers are running trials of many new drugs, hoping to find a more effective treatment. Many patients are drawn to participating in these experiments in the hope that they'll be among the first ALS sufferers to be cured, or that their experiences will help others. People with ALS are also often lured to alternative medicine; many take vitamin E or selenium, for instance. Unfortunately, these therapies have not been shown to be helpful.

The prospect for discovering better treatments for ALS in the coming decades is excellent. In what was once a totally neglected field, neuroscientists are now actively engaged in several lines of work that could lead to therapies. It is worth remembering that doctors once perceived pernicious anemia and its neurological form, combined system degeneration, as inescapably fatal. Once researchers determined that this disease was caused by a deficiency of vitamin B_{12}, the entire picture changed. Now we can measure vitamin B_{12} in the blood and readily correct low levels with injections. That severe disease has virtually disappeared. ALS may not turn out to have such a simple cause, but with hard work and a little luck we will surely find effective solutions. We are confident that ALS will prove to be a treatable disease.

CHAPTER 17

Pain

C54   Headache   540

C55   Migraines   548

C56   Back Pain and Disk Disease   553

C57   Chronic Pain   559

C58   Trigeminal Neuralgia   565

"Doc, it hurts when I do this," says a man in a very old joke. "Well, don't do that," the doctor replies. And in most cases, that is useful advice about pain (**B5**). Pain is the body's way of telling us *not* to grab a hot pan, step on a sharp rock, run another six miles, or do something else that would cause us physical harm. Even a minor, transient pain like a headache can be a sign that a person should change his or her behavior, or (in rare cases) an early alarm about a threat to health. Much as we all want to avoid pain, life would be very hard without its warnings.

This chapter does not address those sorts of pain, from sources we can easily identify and avoid. Instead, most of the sensations discussed in the following pages are recurrent or nearly constant. Such suffering can interfere with sleep, concentration, freedom of movement, and the ability to enjoy life. Sometimes the problem is physical: a spinal disk, blood vessel, or tumor may be pressing directly on nerve tissue. For a few people, the pain system itself seems to have gone haywire, and pain becomes a chronic condition they must manage.

Headache

We don't expect pain to be a part of daily life. So why do so many people suffer from regular headaches? Some of these pains serve a useful purpose as a warning of life-threatening disease, such as meningitis (**C37**) or cerebral hemorrhage (**C60**). But often recurrent and severe headaches seem to serve no obvious purpose. They simply cast a shadow over the enjoyment of life.

Certain people seem especially prone to headaches, and the cause appears to lie in the brain. Our brains are equipped with an internal pain-control system that damps down the perception of unwanted stimuli. These feelings can be leg pain in a long-distance runner, or head pain from dilated blood vessels or excessive contraction of jaw, scalp, and neck muscles. The system depends on chemical neurotransmitters, serotonin (5-hydroxytryptamine) and noradrenaline, to pass the pain-control message from centers in the midbrain (periaqueductal gray matter and the locus ceruleus) downstream to the cells in the brain stem and upper spinal cord that receive pain impulses from the head and neck. It is likely that in people susceptible to headaches this pain-control system is more delicate. Trigger factors

such as excitement, emotional upsets, heat, glare, noise, strong perfumes, missing meals, or sleeping late can bring on undampened pain. This susceptibility is also often inherited.

A person who never suffers from an occasional headache is very lucky indeed. A survey of 1,000 people in Denmark found that over a person's lifetime, the likelihood of ever experiencing a hangover headache was 72 percent, a tension headache 69 percent (including 3 percent in whom headaches recurred nearly every day), a migraine 15 percent, and the pain of sinusitis 15 percent. Disorders of the neck and headaches associated with coughing, exertion, and sexual activity had each affected 1 percent of the people surveyed. This section discusses each of these types of headaches except migraine, which is covered in section **C55.**

Most headaches are not associated with any underlying problem in the head and are thus called benign. If you are subject to an occasional tension headache that disappears with acetaminophen, aspirin, or another over-the-counter pain reliever, you do not need to seek further remedy. But if your tendency to have headaches is recent or your headaches are becoming more frequent or severe, see your doctor. You may be referred to a neurologist for specific diagnosis and treatment. A few types of headache, and only a few, require urgent attention. Most forms can be treated satisfactorily to restore your natural freedom from pain.

"Thunderclaps" and Other Serious Headaches

Any bad headache occurring suddenly for the first time—a "thunderclap headache"—warrants immediate investigation. The sudden onset of a severe headache, particularly if accompanied by neck stiffness, can signal that blood is leaking into the subarachnoid space surrounding the brain, usually from a leaking aneurysm (a blowout of a major cerebral artery). This may lead to a hemorraghic stroke (**C60**). A sudden surge of blood pressure can cause a similar thunderclap headache. Meningitis and other serious illnesses can also appear in this manner (**C37**).

Sex headache. Another, more benign cause of thunderclap headache for some people is sex. As sexual excitement builds up, muscle tension in the head and neck increases. A person may feel this as a dull headache, and, if he or she proceeds to orgasm, may experience a sudden, severe explosive headache at the moment of climax. This feeling may persist for some hours afterward (the headache, unfortunately, not the climax). This variety of sudden, severe headache is caused by the rapid elevation of blood pressure at orgasm. (On occasion, that spurt in blood pressure has even caused some people to suffer a cerebral hemorrhage; **C60**.) Sex headaches bear some relation to the exertional headaches mentioned on page 543, but they may also develop when a person becomes sexually excited even without physical exertion. Naturally, this explosive headache worries people, not to mention how it interferes with the enjoyment of life.

Once imaging and other tests have excluded more serious causes for this problem, people who have recently suffered from sex headache can simply desist from sexual activity when they feel a headache coming on. Fortunately, these headaches are capricious; they may occur a few times and then never again. If the tendency persists, using a noradrenergic beta-blocker like propranolol may prevent them.

Progressive headache. Less-than-severe headaches that grow progressively worse are also cause for worry. Following a blow to the head, even a minor one, bleeding from a cerebral vein can cause increasing pressure on the brain (**C61**). Someone with this symptom should see a physician immediately. In people older than 55, scalp arteries can become inflamed (temporal arteritis); doctors should suspect and treat this condition early because the inflammation can spread to the arteries supplying the eyes and thus cause blindness.

Brain tumors may also cause headaches of progressive severity as the growing tissue presses against the arteries of the brain (**C10, C64**). Fortunately, these are rare compared with the many other types of headaches in life. Pressure within the cranium may also increase without any brain tumor being present. This is called idiopathic intracranial hypertension, and it usually occurs in obese young women. It is usually associated with blurred vision and must be treated before it can cause blindness (**C15**). (The opposite condition, *low* intracranial pressure, is uncommon except after a person has had a lumbar puncture it appears as a headache that starts when the person stands up.)

Cough headache. Headache brought on by coughing, sneezing, or straining can be a serious symptom. It may indicate a valvelike obstruction blocking the normal cerebrospinal fluid channels in the brain (the ventricles), or a displacement of pain-sensitive blood vessels by a brain tumor (**C10, C64**). Once these unpleasant possibilities have been ruled out by computed tomography (CT) scanning or magnetic resonance imaging (MRI) of the brain, the problem is labeled "benign cough headache." People suffering from this condition, usually middle-aged, benefit from having the blood flow in their carotid and vertebral arteries, which feed the brain, checked to ensure that they are not narrowed by fatty material (atheroma). Physicians do not have to inject anything into the arteries to do this; they can use an ultrasound tool instead. Cough headaches usually respond to indomethacin, a medication that reduces inflammation.

Vascular Headaches

Some pains stem from the blood vessels in the head: dilated arteries set up a headache that throbs with each pulse. On occasion, sufferers notice that arteries in their forehead and temple become swollen and tender, and that pressure on these areas may ease the pain. The most common of these headaches is migraine (**C55**).

Cluster headache. An uncommon but intriguing syndrome is cluster headache. This mainly affects males, while migraine and tension headaches affect women more usually. Cluster headaches generally start in a person's teens or twenties, but some cases start in infancy. The name *cluster headache* derives from the unusual pattern of

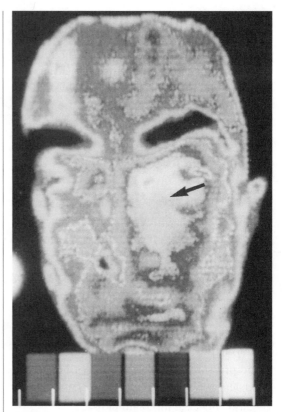

Cluster headache. The arrow in this thermal scan points to a "hot spot" of increased blood flow during a cluster headache. FROM LANCE, J. W., *MIGRAINES AND OTHER HEADACHES*, SIMON & SCHUSTER, SYDNEY, 1998

headaches recurring in bouts lasting for weeks or months, separated by periods of freedom for months or years. During each bout the victim experiences one or more episodes of severe pain for several hours at a time, usually felt behind one eye but often radiating over the head or down the face. The eye on the affected side reddens and waters, the eyelid droops, and the nose becomes stuffy.

Cluster headaches may come on at a particular hour of the day, as though set by an internal alarm clock. If sufferers travel from New York to California, they continue to have their headaches on New York time until their sleep cycles and other internal clocks adapt. This internal timekeeper probably lies in the hypothalamus, where positron-emission tomography (PET) scanning has shown a "hot spot" of increased metabolism during headache episodes.

Bouts of cluster headache can usually be suppressed by such medication as verapamil (Calan SR), methysergide (Sansert), or prednisone (Cortan). Most people can shorten the duration of the pain if they inhale 100 percent oxygen or, if the headaches are truly debilitating, inject the drug sumatriptan (Imitrex).

Exertional headache. Headaches provoked by exercise are quite common in young people because the blood vessels in the cranium swell up and become sensitive to pain. These headaches can often be avoided by taking a vasoconstricting agent such as ergotamine just before one plans to exercise. After the headaches have started, they usually respond well to the anti-inflammatory agent indomethacin.

Hangover. Alcohol can cause headache by dilating blood vessels in the head. Wines contain substances that may precipitate this headache in some unfortunate people. In most countries, drinkers blame red wine for the worst hangovers, but in France, for some obscure reason, headaches are attributed more often to white wine. The "morning after" headache probably results from the breakdown of the alcohol into acetaldehyde and acetate—these chemicals cause a painful relaxation of arteries inside the skull.

Caffeine. Coffee, tea, and many soft drinks contain caffeine, which constricts blood vessels. They can thus help relieve those types of head-

aches in which blood vessels are dilated. But that effect wears off in a few hours, sometimes leading to caffeine withdrawal headaches. Often a person relieves that pain with more caffeine, thus starting a cycle.

Marijuana. Cannabis dilates blood vessels and thus may bring on a mild frontal headache. On the other hand, tension headaches may be relieved because of the relaxation this substance induces. Of course, the legal problems that marijuana possession can create are a different and more troubling sort of headache.

Tension Headaches

The all-too-common tension headache is a constant tight or pressured feeling, like a band around the head or a weight on top of it. It may be brought on by concentration, worry, emotion, fatigue, eyestrain, or exposure to flickering light, glare, or noise. In many cases a tension headache is associated with poor posture, frowning, or jaw clenching; some sufferers recognize that they grind their teeth in their sleep. If a person is also feeling anxious or depressed, the frequency of tension headaches may increase until they occur every day and persist all day.

Another cause of chronic daily headaches is the frequent use of acetaminophen, aspirin, or other medications to relieve tension or migraine headaches; the headaches rebound the next day, leading to a further intake of analgesics, which sets up a vicious circle perpetuating the headache. If people suffering from episodic migraine headaches (C55) become anxious or depressed, or if they overuse pain relievers, their headaches become more frequent and may appear daily (a condition called transformed migraine). People suffering from daily headaches need to avoid any underlying source of stress whenever possible, practice muscular relaxation (with or without some form of biofeedback), maintain a comfortable upright posture ("think tall"), and learn to manage any associated psychological problem or depression.

Interestingly, the most effective treatments for frequent tension headaches are the tricyclic antidepressants amitriptyline, dothiepin, and imipramine taken daily; this treatment often controls these headaches even when a person is not depressed. They probably act on the brain's pain-control pathway by increasing the supply of serotonin and noradrenaline. The newer antidepressants called selective serotonin reuptake inhibitors (SSRIs) are not nearly as effective in relieving headaches as the older tricyclics. In fact, they may sometimes exacerbate the problem.

AVOIDING AN AIR TRAVEL HEADACHE

If you are traveling by air while your nose is blocked, carry a nasal decongestant. Otherwise you may feel intense pain on descent. The rise in air pressure as the plane nears the ground naturally increases the pressure on your sinuses. You may not realize that the sinus openings are blocked by mucus until you feel pain in those parts of your head.

The effect of changing air pressure on sinuses and ears is also the usual reason babies scream as an airplane descends. Keep your small children sucking and swallowing to equalize the air pressure inside their sinuses and middle ear with that of the outside air.

Headaches Arising from Structures in the Face and Neck

Sinusitis. Sinuses are cavities in the forehead (frontal sinuses), behind the bridge of the nose (ethmoid and sphenoid sinuses), and in the cheek bones (maxillary sinuses). Normally they contain air, and they open into the nasal cavity so that any mucus in them can drain freely. If the nostrils or the openings from the sinuses into the nose are blocked, however, mucus accumulates in these cavities under pressure and may become infected. People may then experience pain and tenderness over one or more of the sinus areas.

The treatment for sinusitis involves constricting the swollen vessels in the lining of the nostrils through nose drops and sometimes pills containing pseudoephedrine (Sudafed). This enlarges the airway and allows free drainage from the sinuses into the nose. If you are having headaches and facial pain at regular intervals without a blocked nose, you probably have a vascular headache such as migraine rather than sinusitis.

Temporomandibular joint (TMJ) dysfunction. An irregular bite and a tendency to grind the teeth while sleeping or to clench the jaw during the day can lead to pain and crackling noises in the hinge joints of the jaw. TMJ pain can radiate up or down from the area immediately in front of the ears and cause headache and facial pain. A person with this problem, also called Costen's syndrome, may need to wear protective dental splints at night. Often, however, being aware of the cause, doing relaxation exercises, and taking a small dose of amitriptyline at night to promote muscular relaxation are enough to relieve the trouble.

Neck problems. The back of the head is served by nerves in the second and third cervical roots.

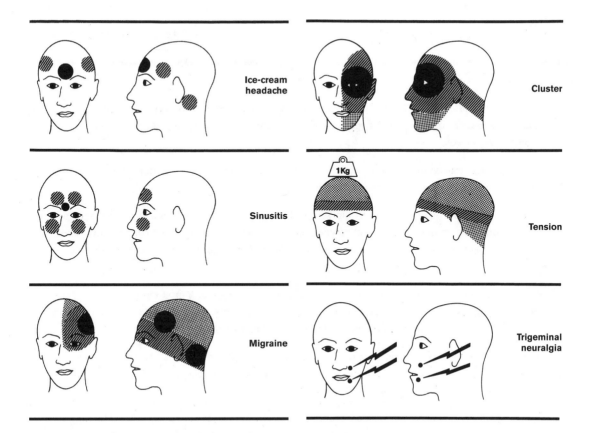

Headache and facial pain have distinctive points of origin and characteristic areas of pain.
FROM LANCE, J. W., *MIGRAINES AND OTHER HEADACHES,* SIMON & SCHUSTER, SYDNEY, 1998

Degeneration of the side joints of these upper cervical vertebrae can produce pain. Because the impulses coming into the spinal cord at this level converge on the same cells that convey sensation from the face and head, a person may end up feeling pain in the eye and forehead on the affected side. This is an example of "referred pain."

In an interesting variation on this condition, a person can feel pain and numbness in the upper neck along with a feeling of numbness or movement in half the tongue on the same side when he or she rotates the neck forcibly. This is particularly common in adolescents playing tennis or any sport in which the neck turns suddenly. It has been called the neck-tongue syndrome and is usually nothing to worry about, but people who notice this problem should avoid extreme neck movements.

Neuralgia. Any disturbance of the cranial nerves conveying pain from within the skull may set up a stabbing or continuous pain, termed neuralgia. The most common type is trigeminal neuralgia, or tic douloureux (C58), a severe jabbing pain in the jaw or cheek. It is usually caused by a small artery touching the trigeminal nerve and can

TREATING HEADACHES

These therapies can potentially minimize the causes of your headaches and significantly decrease the frequency or severity of your attacks.

■ **Relaxation training:** Relaxation training teaches you, first, to recognize your body's involuntary responses to stress (all of which can be measured) and, second, to modify your responses and reduce your body's stress level.

■ **Progressive muscle relaxation:** By contracting and relaxing the different muscle groups of the body in succession, you may feel a sense of deep relaxation.

■ **Guided imagery:** When you draw on your "mind's eye" through guided imagery, you see and take control of your body's stress points and visualize yourself in a relaxed setting in which you let go of tension. Some people have been able to use this technique to stop a migraine early on or to reduce its pain.

■ **Diaphragmatic breathing:** This approach would be used at the first sign of a prodrome, the first phase of a migraine, which occurs days or hours before an attack. It prevents the rapid and shallow breathing that typically follows the onset of migraine and that actually increases head and neck pain.

■ **Biofeedback:** By monitoring your body's involuntary physical responses—such as breathing, pulse, heart rate, temperature, muscle tension, and brain activity—biofeedback equipment helps you refine and perfect your relaxation exercises.

■ **Acupuncture:** This is an ancient Chinese procedure that blocks pain by stimulating nerves. Although it does not affect the cause of chronic headaches, nor is it believed to prevent or cure a headache, acupuncture may offer relief to some headache sufferers.

■ **Physical and massage therapy:** Physical therapy, which stretches and strengthens the muscles, can relieve muscle tension resulting from stress or physical habits. Massages—to the neck, temples, lower skull, and shoulders—may also alleviate tension and tightness associated with headaches.

■ **Counseling psychotherapy:** Although chronic headaches may not be psychosomatic, they can be caused by depression or anxiety. Thus, counseling can help you identify and address emotional concerns and should be considered as part of your treatment.

Adapted from www.headaches.org

generally be controlled with carbamazepine or other medications and cured by a surgical procedure.

Other Benign Headaches

Ice cream. Swallowing a cold drink or ice cream can evoke a sudden pain in the palate, throat, or forehead. Such "ice-cream headaches" are more common in people prone to migraines. They are easy to avoid.

Cold and pressure. Exposure to icy winds or diving into very cold water can rapidly induce a headache through excessive stimulation of the scalp nerves. The same nerves can be squeezed by a tight hat or goggles worn while swimming ("swim-goggle headache").

Foods and fasting. Nitrites are added to some cured meats to maintain their red color. A few people are sensitive to nitrites, even the small amounts used, and thus suffer "hot-dog headache" as the chemicals dilate the blood vessels in their heads. Monosodium glutamate (MSG) is also widely used as a food additive and may cause headaches on occasion. Low blood sugar after missing meals or fasting for a day not uncommonly induces headaches.

As we described at the start of this section, most of the headaches people experience are benign—passing annoyances that home treatment can remedy. Talk to your doctor about any headaches that are sudden, severe, recurrent, or growing progressively worse.

Migraines

Migraine attacks account for the bulk of headache-related visits to physicians. In contrast to other headaches (**C54**), migraine is characterized by episodes of head pain that is moderate to severe, pulsing, and often on only one side. The pain typically lasts 4 to 72 hours and worsens with physical activity. Nausea and vomiting so frequently accompany a migraine headache that these symptoms help define the problem.

About 15 percent of migraine headaches are also preceded by an aura—a neurological symptom that begins gradually over minutes and typically persists less than an hour. Most often an aura appears as a slowly expanding visual disturbance, usually starting at the center of a person's vision and spreading to the edge, with shimmering and wavy images. Severe headache follows the aura. Typically within 15 to 20 minutes, a person suffers nausea, vomiting, and sensitivity to light, sound, and smell, particularly after the aura has disappeared.

Some migraine sufferers, or "migraineurs," sense tingling or numbness on one side, particularly in the arm, hand, and face, that then spreads like the visual aura. Other people may experience difficulties with language, balance, or weakness.

In some cases, euphoria, increased energy, or depression can precede a headache, with abnormal cravings for certain types of food that may last up to 24 hours.

Migraine headaches may be incapacitating, requiring a person to take time off from work or other important activities. Another factor that brings migraineurs to the doctor are the related neurological symptoms. The aura can be disturbing. Sufferers sometimes worry that the symptoms are the first sign of a brain tumor (**C64**), stroke (**C59, C60**), or epilepsy (**C13**). Fortunately, a physician can readily distinguish between epilepsy and migraine and rule out the more sinister diagnoses through brain imaging. Furthermore, it's rare for the neurological symptoms and signs to persist in migraine, but a brain tumor or stroke creates an ongoing dysfunction of the nervous system affecting vision, sensory, or motor activity.

Who Gets Migraines?

Before the age 11, migraine is equally common in boys and girls—which is to say, not

FEMALE HORMONES AS FACTORS IN MIGRAINES

Migraine attacks affect women three times more often than men. That female predominance appears in adolescence at around the same time as menarche. About 60 percent of migrainous women link their attacks to their menstrual periods, and 14 percent report that the migraines begin only within 48 hours of menstrual flow. For these reasons, it is thought that fluctuations in ovarian steroid hormones influence the susceptibility of many women to migraines, but the exact interaction is still not understood.

Female migraineurs have higher estrogen and progesterone levels during the premenstrual phase than other women. However, the headaches may be triggered more by sudden *changes* in hormonal levels than by their absolute levels. Trying to prevent menstrual migraine by taking estrogen delays the attacks but doesn't block them, and many women experience significant worsening after estrogen treatment. The relationship between ovarian hormones and migraine headaches thus remains a frustration. Fortunately, the other side of that relationship is that when certain of a woman's hormones stop flowing after menopause, the migraines become less common.

very common at all. Migraines commonly begin in the second or third decade of life and become less frequent after middle age. In adulthood, migraine headaches both with and without auras occur more commonly in women than in men, in a 3-to-1 ratio. Surveys in industrialized countries show that 10 percent to 12 percent of people suffer migraines in a given year, 15 percent to 18 percent of women and 6 percent of men. Most migraine sufferers experience attacks less than once a month. Typically, about 60 percent of migraineurs suffer fewer than eight attacks per year, 25 percent have eight to fourteen per year, and 15 percent have more than fourteen per year.

There is a widely held impression that migraine occurs more commonly in individuals with greater intelligence, more education, or higher social class. Comforting as this belief may be for a migraineur, it's not supported by data from the general population. In fact, people with lower socioeconomic status appear to be at greater risk, perhaps because the condition is associated with stress.

Perfectionism was also thought to predispose a person to migraines, but a rigorous measurement of obsessionality among people suffering from the problem hasn't shown that to be a risk factor. There is, however, good evidence that migraineurs are at a higher than usual risk for depression (C20) and anxiety and panic disorders (C21). Depression in this instance is not just a response to the headaches; it often appears before the onset of migraine. Of course, the recurrent pain and debility can make depression and anxiety worse.

A wide variety of factors in the environment are thought to trigger migraine attacks, though these are rarely reliable or predictable. Several triggers may have to combine to precipitate a person's headache, possibly during a vulnerable period. Some of the most frequently reported causes include certain foods or food additives, too much or too little sleep, fasting or missing a meal, strong odors, changes in weather (especially barometric pressure), flickering or glaring light, emotional upset, physical exertion, and fluctuation in hormonal levels.

The biological basis for migraine is not well understood but is being carefully studied. Because so many people suffer migraines, the condition may have a lot to tell us about the brain's normal organization and function. New techniques developed over the past two decades are beginning to provide more focused investigations, especially in genetics, the mechanisms of pain generation, and the changes in the brain that occur during the aura.

At present, two theories shape thinking about the biological basis for an attack. The first assumes that the aura is caused by a temporary lack of blood to the brain due to a contraction and narrowing of the blood vessels, and that the headache develops from the subsequent expansion of those vessels, which activates the pain fibers around them. As evidence to support this theory, the drugs most commonly used to stop a migraine attack act to constrict blood vessels. The main competing theory suggests that migraine arises primarily from a disturbance in the brain, and the abnormal brain cell functioning is what disturbs the blood vessels. Proponents of this hypothesis say the narrowing and widening of the vessels are neither necessary nor sufficient to generate the migraine symptoms. There are indeed multiple neurological symptoms during the aura that would be difficult to blame entirely on the blood vessels in a specific region of the head. If applied rigidly, neither theory explains all the features of an attack.

Migraine attacks can be divided into stages, and the initiation stage is the least understood. Some researchers have suggested that there is a migraine generator in the brain stem; this would act as a control switch, rendering people more or less susceptible and conceivably activating an attack itself. Other studies suggest that the attacks start in the cerebral cortex with an event closely resembling a spreading excitation of cells within the brain, not unlike what migraineurs experience during the flashing light of a visual aura. This spreading excitation is then followed by a "quieting" or depression of neuronal activity. Researchers have found evidence for this latter theory by using a variety of imaging techniques on the brains of people suffering attacks. These recent studies confirm that a migraineur's brain is unusually susceptible to slow spreading waves across the cerebral cortex.

A number of twin studies show that identical twins have a higher rate of migraine than nonidentical twins. This hints that there are genetic factors in a person's susceptibility, but no one has identified a clear pattern of inheritance.

A recent study convincingly linked a mutation in a particular gene to a rare variant of migraine in which motor weakness is very common. This disorder, called familial hemiplegic migraine, seems to be due to a mutation on chromosome 19 and relates to problems with a protein that controls the flow of calcium into and out of cells. We know from other studies that calcium flux is very important in determining nerves' excitability and their release of neurotransmitters, and thus affects how cells communicate with one another. Approximately 50 percent of families with this rare form of migraine have an abnormality of this gene, so it seems likely that similar genes and proteins are related to other inherited forms of migraine.

This indication that calcium flux is involved in some migraines has led researchers to focus on the channels that move calcium, potassium, sodium, and other ions into and out of cells. These channels cause occasional transient disturbances, called channelopathies, in muscles and nerves. Neurons are for the most part unaffected, but every so often a disturbance in channel function appears as a neurological problem lasting minutes or hours, after which the nerves resume working normally. Stress seems to be important in inducing these attacks, just as it is in migraines. If we can better understand these ion-flux channels and how they produce transient disturbances, we may be able to develop drug therapies for those problems and possibly migraine as well.

Diagnosis and Treatment

There are no blood tests, urine tests, or X rays to diagnose migraine, though doctors may use such studies to exclude other conditions that masquerade as an attack. Rather, migraine is identified by collecting the symptoms that a person reports and matching them to a list of diagnostic criteria.

Fortunately, migraine can be well treated and controlled by medications. Aspirin-like drugs (nonsteroidal anti-inflammatory drugs) are often effective. Ergotamine is frequently prescribed specifically for debilitating migraines and can be taken orally or with an inhaler. For faster effect, the related drug dihydroergotamine mesylate can be taken by injection. Both of these chemicals cause blood vessels to constrict. A new group of drugs, the triptans, that bind to receptors for the molecule serotonin have also proved useful in treating acute migraine attacks. As many as 80 percent of people find significant relief during attacks by taking these medications.

For people who want to or have to minimize their use of these medications, untreated migraine attacks generally persist for a few hours and rarely more than 72 hours. Sleep is an excellent way to terminate an attack. Relaxation techniques work in some individuals but are less effective than medication. Removing sources of stress or emotional turbulence often reduces the severity and frequency of symptoms, though this may not always be feasible for an individual.

Usually migraines don't require a person to see a headache specialist. When they do, there are physicians and centers specializing in the treatment of migraine. The headache specialist is particularly useful when the disorder no longer responds to medications, and when the migraine changes its character by becoming more frequent and incapacitating. Often when migraine attacks are severe, doctors prescribe medication on a daily basis, not waiting for the headaches to begin; this is meant to lessen the frequency and intensity of attacks when they occur.

Sometimes migraineurs become anxious or depressed, or overuse pain relievers, and start suffering daily headaches without the other symptoms of migraine. This condition, called transformed migraine, is a form of tension headache and should be treated as such (**C54**). The medicines and other treatments for migraine won't be as effective.

At present, there are no cures for migraine, but the natural history for most people is a waxing and waning course. Periods with increasing attacks will be followed by periods in which the attacks become much less common and medication unnecessary. There is no surgical treatment for migraine, and that approach is unlikely in the future.

As we start to understand the neurological events early in a migraine attack, we'll be able to identify additional targets for therapy, most likely including the waves of excitation and depression in nerve cells, and the genes associated with the flux of specific ions into and out of cells. Until the past decade, most drugs for migraine were discovered through serendipity: they decreased attacks when migraineurs happened to be taking them for unrelated disorders. That situation has changed with the introduction of better imaging technology and tools that let us work at a molecular level. Our challenge for the future lies in identifying the genetic and environmental factors that render an individual susceptible to an attack, and in better understanding how those factors alter brain function for a transient but painful time.

Back Pain and Disk Disease

Nearly all of us suffer back or neck pain some-time in our lives. In the United States, that problem is second only to colds as the chief reason individuals see their primary care physicians. When we total up lost productivity and medical costs, backaches are the most expensive chronic illness among Americans 30 to 60 years of age. Fortunately, most people with back and neck pain can return to their usual activities after a few days or weeks of rest and, perhaps, pain-relieving medicines. Most of these cases are probably due to strains and sprains of muscles and ligaments.

Back pain can also herald a serious underlying disease, however, such as cancer, aneurysm, vertebral compression fracture, or infection. Or the problem can arise within the spinal structure, such as a herniated disk or bone spur in the wrong place; these problems can cause severe symptoms (paralysis, sensory loss, and incontinence among them) and eventually irreversible nerve damage. It is important, therefore, to identify the cause of serious back and neck pain. The problems discussed in this section are disk herniation, spondylosis, cervical spondylotic myelopathy, and lumbar spinal stenosis.

Watching Your Back

To understand how pain can arise in the spine, and how problems in the spine can cause you to feel pain elsewhere in your body, it helps to begin with the anatomy of the spine. The spinal column is composed of 30 vertebral bones divided into five regions—cervical, thoracic, lumbar, sacral, and the coccyx (tailbone). Every vertebra is identified according to its place along the spine: for example, L5 is the fifth bone in the lumbar region, and S1 is the first bone in the sacral region. Together the vertebrae form the spinal canal, through which the spinal cord runs from the skull to about the second lumbar vertebra. Below the spinal cord is the cauda equina, a group of nerve roots that innervate our legs and pelvic region. Thus, when doctors perform a spinal tap, or lumbar puncture, the needle enters the spinal canal *below* the spinal cord.

Each vertebra has two facet joints that fit between the facet joints of the vertebrae immediately above and below. This arrangement makes the spine very flexible while still protecting the spinal cord. Nerve roots exit the cord to each side through spaces between pairs of vertebrae. (In the thoracic and lumbar areas, each root is numbered with the vertebra above it: for example, T12, L1, and so on. In the cervical area, each nerve root is numbered with the vertebra below it: for example, C5, C6.) These nerve roots carry sensory impulses from all parts of the body below the head to the spinal cord, which in turn carries them to our brain. These roots also carry all motor impulses to our muscles. Bundled in them are the autonomic nerves that connect to our internal organs, including the heart, lungs, intestines, bladder, and sweat glands. Obviously, proper functioning of these nerve roots is essential to how our bodies work.

This anatomical arrangement also explains how our first sign of a spinal problem can be pain that we feel in other parts of the body, a condition known as referred pain or radicular pain. The best known example is sciatica. A herniated disk or bone spur can put pressure on a low lumbar or sacral nerve root (L4, L5, or S1). When this root is irritated, a person can feel "pins and needles" or pain from the back down through the buttock into the back of the thigh and calf and, at times, even into the foot. A physician can sometimes diagnose the precise nerve root involved from listening to the patient's history of pain and numbness and performing an examination. For example, if the numbness goes into the big toe, the problem is apt to be with the L5 nerve root. If the numbness extends into the little toe and a person's ankle reflex is diminished, the nerve root affected is more likely to be S1.

Similarly, doctors can investigate problems in the cervical area by testing deep tendon reflexes in a person's arms. Our reflex in the biceps muscle depends predominantly on the C5 nerve root, in the triceps on the C7 root, and in the brachiora-

dialis on the C6 root. These tests are done by tapping the tendon for muscle contraction.

Disk Herniation

In the cervical, thoracic, and lumbar regions of the spine, there is a disk between each pair of vertebrae. You can think of these intervertebral

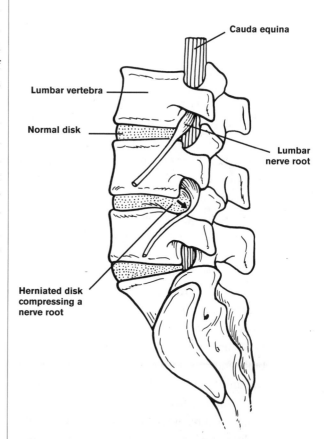

When a disk herniates, a portion of the nucleus pulposus (the gelatinous material in the disk) bulges out of its covering. That material, pressing on a nearby nerve root, may cause pain and nerve damage. Most herniated disks are a result of the wear and tear of daily living. Back pain is second only to colds as the chief reason individuals see their primary care physicians.
ILLUSTRATION © KATHRYN BORN

disks as being like jelly doughnuts. In the middle is a gelatinous material, called the nucleus pulposus, that is surrounded by a fibrous container called the annulus fibrosus. When a disk herniates, a portion of the nucleus pulposus protrudes through its covering. If that material presses on a nearby nerve root or (in rare cases) on the spinal cord itself, it can cause pain and nerve damage. Although severe injuries can cause disks to herniate, more commonly the problem arises from the wear and tear of daily living.

Disk herniations may cause mild to severe pain in the back or neck, muscle spasm, and pain which travels along the course of the nerve root being pinched. Often people feel these symptoms more when they cough, sneeze, or strain.

Most disk herniations occur at the low cervical and low lumbar regions. The problem in the lumbar spine may cause pain to radiate into the buttock and leg (sciatica), or produce numbness or weakness in the leg. If the cauda equina is compressed, a person may suffer bowel and bladder incontinence, leg weakness, sensory loss, and other neurological problems. Sitting may exacerbate the pain of a lumbar disk herniation because that position puts more pressure on the disks than standing or lying down.

Disk herniations in the neck may cause pain that radiates down one arm as far as the hand. If the nerve root is severely compressed, a person may notice arm numbness and weakness. When a herniated disk compresses the spinal cord, the results may be leg weakness, gait difficulties, or bowel and bladder incontinence.

Diagnosis and Treatment

Diagnosis begins with a physician taking a thorough history and conducting a physical examination. Routine X rays of the spine do not show the herniation of a disk but may reveal related problems, such as spondylosis (degenerative disease) and fractures. Magnetic resonance imaging (MRI) and computed tomography (CT) scans may identify the disk herniation and whether it is compressing a nerve root or the spinal cord. Myelography, which requires injecting dye into the spinal canal, is less common since MRI and CT became available.

Neurologists may also conduct electrodiagnostic studies such as EMG (electromyography) to identify damage to the nerve roots. This involves placing a needle in a muscle and measuring the pattern of electrical activity when the muscle is relaxed or contracted. The results help to show if the nerve feeding the muscle has been damaged.

For most people, the symptoms of herniated disks disappear with several weeks of rest and analgesics. In some cases, a supervised exercise and physical therapy program may relieve the acute symptoms and help prevent them from recurring. Pain due to muscle spasm is common, and treatment with ice, heat, massage, stretching, and sometimes traction may be helpful.

A physician may recommend surgery to remove the disk herniation if a person has severe or worsening nerve damage such as weakness or incontinence, or if the pain does not respond to nonsurgical treatments. The surgeon may choose to approach the disk from the back, removing a small piece of bone (laminectomy) and the disk material. Alternatively, the surgeon may choose to approach the disk from the front, especially when it is in the neck; in this case, the doctor often considers fusing the vertebrae on either side of the damaged disk.

NORMAL WEAR AND TEAR

Herniated spinal disks and bone spurs on the vertebrae can cause a lot of pain and other difficulties if they compress nerve roots or the spinal cord. But bulging disks and bone spurs are actually common in our bodies as we grow older.

Many people with no back problems who undergo MRI tests have been found to have bulging disks. Nearly a third of people in middle age show actual disk herniations that cause no neurological symptoms because they do not affect nerves. Recent studies indicate that many herniated disks are reabsorbed spontaneously.

Similarly, most individuals develop cervical and lumbar bone spurs (spondylosis or osteoarthritis) by late middle age. MRI and CT studies find spurs on the spines of most individuals over 50. Such spondylosis seems to be part of our normal aging process, generally beginning in middle age. Unfortunately, the sites of our greatest spinal flexibility—the low cervical and low lumbar regions—are where we are most likely to develop bone spurs.

Because of these conditions, we should not be surprised to experience some back pain or stiffness in our lives. At the same time, one must be careful about ascribing a person's pain or other symptoms to a herniated disk or spondylosis. These conditions certainly can cause such problems, but they can also be completely asymptomatic, and other conditions can produce similar symptoms. Accordingly, it is important for physicians to carefully correlate a person's history of pain and other symptoms with a physical examination and imaging studies such as MRI.

Spondylosis

Spondylosis, also referred to as degenerative joint disease or osteoarthritis, is a condition of normal aging. Cervical and lumbar spondylosis is especially common; nearly all of us have it by late middle age. Bone spurs (osteophytes) form on the edges of the disks and the facet joints where the vertebrae link to each other. These bone spurs commonly result in stiffness, loss of range of motion, and discomfort.

In more severe cases, spondylosis can lead to back and neck pain, muscle spasms or guarding (that is, stiffening of muscles to avoid precipitating pain), and the radiating of pain into extremities. These symptoms are similar to those of disk herniation, but they tend to be less acutely severe and more chronic and intermittent. Spondylosis and disk herniation may also occur together and both may contribute to a person's difficulties.

If bone spurs form between vertebrae, they can irritate the adjacent nerve roots, producing such symptoms as pain in a limb and, less often, loss of sensation or weakness in the area served by that nerve root. If a bone spur forms in the spinal canal, the result can be cervical spondylotic myelopathy or spinal stenosis (discussed on page 557).

Diagnosis and Treatment

Physicians start with a thorough medical and neurological history and examination while considering other diseases that can mimic spondylosis. Imaging the spine with X rays, CT, or MRI may identify bone spurs and whether they are likely to be compressing nerves.

Discomfort from spondylosis usually responds to rest, analgesics such as aspirin, and nonsteroidal anti-inflammatory agents. A physician may also recommend physical therapy and an exercise program of stretching and strengthening. If there is severe nerve or spinal cord compression, however, the doctor may recommend surgery.

Cervical Spondylotic Myelopathy

Cervical spondylotic myelopathy refers to a condition in which spondylosis leads to compression of the spinal cord itself. Usually the first symptom is discomfort in the neck or shoulders and arms over a number of months or years, followed by problems with walking and running, weakness or sensory loss in the legs, or bowel and bladder difficulties. Symptoms may be intermittent over many years or become steadily worse. A person may develop dulled reflexes in the arms when the nerve roots are compressed and spastic "jumping legs" because the compression interferes with the inhibitory impulses from the brain to the legs.

Diagnosis and Treatment

Doctors do a neurological examination, looking for these hypoactive and hyperactive reflexes and other symptoms and signs. They may also test for the Babinski sign: stroking the sole of the foot and watching for an upward movement of the big toe. Diagnosis is usually confirmed by MRI, which can show the offending osteophyte(s) and disk material as well as the spinal cord and nerve roots.

If the spinal cord is significantly compressed, the MRI may even show it as distorted.

At the same time, physicians consider many neurological diseases with similar symptoms, such as multiple sclerosis (**C33**), vitamin B_{12} deficiency (**C65**), amyotrophic lateral sclerosis (**C53**), brain tumors (**C64**), inherited and degenerative diseases of the nervous system, and syringomyelia.

Managing cervical spondylotic myelopathy depends on an individual's particular condition, but in general it includes both surgical and nonsurgical treatments. In some people whose neurological deficits are mild and not worsening, physicians may recommend rest, a collar to stabilize the neck, and neck-strengthening exercises. These individuals are usually followed closely by their doctors in order to identify any changes.

Alternatively, the patient and physician may decide that the best course is surgery to decompress the spinal cord. There are several different procedures possible. These include approaching the spinal area from the front or the rear and spinal fusion. Selecting the most appropriate operation is important.

Lumbar Spinal Stenosis

In lumbar spinal stenosis, a person's lumbar spinal canal becomes narrowed, usually because of bone spurs and sometimes because of disk herniation as well. The initial symptoms are therefore similar to those described above. If the stenosis becomes severe, however, the nerves of the cauda equina may be compressed. This condition is most likely to occur in individuals who are born with a narrow spinal canal and develop spondylosis later in life.

The symptoms of lumbar spinal stenosis are sometimes called neurogenic claudication. They include difficulty in walking, which develops gradually but becomes apparent after an individual has gone some distance. Commonly the signs are discomfort in the back and legs and numbness and tingling in the legs, which gets worse the longer one walks. As the condition progresses, the distance one can walk comfortably diminishes. Characteristically, a person's symptoms improve if he or she bends forward; in this position the spinal canal becomes wider, reducing the nerve root compression. Thus, a person may be able to walk much farther leaning on a shopping cart than walking upright. In advanced cases, people develop symptoms from simply standing for extended periods.

Diagnosis and Treatment

Physicians usually diagnose lumbar spinal stenosis using MRI and CT scanning. Electro-diagnostic studies such as EMG may help identify damaged nerve roots that are causing weakness in the lower extremities. Neurogenic claudication must be distinguished, however, from claudication due to diminished blood circulation to the legs.

In some cases, neurogenic claudication from lumbar spinal stenosis may be alleviated by surgery to stop the nerve compression. If it is decided that the risk of an operation outweighs the possible benefits, doctors may prescribe anti-inflammatory agents, encourage weight loss, and recommend an exercise and conditioning program.

Chronic Pain

Most people have experienced at least one episode of severe pain. You may have done so in breaking a bone, birthing a child, or suffering from acute appendicitis. Your body was confronted with a painful stimulus and your autonomic nervous system (ANS) became hyperactive, producing a fast heart rate, elevated blood pressure, and sweating. But eventually the ANS quieted and the pain went away. Your fracture healed, your baby arrived, your appendix was removed. In each of these examples, pain flared up in response to a known cause. You either received treatment, or your body healed by itself, and you stopped hurting. Doctors call that kind of pain acute pain. It is a normal sensation triggered in the nervous system to alert you to an injury.

In contrast, chronic pain persists for at least three months. For some people, it originates in an episode of acute pain; for others, there is an ongoing cause, such as arthritis or cancer. Most often the cause is musculoskeletal, such as pain in the lower back (**C56**), knees, neck, limbs, and joints. Headache (**C54**), nerve injuries, surgical and postoperative pain, and traumatic injury are also common. And some people suffer chronic pain with no evident past injury or body damage. In all of these cases, the symptoms are less apparent to observers than are those of acute pain because over time the autonomic nervous system adapts. People in chronic pain may not moan or groan, sweat, or experience a high heart rate. Nevertheless, they hurt.

It is estimated that more than 50 million Americans suffer from chronic pain, twice as many as suffer from acute pain at any given moment. Women seem more likely to suffer from some kinds of pain than men. Feeling continual pain can cause significant changes in a person's personality, lifestyle, and ability to function—all of which compromise quality of life. Some people can no longer work, while others lose their appetite or are unable to engage in any physical activities. Many have difficulty sleeping (**C11**); the resulting exhaustion can lead to irritability and depression (**C20**), trapping the sufferer in an endless cycle of weariness, depression, and pain.

Chronic pain affects a person's family members and friends, too. A recent survey found that almost half of American households (43 percent) had someone living with chronic pain due to a specific illness or medical condition. Everyone involved must fight against the emotional stresses caused by this illness.

Identifying Types of Pain

Fortunately, many people with chronic pain can be helped once they understand the cause of their pain. One of the first things sufferers can do is to help their doctors identify what type of pain they are experiencing. There are three types: somatic, visceral, and neuropathic.

Somatic pain results from activation of some peripheral nerves that send information about the body to the brain without injury to the nervous system itself. People with this condition typically describe their pain as either sharp or dull. It is usually well localized, as, for example, a pinprick or a burn from a hot object.

Visceral pain is also caused by an injury or disease outside the nervous system, this time originating in the viscera (abdomen, bowels). It is characterized by an ongoing, deep, aching, cramping sensation. People with visceral pain have greater difficulty localizing their symptoms and may experience the pain at a site quite distant from its actual cause. An example of visceral pain is chronic abdominal pain.

Neuropathic pain results from direct injury to peripheral nerves or the central nervous system (CNS). It is typically described as burning or stabbing pain. People with neuropathic pain may also have an area of numbness or lack of sensation in the neighborhood of the pain. Some individuals complain of worsening pain when the area is brushed, or excessive pain when even a light touch is applied to the region. The pain caused by shingles (**C34**) is a common example of neuropathic pain.

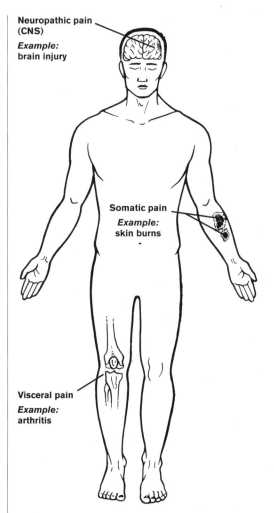

Neuropathic pain (CNS)
Example: brain injury

Somatic pain
Example: skin burns

Visceral pain
Example: arthritis

Chronic pain typically arises from any one of many sources of acute pain but may also begin with another illness, such as cancer or arthritis. Pain is considered chronic when it persists for at least three months. ILLUSTRATION © KATHRYN BORN

We can also classify pains by their causes. One group includes chronic pain associated with structural disease such as metastatic cancer, sickle-cell anemia, or rheumatoid arthritis. This group is usually characterized by prolonged episodes of pain alternating with pain-free intervals, or unremitting pain waxing and waning in severity. In these cases, the successful treatment of the pain is closely allied to treating the disease. But in some instances—for example, in a person with advanced cancer that does not respond to anticancer treatment—relieving pain becomes the physician's only therapeutic goal. For such people, psychological factors may play an important role in exacerbating or relieving the pain. Analgesic (pain-relieving) drug therapy, or pharmacotherapy, is often the mainstay of treatment.

Another group of people suffer from psychophysiologic disorders, meaning those with both physical and mental aspects. These individuals may once have suffered from a structural disease, such as a herniated disk or torn ligament, but psychological factors have caused chronic physiological alterations, such as muscle spasms, which produce pain long after the original injury has healed. Typically, such individuals are physically inactive and spend much of their time thinking and talking about their pain, which often leads to social and emotional isolation. Pain is indeed their major symptom. Such people often respond poorly to analgesic drugs and may suffer from adverse drug reactions and ineffective surgical procedures. Many hospitals have multidisciplinary pain clinics that diagnose and treat these intractable chronic pain syndromes, and such individuals should seek evaluation and treatment at these clinics.

Pain and the Brain

Doctors have focused increasing attention on the interaction between the persistence of pain and a person's psychological state. There is no doubt that ongoing pain can affect people in profound ways. A recent survey found that 40 per-

cent of patients with chronic pain are uncomfortable discussing their pain; 37 percent say it can be isolating, leaving them feeling alone. One third do not believe people understand how much pain they are in, and one quarter say their family is tired of hearing about their pain.

As our understanding of chronic pain has grown over the past several years, we have developed greater respect for a person experiencing pain. Twenty or thirty years ago, a popular myth claimed that debilitating pain without a clear physical cause was "all in the mind," meaning that the person's weak psychological state was what prevented him or her from functioning at a normal level despite the pain. Numerous studies have now shown that the persistence of pain can seriously affect a person's psychological state and immune mechanisms; in fact, animal studies suggest that pain can even kill.

Today we recognize that pain is indeed in the brain, and that pain without a visible cause can be no less agonizing than other types. We have developed a very sophisticated understanding of the neuroanatomy, neurophysiology, pharmacology, and molecular biology of pain.

Imagine, for instance, that you trip and fall, landing hard on your knee. You would experience an acute, localized, painful sensation in your knee, followed by a dull and aching sensation. This is due to two types of fiber systems that conduct pain from the peripheral nerves into the CNS: A-delta fibers, which are myelinated fibers that conduct rapidly, and C-fibers, which are unmyelinated and conduct slowly. These fibers enter the spinal cord and relay information to the brain through very specialized pain-sensory systems. Recent studies using positron-emission tomography (PET) and magnetic resonance imaging (MRI) have identified specific areas in the cortex—

particularly in the anterior cingulate gyrus—that are activated by painful stimuli.

These ascending signals are matched by specific descending inhibitory pathways that help modulate pain. We now think that neurons in the brain release chemicals called endorphins, which might act to turn off the spinal cord's pain cells. Laboratory experiments have confirmed that painful stimulation leads to the release of endorphins from nerve cells. Chronic pain is associated with changes that are believed to take place in the central modulation of pain—for instance, pain after a stroke affecting the thalamus. This is likely due to a loss of the inhibitory systems.

We can see this process clearly when people develop sensitive areas that become painful if they are touched or even brushed against. There is a clear anatomical and neurophysiological basis for this exquisite sensitivity, which occurs especially in neuropathic pain. Neurons in a person's spine become abnormally active after repeated stimulation from the C-fibers. Furthermore, CNS neurons be-come open to more signals, start to activate at lower levels, and sometimes fire spontaneously.

Diagnosing and Treating Pain

Chronic pain is both a disease and a symptom. As a symptom, physicians use it as a clue to an overall illness, such as cancer or sickle-cell anemia. As a disease, it demands its own treatment. Assessing a person in pain demands a detailed evaluation that focuses on that individual's symptoms. Physicians must use a careful physical, neurological, and psychological examination to define the site of the pain, the condition's associated medical and psychological aspects, and the possible causes.

One of the difficulties in treating pain is that its level is subjective. Doctors must rely on their patients' descriptions of pain, and what one person may describe as "unbearable" another might call "uncomfortable." Doctors use several methods to help their patients express how much pain they feel:

- Categorical scales, which use a variety of words, such as *mild, moderate,* and *severe.*

- Numerical scales, which ask individuals to rate their pain as a number from zero to ten, with zero representing no pain, and ten representing the worst pain possible.

- Visual analog scales, which consist of a four-inch line whose ends are labeled "no pain" and "worst possible pain"; an individual marks on the line the intensity of his or her pain. For young children, similar scales use a series of cartoon faces, from crying to smiling broadly.

These pain-intensity scales have been validated by large studies. The Joint Commission on Hospital Accreditation has now mandated that health care facilities use such scales, meaning each patient must be asked routinely about his or her pain intensity. A physician can use the results to assess a person's pain and to map how it changes, thus helping doctor and patient plan appropriate treatment together.

Many different types of treatment are available for pain. The most common over-the-counter painkillers are aspirin and acetaminophen (Tylenol is an example). Anti-inflammatory drugs include ibuprofen and naprosyn. Newer anti-inflammatory drugs include cyclooxygenase-2 (or COX-2) inhibitors. Examples of these are Celebrex

---

CHRONIC PAIN

Making the journey from patient to person takes time. The isolation and fear that can overwhelm a person who has chronic pain grow over time. And the return to a fuller, more rewarding life also takes time. Here are some suggestions to make the transition smoother.

- **Learn all you can about your physical condition. Understand that there may be no current cure and accept that you will need to deal with the fact of pain in your life.**

- **Look beyond your pain to the things that are important in your life. Setting priorities can help you find a starting point to lead you back into a more active life.**

- **Emotions directly affect physical well-being. By acknowledging and dealing with your feelings, you can reduce stress and possibly decrease the pain you feel. It is normal to feel angry, helpless, hopeless, and alone. It is important, though, to seek help in dealing with these feelings. You can get professional help at pain centers and from mental health professionals.**

- **Pain increases in times of stress. Relaxation exercises are one way of reclaiming control of your body.**

- **Reach out and share what you know. Living with chronic pain is an ongoing learning experience.**

- **Be good to yourself. Nurture supportive friendships, exercise, and eat healthfully.**

Adapted from www.theacpa.org (The American Chronic Pain Association)

and Vioxx; they cause less gastrointestinal disturbance or irritation than aspirin or other anti-inflammatory drugs. Antidepressants such as Elavil (amitriptyline) can be useful, as well as such anticonvulsants as Neurontin (gabapentin). For severe intractable pain, neurosurgical procedures such as dorsal column stimulators, lesioning of pain pathways, and cingulotomy are sometimes used.

It has long been known that drugs derived from opium poppies—morphine, heroin, codeine, and demerol (synthetic)—are quite effective in relieving pain. However, fears of addiction and physicians' lack of knowledge impede many people from receiving the benefits of these opioid medications. More recently, researchers have given renewed attention to their role and use. Many studies have shown that doctors can manage these drugs to help people with cancer, without the feared side effects. Individuals suffering from chronic pain can gain relief for months and years with ongoing opioid therapy. In some patients with pain, opioid medications can be injected directly into a person's cerebrospinal fluid and can work alongside their chemical relatives, the endorphins.

Research suggests that the wide variation in people's responses to pain treatment with analgesic drugs may be genetically based. For example, 10 percent of the population cannot metabolize codeine in the body to the active agent morphine. Such individuals therefore do not obtain effective pain relief with standard doses of codeine. Animal studies have found a wide variation in the distribution and type of opiate receptors; that finding suggests that similar genetic variations in opiate receptors may occur in humans, though that has not yet been demonstrated.

Some researchers are exploring ways of taking advantage of our understanding of the molecular biology of pain. New drug development is focusing on N-methyl-D-aspartate (NMDA) antagonists, calcium channel blockers, nerve growth factors, and new anesthetic agents for pain relief, but the challenges are varied and complex. Another area of research begins with the knowledge that there are particular types of opioid receptors located in specific areas of the brain, spinal cord, and peripheral nervous system. We might thus be able to develop new analgesics targeted for specific receptors in the brain. The symptom of chronic pain can cause people to feel helpless, but our ability to treat the condition is improving all the time.

Trigeminal Neuralgia

Trigeminal neuralgia, formerly called tic douloureux, is a terrible shooting pain in the face. People usually remember their first attacks in great detail because they are so severe. Some individuals may feel a prodrome, or early symptom, of mild pain or "pins and needles" (paresthesia). Once the pain appears, it can recur at any time. It may last a fraction of a second or, like repetitive bolts of lightning, strike over and over again for up to an hour. An attack may be precipitated by many things: talking, chewing, feeling a cold breeze, brushing the teeth, applying makeup, kissing, and shaving. A person may set off the pain by lying down on the affected side, turning into a particular position, or turning the head. Or there may be no regular trigger.

The pains of trigeminal neuralgia are somewhat more common on the right side of the face than the left, by a ratio of 3 to 2. They are much more common in the central and lower face; the forehead, eye, and top of the head are involved in only 5 percent of cases. For most people, trigeminal neuralgia attacks can start in any area and gradually spread to the whole face, though occasionally one entire side of the face is involved from the onset.

As time passes, the pains become more frequent and more prolonged. It may no longer take being in certain positions to set off an attack; they may occur at any time. Many people find the attacks to be more severe in the winter and fall, though better pain medications have made that change harder to measure. There are rarely any other symptom than pain. A few people develop some redness of the cheek or the eye, and some develop mild numbness after many years or a serious episode.

Trigeminal neuralgia is usually a problem of middle age and later: most people are in their sixth or seventh decade when the onset occurs. The problem may occur at any age, however; when it appears in young women, they are very prone to have pain in the cheek only. There has even been a case of a thirteen-month-old baby suffering an attack.

Often people having trigeminal neuralgia attacks think they have a dental problem. They may go to a dentist to have teeth extracted, root canal surgery, or other well-intentioned procedures that do nothing for the pain. Sometimes one dentist will refuse to remove a healthy tooth, and a person in pain will shop around to find another. People may also worry that the pains are a symptom of such dire problems as strokes (**C59, C60**) or a fatal disease. Often people have gone to three or more dentists and one or two physicians before their real problem is diagnosed.

Trigeminal neuralgia is not a fatal condition, but it can be debilitating. People state that its pain is the worst they have ever had and that waiting for the next attack is almost as bad as having one. The pain can take over people's lives, making them afraid to do things they enjoy. They can also become dependent on medications to control the pain, or be harmed by their side effects. People have even been known to commit suicide, especially before we understood the problem and developed current treatments.

Mechanisms

Trigeminal neuralgia, we now know, is caused by an abnormality of the trigeminal nerve, which is adjacent to the area of the brain stem called the pons. Usually a blood vessel, either an artery or a vein or both, is compressing and distorting the nerve in that area. There is a clear correlation between the site of the pressure and the part of the face that is in pain. Normally the myelin sheath around the nerve protects it from "short circuits," but there may be scattered abnormalities in that coating in patients with trigeminal neuralgia.

Occasionally something besides a blood vessel is what puts pressure on the trigeminal nerve. About 5 percent of people with trigeminal neuralgia turn out to have benign tumors (**C64**) pushing

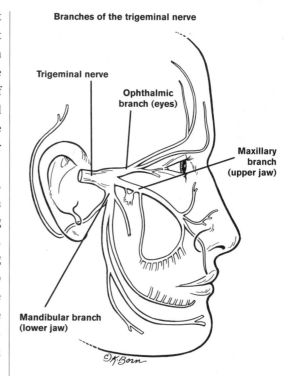

Branches of the trigeminal nerve

Trigeminal nerve

Ophthalmic branch (eyes)

Maxillary branch (upper jaw)

Mandibular branch (lower jaw)

©K.Born

Trigeminal pain is a sharp, stabbing pain on one side of the face that some people describe as the "worst pain of my life." It most typically develops in a person's 60s or later. Illustration © Kathryn Born

the nerve and blood vessel together. People with multiple sclerosis (**C33**) may develop the pains if a plaque is located in this area of the trigeminal nerve.

The true prevalence of trigeminal neuralgia is unknown because there have been very few studies. Experts estimate that there are anywhere from 10,000 to 25,000 new cases every year. Sixty percent of people with the disorder are women. It seems to be more common among Caucasians than among African Americans and Asian Americans, but this is not clear. There is a small genetic component, and individuals whose parents and grandparents were prone to trigeminal neuralgia tend to develop it at an earlier age.

Physicians once thought that viruses were involved, but they have nothing to do with the condition.

Diagnosis and Treatment

A doctor's first step in diagnosing the cause of a person's shooting facial pains is to ask for the history of those pains. As noted earlier, most people have a vivid memory of their first attack. The major diagnostic tests are to check hearing, because benign tumors may be present that cause hearing loss. The doctor will order a magnetic resonance imaging (MRI) scan to look for abnormal blood vessels, benign tumors, or the plaques of multiple sclerosis.

For most people, the best first treatment is pain medication, with the caution that the doctor and patient must carefully monitor the side effects of the prescribed drug. A number of medications have been used. The benchmark treatment is carbamazepine (Tegretol), but not all physicians know how to prescribe it. One must start with a small dose, such as 100 milligrams twice a day, and increase the dose by 200 milligrams every 48 hours until the pain is relieved. Trileptal is a new variation of Tegretol and has been useful. Gabapentin and baclofen may also be effective, and phenytoin (Dilantin) has been used.

In the long run, people with trigeminal neuralgia have to increase their medications gradually or combine them, making their side effects more worrisome. As individuals become older, furthermore, they may become less able to have surgery to fix the underlying cause of the pain. For those reasons, many people who develop trigeminal neuralgia early or in middle age may do best to have an operation to relieve pressure on the cru-

cial nerve. All operations carry some risks: possible bad reaction to anesthetics, infection, and in this case the potential of damaging the nerve and causing permanent numbness or weakness in some parts of the face. An individual and his or her doctor must balance those risks against the potential benefits of stopping the pain.

There are a range of operative procedures available for treating trigeminal neuralgia. A person should consult with a neurosurgeon who can do various operations so that together they can choose the approach best suited to the case. As always, it is valuable to have an experienced surgeon perform an operation—especially so when working around the trigeminal nerve.

The benchmark operative procedure is the microvascular decompression, a procedure lasting about two hours. Using a small incision behind the ear, a surgeon moves the blood vessel causing the problem and inserts soft plastic implants to hold it away from the nerve. This is a very small-scale procedure, but microsurgical techniques have enabled surgeons to perform it safely and effectively. When performed using the latest techniques, this procedure has a recurrence rate of only 0.5 percent per year after the first two years.

A second procedure, appropriate for multiple sclerosis plaques, is a percutaneous radio-frequency rhizotomy. The doctor puts a needle through the cheek into the trigeminal ganglion and burns the nerve. The more severe the burn, the more pain it relieves and the longer the relief lasts. Unfortunately, there is a high incidence of side effects that are difficult to treat, including anesthesia dolorosa, or painful numbness. Up to 20 percent of people undergoing this operation develop disordered sensations, including numbness, which in some cases are worse than the initial pain.

In people too frail for surgery, the treatment of choice may be injecting glycerol into the nerve. This is a needle procedure done with the patient awake but sedated in the operating room. It produces good short-term results, and an experienced surgeon is unlikely to bring on the side effect of numbness. Unfortunately, up to half of people who undergo the procedure suffer recurrent pains within two years.

Another procedure, which has come into use only recently, is focused high-energy radiation to the nerve. This is the most costly procedure. We await long-term studies on its efficacy and whether it is followed by recurrences of pain.

Older treatments, no longer recommended, include injecting the trigeminal nerves with alcohol and cutting (sectioning) those nerves.

The promising paths of research into trigeminal neuralgia involve changing the basic metabolism of a person's myelin to make the nerve sheaths less sensitive to compression, and, of course, developing better medical therapy.

CHAPTER 18

Nervous System Injuries

C59   Ischemic Stroke   570

C60   Hemorrhagic Stroke   576

C61   Brain Trauma, Concussion, and Coma   581

C62   Spinal Cord Injury   591

C63   Paraneoplastic Syndromes   600

C64   Brain Tumors   604

C65   Nutritional Disorders   610

C66   Chemicals and the Nervous System   617

Injuries to the central nervous system are among the most devastating we can suffer. A severe injury can affect nearly every function of the brain, including those that keep us alive. The most common brain injuries—indeed, among the most common causes of death and disability in the United States—are strokes, which come in two forms: loss of blood circulation to part of the brain (ischemic), and bleeding into the brain (hemorrhagic). Other serious injuries include blows to the head (traumas), abnormal growths within the brain (tumors), and harm to the spinal cord.

The most effective way to avoid these injuries is preventive medicine. A healthy diet, exercise, and not smoking minimize an individual's risk of stroke. Caution when driving and performing risky physical activities can save you from badly harming your brain or spinal cord. We can't do anything about our genetic vulnerability to cancerous growths, aneurysms, and other conditions, but we can choose a lifestyle that does not help these dangers along.

Ischemic Stroke

Each year in the United States, nearly 750,000 individuals have a stroke. Of those people, 150,000 (90,000 women and 60,000 men) die from the resulting brain injury. Strokes are the country's third leading cause of death, and the number one cause of persistent disability. The chance that you will have some type of stroke during your lifetime is about one out of seven. All told, there are about 2 million stroke survivors in the United States today. In other parts of the world, strokes are even more common. In China, for instance, 1.5 million people die annually because of strokes.

There are two major kinds of stroke. Four strokes out of five are due to ischemia, meaning that part of the brain stops receiving enough blood. The other 20 percent are caused by bleeding, or hemorrhage, into the brain or the fluid surrounding it; these hemorrhagic strokes are discussed in section **C60**.

In a brain ischemia, the blood flow to part of your brain is cut off, and the cells in that region do not receive the oxygen and fuel (sugar) they need. The neurons stop functioning and die unless the blood flow is restored quickly. The brain damage caused by deprivation of blood is called ischemic stroke, and the region of damage is called a brain infarct.

Brain ischemia usually develops abruptly, most often in the morning. The symptoms depend on the area of the brain that stops receiving blood. Sometimes a person notices vision loss or problems in one eye, or in the left or right half of the visual field in both eyes (**C15**). A person may notice weakness or diminished feeling in the face, arm, hand, and leg on one or both sides of the body, or have trouble walking (**C46**). He or she may suddenly have difficulty with memory (**C68**, **C69**), or with speaking, understanding speech, reading, or writing (**C70**). Some people notice dizziness (**C14**) and double vision. The symptoms can also fluctuate in severity for hours and even days.

These same symptoms can also appear temporarily, lasting a few minutes or hours only, in which case they are called transient ischemic attacks (TIAs). For instance, you might sense a gray shade blocking the vision in your right eye for a couple of minutes, or feel your left hand and arm suddenly becoming numb and weak for an hour. Such problems indicate a temporary halt in blood flow to particular parts of your brain. Some peo-

BE PREPARED IN CASE OF STROKE

■ Keep a list of emergency rescue service numbers next to the telephone and in your pocket, wallet, or purse.

■ Find out which area hospitals have 24-hour emergency cerebrovascular care.

■ Know (in advance) which hospital or medical facility is nearest your home or office.

THE WARNING SIGNS OF STROKE

■ Sudden numbness or weakness of the face, arm, or leg, especially on one side of the body.

■ Sudden confusion, trouble speaking or understanding.

■ Sudden trouble seeing in one or both eyes.

■ Sudden trouble walking, dizziness, loss of balance or coordination.

■ Sudden, severe headache with no known cause.

■ Not all the warning signs occur in every stroke. Don't ignore signs of stroke, even if they go away.

■ Check the time. When did the first warning sign start? You will be asked this important question later.

■ If you have one or more stroke symptoms that last more than a few minutes, don't delay!

If you're with someone who may be having stroke symptoms, immediately call 9-1-1 or the EMS. Expect the person to protest—denial is common. Don't take no for an answer. Insist on taking prompt action.

Adapted from www.americanheart.org

ple try to ignore these problems—after all, they go away—but that is unwise. TIAs signal the possibility of a longer loss of blood supply. As troubling as these symptoms are, people who have them are actually lucky. Other people who have strokes lose brain functions with no such warning.

The symptoms of a stroke or TIA demand immediate medical attention. Any possible stroke is an *emergency.* The sooner a person having a stroke arrives at a hospital, the more likely that treatment will be effective. The more time it takes for a person to seek care, the more damage the brain undergoes. That has given rise to this medical reminder: Time = Brain.

What Causes Ischemia?

Brain ischemia is most often caused by blockage of an artery that brings oxygenated blood to some portion of the brain. The obstruction can occur where arteries pass through the neck or within the skull, with varying results.

Sometimes the clog develops in the artery itself, a process called thrombosis. Most commonly, this starts with plaques forming inside an artery due to atherosclerosis, or a hardening of the arterial walls. These plaques are composed of cholesterol and fibrous and connective tissue. They grow in and under the inner lining of arteries and jut out into the space where blood should flow. Other vascular diseases can also narrow the artery, decreasing blood flow. These conditions include overgrowth of muscle and fibrous tissue in arteries (fibromuscular dysplasia), the tearing of arterial walls, and inflammation (arteritis). Plaques and other abnormalities of arteries' inner lining also release chemicals that make blood platelets stick together and adhere to irregular crevices in the plaques. Whatever the cause, narrowing of the artery impedes blood flow and causes a clot (thrombus) to form, perhaps completely clogging the artery.

Alternatively, an artery can be blocked by material that originates elsewhere in the cardiovascular system and travels there. This process is called embolism. The material (an embolus) is usually a clot that originates in the heart, the aorta, or other blood vessels and then moves through the circulatory system. Sometimes illnesses like cancer and infections can start the clotting process. Occasionally, abnormalities in a person's clotting system can lead to a thrombus in an artery that has no major disease. An embolus travels until it gets stuck in, and blocks, the first artery too small for it to pass through.

Doctors customarily divide brain ischemias by location. What we call vertebrobasilar strokes, or posterior circulation strokes, occur when the clog is in the vertebral arteries in the back of the neck, in the basilar artery formed in the head where the two vertebral arteries join, or in their branches. This type of ischemia affects the brain stem, cerebellum, or the very back of the cerebral hemispheres. It can result in loss of memory, dizziness, slurred speech, difficulty swallowing, abnormal gait, and impaired vision on one or both sides.

When blood is blocked in the carotid arteries or their branches in what we call the anterior cir-

culation, a person can lose function in the cerebral hemisphere on the side of the blockage. The symptoms produced by such ischemia often include loss of vision in the eye on that side, and weakness, numbness, and loss of vision on the opposite side of the body. When a stroke develops in the left anterior circulation, a person often loses spoken and written language skills because those are centered on the left side of the brain. When the damage is to the right carotid artery system, people have difficulty with visual-spatial skills and with giving and understanding emotional messages.

Both genes and lifestyle can promote the formation of atherosclerotic plaques and lead to degenerative changes in the heart and blood vessels that bring on ischemic stroke. Risk factors for stroke include a strong family history of heart disease and stroke, hypertension (high blood pressure), diabetes, high levels of cholesterol in the blood, cigarette smoking, obesity, a sedentary lifestyle, and high blood homocysteine levels. You can take steps to counteract all those factors but the first.

Diagnosis and Treatment

Physicians diagnose ischemic stroke and brain ischemia based on people's descriptions of their symptoms, physical and neurological examinations, and the results of blood tests, brain images, and blood vessel tests. If a stroke seems to have occurred, a neurologist should usually direct diagnosis and treatment.

Brain images (computed tomography, or CT, and magnetic resonance imaging, or MRI, scans) can differentiate between the two types of stroke—ischemia and hemorrhage. This is impor-

PREVENTIVE MEDICINE

It is much easier to prevent a stroke than to recover from one. Many of us do not like to think ahead to such a dire possibility, but it is wise to do so. Strokes can occur without warning. A relatively short period of ischemia can produce years of disability and frustration. Indeed, a stroke may be so damaging that a survivor can never recover, or even recognize his or her losses.

The most important steps you can take to lower your chance of having a damaging ischemic stroke are:

- not smoking

- controlling your blood pressure

- lowering your blood cholesterol

- losing excessive weight

- exercising regularly

These actions also help lower your risk for hemorrhagic strokes (**C60**). Many of them benefit other parts of your health as well, and let your brain function at its best. But they require long-term, dedicated effort.

Some people resist that commitment, or other advice they hear from doctors. For instance, people who develop an abnormal heart rhythm (atrial fibrillation) face a higher risk of the embolisms that can lead to strokes. Physicians often prescribe the blood-thinning drug Coumadin to prevent these clots from forming. Some people decline to take this medicine because it requires frequent blood tests and carries a risk of increased bleeding. Coumadin is also used in some rat poisons, so it sounds dangerous. (In fact, the human cardiovascular system is much more robust than a rat's, and carefully monitored doses of Coumadin rarely cause problems.) For many people, aspirin seems like a safer alternative.

The problem is that studies have shown that Coumadin is twice as effective as aspirin in preventing embolism in people with atrial fibrillation. Choosing the weaker drug may lower your risk of small problems but raise your risk of a much bigger one. Talk with your physician about the trade-offs involved. Learn all that you can about your options. Then make an informed decision.

---

tant because the two conditions are treated differently (**C60**).

Brain imaging technology can also show the regions of the brain damaged by ischemia and yield information about blood flow to those areas. CT and MRI are now sophisticated enough to produce images of a person's arteries; these techniques are called CT angiography (CTA) and MR angiography (MRA). Sometimes it is necessary to inject a dye into the arteries to obtain clear pictures. Ultrasound checks of the neck and head can also provide important information about arterial blockage and blood flow. Since the heart and aorta are often the source of emboli, doctors use electrocardiograms (ECGs) and echocardiograms of the heart to identify the cause of the brain is-

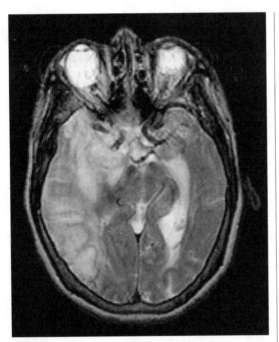

Ischemic stroke results when blood flow is obstructed to an area of the brain, resulting in the death of brain tissue. The white area on the left-hand side of this MRI shows damage from an ischemic stroke. Scan courtesy of Keith Johnson, *The Whole Brain Atlas*, www.med.harvard.edu/AANLIB/home.html

chemia. Blood tests can determine whether a person's system contains too many or too few red blood cells or platelets, and whether the blood is clotting normally.

As noted earlier, fast diagnosis and treatment of strokes are vital to helping a person recover successfully. The sooner the patient comes to the hospital to be examined, the more effective any therapy is likely to be. The treatment of patients with brain ischemia depends very much on what caused the problem. Blocked arteries can sometimes be opened by surgery, by placing balloons or tubes in these blood vessels to push back their walls, or by administering drugs that break up clots, such as recombinant tissue plasminogen activator (rt-PA) and urokinase.

To prevent further brain damage and strokes, doctors often prescribe drugs that change how platelets work (such as aspirin, clopidogrel, and dipyridamole), or anticoagulant drugs (such as heparin and Coumadin), which decrease the formation of red-blood-cell clots. Controlling blood pressure while ensuring an adequate volume of blood within the body is also helpful in minimizing brain damage. Strokes are usually signs of suboptimal cardiovascular health, so doctors and patients must take steps to avoid heart attacks and related problems.

People who have had strokes often lose some physical abilities, such as eating, walking, or using a limb as easily as they once did. Sometimes they must lie in bed for extended periods. These physical disabilities can lead to complications that prolong recovery from the stroke and even endanger a person's life. Such problems include:

- lung and urinary tract infections
- blood clots in little-used legs, which can travel to the lungs (pulmonary embolism)
- joints rendered stiff or weak by immobility
- loss of bone on the paralyzed side because of lack of exercise
- breathing food or throat contents into the lungs (aspiration)

Therefore, part of therapy after a stroke involves teaching the person and any caregivers ways to prevent those problems, and to recognize and treat them quickly if they do develop.

Some people sustain such damage from strokes that they do not even realize how badly

RECOVERY FROM ISCHEMIC STROKE

Most gains in a person's ability to function in the first 30 days after a stroke are due to spontaneous recovery. Further rehabilitation depends on:

- **the extent of the brain injury**

- **the patient's attitude**

- **the rehabilitation team's skill**

- **the cooperation of family and friends**

The success of rehabilitation therapy often depends on both the location and the extent of damage to the brain, but the determination of the patient can be no less important. Studies have shown that the brain has plasticity: the lifelong ability to adapt to change, overcome injury, and compensate for loss of function in one portion of the brain by working harder in another area. Complete recovery may not be a reasonable expectation, but the goal of rehabilitation therapy is *some* level of improvement. Improvement in function after stroke can make the difference between hospital stays and home recovery. For a stroke survivor, the goal of rehabilitation is to be as independent and productive as possible, given the limitations resulting from the stroke.

they have been impaired. Others know that they have lost some mental or physical ability—to express themselves as they did before, to walk, to do detailed work—and this can be very frustrating. A person's outlook for recovery depends mostly on the cause of the brain ischemia and the amount of the damage. Rehabilitation specialists can help people relearn tasks, or learn to do them in a different way, perhaps using different parts of the body. The brain's plasticity is a great asset in this process. If the damaged area is not too large, the neurons can often create new channels for their electrochemical signals and restore functions a person enjoyed before a stroke.

Hemorrhagic Stroke

A sudden, severe headache—"like a thunderclap"—is a very serious neurological sign. There are several possible reasons for this pain, but by far the most critical is a hemorrhagic stroke. (The other reasons are discussed in section **C54.**) If the headache is accompanied by nausea, vomiting, a stiff neck, or loss of mental or physical functions, it definitely requires immediate medical attention. Indeed, any possible stroke is an *emergency,* and swift diagnosis and treatment are essential.

A hemorrhagic stroke is caused by a sudden bleeding, or hemorrhage, into or next to the brain. This problem accounts for about 20 percent of all people admitted to hospitals for strokes. (The rest of these cases are ischemic strokes; see **C59.**) Most hemorrhagic strokes occur in the brain itself and are called intracerebral hemorrhages. Smaller groups of people suffer bleeding into the fluid-filled spaces located deep in the brain (intraventricular hemorrhage) or into the small space between the brain and the membranes that cover it (subarachnoid hemorrhage).

Any hemorrhage affecting the brain or its adjacent spaces is a very serious condition. Depending on the location and size of the mass of loose blood (called a hematoma), it may even be life-threatening. Many hemorrhages in or close to the brain stop spontaneously within the first hour. But bleeding can continue until the accumulated fluid disrupts vital brain structures or compresses otherwise healthy parts of the brain, and the person dies.

Bleeding into the Brain. In an intracerebral hemorrhage, the rapidly developing mass of blood in the brain usually causes symptoms resembling those of ischemic strokes. These include sudden weakness or numbness in one part or side of the body, difficulties speaking or understanding language, abrupt confusion, and problems seeing in one eye or in half the visual field. A person may be unaware of his or her impairment, which is another form of impairment. Unlike ischemic strokes, however, an intracerebral hemorrhage is more likely to cause a steady *worsening* of the initial symptoms, as blood continues to accumulate. A person who has had a hemorrhagic stroke is also more likely to have a headache, feel nauseous, or vomit in the minutes after onset.

Which brain functions are impaired and how badly depend mainly on the size and location of the bleeding. A hemorrhage involving the deep structures of one brain hemisphere might result in weakness on the other side of the body, and at times numbness and visual problems on the same side. If the hemorrhage occurs in the brain stem, the person may immediately plunge into a coma (C6l), with weakness in both arms and legs and impaired movements of the eyeballs.

In hemorrhages involving the cerebellum, symptoms usually begin abruptly with vomiting and such severe loss of coordination that a person cannot stand or walk. These signs are occasionally accompanied by slurred speech and double vision (C15). The growing mass of blood does not change the symptoms until it starts to compress the adjacent brain stem; that might bring on coma, at which point it is too late for surgeons to drain the hematoma and reverse the damage. That small margin of time between an alert state and an irreversible coma makes it imperative for people with stroke symptoms to get medical help quickly, and for doctors to consider the possibility of a stroke in all people showing sudden vomiting and incoordination. Prompt brain scans can settle the diagnosis and allow doctors to start treatment.

Bleeding Around the Brain. Individuals undergoing either intraventricular or subarachnoid hemorrhage commonly complain about "thunderclap" headaches. Usually they also experience nausea and vomiting, or a stiff neck. In these two conditions most of the blood leaks into a fluid cavity and not directly into the brain (at least initially). People may therefore not notice the problems associated with bleeding into the brain and ischemic strokes. However, not everyone stays awake to describe their symptoms. An

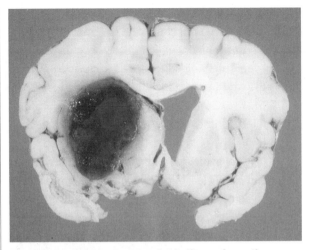

The dark area on postmortem brain tissue shows the results of a hemorrhagic stroke, sudden bleeding, or hemorrhage, into the brain. Photo courtesy of Christian Stapf, M.D., Stroke Center, The Neurological Institute, Columbia University College of Physicians and Surgeons

abrupt displacement or compression of vital brain structures may lead to sleepiness, loss of consciousness, and coma. Weakness or numbness in one side of the body and impaired vision, speech, or awareness of the disorder also tend to be bad signs; they indicate that important brain tissue is being disrupted.

How Hemorrhagic Strokes Occur

Intracerebral hemorrhages can happen in any of the cerebral lobes or the cerebellum, but they are most likely to occur in the deeper brain structures: the basal ganglia, thalamus, and brain stem. Most commonly the problem arises at weak spots in the walls of small arteries inside the brain, which have been caused by disease. These tiny blood vessels start to leak. Because the actual source of the bleeding is often small, it can take time for the loose blood to build up. That is why the symptoms of an intracerebral hemorrhage often increase over minutes or hours.

Intraventricular hemorrhage occurs when the source of the bleeding is located close to or within the wall surrounding one of the brain ventricles. In these cases, the blood drains into the fluid-filled ventricular system, often sparing healthy brain tissue.

The source of subarachnoid hemorrhage is commonly located on the surface of the brain. In 80 percent of cases, the problem starts with a congenital weak spot on the wall of a major brain artery, most often where the large arteries divide at the base of the brain. This defect grows into a thin-walled pouch bulging out of the artery's side, shaped something like a berry. Such a condition is called an aneurysm. When the walls of the pouch grow too weak to hold the blood inside, it ruptures. The leaking blood may drain not only into the small space surrounding the brain but occasionally directly into brain tissue. The mass of the growing hematoma may also displace or compress vital brain structures.

As the brain itself is not sensitive to pain, headaches from hemorrhagic strokes are believed to be due to either the stretching of the arterial wall when an aneurysm ruptures, the sudden increase of pressure within the skull, or the stretching of the membranes surrounding the brain.

Hemorrhagic strokes that stop shortly after they begin may not cause the steady progression of symptoms that helps doctors distinguish them from ischemic stroke. But it is very important to identify which type of stroke a person has had. Treatment to declog an artery (the proper response to ischemia) may cause or contribute to another hemorrhage. Separating hemorrhage from brain ischemia requires emergency brain imaging.

Diagnosis and Treatment

Any stroke symptoms require immediate workup in a hospital. The diagnosis of a hemorrhagic stroke is based on the person's history, a neurological exam, and brain imaging. A computed tomography (CT) scan shows fresh blood in the skull as a white spot on the film.

Sometimes a person's symptoms and clinical exam point to a subarachnoid hemorrhage, but the CT scan cannot confirm the diagnosis because there is only a small amount of blood in the space between the brain and the surrounding membranes. In this case, the physician usually undertakes a lumbar puncture, or spinal tap, in order to detect any fresh blood cells in the cerebrospinal fluid.

Magnetic resonance imaging (MRI) may also detect fresh bleeding in the brain, but it is even more useful in the search for possible underlying causes. It can detect vascular malformations, tumors, evidence for congophilic amyloid angiopathy, and even aneurysms. A specialized type of ultrasound called transcranial Doppler ultrasonography is another useful tool for spotting larger malformations of blood vessels—it's often used for follow-up evaluations of people who have had a subarachnoid hemorrhage. The most reliable technique to confirm or rule out the presence of aneurysms and other malformations of the blood vessels is a cerebral angiogram; physicians inject contrast dye into the blood system to make arteries stand out on X-ray films.

People having a hemorrhagic stroke should usually be kept under close observation in the acute phase of the disease and may even require the support of an intensive care unit. Balancing conservative treatment (administering pain and comfort medication, stabilizing vital signs, lower-

RISK FACTORS IN HEMORRHAGIC STROKES

The most common cause of a spontaneous intracerebral hemorrhage is chronic hypertension, or high blood pressure, which leads to harmful changes in the walls of tiny arteries. Other established risk factors include increasing age, cigarette smoking, drinking alcohol, and low levels of serum cholesterol. We cannot do anything about aging, but we can take steps to minimize the rest of those risk factors.

In the United States, individuals of African, Hispanic, and Asian origin show a higher risk for brain hemorrhage than do whites. Global figures hint that at least some of this difference is rooted in biology. Each year cerebral hemorrhages affect about 7 people out of every 100,000 in the West, but 220 out of every 100,000 in Asia.

Other factors are known to contribute to intracerebral hemorrhages, but not as often. In younger individuals, the causes include poorly formed blood vessels and drug abuse (especially cocaine and amphetamines). In elderly people, a number of intracerebral hemorrhages arise from a degenerative disorder called congophilic amyloid angiopathy, which affects smaller arteries in the brain. People taking blood-thinning medications face a higher risk of hemorrhage as their doses increase. Brain tumors, clotting disorders, and clots blocking one or more veins in the brain are other possible causes of intracerebral hemorrhages. Finally, in some people who have had an ischemic stroke, the infarcted brain area may undergo so-called hemorrhagic transformation as the blood in a formerly clogged artery finds a new channel; this mimics the picture of an intracerebral hemorrhage.

Each year in the United States, 7 to 8 individuals in 100,000 have a subarachnoid hemorrhage. Women tend to be affected more than men by a ratio of 3 to 2, and the risk seems to increase in the fifth and sixth decades of life. High blood pressure, alcohol consumption, and smoking are known risk factors. But heredity also plays a big role—about 80 percent of people suffering this problem are thought to have been born with weak spots in their major brain arteries.

Other possible sources are aneurysms due to arteriosclerosis, infection, or tumors; malformations in blood vessels located on the brain surface; the tearing of an artery within the cranium; blood-clotting disorders; and drug abuse (again, predominantly cocaine and amphetamines). In up to 15 percent of cases, however, no clear source for the subarachnoid hemorrhage can be determined.

You can take individual action to lower your risk for strokes, regardless of your genetic heritage and other unavoidable factors, by following the preventive steps listed in section C59.

ing the pressure inside the head, and so on) against the need for invasive treatment options such as surgery is influenced by a complex variety of factors. Some cases of intracerebral hemorrhage may require removing the blood in order to relieve otherwise healthy brain areas from pressure. In some instances of intraventricular hemorrhage, surgeons may relieve pressure by inserting a small tube into the ventricles to drain the system (a "shunt" operation).

Whether an aneurysm that caused a subarachnoid hemorrhage is treated immediately or after the acute phase depends on the individual's condition and on the treatment chosen. Options include "clipping" the aneurysm surgically or blocking it with metal coils inserted through a very small tube (catheter) during the angiogram.

Hemorrhagic strokes tend to be more deadly than ischemic strokes. Subarachnoid hemorrhage is the most life-threatening, with an average mortality of 40 percent within the first month after the bleeding. Overall, a person's prognosis tends to be worse if there is more blood around the brain. But an individual's chances also depend on the exact location of the hematoma and on how severely he or she has been affected.

These types of strokes may also cause secondary complications for people after the initial bleeding. Impaired circulation or resorption of the cerebrospinal fluid may lead to hydrocephalus (**C8**); this often requires a shunt operation. One third of people with such strokes have epileptic seizures, which are usually managed with medication (**C13**). Other direct effects of the hemorrhage on the brain include irregular heartbeat (cardiac arrhythmia), fluid in the lungs, impaired electrolyte balance, and fever.

The most feared acute complication is more bleeding from the original hemorrhage source. Up to 20 percent of people with ruptured aneurysms have this trouble. Another serious complication, particularly in cases after subarachnoid hemorrhage, is the occurrence of spasms in the basal brain arteries. This condition, called vasospasm, usually occurs between the third and fifth day after the hemorrhage. When these arteries narrow, there is a risk of an additional, ischemic stroke (**C59**).

People who survive a hemorrhagic stroke and the critical period that immediately follows often make a remarkable recovery. As the mass of the hematoma slowly decreases, the actual disruption of brain tissue can turn out to be smaller than what doctors or family members had feared. Early rehabilitation after strokes benefits most people.

Brain Trauma, Concussion, and Coma

Head trauma and the resulting brain injuries are one of the leading causes of death and disability in the industrialized world. In the United States, more than 50,000 people die every year as a result of traumatic brain injury. Furthermore, it is estimated that a head injury occurs every seven seconds, and hospital emergency rooms treat 1 million people for brain injuries every year. Currently about 5.3 million Americans—a little more than 2 percent of the U.S. population—live with disabilities resulting from such injuries.

Traumatic brain injury may occur at any age, but the peak incidence is among people between the ages of 15 and 24. Men are affected three to four times more often than women. Motor vehicle accidents are the leading cause, accounting for approximately 50 percent of all cases. Falls produce the most brain injuries in people older than 60 and younger than 5. Other causes include violent assault and firearms misuse. It has been estimated that after one brain injury, the risk of a second injury is three times greater, and that after a second injury, the risk of a third is eight times greater.

There are many head injury symptoms, ranging in seriousness. Minor injuries will cause mild or no symptoms, while severe injuries will cause major derangement of function. The most common symptom of brain injury after head trauma is a disturbance of consciousness; some people remain awake, but others are confused, disoriented, or unconscious. Headache, nausea, and vomiting are other common symptoms.

Anyone who sustains a head injury should be examined by a physician. Symptoms of brain trauma can be initially subtle, seemingly unrelated to the head, and not immediately apparent. A person who has sustained a serious head injury should not be manipulated or moved by people who are not trained to do so, because this may aggravate an injury.

Diagnosing Brain Trauma

The first thing doctors do when assessing a head injury is determine whether the person is in imminent danger of death. Once the person's vital functions are stabilized, physicians examine the individual from a neurological perspective, checking:

- level of consciousness

- function of the cranial nerves (through pupillary responses to light, eye movements, and facial symmetry)

- motor function (strength, symmetry, and any abnormality of movements)

- breathing rate and pattern (linked to brain stem function)

- deep tendon reflexes, such as the knee jerk

- sensory function, such as response to a pinprick

- external signs of trauma, fracture, deformity, and bruising in the head and neck

Each of these parts of the physical exam will give a physician clues about the extent and location of any brain injury.

Doctors also need to know about the person's behavior before, during, and after the injury. All of these points yield clues about what might have happened and how best to treat the person. Family members or people who witnessed the accident can usually provide helpful information. They can help medical professionals provide the best care possible by taking note of certain symptoms:

- unusual sleepiness or difficulty awakening

- mental confusion

- convulsions

- vomiting that continues or worsens

- restlessness or agitation that continues or worsens

- stiff neck

- unequal pupil size or peculiar eye movements

- inability to move arms and legs on either side

- clear or bloody drainage from the ears or nose

- bruising around the eyes or behind the ears

- difficulty breathing

This is a partial list.

Physicians can use a variety of radiological tests to assess a person with head trauma. Most hospital emergency departments can now do computed tomography (CT) scans. CT provides more information, and is excellent for diagnosing skull fractures, bleeding, or other important lesions in the brain. CT also helps doctors follow people with head trauma as they recover. Magnetic resonance imaging (MRI) currently has little involvement in diagnosing and treating an emergency, but once a person's condition is stable an MRI may provide useful information that a CT cannot, such as evidence of white matter damage.

Different types of injuries require particular treatments. Surgery is needed to remove blood or foreign material, or to reconstruct parts of the skull. Very often brain trauma causes tissue to swell against the inflexible bone. In these cases, a neurosurgeon may relieve the pressure inside the skull by placing a ventriculostomy drain that removes cerebrospinal fluid. If the swelling is massive, a neurosurgeon may remove a piece of the skull so that the brain has room to expand; the surgeon keeps and reimplants the bone after the swelling has gone down significantly. Often during these procedures, the surgeon places a small pressure valve inside the skull to measure pressure on a moment-to-moment basis.

Most nonsurgical management of brain trauma involves close monitoring, often in an intensive care unit, to prevent further injury. Physicians will conduct further neurological exams in order to assess whether the person is improving or worsening. Doctors have no "miracle drug" to prevent nerve injury or improve brain function immediately after trauma, but they can use medication to modify a person's blood pressure, optimize the delivery of oxygen to the brain tissue, and prevent further brain swelling.

Specific Injuries in Head Trauma

Trauma to the head can produce many problems because so many components may be injured. Brain tissue is surrounded both by the skull and by a tough membrane called the dura, which is right next to the brain. Within, and surrounding, the brain tissue and dura are many arteries, veins, and important nerves (the cranial nerves). Therefore, trauma to the head may damage the skull, the blood vessels, the nerves, the brain tissue itself, or all of the above. Depending on the nature and severity of their injuries, people may exhibit a very wide range of symptoms: from absolutely none to coma.

Injuries to the Skull

Fractures of the skull can be divided into linear fractures, depressed fractures, and compound fractures. Linear fractures are simple "cracks" in the skull. Most require no treatment. The concern with these fractures is that a force large enough to break the skull may have damaged the underlying brain or blood vessels. This is especially true for fractures of the bottom, or "base," of the skull.

Depressed skull fractures are those in which part of the bone presses on or into the brain. The extent of the damage depends on what part of the brain the depressed skull overlies, as well as the nature of any associated injuries to other tissues.

In compound fractures, the trauma is severe enough to break the skin, bone, and dura and expose the brain tissue. These types of fractures are usually associated with severe brain damage.

Treating skull fractures depends on the extent of damage to structures beneath the bone. Most linear fractures will not damage other structures unless the fractured bone becomes displaced and presses on the brain. In this case a surgical repair may be necessary to restore the bone to its normal position. Depressed skull fractures are usually also treated surgically in order to restore normal anatomy and prevent damage to underlying tissues by bone fragments.

Compound fractures are a special case since, by definition, there has been contact between the brain tissue and the outside air. These fractures therefore bring the possibility of infection from environmental debris. The fracture site is therefore vigorously cleaned and decontaminated before repair. In addition, these fractures are usually associated with severe injuries to the brain, blood vessels, and nerves, and repairing these structures may also be necessary.

Injuries Involving Vessels

Injuries to the blood vessels within the skull may lead to the collecting of blood in abnormal places. A collection of blood outside a vessel is called a hematoma. In all of the following types of hematomas, individuals are in danger if there is enough accumulating blood to press on the brain or other important structures within the skull. (In this respect, a head injury can resemble a hemorrhagic stroke; **C60**.) In these cases, the hematoma may compress the brain and shift it from its normal position. Too much shifting can damage the crucial brain stem. Bleeding may also raise the pressure inside the skull to the point that it shuts off the blood supply to the brain (as in an ischemic stroke; **C59**). These conditions can be very serious and require emergency surgery.

Epidural hematomas occur between the skull and the dura. These are usually caused by a direct-impact injury that causes a forceful deformity of the skull. Eighty percent are associated with skull fractures across an artery called the middle meningeal artery. Because arteries bleed quickly, this type of injury can cause significant bleeding within the skull and require emergency surgery. Although uncommon (affecting only 0.5 percent of all head-injured individuals), epidural hematomas are a surgical *emergency*, and people with this type of injury must have the damage immediately repaired in the operating room.

Subdural hematomas appear between the dura and the surface of the brain. These are more common than epidural hematomas, occurring in about 30 percent of people with severe head trauma. They are produced by the rupture of small veins, so the bleeding is much slower than in epidural hematomas. A person with a subdural may have no immediate symptoms. As blood slowly collects within the skull, however, it compresses the brain and increases the intracranial pressure.

There are three types: acute, subacute, and chronic. The acute subdural may cause drowsiness or coma within a few hours and requires

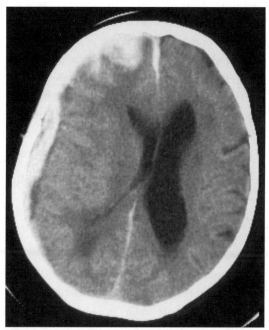

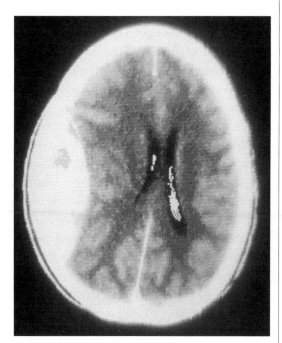

Epidural hematoma is bleeding between the skull and the dura, the tough outer layer covering the brain. These injuries are usually caused by a blow to the skull. Bleeding in this area can press brain tissue inward, causing damage. Scan © Mehau Kulyk/SPL/Photo Researchers, Inc.

Subdural hematoma is bleeding between the dura and the surface of the brain. These are more common than epidural hematomas, occurring in about 30 percent of people with severe head trauma. They are produced by the rupture of small veins. As blood slowly collects within the skull, it compresses the brain. Scan © Department of Clinical Radiology, Salisbury District Hospital/SPL/Photo Researchers, Inc.

urgent treatment. A subacute subdural should be removed within one to two weeks. The most treacherous is a chronic subdural hematoma. It is not uncommon for such an injury to go undiagnosed for several weeks because individuals or their families do not recognize subtle symptoms. A person may appear well but nonetheless have a large subdural. That is why it is important for a heath professional to evaluate all individuals with head injuries. Depending on the symptoms and size of the subdural, treatment may involve careful monitoring or surgical removal of the blood.

Scans should be done on any person with prolonged headaches or other symptoms after head injury.

Intracerebral hematoma. Injuries to small blood vessels in the brain may also lead to bleeding within the brain tissue, called an intracerebral hematoma. The effect of this hematoma depends on how much blood collects, and where, and whether the bleeding continues. Doctors may respond conservatively, finding no need for treatment, or treat the problem as an emergency. More than half of people with intracerebral hematomas lose consciousness at the time of injury. There may be associated brain contusions with this hematoma.

Subarachnoid hemorrhage. Bleeding may occur in a thin layer immediately surrounding the brain (the subarachnoid space). In head trauma, it is common to have some degree of subarachnoid hemorrhage, depending on the force applied to the head. In fact, subarachnoid hemorrhage is the most commonly diagnosed abnormality after head trauma. CT detects it in 44 percent of severe head trauma cases. Fortunately, individuals with subarachnoid hemorrhage but no other associated injuries usually do very well. However, they may get delayed hydrocephalus as a result of blockage of the flow of cerebrospinal fluid.

Injuries to the Brain Tissue

Our brains are somewhat mobile inside our skulls, which can give rise to other injuries. There are some spiny contours on the inside of the skull, but under normal circumstances a barrier of cerebrospinal fluid surrounds the brain and cushions it from direct contact with the hard bone. However, when a person's head is subjected to violent forces, the brain may be forcibly rotated and battered within the skull. During such episodes brain tissue may be ripped, stretched, battered, and bruised. Bleeding, swelling, and further bruising of brain tissue usually follows. In these cases, people usually sustain permanent damage.

Injuries to the brain are classified according to the degree of tissue damage that they cause. It is important to remember that the different types of brain injuries are part of a spectrum. There may not be a clear distinction in every case, and one person may suffer multiple types of injuries.

Concussion. A concussion is a temporary and fully reversible loss of brain function caused by direct injury to the brain. It is the mildest form of brain injury, usually resulting from minor trauma to the head. In concussions, it is not possible to identify any structural damage to the brain tissue. People who suffer a concussion usually lose consciousness, but only for a brief time; their long-term outcome is excellent.

Contusion. Contusions are localized areas of "bruising" of the brain tissue. They consist of areas

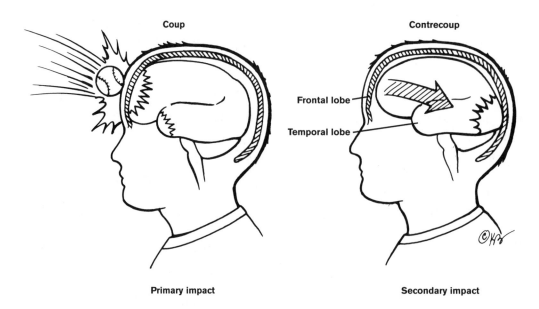

A blow to the head may cause the brain to suffer two separate hits: first at the point of impact, and then as it is thrown against the back of the skull. ILLUSTRATION © KATHRYN BORN

of swollen brain and blood that has leaked out of small arteries, veins, or capillaries. Contusions will often occur under the impact point on the skull (coup). They may also, in the same incident, occur on the side directly opposite the impact because the brain may rock away from the blow and strike the inside of the skull (contrecoup). Sometimes the skull is broken at the site of a contusion, but not always. Whatever the cause, contusions are likely to be most severe in the tips of the frontal and temporal lobes, after trauma forces these areas of the brain against bony ridges inside the skull.

Lacerations. Lacerations are actual tears in the brain tissue. They can be caused by shear forces placed on the brain, or by an object (such as a bullet) penetrating the skull and brain. The degree of damage depends on the depth and location of the laceration, as well as on whether associated blood vessels and cranial nerves suffer damage.

Diffuse axonal injury. Diffuse axonal injury (DAI) refers to impaired function and eventual loss of axons (the long extensions of nerve cells, which enable them to communicate with one another). It is caused by the acceleration, deceleration, and rotation of the head during trauma, as in a car crash, probably the most frequent cause of this type of injury. These forces can stretch and shear axons. DAI is a microscopic injury that does not show up on a CT scan. Therefore, diagnosing DAI depends on physicians' observations. Individuals with this sort of injury are usually unconscious for longer than six hours and, depending on the degree and location of axonal injury, may remain this way for days or weeks. DAI may be mild and reversible or, if extensive, may lead to severe brain damage or death. This is the most common cause of injury from high-velocity trauma and has no treatment.

Brain swelling and ischemia. Often, a person's immediate injury may not be the worst. Usually, there is additional secondary injury to the brain that occurs hours to days later. The damage to the brain tissue, blood vessels, and nerves causes the brain to swell. If that swelling is severe, the blood supply to the brain may be blocked (ischemia), leading to tissue death. Also, since the brain is encased in a hard skull, the swelling may actually compress the tissue against bone. Excessive compression of areas such as the brain stem, which is responsible for regulating our breathing and consciousness (among other vital functions), can lead to severe disability and death.

Long-Term Outcome

Perhaps the most widely used system to predict outcome after head injury is the Glasgow Coma Scale (GCS). The individual is evaluated in each of three parameters, and the sum of the three parts provides the total score.

People with mild head injury, usually defined as Glasgow Coma Score 13–15, tend to do very well. These individuals have often suffered concussions or minor degrees of brain swelling or contusion. Although headaches, dizziness, irritability, or similar symptoms may sometimes trouble them, most suffer no residual effects. For people with a simple

GLASGOW COMA SCALE

ACTION	POINTS	EXPLANATION
Eye opening		
Spontaneously	4	
Responding to verbal command	3	
Responding to pain	2	
None	1	
Verbal response		
Converses and oriented	5	
Converses but confused	4	
Inappropriate words	3	
Incomprehensible words or sounds	2	
No response	1	
Motor response		
Obeys verbal commands to move	6	
Localizes to painful stimuli	5	Moves limb in an effort to remove painful stimuli
Flexion withdrawal	4	Pulls away from pain by bending limbs
Decorticate posturing	3	Abnormal bending of extremities
Decerebrate posturing	2	Abnormal extension of extremities
No response	1	

COMA AND PERSISTENT VEGETATIVE STATE

The word *coma* simply means loss of consciousness. Medically, coma is a sleeplike state from which people cannot be aroused even if you vigorously stimulate them. It can arise from many causes, including infections, toxins, medications, seizures, and injury to the brain from trauma.

In the case of brain trauma, a person may lose consciousness for only a few seconds, or for hours or even days. The duration of such a coma usually relates to the severity of the injury to the brain. Some investigators have set a dividing line at six hours. A loss of consciousness for less than six hours usually means that the injury is limited to a concussion, and the long-term outcome for these individuals is usually excellent. If coma lasts longer than six hours, there may be significant brain tissue injury.

People who survive brain trauma and are in a coma may regain consciousness to a varying degree. But between complete recovery and death lies a broad spectrum of consciousness.

The worst form of coma is known as persistent vegetative state (PVS). In the United States 10,000 to 25,000 adults and 4,000 to 10,000 children are in PVS. Whereas people in comas are neither awake nor aware of their surroundings, people in PVS are awake but not aware. They may open their eyes and look around the room. They may yawn, chew, swallow, and (in rare cases) make guttural noises. All of these actions can be very distressing to family members, since their loved one seems to be having "normal" functions. However, these are all reflexes mediated at the level of the brain stem—not the brain cortex, where our centers for thought, reasoning, speech, and language processing are located. A person is diagnosed as being in PVS after sustaining brain trauma and showing no detectable awareness of the environment for one month.

Individuals in PVS rarely show any improvement, and none regain completely normal function. Partial recovery to the point where the person can communicate and comprehend has been reported in only 3 percent of individuals after five years, and recovery to the point where the person can carry out the activities of daily living is even more rare.

The care of people in coma is mostly supportive and aims to prevent further complications. These individuals must be monitored closely and will usually remain in an intensive care unit under 24-hour supervision. Since a person in a coma has a severely injured brain, medical personnel and machines must take care of many of the brain's normal functions. Doctors may prescribe medications to control and treat seizures, infections, brain swelling, and changes in blood pressure, among other things. Nurses and other health care workers will monitor the person's vital signs (blood pressure, pulse, respiration, and temperature) and optimize nutrition and fluid intake. Breathing will usually be regulated by a machine.

concussion, the mortality rate is zero. Of people with mild brain swelling, fewer than 2 percent die.

People with moderate head injuries (GCS 9–12) do less well. Approximately 60 percent will make a good recovery, and another 25 percent or so will have moderate degrees of disability. Death or persistent vegetative state (PVS) will be the outcome for 7 percent to 10 percent. The remainder are usually left with severe disability.

People with severe head injuries (GCS under 8) have the worst prognoses. About 25 percent to 30 percent of these individuals have good long-term outcomes, 17 percent have moderate to severe disabilities, and 30 percent die. A small percentage remain in PVS.

In penetrating head injuries, such as those inflicted by bullets, the statistics are a bit different. Over half of all people with gunshot wounds to the head who are alive when they arrive at a hospital later die because their initial injuries are so severe. But the other half, with more mild injuries, usually do fairly well.

The outcome for people in coma after brain injury depends in part on their age. People under 20 are three times more likely to survive than those over 60. One study found that people who showed no motor response to painful stimuli and no pupillary response to light (normally our pupils get smaller when light is shone on them) 24 hours after brain injury were likely to die. However, the presence of both of these responses was a very positive finding, especially in young people.

Rehabilitation After Brain Injury

People who have suffered head trauma and resultant brain injury will often benefit from some physical therapy during their hospital stay or after they leave the hospital. If they are not acutely ill, moving to a rehabilitation program may speed any further recovery. These centers usually teach individuals strategies for reaching the maximum level of functioning their impairments allow. People sometimes have to relearn skills essential for everyday activities. Another major goal of these centers is to work with families to educate them about realistic future expectations and how they can best help their injured family member.

After brain trauma, individuals may have persistent cognitive or emotional disabilities that include:

- short-term memory loss (**C68**)
- long-term memory loss (**C68**)
- slowed ability to process information
- trouble concentrating or paying attention for periods of time
- difficulty keeping up with a conversation
- problems finding words (**C70**)
- spatial disorientation
- organizational problems and impaired judgment (**C71**)
- inability to do more than one thing at a time (**C71**)

Physical consequences can include:

- seizures (**C13**)
- muscle weakness or spasticity
- double vision or impaired vision (**C15**)
- loss of smell or taste (**C17**)
- speech impairments such as slow or slurred speech

SUGGESTIONS FOR FAMILY MEMBERS AFTER BRAIN INJURY

For the person with a brain injury, learning more about the type of injury, identifying the mental or physical changes the injury may have caused, and, ultimately, adjusting to the limitations resulting from the brain injury can be a challenging, difficult, but necessary process. Family members of the person with an injury have the dual challenge of changing their vision of the person with the brain injury while at the same time accepting that the dynamics of the family and each person's role in it may be altered as well.

Seven things families need to remember:

■ Reinforce the behaviors you would like to promote.

■ When safety is not an issue, ignore the behaviors you would like to minimize.

■ Model the behaviors you would like to see.

■ Avoid situations that provoke behaviors you are trying to reduce.

■ Structure the environment; use cues for positive behaviors.

■ Redirect the person rather than challenging him or her.

■ Seek professional help sooner rather than later.

Adapted from www.biausa.org (Brain Injury Association). Additional site: www.comarecovery.org (Coma Recovery Association)

■ headaches or migraines (**C54, C55**)

■ fatigue, increased need for sleep (**C11**)

■ balance problems

Long-term recovery from brain injuries depends on many factors, including the severity of the trauma, associated injuries, and a person's age. Unlike in the movies, people rarely recover their preinjury level of functioning after severe head trauma. Rather than emphasizing complete recovery, treatment aims to improve function, prevent further injury, and rehabilitate individuals and their families physically and emotionally.

Spinal Cord Injury

An injury to the spinal cord disconnects the body below the injury site from the brain. Thus, an injury to the cervical spinal cord, at the level of the neck, produces quadriplegia, or loss of function in all four limbs, while an injury to the thoracic spinal cord, at chest level, causes paraplegia, or loss of function in the legs.

Spinal cord injury, however, does much more than cause loss of sensation to, and paralysis of, the arms and legs. The spinal cord also carries autonomic signals for the bowel, bladder, lungs, and other organs to and from the brain. Spinal cord injury interrupts brain control and sensation of these organs. An injury to the upper part of the neck will stop breathing, and the person must be artificially respirated. Most spinal cord injuries affect the bowel and bladder.

The part of the spinal cord that is separated from the brain by the injury usually becomes hyperexcitable. The paralyzed parts of the body often show increased reflexes or spasticity and can even produce spasms violent enough to throw the person out of a wheelchair. Likewise, bladder and bowel become spastic. Bladder spasticity is a particular problem, since it can cause urine reflux and kidney damage. The autonomic system becomes similarly hyperexcitable and can produce life-threatening increases of blood pressure.

Most people with spinal cord injury suffer from abnormal sensations and pain below the injury site. Closely akin to "phantom limb" pain that people suffer after amputations, the abnormal sensations are often "burning" or "freezing," and are localized to areas below the injury site. Called neurogenic pain because these sensations originate from the spinal cord, this kind of pain is typically unresponsive to conventional painkilling drugs.

Paralyzed muscles shrink and become atrophied. If the injury damages the spinal cord where the motoneurons—the neurons that send movement commands to, or innervate, the muscles—are situated, the person will develop severe atrophy of the muscles innervated by the motoneurons. This will result in flaccid limbs, incompetent bowel and bladder sphincters, and dysfunctional sexual organs. These consequences of spinal cord injury can be devastating, particularly for young men, who are the most frequent victims of spinal cord injury.

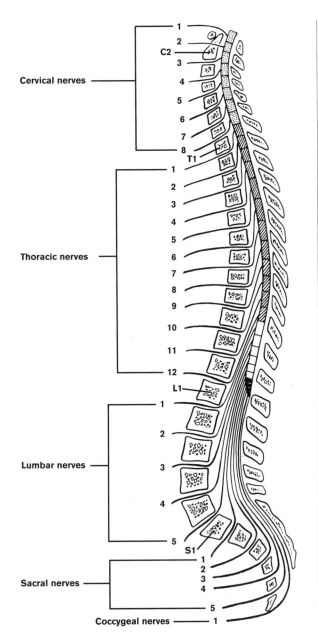

Cervical nerves

1
2
C2
3
4
5
6
7
8
T1

Thoracic nerves

1
2
3
4
5
6
7
8
9
10
11
12
L1

Lumbar nerves

1
2
3
4
5
S1

Sacral nerves

1
2
3
4
5

Coccygeal nerves — 1

The nerves of the spinal cord are divided into five levels. Illustration © Kathryn Born

For much of human history, spinal cord injury was considered to be an incurable condition. The standard clinical approach emphasized prevention of further injury, acceptance of the condition, and learning to use remaining function, rather than restoring function. Several recent developments, however, provide hope that curative therapies of spinal cord injury are not only possible but also imminent.

Diagnosis and Treatment

Diagnosis of spinal cord injury is relatively straightforward. Because the injury causes a loss of motor and sensory function below the injury site, a careful neurological examination suffices to identify and characterize the level and severity of injury. The American Spinal Injury Association has developed a spinal cord injury classification system and a neurological outcome scale that are internationally accepted. The spinal cord and spinal column can be readily studied by magnetic resonance imaging (MRI) and computed tomography (CT) scans, which show soft tissue and bone and their impingement on the spinal cord.

Medical treatment of spinal cord injury is also straightforward. In 1990 the National Acute Spinal Cord Injury Study (NASCIS) reported that high-dose methylprednisolone, a potent synthetic steroid, improves neurologic recovery by about 20 percent in people when it is administered within eight hours after injury. This was the first therapy that improved recovery of function in people when given after spinal cord injury. This discovery opened the doors to the concept of secondary tissue damage in the spinal cord and brain, leading to the new field of neuroprotective therapies. Although several recent studies have criticized several aspects of the NASCIS trial, methylprednisolone is now routinely given to all patients with acute spinal cord injury in the United States and around the world.

Surgical treatment of spinal cord injury, however, is split between two camps. The first, and more conservative group, holds that if the patient has no function below the injury site and therefore has a "complete" injury, surgical decompression of the cord will not restore function. Therefore, a common practice is to delay the surgery for a week or more after injury, so that the surgery can be carried out electively. The second group comprises surgeons who will decompress the spinal cord immediately, believing that there is a small window of opportunity. Most surgeons will now stabilize the spinal column with titanium plates or rods that allow immediate immobilization of the fracture and more rapid rehabilitation of patients, in contrast to years past when patients had to remain in traction or external devices that required prolonged bed rest and limitations of activity for many months.

Rehabilitative therapy focuses on teaching patients, families, and caretakers techniques to manage the most serious consequences of spinal cord injury: impaired bladder function and infections, skin care, spasticity, neuropathic pain, paralysis, and sensory loss. Although the goal of rehabilitation remains constant—making the most of residual function—the techniques for achieving this goal have shifted dramatically. In addition to standard physical therapy, urological and skin care, and help dealing with social and environmental barriers, many rehabilitation centers are now emphasizing novel exercise and pharmacological and electrical stimulation.

Perhaps the most important research advance in spinal cord injury care was the recent discovery that many people who have never walked after injury can recover independent locomotion through intensive supported ambulation training. This has led to a popular theory that neuronal circuits in the spinal cord may turn off if they are not used for a period of time. The good news, however, is that intensive forced-use exercise and training can restore function, sometimes many years or even decades after injury.

Recovery After Spinal Cord Injury

Contrary to popular belief, recovery is the rule and not the exception in spinal cord injury. If a person has even a trace of voluntary movement or touch sensation below the injury site shortly after injury, that person has a good prognosis for substantial recovery. In the United States about 10,000 people every year have traumatic spinal cord injuries of sufficient severity to require hospitalization. More than 60 percent of people who are admitted to hospitals with the diagnosis of spinal cord injury have "incomplete" injuries. A much larger number of people suffer a milder form of spinal cord injury called whiplash, which causes temporary loss of arm or leg function. An estimated 4 out of 1,000 people, or about a million a year, are treated for whiplash. Thus, many people walk away from spinal cord injury. On the other hand, about 250,000 people in the United States have had severe traumatic spinal cord injury from which they did not recover.

The Science of Spinal Cord Recovery

A majority of people recover to some extent after injury. Many recover substantially more

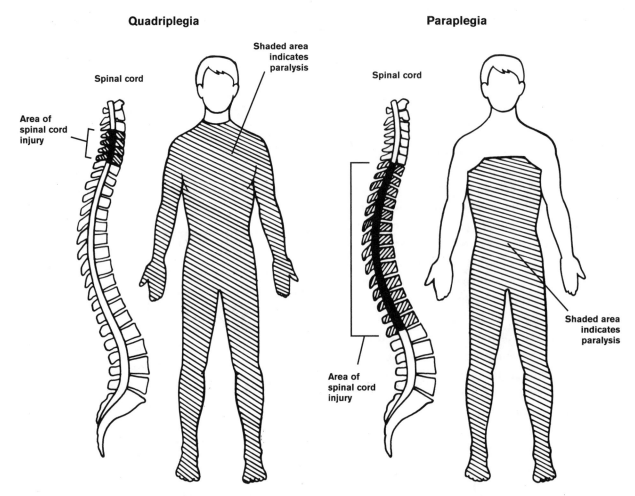

Quadriplegia

Spinal cord

Area of spinal cord injury

Shaded area indicates paralysis

Paraplegia

Spinal cord

Area of spinal cord injury

Shaded area indicates paralysis

An injury to the spinal cord at the cervical nerve level can result in quadriplegia—complete loss of movement below the neck. Persons with this injury often require a respirator to breathe. ILLUSTRATION © KATHRYN BORN

An injury in the thoracic nerve region of the spinal cord can cause paraplegia—paralysis from the chest down, with arm mobility intact. ILLUSTRATION © KATHRYN BORN

than expected by their doctors. How is it possible that some people recover so well from spinal cord injury while others do not? Two factors may influence recovery. First, the spinal cord has redundant pathways for achieving the same function. Both humans and animals can recover locomotor function even after injuries that damage as much as 90 percent of the pathways. The spinal cord is quite plastic and can continue to function with relatively few connections with the brain. Second, while the spinal cord turns off neuronal circuits that are not used for a period of time, intensive forced-use therapy may be able to restore them.

The Spinal "Brain"

The spinal cord is capable of remarkably complex motor behavior on its own. It not only contains the neuronal circuitry and reflexes necessary for complex motor activities and sensory processing, but also can adjust its circuitry to perform in a wide variety of environments and situations. It does this with little or no input from the brain. For example, locomotion is controlled by, a neural center in the lower spinal cord called a central pattern generator (CPG). To walk, the brain sends a signal to the CPG to initiate walking. Once the program starts, the brain just manages the movements. Relatively few connections are required.

Animals and people with no voluntary motor control can be trained to stand, walk, and even perform complex behaviors such as walking on a treadmill. Several studies have reported that the isolated spinal cord is capable of learning complex behaviors. For example, researchers recently reported that cats and rats with completely cut spinal cords not only can learn to walk on a treadmill but can adjust their walking behavior in response to sensory cues. While the animals do not have voluntary control over the muscles and do not have sensory feedback to the brain, training can produce remarkably coordinated locomotion that outlasts the training period. The ability of the spinal cord to function with relatively little input from the brain probably accounts for the remarkable recovery of many people who have so-called incomplete spinal cord injuries.

However, recovery of control and sensation in the limbs and organs affected takes months, or even years, after spinal cord injury. During that period, several developments may limit recovery. Muscles undergo atrophy when they are not used. Such atrophy can be partly reversed with electrical stimulation; and spasticity, even though it is troubling to the patient and family, can help maintain muscle bulk. Thus, it is important that

antispasticity drugs not be overused during the recovery phase of spinal cord injury. Several recent studies have suggested a novel approach to preventing atrophy and perhaps restoring muscles: researchers showed that implantation of embryonic neurons into muscles can prevent the atrophy that occurs in denervated muscles.

Learned Nonuse

Atrophy may also occur in the central nervous system. In the 1970s researchers showed that monkeys would stop using a hand when the sensory nerve to the hand was cut. Over time, the unused hand became effectively paralyzed, even though motor nerve connections were still intact. In other words, failure to use a limb due to sensory loss may lead to paralysis of the limb. Called learned nonuse, this phenomenon may account for much of the lack of recovery after stroke, traumatic brain injury, and spinal cord injury. For many years, clinicians considered this condition to be irreversible, and few attempts were made to restore function. Patients have been told not to even try to use their paralyzed limbs, and the loss of function was attributed to loss of neural connections. Most clinicians and scientists believed that regeneration would be necessary to overcome the paralysis.

Recent studies, however, indicate that learned nonuse can be reversed, even after many years of paralysis. Researchers have reported that forced-use training programs can reverse learned nonuse in people even many years after stroke. In the mid-1990s several groups in Germany reported that they were able to use intensive supported treadmill walking to restore locomotion in as many as 50 percent of people five years or more after their spinal cord injuries. Several preliminary trials in the United States have confirmed these results. The National Institutes of Health is funding a clinical trial

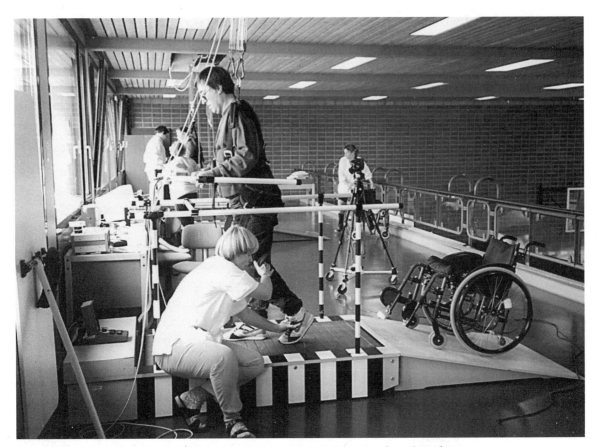

Spinal cord injury can result in impairments to movement because of a variety of complications that can arise at the site of the injury: scar tissue can interrupt nerve impulses needed to complete a movement, and axons that have lost their myelin sheath (the white fatty insulation) do not carry impulses as efficiently as normal nerves. A few fibers may be spared, however, and rehabilitation training focuses on preserving and improving the functioning of those fibers. PHOTO COURTESY OF ANTON WERNIG

to assess supported ambulation training, and preliminary data suggest that such training can restore locomotion in chronic spinal cord injury.

The discovery that locomotor function can be restored even after years of functional loss has profound implications for the biology of functional recovery. First, it means that central neural circuits can remain silent for years, even decades, and can then be reactivated. Most clinicians have hitherto assumed that absent function means absent circuits. Second, activity is important for maintaining and restoring function. The old maxim "Use it or lose it" may apply to both muscle and neurons. These findings have important implications for clinical care and trials of therapies. Clinical trials must take the post-treatment rehabilitation seriously. Without programs to reverse learned nonuse, regenerative and remyelinative therapies may well fail.

Training programs to reverse learned nonuse

are laborious and expensive. Several groups are developing computerized robots to substitute for the manual labor required for such training. Much research is required to validate, improve, and define the most effective timing, duration, and intensity of forced-use training. However, if these techniques do restore function, such training will be well worth the expense. People who survive spinal cord injury live an average of 40 years, at the cost of more than $22,000 a year. Current care costs for spinal cord injury exceed $10 billion a year. Restoring function will yield recurrent lifetime savings, saving government and society many billions of dollars.

From Bench to Bedside

A majority of scientists and clinicians believe that regenerative therapies are both possible and imminent. Many promising spinal cord injury therapies have been discovered in animals, and a few have entered clinical trial. Reliable animal models of spinal cord injury have been established and well-standardized outcome measures are available for both animal and clinical trials. These advances made it possible for spinal cord injury research to show methylprednisolone to be the first effective neuroprotective therapy for the central nervous system. Likewise, the first studies showing functional regeneration were done in spinal cord injury models. For these reasons, the first regenerative therapies will probably be demonstrated in human spinal cord injury.

Future Therapies for Recovery of Movement

Scientists and clinicians have long known that the survival of only a remarkably few spinal axons (nerve fibers) is necessary for a person to recover most functions. Nearly 50 years ago, studies in cats showed that only 10 percent of spinal axons are necessary and sufficient to support substantial motor and sensory recovery, including locomotion. Rats are able to walk with only 10 percent of their spinal axons. Much clinical experience suggests that people with as much as 90 percent damage of the spinal cord will walk out of the hospital. Thus, therapies do not have to restore or regenerate many axons to restore function.

Spinal cord injury not only disconnects axons but also damages the cells that myelinate spinal axons. Myelin, the white fiber coating around axons, helps them conduct electrical signals efficiently, and thus the loss of myelin through crushing or bruising of the cord causes further neurological deficits in spinal cord injury. Implantation of myelinating cells, such as Schwann cells, cells that contribute to the formation of myelin (called oligodendroglial precursors), and neural stem cells can remyelinate spinal axons. A drug called 4-aminopyridine (4-AP) increases the ability of myelin-damaged axons to conduct and was in clinical trial as of 2001. Another drug, called M1, with similar action, was being readied for clinical trial as this book went to press.

The Outlook for Regeneration

Early studies indicated that damaged spinal axons will engage in short-distance sprouting, but long-distance regrowth of axons did not occur. Thus, most scientists believed that the spinal cord could not regenerate. However, studies in the 1990s decisively overturned this dogma, such that a majority of scientists now believe that the spinal cord can regenerate.

Healing with the Immune System

Recent studies suggest several novel approaches to regenerating the spinal cord. Some of the most provocative involve the immune system: scientists have reported that vaccinating mice with parts of the spinal cord can induce antibodies that promote spinal cord regeneration. Other researchers have found that macrophages or lymphocytes activated by exposure to certain proteins can protect the spinal cord and improve recovery. The former are currently being tested in clinical trial. These findings suggest that the immune system may play an important role in the recovery of the spinal cord.

Electrical Stimulation

Scientists have long suspected that electrical current can enhance regeneration. Several groups of researchers have reported that electrical currents produced spinal cord regeneration in rabbits and dogs. A study in 2001 revealed that electrical currents increase an intracellular messenger molecule, called cAMP (cyclic adenosine monophosphate), that stimulates growth of axons. Although studies over many years have shown that electrical currents stimulate axonal growth, the mechanism was not well understood until this discovery. A clinical trial has started testing the effects of implanted devices that deliver alternating electrical currents to the spinal cord.

Cell Transplantation

Cell transplant therapy for spinal cord injury began with fetal cells. Researchers showed that transplanted fetal cells survive and integrate into injured spinal cords, altering the behavior of rats after injury. In addition, a clinical trial of fetal cell transplants has shown the safety and feasibility of these transplants in human spinal cord injury.

Fetal cells, however, may soon be supplanted by embryonic stem cells, cells that can produce many cell types. Scientists recently discovered that embryonic stem cells will remyelinate the spinal cord and improve function recovery in rats.

Until recently, scientists believed that certain cells in the brain and spinal cord could not be replaced. For example, the neurons that we die with were believed to be the same neurons that we were born with. However recent studies have shown that the human brain and spinal cord contain stem cells that can produce additional neurons and glial cells. In other words, the brain and spinal cord appear to be capable of producing new neurons to replace those that have been lost due to injury, disease, or aging. Furthermore, implantation of stem cells into an injured brain and spinal cord may restore function. Animal stem cells taken from bone marrow can also myelinate the human spinal cord. Neural stem cells from pigs are now being implanted into people with chronic spinal cord injury in a clinical trial.

Animal studies have shown that other cell transplants can stimulate regeneration and improve recovery. For example, olfactory ensheathing glia (OEG) are special cells that reside in the olfactory nerve and bulb, the nerve inside the nose and the related brain structure that mediate our sense of smell. The OEG cells are believed to be responsible for the mammalian olfactory nerve's unusual ability to regenerate continuously throughout adult life. OEG transplants into rat spinal cords have stimulated functional regeneration. Several groups are considering implanting OEG cells into patients, and trials have already begun in Russia.

Recent studies in animals have suggested that it may not even be necessary to breach the spinal cord in order to implant cells to prompt regenera-

---

SPINAL CORD INJURY REHABILITATION

Rehabilitation will enable the person with an injured spinal cord to return to the environment of social and vocational functioning as best as can be managed. Before returning to the world outside the rehabilitation center, however, the spinal-cord-injured (SCI) patient must learn a number of things to aid him or her in this step toward independence.

- During the initial phase of rehabilitation the strongest emphasis is on the SCI patient's regaining as much strength and movement as possible in the arms or legs, depending on the locality and severity of the injury. A full understanding of spinal cord injury and what it entails is another aspect emphasized during the beginning stages of rehabilitation.

- The two most important areas of function for the SCI patient are in mobility and transportation and in communication. The person must also adjust psychologically to major loss. He or she has lost some part of physical function but may also have experienced other losses, such as employment, housing, and future dreams.

- Other types of rehabilitation include physical and occupational therapy. Physical therapy includes an exercise program geared toward muscle strengthening, while occupational therapy involves the redevelopment of fine motor skills.

- As with any type of physical injury, medications are needed to keep the fine motor and leg and arm motor systems regulated and for preventive measures of other conditions that can be brought about from the initial injury, such as pressure sores and bladder damage. A person may need to use a variety of medications to counteract conditions caused by the injury.

Adapted from www.users.sgi.net/~ozzy/scirehab.htm (Rehabilitation Process of Persons with Spinal Cord Injury); another useful link is www.spinalcord.org (National Spinal Cord Injury Association)

---

tion. For example, several research teams showed that bone marrow stem cells injected into a vein or into the space around the gut migrate to the brain and produce neurons. Similarly, another team found that embryonic stem cells injected into the cerebrospinal fluid surrounding the spinal cord migrated into the spinal cord and replaced neurons that had degenerated in a mouse model of amyotrophic lateral sclerosis. Thus, future clinical trials of cell transplants may not require surgery to place the cells in the spinal cord.

A dazzling array of promising therapies are or will soon be available for experimental clinical studies. Initial clinical trials have already shown the safety and feasibility of some of these therapies. These are the first generation of therapies for spinal cord injury that may help restore some function to some people. In a few years, a second generation of optimized first-generation therapies should begin, which should restore more function to more people. Third-generation "curative" therapies should be available by the year 2010.

Paraneoplastic Syndromes

Paraneoplastic syndromes are disorders of an organ or tissue caused by a cancer but *not* due to spread of the cancer to that organ or tissue. The term *paraneoplastic* comes from the Greek roots *para* (alongside or near), *neo* (new), and *plastic* (being formed or shaped), and thus means "beside a new formation, or cancer." These syndromes can affect any organ or tissue, including the liver, skin, and muscles, but the nervous system itself is a common site. A paraneoplastic disorder may affect only one part of the nervous system, such as the cerebellum, or multiple areas at once. When more than one part of the nervous system is affected, the disorder is often called encephalomyelitis associated with cancer. See the list of well-known paraneoplastic syndromes on page 601.

Paraneoplastic syndromes are rare, affecting fewer than 1 percent of patients with cancer. Nevertheless, they are important for several reasons. They usually precede identification of the cancer, so recognizing them may lead to early diagnosis and treatment of that cancer. The presence of a paraneoplastic syndrome may also predict slower growth of the cancer. Sadly, a paraneoplastic syndrome can cause severe neurological disability, incapacitating a person whose cancer is small and curable.

The Underlying Cause

Current evidence suggests that most paraneoplastic syndromes are the result of the way in which our immune systems respond to cancer. According to this hypothesis, the process starts with proteins normally present only in nerve cells. These proteins are also found, for unknown reasons, in some cancers. In nerve cells the proteins are probably essential for growth and maintenance, so they may also be essential for those cancers' growth. When a person's immune system senses a tumor growing in the body, it can respond by identifying those cancerous cells and the crucial protein or proteins within them as foreign, or "nonself." The immune system thus responds with an attack on each protein and all the cells that contain it. The immune attack, if it is vigorous enough, can slow the growth of the tumor, but it also attacks the nerve cells that normally

EXAMPLES OF NERVOUS SYSTEM PARANEOPLASTIC SYNDROMES

INVOLVED AREA	SYMPTOMS	DIAGNOSIS
Brain	Memory loss	Limbic encephalitis
Cerebellum	Loss of coordination	Paraneoplastic cerebellar degeneration (PCD)
Retina	Blindness	Carcinoma-associated retinopathy (CAR)
Spinal cord	Paralysis	Motor neuron disease (amyotrophic lateral sclerosis, see C53)
Dorsal root ganglion	Loss of sensation	Sensory neuropathy
Peripheral nerve	Weakness, loss of sensation	Sensorimotor neuropathy
Neuromuscular junction	Weakness	Lambert-Eaton myasthenic syndrome (LEMS), myasthenia gravis
Muscle	Weakness, pain	Dermatomyositis
Multiple	Combined	Encephalomyelitis

contain the protein(s). As a result, a person can develop severe nervous system problems, such as memory loss, lack of coordination, and weakness. Meanwhile, the growth of the cancer may be slowed so successfully that it becomes small and difficult to detect by conventional means.

The blood of many, but not all, people suffering from paraneoplastic syndromes contains antibodies that the immune system has produced in response to specific proteins. The presence of such antibodies can tell physicians that a person's neurological disorder is paraneoplastic; it can also indicate the probable site of the cancer that is at the root of the trouble. For example, an antibody called anti-Yo causes paraneoplastic cerebellar degeneration (PCD), which results in severe loss of coordination while walking and moving one's ex-

tremities. Most people with the anti-Yo antibody are also suffering from either breast or ovarian cancer. Another example is the anti-Hu antibody, associated with both encephalomyelitis and small-cell cancer of the lung.

As you can see, nervous system problems can arise from a tumor in a seemingly unrelated part of the body, as when testicular cancer causes lapses in memory. Although paraneoplastic syndromes affecting the nervous system can cause a bewildering variety of symptoms, they tend to share certain characteristics that help doctors identify them:

1. The neurological signs and symptoms usually appear rapidly—within a matter of days, weeks, or a few months. In contrast, degenerative dis-

ANTIBODIES

Doctors refer to all antibodies with the prefix "anti-," indicating that the body produces them to attack some substance within it. Some paraneoplastic antibodies get their names from the first two letters of the last name of the person who supplied the tissues in which the substances were first identified: for example, anti-Hu and anti-Yo. Other names indicate the functions of the proteins these antibodies attack: the anti-VGCC antibody, for instance, attacks the voltage-gated calcium channels. When discussing the immune system, the substance that an antibody is built to attack is called an antigen, even though it can be a protein that serves a useful puropose in some other part of the body.

eases like Parkinson's (**C41**) and Alzheimer's (**C67**) develop gradually, over years.

2. The neurological signs usually precede those

of the cancer, which is often extremely small and difficult to detect.

3. The neurological disorder usually causes severe disability. Many people with cerebellar degeneration become unable to walk. Many people with limbic encephalitis cannot function because they cannot remember ongoing events. While the cancer may still be restricted to one corner of the body, the immune response to that cancer is thorough and systematic.

Certain disorders have a high probability of being caused by a paraneoplastic syndrome. One example is Lambert-Eaton myasthenic syndrome (LEMS), characterized by muscles that are weak and easily fatigued. LEMS is caused by antibodies aimed at the voltage-gated calcium channel (VGCC) antigen, which binds to the junctions between nerves and muscles and prevents the release of acetylcholine, the chemical that causes muscles to contract. In about two thirds of pa-

SOME ANTIBODY-ASSOCIATED PARANEOPLASTIC DISORDERS

ANTIBODY	USUAL CANCER	USUAL NEUROLOGICAL DISORDER
Anti-Yo	Ovary, breast	Cerebellar degeneration
Anti-Hu	Lung	Encephalomyelitis, sensory neuropathy
Anti-CAR	Lung	Photoreceptor degeneration
Anti-amphiphysin	Breast	Stiff person, encephalomyelitis
Anti-VGCC	Lung	Lambert-Eaton myasthenic syndrome (LEMS)
Anti-Ta	Testicle	Limbic encephalitis
Anti-Tr	Hodgkin's lymphoma	Cerebellar degeneration
Anti-CV2	Lung	Encephalomyelitis, cerebellar degeneration

tients who have this problem, the disorder is paraneoplastic, usually caused by small-cell lung cancer. Another example is PCD, a disorder of coordination. People with PCD cannot control fine movements of their extremities or even their tongues, and thus develop slurred speech, inability to walk, and often inability to feed themselves. This disorder can occur in adult life as a degenerative disease unrelated to cancer, but when it develops rapidly, about half of the sufferers will be found to have cancer.

Treatment

The treatment of paraneoplastic syndromes has two components. First, doctors try to remove the source of the antigens—in other words, they treat the cancer. Because the protein causing the immune reaction is in the tumor, treating the tumor sometimes reverses the neurological disease. The second measure doctors can take is to suppress the immune reaction. Various agents and techniques suppress immunity, including administering adrenocorticosteroids (such as cortisone), providing immunoglobulin through an IV, and even taking some of a person's blood plasma, physically removing the troublesome antibody from it, and putting the plasma back in. These techniques help some people and do not seem to have the unwanted effect of promoting growth of the tumor.

Unfortunately, most paraneoplastic syndromes do not respond to treatment of either the tumor or the immune system. A person with such a condition may remain substantially disabled even when the tumor that created the problem has been treated effectively. The paraneoplastic syndrome may have brought that cancer to light and allowed early treatment of it, but the neurological problem itself remains, and the person must usually learn to deal with it as a chronic condition.

Brain Tumors

We use the term *brain tumor* to describe any tumor growing within the skull, though a more accurate term might be *intracranial tumor.* Only some of these growths arise directly from brain tissue. Others grow from the other tissues inside the skull, such as pituitary tumors. In contrast to these *primary* brain tumors, which arise within the skull, another group consists of tumors that spread to the head from another source, such as lung or breast cancer; these are *secondary* brain tumors, and they are much more common. There are a great many different types of brain tumors, each with its own specific biology and treatment, but all cause similar symptoms.

Both primary and secondary tumors exist on a spectrum, from high to low grade. In most high-grade tumors, also called malignant, or cancerous, the cells are very different from normal cells, grow relatively quickly, and can spread (metastasize) easily to other locations. However, malignant brain tumors differ from malignant tumors that arise elsewhere in the body because they do not spread to other organs.

Tumors are usually called low-grade, benign, or noncancerous if their cells are similar to other, normal cells in the body, grow relatively slowly, and remain confined to one location. In most areas of the body, these growths cause little damage, and surgical removal is usually a cure. The same is true for many benign intracranial tumors that arise outside the brain, such as meningiomas and pituitary tumors. However, benign tumors arising within the brain can quickly become harmful and are very difficult to treat or cure. Most of the human body is soft and yielding, but our hard skulls mean that any abnormal growth inside can squeeze sensitive tissues. A benign tumor growing next to vital brain structures does not have to grow very large before it can seriously impair function and threaten health. Furthermore, if a benign tumor is growing deep inside the brain, surgeons have to cut through important areas, causing irrevocable damage, to remove it. Over time, some benign tumors can also become malignant.

Symptoms of Brain Tumors

A common feature of many intracranial tumors is the swelling that they incite in the surrounding brain. The growth irritates the brain and triggers a process called edema, in which fluid from the blood leaks into the surrounding tissue. This fluid can disrupt brain function, and the symptoms caused by a brain tumor are usually due to the combination of the tumor itself and the edema surrounding it. The fluid causes pressure that disrupts the function of surrounding brain regions. Shrinking the edema with steroids will frequently relieve symptoms such as weakness, numbness, or impaired speech.

Seizures (**C13**) are a common initial symptom of brain tumors. They may be either generalized (grand mal), in which case an individual loses consciousness, or limited to only a portion of the body (for example, involuntary shaking of one arm or leg). Other symptoms of a brain tumor may include progressive weakness of one side of the body, or such language difficulties as trouble finding the correct words to express one's thoughts (**C72**). People may display personality changes, such as loss of initiative, or apathy; loved ones may mistake this change as depression (**C20**), but it can be related to a brain tumor. Nausea and vomiting, vision or hearing difficulties, balance problems, and other behavioral and cognitive symptoms, such as trouble with thinking and memory or psychotic episodes, can all occur. About 40 percent of patients with brain tumors suffer headaches (**C54**); however, they almost always accompany other symptoms.

With the exception of abrupt seizures, these symptoms all usually develop slowly over several weeks or even months. This contrasts with the same symptoms when caused by other common neurological problems. In a stroke, symptoms appear suddenly (**C59, C60**). In Alzheimer's disease, they take many years to develop (**C67**).

What Causes Brain Tumors?

Each year, doctors in the United States diagnose approximately 17,000 new primary brain tumors, and 100,000 new secondary brain tumors. Overall, brain tumors are slightly more common in men than in women—except for meningiomas, which are more common in women. There is no known ethnic predisposition for the most common types of brain tumors. In adults, the incidence of brain tumors increases with age. There is concern that the incidence of brain tumors has been rising, but it is difficult to know whether that indicates a real increase in tumors or is the result of better diagnosis with modern imaging techniques.

There is no known behavioral or environmental factor that leads to brain tumors. Fears about cellular phones, microwave ovens, foods or food additives, and other rumored brain carcinogens have no scientific basis. The only definitive risk factor is having had radiation therapy to the head, usually for another condition; this can increase the risk of most common types of brain tumors, but it may take one or two decades before a brain tumor appears. Dental X rays do not carry an increased risk. Brain tumors are associated with some genetic syndromes, such as neurofibromatosis (**C7**), but these conditions account for a small fraction of all brain tumors in the United States.

Diagnosing a Brain Tumor

The best way to establish the diagnosis of a brain tumor is with an imaging test, such as a computed tomography (CT) or magnetic resonance imaging (MRI) scan. In general, MRI is su-

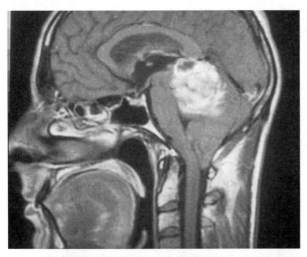

This MRI scan shows a cerebellar glioma. About half of all primary brain tumors are gliomas, meaning that they grow from glial cells, which usually occur in the cerebral hemisphere but also—particularly among children—develop in the cerebellum. Scan © Simon Fraser, Photo Researchers

perior to CT, but in many instances a CT scan can accurately reveal the underlying problem. For the most part, imaging is the only test necessary to diagnose a brain tumor.

Neurologists are the specialists who typically diagnose brain tumors. A subspecialty of neurology is neuro-oncology. Neuro-oncologists are doctors who specialize in the treatment of brain tumors; they should be consulted by most patients with brain tumors.

The next step is figuring out what sort of brain tumor a person has. How malignant is it? From what sort of cells did it grow? Answers to these questions are crucial to planning treatment. In many cases, this identification process requires removal of the tumor or a small piece of the tumor for biopsy, which can require surgery. Frequently this can be done with a needle through a small hole in the skull using radiologic

coordinates, a procedure known as stereotactic biopsy.

Occasionally, physicians use other tests to plan treatment. For instance, before surgery to remove a meningioma, they may do an angiogram, injecting a dye into the blood vessels to outline the tumor. A functional MRI may reveal how close a tumor is to critical brain areas—for example, those that control language. These examinations enable surgeons to operate aggressively but safely. Doctors may also test a person's functioning to determine how much harm a tumor is causing; for example, visual-field testing can reveal impairment from tumors pressing on the optic nerve (**C15**).

Types of Brain Tumors

The most common types of primary brain tumors in adults are gliomas and meningiomas. (Tumors most likely to occur in children are discussed in section **C10**.) Cures for gliomas are almost nonexistent, unless they are extremely low grade—and these typically evolve to become malignant.

Gliomas

About half of all primary brain tumors are gliomas, meaning that they grow from glial cells. Within the brain, gliomas usually occur in the cerebral hemispheres but may also strike other areas, especially the optic nerve, the brain stem, and—particularly among children—the cerebellum. Gliomas are classified into several groups because there are different kinds of glial cells.

The most common type of glioma is the astrocytoma, named for its star-shaped cells. Tumors of this sort are usually classified in one of four grades, depending on their growth rate and ease of treatment. A grade I astrocytoma is a rare type of tumor called a pilocytic astrocytoma and is usually seen in children (**C10**). Grade II astrocytomas are also called "well-differentiated," grade III "anaplastic," and grade IV "glioblastoma multiforme." Lower-grade astrocytomas can be treated with surgery, sometimes followed by radiation or chemotherapy. In contrast, glioblastoma multiforme is among the most common and devastating primary brain tumors that strike adults. It grows rapidly, invades nearby tissue, and contains very malignant cells. It is usually treated with the same methods, but has a lower success rate.

Among other types of gliomas, ependymomas develop from glial cells that line the hollow cavities of the brain and the canal of the spinal cord. They usually occur in children, and about 85 percent are benign. Treatment usually includes surgery followed by radiation therapy.

Oligodendrogliomas, which make up about 5 percent to 15 percent of all gliomas, occur most often in young adults, within the brain's cerebral hemispheres. Doctors often treat these tumors with surgery followed by radiation therapy or chemotherapy.

The rarest form of glioma, ganglioneuroma, grows relatively slowly and may arise in the brain or spinal cord. These tumors are usually treated with surgery.

Brain stem gliomas are most common in children and young adults. Surgeons usually cannot treat brain stem gliomas because of their vulnerable location. Radiation therapy sometimes helps to reduce symptoms and improve survival by slowing tumor growth.

Optic nerve gliomas are found on or near the nerves that travel between the eye and the brain's vision centers. They are particularly common in individuals who have neurofibromatosis (**C7**) and are usually treated with surgery or radiation.

Mixed gliomas contain more than one type of glial cell, usually astrocytes and other glial cells. Treatment focuses on the most malignant type of cell found within the tumor.

Meningiomas

Meningiomas develop from the thin membranes, or meninges, that cover the brain and spinal cord. They account for about 15 percent of all brain tumors. They affect people of all ages, but are most common among those in their 40s. Meningiomas usually grow slowly, generally do not invade surrounding normal tissue, and rarely spread to other parts of the body or central nervous system. Surgery is the preferred treatment for accessible meningiomas and is more successful for these tumors than for most others.

Other Types of Brain Tumors

Tumors involving tissue from the pineal and pituitary glands are often treated by surgery, and pituitary tumors may be treated with the drug cabergoline.

Primitive neuroectodermal tumors (PNETs) usually affect children and young adults. PNETs are very malignant, and because their cells spread in a scattered pattern, they are difficult to remove through surgery. Thus, surgery is followed in most cases by high doses of radiation and chemotherapy.

Schwannomas are tumors that arise from the cells that form a protective sheath around nerve fibers. Usually benign, they are surgically removed when possible.

Vascular tumors are rare, noncancerous tumors that arise from the blood vessels of the brain and spinal cord. The most common vascular tumor is the hemangioblastoma, which rarely spreads and is usually treated by surgery.

Treatment

Treatment varies from one tumor type to the next but often involves a combination of surgery, radiotherapy, and chemotherapy. Early treatment improves the chance of a good outcome for some types.

Some tumors, such as meningiomas, can be completely cured by surgical removal. Others can be better controlled for a time if the surgeon removes all of the area that appears diseased on an MRI. This is true for almost all of the gliomas, but these tumors are rarely cured by surgery alone. Even low-grade gliomas cannot be cured by surgery alone because individual cells migrate great distances within the brain tissue, and a surgeon cannot remove large portions of the brain without causing unacceptable damage.

Depending on the type of tumor, therefore, oncologists may recommend radiation after surgery. For most tumor types, radiation is administered only to the involved area of the brain. Occasionally, the entire brain must be irradiated because there are multiple tumors. Radiation often controls tumor growth for a period and can

---

CHALLENGES OF A BRAIN TUMOR TO PATIENT AND FAMILY

Brain tumors, regardless of type, force the individual and his or her family to face a spectrum of feelings and issues. Some include:

■ Seizure management: brain tumors sometimes interfere with nerve pathways and cause seizures. The individual and his or her family members should receive training from a medical expert in how to recognize the warning signs of seizures and how to handle seizures if they occur.

■ Depending on the size and location of the brain tumor, any number of functions may become impaired: memory, motor skills, communication skills. Different therapies can address different challenges, with various degrees of success.

■ Emotional stress: a brain tumor can take an emotional toll on both the individual and family members. Stress, depression, frustration, and feelings of loss are just some of the challenges the family may face. The person with the tumor may need to make plans for hospice care or end-of-life arrangements while dealing with the effects of the tumor and the aftereffects of different treatments, including surgery and chemotherapy. Even when the tumor is successfully eliminated, the person and his or her family may have to face challenges of motor or cognitive impairment, possible inability to work, or perceived personality changes. Doctors and mental health professionals can help both patient and family deal with the emotional strain.

Adapted from www.abta.org (American Brain Tumor Association). Additional sites: www.btfcgainc.org (Brain Tumor Foundation for Children); www.makingheadway.org (family support); www.tbts.org (The Brain Tumor Society)

occasionally cure tumors. The short-term side effects are nausea and vomiting; in the long term, there may be cognitive dysfunction.

Chemotherapy, or drug treatment, is given to improve survival or, in the case of lymphoma, cure the tumor. However, drug treatments for brain tumors can be hampered by the blood-brain barrier—the combination of physical and functional characteristics that prevent most chemicals in the bloodstream from reaching the brain. This is a normal protective mechanism that prevents many toxic substances from harming our brains (C66). Fortunately, there are several chemotherapeutic agents whose normal properties allow them to penetrate the barrier. In addition, many tumors have an abnormal blood-brain barrier, allowing agents to enter them but not to reach areas of normal brain. These characteristics permit us to use chemotherapy to treat some brain tumors. The side effects are nausea, vomiting, bone marrow suppression, and fatigue.

A number of medications are available to treat the symptoms of brain tumors. For seizures, there are a variety of anticonvulsants; some people require more than one. Glucocorticoids (steroids) help reduce the swelling, or edema, around brain tumors. This often results in improved function within one or two days. Such steroids as dexamethasone (Decadron) are very beneficial, but their prolonged use often leads to side effects: weight gain, insomnia, muscle weakness, and diabetes.

Research on genetic abnormalities in brain tumors has identified persistent activation of growth factor receptors in brain gliomas. There also appears to be activation of some oncogenes. This has led to the development of experimental models of brain gliomas, which should hasten the development of new therapies.

Over the years scientists and doctors have found many ways to improve tumor treatments, resulting in longer and healthier lives for many people. Continuing research into the unique traits of brain tumors will lead us to more answers and improved treatments for the thousands of people facing this frightening disease.

Nutritional Disorders

Nutritional deficiency can adversely affect the nervous system, both centrally and peripherally, leading to problems in thinking and other brain functions as well as in the brain's regulation of the body. In developing countries such deficiency is usually the result of starvation or dietary restriction. In developed countries, the major causes of nutritional deficiency are alcoholism (**C30**), diseases that cause malabsorption of particular nutrients, chronic illnesses that involve general physical wasting, psychiatric illnesses, food faddism, infantile malnutrition, and, rarely, genetic disorders.

The most clearly defined nutritional deficiencies producing neurological symptoms and signs involve vitamins—organic compounds required for normal metabolic functions but not synthesized in the body. The signs and symptoms of vitamin deficiencies that may prompt a person to seek medical attention differ, depending on the particular vitamin. These symptoms are described in detail in this section.

Because vitamins are not produced in the body, they must either be provided in sufficient amounts in your daily diet or be taken as dietary supplements. Vitamins are classified as water soluble or fat soluble (see table). Deficiency of fat-soluble vitamins is often a result of malabsorption associated with liver, pancreatic, or gastrointestinal disease. With the exception of vitamin B_{12} (cobalamin), deficiency of water-soluble vitamins is usually the result of inadequate intake. Malnutrition (including that associated with alcoholism) seldom produces a deficiency of just one or two vitamins; the symptoms and signs are likely the result of multiple deficiencies.

A popular misconception is that if some vitamins are good, then more must be better. However, excessive intake of certain vitamins can be neurotoxic—the medical term for the effects of such an excess is hypervitaminosis. Because water-soluble vitamins are rapidly excreted from the body, symptomatic hypervitaminosis usually involves fat-soluble vitamins. (This risk is discussed in the sections that follow for the relevant vitamins.)

Water-Soluble Vitamins

Thiamine (Vitamin B₁)

Thiamine works together with a number of enzymes to metabolize glucose. Because body

VITAMINS

WATER SOLUBLE	MINIMAL DAILY REQUIREMENT FOR NONPREGNANT, NONLACTATING ADULTS
Thiamine (vitamin B₁)	1.5 mg
Niacin (nicotinic acid, nicotinamide)	20 niacin equivalents (1 mg of niacin or 60 mg of dietary tryptophan)
Pyridoxine	2 mg
Riboflavin	1.8 mg
Pantothenic acid	7 mg
Biotin	100 mg
Ascorbic acid (vitamin C)	60 mg
Cobalamin (vitamin B₁₂)	2 mcg
Folic acid (folate)	200 mcg
FAT SOLUBLE	
Vitamin A (retinol)	100 retinol equivalents (1 mg of retinol or 6 mg of beta-carotene)
Vitamin D (calciferol)	10 mcg of cholecalciferol (400 IU of vitamin D)
Vitamin E (tocopherols)	10 mg alpha-tocopherol equivalent
Vitamin K (phytonadione menaquinones)	80 mcg

stores of thiamine are limited, symptoms of deficiency can appear after only a few weeks of inadequate intake. In developing countries, thiamine deficiency is most likely to produce beriberi, with cardiac failure and peripheral neuropathy. In Europe and North America, thiamine deficiency, especially in alcoholics, is more often associated with symptoms indicating harm to the central nervous system—namely, Wernicke-Korsakoff disease, which is really two disorders arising from the same cause.

Wernicke's syndrome has three clear characteristics: altered mental function, disordered eye movements, and loss of balance (gait ataxia). Mental symptoms include drowsiness, inattentiveness, impaired memory, and slowed thinking, which, if untreated, can progress to coma and death over days. Abnormal eye movements include rhythmic jerking, usually from side to side (nystagmus), and restricted eye movements, which can progress to complete immobility (ophthalmoplegia). Gait ataxia can progress to an inability to walk or stand unaided.

Treatment of Wernicke's syndrome includes 50 to 100 milligrams of thiamine given intravenously or intramuscularly daily for several days to saturate body stores, plus multivitamins. Thereafter, doses of more than a few milligrams daily will simply be excreted. Symptoms usually improve over days, but treatment delay can result in permanent neurological impairment. Some mental symptoms may remain; these most often consist of a relatively selective memory loss (Korsakoff syndrome) in both learning new memories (anterograde) and retrieving old memories (retrograde), sometimes with confabulation (filling in amnesic gaps with false memories). Eye movements may return but nystagmus is often persistent, and gait may improve but with a continuing unsteadiness and a tendency to fall.

In diagnosing Wernicke-Korsakoff disease, a physician may order blood tests. These can show thiamine deficiency because it causes elevated levels of two blood chemicals, lactate and pyruvate, and, more specifically, decreased levels in red blood cells of an enzyme called transketolase. The diagnosis is usually based on symptoms and signs, however, and it is standard practice to give thiamine and multivitamins to any hospitalized alcoholic.

In autopsied brains of patients with Wernicke-Korsakoff disease, there are characteristic pathological abnormalities of neurons, glia, and blood vessels in deep regions of the cerebrum (thalamus and hypothalamus) and in the brain stem and cerebellum. In some patients, cerebellar damage and gait ataxia occur without other features of Wernicke's syndrome; the relative contribution of thiamine and other vitamin deficiencies to this more restricted cerebellar disorder is unclear. Similarly uncertain is the role of specific vitamin deficiency in alcoholics with optic neuropathy (impaired vision caused by degeneration of the optic nerve) and peripheral neuropathy (**C48**), which causes pain and sensory loss in the feet and hands and sometimes weakness of the arms or legs, and autonomic symptoms—for example, light-headedness on standing and palpitations.

Niacin

Also called nicotinic acid (and having no chemical relationship to tobacco), niacin is converted in the body to active forms that are involved in tissue respiration. Deficiency causes pellagra, a disease that affects the skin, the gastrointestinal tract, and the central and peripheral nervous systems. Pellagra is so dramatically debilitating that before it was understood to be a niacin deficiency, people suffering from this disorder were confined to institutions. A sunburnlike rash on light-exposed areas can progress to darkening and even scarring. The tongue becomes red and sore, and nausea, vomiting, and watery or bloody diarrhea result in weight loss. Neurological manifestations include mental change (anxiety, irritability, insomnia, fatigue, depression, and impaired memory, progressing to dementia or psychosis with delusions and hallucinations, and then to delirium or coma), sensorimotor peripheral neuropathy (weakness and sensory loss in the arms or legs), spinal cord damage (weakness in both legs and loss of bladder and bowel control), optic nerve and retinal damage (impaired vision), and seizures.

Diagnosis can be confirmed by measuring niacin metabolites in the urine but is usually based on history and examination. Treatment is with 50 to 150 mg a day of niacin (or a precursor compound, nicotinamide), given orally, plus other vitamins. Symptoms usually improve, but mental abnormalities may be permanent.

Niacin is used to treat hyperlipidemia (elevation in the serum of cholesterol and other fats), and high doses cause flushing, vomiting, diarrhea, liver dysfunction, delirium, and retinal damage. In 1989 several thousand people taking tryptophan (a niacin precursor) obtained in health food stores developed muscle pain, weakness, impaired memory, peripheral neuropathy, and elevations of particular white blood cells in their blood. The disorder is believed to have been caused by a contaminant rather than by tryptophan (or niacin) itself.

Pyridoxine (Vitamin B₆)

Vitamin B_6 consists of three compounds—pyridoxine, pyridoxal, and pyridoxamine—each of which is converted in the body to a common metabolite that works with a number of enzymes. Pyridoxine deficiency causes seizures and sensorimotor peripheral neuropathy, but ascribing particular symptoms in a malnourished person to pyridoxine deficiency alone is difficult because an affected individual is nearly always deficient in other nutrients as well. More specific are "pyridoxine dependency" diseases. For example, the drugs isoniazid, used to treat tuberculosis, and hydralazine, which may be prescribed to treat hypertension, inactivate pyridoxine, requiring dietary supplements to prevent the development of sensory peripheral neuropathy. For reasons that are unclear, some newborns develop seizures that respond to pyridoxine only in doses several times the standard daily requirement.

Pyridoxine taken in megadoses (2 to 6 grams daily for months) also causes severe sensory peripheral neuropathy, including loss of distal limb proprioception (the ability to sense the position of one's feet when walking), resulting in gait ataxia. Improvement following pyridoxine withdrawal may take months or years.

Cobalamin (Vitamin B₁₂)

Cobalamin is obtained from meat, fish, liver, milk, and eggs. Strict vegetarians therefore require supplementation. In the body, active forms of cobalamin work with enzymes involved in carbo-hydrate and amino acid metabolism; in the process, folic acid is activated. When folic acid is not activated, the result is anemia. Considerable cobalamin is stored in the body, mostly in the liver, so deficiency states can exist for years before symptoms appear. Cobalamin deficiency has several causes (see table on page 614). In pernicious anemia, loss of "intrinsic factor," a compound normally present in the stomach lining, results in malabsorption of cobalamin. Nitrous oxide, popular among recreational "sniffers," inactivates cobalamin (without lowering blood levels), so habitual sniffers develop symptoms of deficiency. Estimates of cobalamin deficiency in the elderly are as high as 20 percent, the result of changes in the gastrointestinal tract associated with aging.

Systemic symptoms of cobalamin deficiency include a red, sore tongue, anorexia, vomiting, diarrhea, weight loss, and, secondary to severe anemia, generalized weakness and fainting. Specific neurological damage involves the spinal cord and the peripheral nerves, causing numbness or tingling, most often in the legs; with progression, there is impaired proprioception and gait ataxia. Leg weakness is less common. Less often a person may have impaired memory, psychiatric symptoms, and decreased vision. Significantly, more than one fourth of patients with cobalamin deficiency and neurological symptoms do not have anemia.

The diagnosis of cobalamin deficiency is based on low blood levels of the vitamin. Borderline levels may be difficult for a physician to interpret, however, and confirmation of true deficiency can be made by the finding of elevated blood levels of metabolites—homocysteine and methylmalonic acid—dependent on cobalamin.

Treatment of cobalamin deficiency is with vitamin B_{12}, which, in the presence of pernicious anemia or malabsorption, is given intramuscu-

---

CAUSES OF COBALAMIN DEFICIENCY

DECREASED INGESTION

Malnutrition

Strict vegetarianism

IMPAIRED ABSORPTION

Pernicious anemia

Inability to release cobalamin from food

Gastrectomy

Ileal resection, ileitis, ileal lymphoma, scleroderma

Sprue, or celiac disease

Fish tapeworm (*Diphyllobothrium latum*)

Bowel diverticula, or blind loops

Pancreatic disease

IMPAIRED USE

Hereditary enzyme deficiencies, abnormalities of serum-binding proteins

Nitrous oxide administration

INCREASED REQUIREMENT

Pregnancy

Neoplasm

Hyperthyroidism

---

larly. Most patients improve with treatment, but improvement may not be evident for a few months and may then continue for years.

Folic Acid (Folate)

Unlike cobalamin, folic acid is present in nearly all foods. Folate deficiency can result from malnutrition (again, especially in alcoholics), malabsorption, or liver disease. Some prescription drugs, such as phenytoin (to treat epilepsy), barbiturates, and oral contraceptives, interfere with folate absorption and storage. Another drug, methotrexate, which a person may be taking for certain cancers or disorders of the immune system, inactivates folate.

Whether folate deficiency in adults causes either peripheral or central nervous system disease is a matter of debate among scientists. Most findings of deficiency in adults are probably based on inadequately treated deficiency of cobalamin or other vitamins. Low folate levels have been associated with depression and cognitive impairment in the elderly, but nutritional status is often inadequate in such individuals, making cause and effect unclear.

Taking folate supplements during pregnancy prevents the occurrence of neural tube defects such as spina bifida and anencephaly, and the U.S. Public Health Service recommends a daily dose of 0.4 mg in women capable of becoming pregnant. (Doses higher than 1.0 mg daily are not a good idea: because of the interaction of folate and cobalamin, higher doses might mask the diagnosis of cobalamin deficiency.)

As with cobalamin, folate deficiency is associated with high blood levels of homocysteine, a risk factor for coronary artery and cerebrovascular disease. Studies are currently under way to determine whether folate and cobalamin supplementation reduces the risk of stroke or heart attack in people who are not deficient in cobalamin or folate but who have high blood homocysteine levels.

Ascorbic Acid (Vitamin C)

Ascorbic acid is essential in the body's synthesis of collagen and other components of body tissues. Vitamin C deficiency causes bleeding, and neurological disease results from hemorrhage into muscles, peripheral nerves, or the brain. Megadoses of vitamin C do not seem to produce adverse consequences other than nausea and diarrhea.

Riboflavin, Pantothenic Acid, and Biotin

Multiple vitamin deficiencies are nearly always present in malnourished individuals, and the association of these vitamins with specific symptoms is usually uncertain. The medical literature has described sensory peripheral neuropathy, impaired vision, and deafness with riboflavin

deficiency. A rare genetic disorder of biotin dependency produces altered thinking, abnormal eye movements, muscle rigidity, and weakness. These symptoms respond to biotin and reappear if treatment is discontinued.

Fat-Soluble Vitamins

Vitamin A

Several forms of vitamin A are derived from plant and animal tissues. Liver disease and malabsorption both lead to deficiency. Hypothyroidism and diabetes mellitus impair conversion of vitamin A in the body to its active form, and kidney failure or sustained fever reduces the body's stores of the vitamin. In developing countries, deficiency of vitamin A is a major feature of generalized malnutrition.

Deficiency affects the skin and eyes, producing night blindness, clouding of the eyes' corneas, dry skin, and thickening of oral, nasal, and respiratory mucous membranes with impaired smell and taste, and lung dysfunction.

Adolescents taking megadoses of vitamin A for acne (usually more than 40,000 IU daily) develop toxicity, including anorexia, weight loss, dry skin, hair loss, muscle soreness, and raised intracranial pressure, which in turn can cause headache, double vision, and decreased visual acuity.

Vitamin D

In the presence of ultraviolet light, vitamin D is synthesized in the skin and is not required in the diet. Further metabolism in the liver and kidney produces its active form. Deficiency can result from liver disease and malabsorption, malnutrition, chronic kidney disease, or lack of sunlight. Phenobarbital and phenytoin reduce blood vitamin D levels, and there are hereditary disorders of vitamin D resistance.

Vitamin D deficiency causes bone disease—rickets in children and osteomalacia (bony softening) in adults—which in turn can cause spinal cord or nerve root compression with pain, weakness, and sensory loss. Low blood levels of calcium produce muscle spasms (tetany), spasm of the vocal cords with airway obstruction (stridor), seizures, and altered thinking, including psychosis.

Repeated ingestion of large doses of vitamin D (usually more than 50,000 IU daily) produces potentially lethal elevations of blood calcium levels. Symptoms include osteoporosis (bone thinning); kidney stones; calcification of the heart and blood vessels with congestive heart failure and arrhythmia; anorexia, nausea, vomiting, and constipation; and neurological symptoms that include weakness, impaired memory, depression, psychosis with hallucinations, delirium, and coma. Treatment includes withdrawal of vitamin D, a low-calcium diet, saline, and the diuretic furosemide.

Vitamin E

Vitamin E, which comprises several compounds of a substance called tocopherol, reduces tissue free-radical production. Deficiency oc-

curs in malabsorption disorders, including the hereditary disease Bassen-Kornzweig syndrome. Symptoms include fatty stool (steatorrhea), acanthocytosis (burrlike deformities of red blood cells), decreased blood cholesterol and triglyceride levels, pigmentary degeneration of the retina with impaired vision, degeneration of the cerebellum and spinal cord (causing ataxia, weakness, and sensory loss), abnormal eye movements, and sensory peripheral neuropathy. Treatment is with large oral doses of vitamin E; for severely affected patients, the vitamin can be administered by injection.

Trials testing the efficacy of vitamin E in degenerative disorders such as Alzheimer's disease and Parkinson's disease are currently under way. Vitamin E is widely available in health food stores, and very large doses have been associated with impaired blood coagulation, raising the risk of hemorrhage into the brain and other tissues.

Vitamin K

Vitamin K, a group of compounds, is involved in the synthesis of coagulation factors. Deficiency is a feature of liver disease and malabsorption, and, less often, of malnutrition or antibiotic use. The result is bleeding, including intracranial hemorrhage.

Chemicals and the Nervous System

Neurotoxicology is the medical specialty that deals with the unwanted effects of chemicals on the nervous system. In the United States and Canada, most adults with serious neurotoxic disease are showing the side effects of either prescribed drugs, substance abuse (**C29**), or suicide attempts involving neurotoxic chemicals (**C32**). People can also contract neurotoxic disease from biological poisons (venoms, fish toxins, toxic plants) and from occupational and environmental chemicals, but such illnesses are uncommon in North America. For children, most neurotoxic problems arise from unknowingly ingesting hazardous household substances. (Neurotoxicology is also a specialty of veterinary medicine, and in that field the most common toxins are plants.)

The Many Types of Neurotoxic Diseases

A substance's potential damage to our nervous system depends on its chemical makeup. Toxins that are fat soluble or have certain ionic structures readily penetrate our brains and nerves. Others, especially large complex molecules, can-

not easily pierce the blood-brain barrier. Some neurotoxic chemicals, once they have entered the nervous system in large amounts, spread widely and produce generalized effects; for example, strychnine causes epileptic seizures (**C13**), and many organic solvents cause coma (**C61**). Other neurotoxic agents attack only specific groups of cells or fibers and produce local effects; the designer drug MPTP destroys the pigmented nerve cells of the midbrain and causes a form of Parkinson's disease (**C41**), while vincristine and other anticancer drugs primarily affect nerve ends and cause numbness of the hands and feet (peripheral neuropathy; **C48**). Stated simply, there is no single type of neurotoxic disease.

Many toxins disrupt the chemical balance and functioning of nerve cells without actually destroying their architecture. Some of these substances cause problems primarily in the central nervous system (CNS): people may become confused and delusional (as with phencyclidine, better known as PCP), turn drowsy or even comatose (heroin), display cognitive impairment (bromine), or have seizures (tetanus). Other toxins of this sort act primarily on the peripheral nervous system

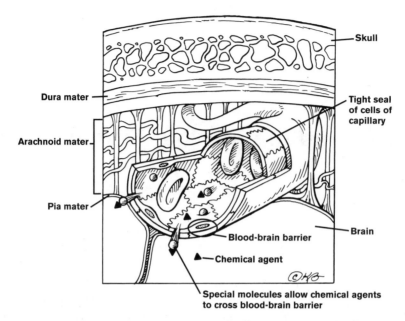

Skull

Dura mater

Arachnoid mater

Pia mater

Tight seal of cells of capillary

Brain

Blood-brain barrier

▲—Chemical agent

Special molecules allow chemical agents to cross blood-brain barrier

The blood-brain barrier prevents most harmful substances from entering the brain. The barrier is formed by the special structure of the blood vessels, which allows only particular sizes and shapes of molecules to cross into the brain. However, a variety of undesirable substances, ranging from drugs of abuse to toxic chemicals, are able to get through this screen. ILLUSTRATION © KATHRYN BORN

and produce paralysis (botulism) or abnormal sensations (ciguatera fish toxin).

Another class of neurotoxins actually degenerates the structure of nerve cells. This damage can occur in the CNS (as with mercury) or peripheral nerves (acrylamide monomer). However, neurotoxins rarely destroy large focal areas of the nervous system. Most chemicals that trigger structural damage to the nervous system produce a consistent pattern of disease that closely matches the dose and duration of exposure.

A person may develop different neurotoxic illnesses from exposure to the same chemicals at different levels. Short-term inhalation of large amounts of the solvent *n*-hexane may end in a fatal coma, while exposure to lower levels for weeks can cause severe peripheral neuropathy

with no CNS symptoms. A few substances produce multiple illnesses following one exposure; for example, exposure to some organophosphates may produce a sudden (sometimes fatal) paralysis by inhibiting the action of acetylcholinesterase and, two weeks later, peripheral neuropathy.

We cannot reliably predict a substance's neurotoxic potential from its chemical formula. Substances with similar chemical structures may have very different effects on our nervous system. Physicians familiar with the side effects of acrylamide monomer, a potent neurotoxin, have needlessly alarmed workers who handle acrylamide polymer, an innocuous substance. Each new chemical created for the workplace or environment must therefore undergo rigorous laboratory testing in tissue culture or experimental animals before it is marketed. Sometimes this screening does not detect neurotoxicity, however, and there are unexpected outbreaks of disease. Failure to detect toxicity in the laboratory usually happens because the experiments were not conducted at the appropriate dose and duration or because of biological differences between humans and animals.

To further complicate matters, a chemical with no known neurotoxic effects may either enhance or depress the toxicity of a neurotoxic agent. This phenomenon was exemplified by a mini-epidemic of peripheral neuropathy among paint sniffers in Berlin. The solvent these people inhaled originally contained the potent neurotoxin n-hexane, but at a harmless level. The manufacturer reformulated the solvent, introducing another nonneurotoxic chemical, methyl ethyl ketone, and lowering the amount of n-hexane further. Several sniffers then developed severe neuropathy. Subsequent animal studies disclosed that while methyl ethyl ketone did not itself cause neuropathy, it made n-hexane more toxic. Such chemical interactions have become an emotional issue, as many fear the mixtures at hazardous waste sites. However, any modulation of a neurotoxin's effect by another chemical should be reproducible in a laboratory.

Specific Chemicals and Their Effects

Many people worry about the effects of substances they encounter at work or in their other environments. Some of these chemicals can indeed be toxic to our nervous systems, but only after unusually high-level or prolonged exposures. Casual contact with solvents, pesticides, and heavy metals is not associated with nervous system dysfunction.

Some medications can cause neurotoxic ef-

fects at customary doses (anticancer and psychiatric drugs), while others can do so only after being administered at unusually high levels (antiepilepsy, antibiotic, and anti-HIV agents). Megadoses of vitamins can also be neurotoxic (C65). In contrast, minute doses of some venoms and potent microbiological agents, such as a form of botulinum, can cause severe, sometimes fatal, nervous system dysfunction.

The list of proven or presumed neurotoxins numbers more than 440 chemicals, and we will doubtless identify more. The table on page 621 includes some of the most common. In looking at these substances, you must remember that in most cases a person must take in a high dose to suffer damage. And all the artificial chemicals listed have their uses, often important ones.

Diagnosis and Treatment

When a person seeks help for a neurological problem, the physician's first task is to minimize any acute symptoms or immediate danger. The second step is to determine the reason for the problem. In diagnosing a neurotoxic disorder, doctors must rule out other conditions that can cause the same symptoms. The signs and symptoms of neurotoxic diseases may mimic naturally occurring diseases, such as uremia from kidney failure, Parkinson's (C41), vitamin deficiency (C65), and diffuse demyelinating diseases (leukodystrophy; C6).

The key to diagnosis is a complete and accurate history of the person's symptoms—when they appeared, how strongly, and with what connection, if any, to neurotoxins. Doctors who have prescribed medications that can affect the nervous system are usually on the alert for their side effects. Similarly, physicians are reasonably famil-

THE DOSE-RESPONSE EFFECT

Few neurotoxic diseases have an allergic or genetic basis; that means that most of us will suffer the same reactions to the same doses of chemicals. Age may be a factor in determining vulnerability. The fetal nervous system is extremely susceptible to toxic exposure, particularly during major cellular migrations. Older individuals may display heightened vulnerability, especially if they have underlying disease of the nervous system. But for most adults, there is a strong relationship between the amount of chemical exposure and the body's response.

That dose-response relationship is the reason we have little cause to worry about neurotoxic injury from pesticide spraying. Current pesticides are potentially lethal if a person ingests them in high concentrations, but innocuous when sprayed in diluted solutions. (There is, of course, considerable risk to individuals with asthma or severe upper airway disease who are directly sprayed with a foreign chemical, but that is not a neurological danger.)

In addition, neurotoxic illness usually occurs while a person is being exposed or shortly afterward. There is rarely a multiyear delay as in, for instance, the development of lung tumors after inhaling asbestos. A few substances may produce delayed neurotoxic effects because they are stored somewhere in the body and slowly released (for example, chloroquine in the eye), or suddenly released during illness or chelation therapy (lead in bones).

However, even though most neurotoxins take effect immediately, people may not recognize the damage right away. Unless an individual performs an unusually skilled job or requires consistent high-level intellectual activity, he or she may not notice a mild decline in performance. Workers exposed to agents that affect their peripheral nerves may gradually experience a subtle loss of sensation in their hands. When people finally notice such a problem, they may feel that the toxin has been building up in their bodies, but in fact they have been undergoing nerve damage since the initial exposure.

iar with the syndromes of exposure to well-known industrial chemicals.

A more trenchant problem is posed when a person's history of chemical exposure is unclear. For example, cognitive impairment and jerking movements are characteristic of Creutzfeldt-Jakob disease (C39), a naturally occurring prion disorder. The same symptoms may also result from taking long-term doses of antacid preparations containing bismuth. A person suffering these symptoms may not mention a common over-the-counter antacid to his or her doctor.

Special toxicology tests are helpful in confirming some diagnoses, especially those involving heavy metals (mercury, lead, arsenic) and overdoses from substance abuse (alcohol, cocaine, heroin). For many pharmacological and industrial agents, however, there are no tests. Also, relatively few neurotoxins stay in the body for weeks, so by the time a person sees a doctor the exposure may be long over. Because most neurotoxins do not cause large areas of destruction, brain imaging techniques usually show nothing amiss; these tests are most useful for ruling out other conditions.

COMMON NEUROTOXINS AND THEIR EFFECTS

CLASS	EXAMPLES	EFFECT
Heavy metals	Arsenic	Peripheral neuropathy
	Mercury	Tremor, visual impairment, dementia
	Lead	Peripheral neuropathy in adults; seizures and cognitive dysfunction in children
Organic solvents	Toluene	Tremor, spasticity, dementia
	n-Hexane	Peripheral neuropathy
Pesticides	Organophosphates	Paralysis, cholinergic reaction, delayed peripheral neuropathy
	Pyrethroids	Abnormal sensations, seizures
	Carbamates	Paralysis, cholinergic reaction
Anticancer drugs	Vincristine	Peripheral neuropathy, delirium, muscle disease
	Taxol	Peripheral neuropathy
	Cisplatin	Peripheral neuropathy (sensory)
Epilepsy drugs	Phenytoin (Dilantin)	Unsteady gait, erratic eye jerks, birth defects, cognitive loss
	Carbamazepine (Tegretol)	Unsteady gait, sedation, birth defects
	Vigabatrin	Visual dysfunction
Antibacterial, anti-TB drugs	Penicillin	Seizures
	Aminoglycosides	Weakness, hearing loss
	Isoniazid (INH)	Peripheral neuropathy, seizures
Anti-HIV agents	Nucleosides (ddC, ddl)	Peripheral neuropathy
	Zidovudine (AZT)	Muscle disease
Occupational agents	Acrylamide monomer	Peripheral neuropathy, delirium
	Ethylene oxide	Peripheral neuropathy, cognitive dysfunction
	Methyl isobutyl ketone	Cognitive dysfunction
	Trichloroethylene	Facial numbness, cognitive dysfunction

(continued)

COMMON NEUROTOXINS AND THEIR EFFECTS (continued)

CLASS	EXAMPLES	EFFECT
Psychiatric drugs	Chlorpromazine (Thorazine) and haloperidol (Haldol)	Parkinsonism, dystonia, tardive dyskinesia
	Benzodiazepines (Valium, Xanax)	Sedation, cognitive dysfunction, myoclonic seizures
	Tricyclic antidepressants (Elavil, Endep)	Tremor, dyskinesia
Bacterial toxins	Diphtheria	Peripheral neuropathy
	Botulism	Paralysis
	Tetanus	Seizures, spasms
Marine toxins	Ciguatera, found in grouper and snapper	Abnormal sensation, weakness
	Tetrodotoxin, found in puffer fish	Paralysis
	Saxitoxin ("red tide"), found in clams and mussels	Abnormal sensation, paralysis
	Scombroid (histamine), found in tuna and mackerel	Headache, hypotension, stroke
	Domoic acid, found in mussels	Delirium, seizures, cognitive dysfunction
Venoms	Black widow spider	Weakness
	Cobra	Paralysis
Plants	*Lathyrus* (a legume)	Spastic gait
	Cassava	Visual loss, peripheral neuropathy
	Hemlock (*Conium*)	Paralysis
	Jimsonweed (*Datura*)– scopolamine	Delirium, hallucinations

PSEUDONEUROTOXIC ILLNESS

Sometimes people have an everyday exposure to an environmental chemical or pharmacological agent, followed by a naturally occurring illness. It is tempting to blame the illness on the substance. In most cases, however, that connection is a mistake. Sometimes the substance is not a neurotoxin at all. In other cases, the substance has genuine neurotoxic potential, but the person has not been exposed at a level that normally causes disease. For instance, adults with unexplained peripheral nerve disorders are sometimes found to have mildly elevated levels of lead or mercury in their bodies. Both lead and mercury have serious toxic effects on children's brains but almost never affect an adult's peripheral nervous system without egregious environmental exposure.

Such cases of pseudoneurotoxicity can come in individual cases or in epidemics. Many veterans of the 1990–1991 Gulf War have reported a syndrome of malaise, cognitive impairment, joint pain, headache, and muscle ache. This has been attributed to, among other causes, a few small oral doses of pyridostigmine bromide (given to protect soldiers from nerve gas). But that chemical does not cross the blood-brain barrier in significant amounts, and has been used in larger quantities for decades to treat myasthenia gravis (C52) with little consequence. Therefore, the connection to pyridostigmine seems untenable, and government and academic researchers have continued to investigate a variety of possible biological sources for these and other symptoms in the Gulf War veterans.

People's complaints of multiorgan intolerance (sinus congestion, coughing, headache, poor attention span, joint pain) after low-level exposure to hydrocarbon solvents or pesticides of any type are another case of pseudoneurotoxicity. Some people attribute their symptoms to minute amounts of these chemicals and have diagnosed themselves as suffering from "multiple chemical sensitivity (MCS) syndromes." They report that subsequent exposure to the original substance or even unrelated chemicals (for example, gasoline fumes, cigarette smoke) triggers many physical symptoms and psychological distress. The people's symptoms and distress are real. Furthermore, they may become disabled by their symptoms or by fear of another attack; some feel compelled to undergo laborious detoxification or make radical changes in their lifestyle. However, their problems cannot be blamed on chemicals, because they do not exhibit dose-response relationships or other characteristics of neurotoxicity. Focusing attention on toxins can distract people and their physicians from identifying the real roots of their problems. Among the possible basic or accompanying disorders that people should discuss with their doctors are post-traumatic stress disorder (C28), panic disorder (C21), and depression (C20).

Neurotoxic illness generally improves after a person stops being exposed. Improvement can be rapid (in hours or days) if the toxin caused only biochemical or pharmacological changes, as in snakebites and illegal-drug overdoses. If structural alterations have occurred only in the peripheral nervous system, as with many anticancer drugs, recovery may be slow and incomplete because nerves regenerate at the rate of only eight hundredths to one tenth of an inch each day. If CNS cells have been damaged or destroyed, the recovery will be poor and incomplete.

CHAPTER 19

Disorders of Thinking and Remembering

C67 **Alzheimer's Disease** 625

C68 **Amnesias** 635

C69 **Dementia** 639

C70 **Trouble with Speech and Language** 643

C71 **Apraxias** 648

C72 **Agnosias** 651

The amount of our brain tissue devoted to processing and remembering information grants us a large capacity for learning. It also means that we can suffer very broad or very particular losses of cognitive function. People with amnesia cannot remember certain facts, and in rare cases cannot learn new facts. In contrast, aphasia is trouble with speaking or understanding language. Apraxia is an inability to remember how to do things, and agnosia an inability to recognize things or people. Finally, dementia is the loss of mental coordination in such severe ways that a person's thinking no longer reflects reality.

Alzheimer's disease is the best known of the disorders that affect memory, producing amnesia and dementia. Many people worry about it, so this chapter has a full section devoted to it. Amnesia, aphasia, and the other memory disorders are each a symptom of an underlying problem, and they can arise from many disorders: advanced Alzheimer's, strokes and other injuries, and diseases that affect particular portions of the brain. These symptoms can be temporary or they can become chronic, depending again on how they affect brain tissue.

Alzheimer's Disease

Alzheimer's disease is a progressive brain disorder that causes a gradual and irreversible loss of higher brain functions, including memory, language skills, and perception of time and space, and, eventually, loss of the ability to care for oneself. The disease was first identified in 1906 by the German psychiatrist Alois Alzheimer. He thought it was a relatively rare disorder, but today we recognize Alzheimer's as the most common cause of the loss of mental function in people over the age of 65. As many as 4 million to 6 million people in the United States have the disorder. Among individuals around the age of 65, 5 percent to 10 percent have Alzheimer's, and this proportion increases to about 10 percent to 15 percent among those in their 70s and to 30 percent to 40 percent among people 85 years of age or older. Given our aging population, it has been estimated that 14 million Americans will have Alzheimer's disease by the middle of this century unless we find a cure or preventive measures.

Alzheimer's is a devastating disease. Those who suffer from it experience frustration, anger, and fear as the disorder begins to strip away their abilities and memories. Those who love and care for people with the disease experience the stress and pain of watching someone they love slowly slip away. Unfortunately, we still do not know what causes Alzheimer's, nor do we know how to cure it.

Symptoms of Alzheimer's Disease

Most cases of Alzheimer's disease occur in people over 65 and are referred to as late-onset Alzheimer's. Early-onset Alzheimer's, which occurs in people who are in their 30s, 40s, or 50s, is much less common; only about 2 percent of Alzheimer's cases are early-onset. The symptoms and manifestations of the two types are identical.

Alzheimer's disease evolves slowly, with occasional plateaus. Memory loss is usually one of the first noticeable symptoms, and can be quite mild. It often begins with difficulty recalling people's names, telephone numbers, and the details of events or conversations during the day. Memories from the remote past and, for some people, previously learned facts tend to remain relatively intact at the beginning of the illness, but will fade later. A person in the beginning stages of the disease might discover that it is difficult to find the right word, or sense a decline in his or her reading comprehension and ability to write. Later the memory loss becomes more notable: a person may have difficulty remembering what day or month it is, or become unable to find his or her way around familiar surroundings.

As Alzheimer's disease progresses, depression becomes more frequent: 5 percent to 8 percent of people suffer serious depression (**C20**) with insomnia (**C11**) or anorexia (**C27**). Muscular rigidity, slowed movements, shuffling gait, and stooped posture are also relatively frequent in people with Alzheimer's disease. Delusions, psychotic behavior, agitation with aggressive behavior, and hallucinations may occur, but only in 20 percent of individuals. People in the final stages of the disease become completely unable to care for themselves and must be helped with all their basic needs.

The average length of time between the appearance of the first symptoms of Alzheimer's and death seems to range from 4 to 16 years. Women with the disease generally survive longer than men. Most Alzheimer's patients die of complications such as pneumonia.

Diagnosing Alzheimer's Disease

It is essential to note that memory loss does not necessarily presage Alzheimer's disease. All of us forget things once in a while. Furthermore, some slowing of memory is a normal consequence of aging. If you experience memory loss, but not at a level that interferes with the activities of daily life, you probably do not have the disease. The vast majority of people past the age of 65 do *not* have Alzheimer's disease.

Furthermore, many conditions besides Alzheimer's can cause memory loss and dementia, a term used to describe impairment of other mental functions, such as language or the ability to think abstractly, along with memory. These conditions include hypothyroidism, depression (**C20**), adverse drug reactions (**C66**), and nutritional deficiencies (**C65**). Some of these problems can be treated or cured, so it is critical to obtain an early and accurate diagnosis of dementia.

Only after doctors rule out other neurological or medical problems do they focus on the diagnosis of Alzheimer's disease. Then they use neuropsychological testing, brain imaging, and other techniques, such as blood tests and neurological and physical examination and history, to place people on two levels of diagnostic certainty:

QUESTIONS FROM THE MINI-MENTAL STATE EXAM

- What is today's date?

- What is the month?

- What is the year?

- Who is the president of the United States?

- Who was the first president of the United States?

- Name another U.S. president.

- Spell the word *world* backward.

- Begin with 100 and count backward by 7. Stop after 5 subtractions.

- probable Alzheimer's disease—the person has no other illnesses that may contribute to the symptoms

- possible Alzheimer's disease—the person meets the criteria for other illnesses that may contribute to his or her mental problems, such as hypothyroidism or cerebrovascular disease

We must reserve the designation of *definite* Alzheimer's disease for cases confirmed by autopsy; we can be sure of the diagnosis only after examining brain tissue under a microscope after the person dies.

Alzheimer's Disease and the Brain

An autopsy of a brain affected by Alzheimer's reveals distinctive changes that we now recognize as hallmarks of the disease. A key step in the progression of the disorder appears to be the accumulation of a protein substance in the form of plaques, or clumps of fibers, in the brain's gray matter. These plaques contain beta-amyloid peptide, a hard, waxy deposit that results from the breakdown of the protein amyloid. Beta-amyloid is also deposited in the walls of the blood vessels in and around the brain. Another characteristic of brains affected by Alzheimer's disease is neurofibrillary tangles within neurons, composed of an abnormal form of the protein tau. There is also a substantial loss of neurons and of the synapses connecting them throughout the neocortex.

Scientists believe that the plaques and tangles cause neurons to shrink and eventually die, first in the memory and language centers of the brain, and finally throughout the brain. Degeneration in the basal forebrain also profoundly reduces the

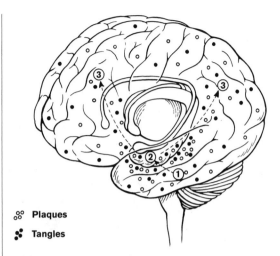

°°° **Plaques**

•• **Tangles**

1. Plaques and tangles develop in entorhinal cortex.
2. Over time they spread into the hippocampus.
3. Finally, the plaques and tangles reach the top of the brain, the neocortex.

The "plaques" of Alzheimer's disease are formed by the peptide beta-amyloid, which is considered the cause of brain cell degeneration in the disease. At the earliest stage, plaques are believed to develop in the entorhinal cortex. As the disease progresses, the hippocampus is affected, producing the memory symptoms most often associated with the disease. In time, however, many areas of the brain are affected, leading to a person's inability to care for himself or herself. ILLUSTRATION © KATHRYN BORN

supply of some brain chemicals, including the neurotransmitter acetylcholine, which is known to influence memory.

We do not know what causes these alterations in the brain, but animal studies suggest that immunizing mice with a synthetic form of the amyloid protein can prevent the accumulation of amyloid plaques. This suggests that treatment directed at the amyloid protein might be an effective way to prevent the disease in individuals at risk or in the early stages of illness. But research teams are investigating many avenues of treatment, in-

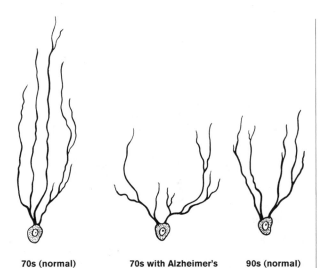

70s (normal)   70s with Alzheimer's   90s (normal)
                            disease

Between age 70 and age 90, some loss of brain cell connections is normal. However, in Alzheimer's disease this loss is extensive; in the brain of a 70-year-old, it is even greater than would be normal at age 90. ILLUSTRATION © KATHRYN BORN

cluding drugs to block the generation of the amyloid protein, anti-inflammatory drugs, and antioxidants.

What Affects the Risk for Alzheimer's Disease?

While we do not know what causes Alzheimer's disease, we can point to a number of factors that determine an individual's risk. Genetics appears to play a key role. First-degree relatives of people with Alzheimer's have more than twice the chance of developing the disease than do individuals without a family history.

Researchers have discovered that mutations in three genes—the amyloid precursor protein (APP) on chromosome 21, presenilin 1 (PS1) on chromosome 14, and presenilin 2 (PS2) on chromosome 1—result in rare autosomal-dominant and familial forms of Alzheimer's disease beginning as early as the third decade of life. The autosomal dominance means that all living children of an affected parent have a 50 percent chance of developing the disease. Both men and women can pass on the mutations, and this form of the disease seldom skips a generation.

Researchers have also associated a polymorphism on chromosome 19 with Alzheimer's disease, but in a different way. Unlike genetic mutations, which usually dramatically change how a protein works, polymorphisms represent normal variations in our genes. Polymorphisms probably account for our subtle differences in eye color, hair color, and height and are seldom associated with disease. Nonetheless, the epsilon 4 polymorphism of the apolipoprotein E (ApoE) gene has been strongly and consistently associated with Alzheimer's disease beginning at age 60 and older. It is not clear how ApoE-4 increases the risk of Alzheimer's disease, but it is known that ApoE participates in amyloid accumulation. Genetic testing is usually not recommended for ApoE or the other markers, because even if these genes are found, the current incomplete knowledge of their role does not allow doctors to offer a reliable analysis of their significance for an individual.

Several other factors also appear to influence Alzheimer's disease. Adults with Down's syndrome, a form of mental retardation (**C3**), develop the plaques and tangles of Alzheimer's disease by age 40, but not all develop dementia. For people who have blood relatives with Down's syndrome, the risk of Alzheimer's disease increases two or three times, suggesting a genetic link.

A history of depression (**C20**) has also been associated with Alzheimer's disease. Whether depression represents incipient disease or is an early symptom remains to be determined, but some studies have found a significant link between the two conditions even when the depression occurred ten years earlier. Although results are not consistent, there is also a suggestion that a head injury (**C61**) can increase a person's risk of Alzheimer's, perhaps by activating amyloid production. This effect may be especially strong among people who already have the ApoE-4 polymorphism.

While popular reports periodically circulate about dietary (for example, zinc) and other environmental factors (such as aluminum), none of these suspects have yielded anything definitive under investigation.

People's educational achievement appears to have a profound influence on their likelihood of developing Alzheimer's disease. Those who are illiterate or who have had little formal education are at higher risk for developing the disease. In one study of nuns, the women's linguistic ability at age 20 predicted their level of cognitive impairment and Alzheimer's disease at age 70. This has led some theorists to propose that having more education helps people develop a "cognitive reserve" that works against the effects of Alzheimer's disease. Other researchers suggest that genetic or environmental factors play a role in both educational achievement and the disease.

On the other hand, some factors seem to lessen the risk of Alzheimer's disease. The use of estrogen replacement therapy by women after menopause has been associated with a decreased risk of Alzheimer's disease. For women who took estrogen, the age at which they developed Alzheimer's disease was significantly later, and their relative risk was significantly lower than it was for other women, even after researchers adjusted for differences in education, ethnic group, age, and ApoE-4. A study is now in progress to assess the effectiveness of estrogen replacement in delaying or preventing Alzheimer's disease.

People who develop Alzheimer's disease tend to use anti-inflammatory agents like aspirin and acetaminophen less often than their peers. Because chronic inflammation has been associated with amyloid deposition, anti-inflammatory agents could play an important role in slowing or inhibiting the disease. Several large studies are now in progress to test whether or not these drugs can prevent Alzheimer's disease.

Cigarette smoking was once purported to protect people from Alzheimer's disease, but studies have not borne out that idea. In fact, there is a clear link between smoking and dementia associated with strokes (**C59, C60**).

Drug Treatments for Alzheimer's Disease

Since there is no cure for Alzheimer's, current treatment focuses on lessening its symptoms. Some researchers consider the loss of acetylcholine to be the reason for declining memory, so they have adopted the strategy of enhancing the brain's acetylcholine production. A class of drugs called cholinesterase inhibitors has a modest but positive effect on the memory-loss symptoms of the disease.

A handful of medications have been approved for treating Alzheimer's disease itself. Physicians may begin prescribing these drugs at any time after a person is diagnosed because they are modestly effective at delaying problems in both mild and moderate stages of disease. Whether people develop a tolerance to their effects after long-term use is unknown. Because higher doses of these drugs have both the greatest benefits and the most adverse effects, physicians usually begin with a small dose and increase it gradually while they and their patients watch for adverse reactions. Treatment can be continued indefinitely, but doctors often recommend discontinuing the drugs because their effects have declined or because the person with Alzheimer's is no longer so able to tolerate their adverse effects. Individuals with Alzheimer's disease and their families should be alert to the possibility of deterioration after drug treatment is stopped.

Tacrine (tetrahydroaminoacridine), sold as Cognex, was the first drug approved in the United States specifically for treating Alzheimer's disease. People must take it four times daily, and eating at the same time decreases the amount the body absorbs. Studies have found that this drug helps people improve their performance on tests of memory, but there is little to no change in overall function. Tacrine can cause a number of side effects, including nausea and vomiting in 28 percent of patients, so few people use it now.

Donepezil (Aricept) was approved for Alzheimer's disease in 1996. Compared with tacrine, it has minimal side effects (nausea and vomiting in 15 percent of people, insomnia in up to 14 percent) and a longer life in the bloodstream, allowing people to take it only once a day. As with tacrine, the efficacy of donepezil is modest, but its relative convenience has caused it to be widely used.

Rivastigmine (Exelon) is similar to tacrine and donepezil in efficacy. It lasts up to ten hours. Because of its side effects, however, people must start taking this drug at a low dose and slowly build up the amount. At high doses, about 35 percent of people suffer nausea; other dose-related adverse effects include vomiting, diarrhea, and anorexia. Nearly 20 percent of people taking high doses of rivastigmine experience weight loss.

Galantamine (Reminyl) will soon be available in the United States. Two studies suggest benefits in the same range as the preceding similar drugs, and its side effects are similar to those of donepezil.

Although there has been some indication that antioxidants can protect against memory loss, none has been shown to prevent Alzheimer's disease. People with Alzheimer's disease given vitamin E (2000 IU per day) lived longer than those taking a placebo, but showed no improvement in their mental function. Ginkgo biloba, an extract from the leaves of a subtropical tree, was found to provide a small benefit on cognitive testing in people with Alzheimer's disease, but the large number of dropouts in that trial has raised concerns about the validity of the results.

Other Treatments

Many people with Alzheimer's suffer from a variety of symptoms beyond memory loss, and many of these symptoms can be treated. As noted above, depression is common and can make the mental losses appear worse than they are. People with Alzheimer's disease can take almost all of the approved antidepressant drugs; studies have shown them to have comparable results, so the choice of one over another should depend on an individual's response. Some tricyclic antidepressant drugs, such as amitriptyline, can result in confusion or orthostatic hypotension (low blood pressure on standing up) in 10 percent to 15 percent of people. Selective serotonin reuptake inhibitors (SSRIs) are better tolerated but can cause insomnia, anorexia, or, in men, ejaculatory failure in up to 5 percent.

Delusions and psychotic behavior increase as

FAMILY CONCERNS

The family members and friends who surround a person with Alzheimer's are deeply affected by the disease. Family-education programs and counseling can help ease the burden of caring for a person suffering from Alzheimer's, and can provide strategies for some of the day-to-day concerns.

One of caregivers' biggest concerns about people with Alzheimer's disease who are still in good physical health is that they might wander away from their homes or health care facilities. Caregivers may therefore feel they must be on alert all the time. Strategies such as concealing doorways and encouraging such activities as walking with a companion for exercise may limit wandering. Caregivers must also be psychologically ready to ask for help when they need it, and to move their loved one to a nursing home or other facility with 24-hour care if that becomes the best option.

If a person does wander off, the Alzheimer's Association has created a nationwide network called Safe Return. The person with the disease wears a Safe Return identification item, which displays a nationwide toll-free number that connects callers to operators 24 hours a day, 7 days a week. If people with such identification are found wandering or sitting away from their homes and in a confused state, the authorities can find out who they are and where they live and return them to their homes.

Alzheimer's disease progresses; once people display these symptoms, about 20 percent have them persistently. Symptoms disappear or diminish in 18 percent of people treated with neuroleptics such as haloperidol (Haldol) and atypical antipsychotic agents such as risperidone. Haloperidol may cause tardive dyskinesia (involuntary facial movements), persisting even after the drug is withdrawn. Parkinsonism, with shuffling gait and stooped posture (C42), and drowsiness are rare side effects of all these medications.

People with Alzheimer's-related psychosis may also become aggressive and agitated, posing a threat not only to themselves but to those around them. Many different drugs have been tried for this problem, with little consistent benefit. Antidepressants, beta-adrenergic antagonists, lithium, benzodiazepines, and anticonvulsant drugs all show inconsistent results but are worth trying because they can help some individuals. In addition to sedating the person, many of these drugs worsen cognitive function; they have also been associated with falls and fractures.

Treatment for sleep disturbances ranges from antipsychotic drugs to antidepressants and sedatives, all of which have adverse effects, so physicians try to use these medications for short periods only. Reducing daytime naps, restricting one's time in bed, and exposure to bright light during waking hours may also be helpful.

The Late Stages of Alzheimer's Disease

In the last stages of illness, people with Alzheimer's disease are often unable to care for their most basic needs. Many individuals need round-the-clock care and are placed in nursing homes. People at this stage of illness may require tube feedings to maintain nutrition and decrease

CONSIDERATIONS FOR FAMILY AND FRIENDS COPING WITH ALZHEIMER'S DISEASE

The ways that families and friends cope with Alzheimer's disease in someone they love are as distinct as the patients and families themselves, but certain considerations are always important. The following brief summary is adapted from the outstanding Caregiver's Guide on the Alzheimer's Association Web site, www.alz.org. In addition to the site's hundreds of helpful suggestions, several books in the reading list at the back of this book offer practical advice, and most people benefit greatly from sharing experiences in support groups.

LEGAL AND FINANCIAL PLANNING: A person with Alzheimer's may be able to manage his or her legal and financial affairs when the disease is diagnosed, but as it advances others will need to begin taking care of these matters. Thus, legal and financial planning should start soon after a diagnosis has been made. Particularly important are:

■ Legal documents securing your loved one's decisions about health care and finances: you should consult an attorney about what documents are advisable. These may include a power of attorney, by which a person authorizes someone to make legal decisions when he or she is no longer competent; a power of attorney for health care; a living will, which allows a person to express his or her decision on the use of artificial life support systems; a living trust, to manage assets when a person becomes unable because of cognitive impairment; and, if the person with the disease does not already have one, a will. If your loved one is no longer able to sign such documents legally, a court may need to appoint a family member or friend as guardian or conservator to make the decisions about care and other matters.

■ A good analysis of the financial situation is the first step in planning how to pay for your loved one's future medical and living expenses. Documents such as bond certificates, bank account statements, real estate deeds, and insurance policies will provide a clear picture of the person's assets. Work with a professional, such as a financial planner, estate planning attorney, or accountant, to coordinate financial strategies. Identify expenses you may encounter. Some help with these costs may be available from Medicare, Medigap, Medicare HMO, Medicaid, tax credits, Social Security disability, supplemental security income, retirement benefits, and personal savings, investments, and property.

DAY-TO-DAY CARE: The abilities, personality, and moods of a person with Alzheimer's may change as the disease advances. Some areas that may test family and friends' skill and creativity are planning activities, improving communication, understanding unusual or unpredictable behavior, recognizing depression, handling safety issues, and providing long-distance or late-stage care.

HYGIENE AND PERSONAL CARE: People with Alzheimer's may need help with grooming and hygiene routines, such as bathing, toileting, dental care, and dressing. The need for assistance can be very difficult for them because it signifies a loss of independence and privacy. It is also difficult for caregivers, especially when a person resists help with private routines that he or she is becoming unable to perform.

CHOOSING HEALTH CARE PROVIDERS AND FACILITIES: The three main categories of services are respite care, residential care, and hospice. The costs differ by service and community. You should carefully interview and compare providers of the service you want before settling on one. Government agencies, insurers, and various Alzheimer's organizations all publish helpful guidelines and checklists to help you with this research.

- Respite care—provided mainly by community organizations or residential facilities—offers temporary relief for caregivers and gives the person with the disease opportunities to socialize with others and live in the community longer. The most common respite programs are in-home care (companion services, personal care, household assistance, or skilled care to meet specific needs) and adult day services in a community center or facility that provides staff-led programs such as musical entertainment and group discussions.

- Residential care facilities include retirement housing, which generally provides each resident an apartment or room with cooking facilities and may be appropriate for persons in the early stage of Alzheimer's; assisted living (board and care homes), which typically combine housing, personalized assistance, and health services; and skilled nursing facilities, which may be the best choice when a person with Alzheimer's needs round-the-clock care or ongoing medical treatment. Certain retirement communities (continuum care retirement communities or CCRCs) provide all three types of living arrangements.

- Hospice programs provide care to persons in the late stages of Alzheimer's and emphasize comfort and care without heroic lifesaving measures. This type of service is available through local hospice organizations and some home care agencies, hospitals, and nursing homes, and the person with Alzheimer's may be eligible for benefits through Medicare, Medicaid, and even some private insurance.

COPING: Caring for someone who has Alzheimer's disease can be overwhelming, exhausting, and stressful. It's critical that caregivers watch their physical and mental health. Depression, changes in relationships, a sense of loss, and helping children and teens understand are just a few of the challenges caregivers may face. Some tips for caregivers:

- See your doctor regularly.
- Get screened for stress and depression.
- Get plenty of rest.
- Eat well-balanced meals.
- Exercise regularly.
- Be realistic about what you can do, give yourself credit for what you accomplish, and don't feel guilty if you lose patience or can't do everything on your own.
- Accept help from others.

Informative Web sites include www.alz.org (The Alzheimer's Association), www.alzheimers.org (Alzheimer's Disease Education and Referral Center), www.alzwell.com (ALZwell Caregiver Support), and www.caregivers.com (Solutions for Better Aging).

the risk of aspiration or choking. Skin care to prevent bedsores is important, as is bowel care. Because people at this stage of the disease are regularly incontinent, they may need frequent checks and adult diapers. Maintaining the dignity of the individual is still important: dressing, bathing, feeding, and grooming a person with Alzheimer's each day is essential even though that person may appear unaware of his or her surroundings.

When making end-of-life decisions, it is desirable to follow an individual's wishes, but that may not be possible if the person has not made appropriate legal decisions. Some people make out documents authorizing certain life-support measures and not others, called Advance Directives, before they succumb to dementia. For people who have not put these choices in writing, the decision is usually up to the next of kin or legal guardian. Disagreements within the family can cause a great deal of difficulty, particularly when a rapid medical decision is required. Counseling can be of help.

Although we have made significant progress in understanding some of the factors leading to Alzheimer's disease, it is likely that the disease will continue to be a major health problem for a long time. Our gains in the ability to diagnose the disease and improvements in its treatment offer hope. Over the next decade treatments based on the known pathogenesis of the disease will become available. Grounded in the remarkable scientific achievements in the past decade, scientists remain hopeful that a cure or preventive treatments will emerge.

Amnesias

Amnesia refers to a significant and selective impairment of a person's memory, either in learning new information or in remembering the past. Since memory is a major brain function (**B13**) and one of the qualities that defines who we are, loss of that capacity can be devastating. Amnesia most commonly occurs as a symptom of another disease, such as Alzheimer's (**C67**) or encephalitis (**C38**), but can also occur by itself, in the absence of any other cognitive deficits.

There are many different types of amnesias, but they fall into two major categories, according to their cause:

- Organic amnesia involves memory loss caused by specific malfunctions in the brain.

- Functional amnesia refers to memory disorders that seem to result from psychological trauma, not injury or disease.

Organic Amnesias

The memory loss of organic amnesia is typically produced by such brain disorders as tu-mors (**C64**), strokes (**C59, C60**), head injury (**C61**), and degenerative diseases, such as Alzheimer's (**C67**). However, certain drugs affecting mood or behavior (**C66**) and alcoholism (**C30**) can also cause amnesia, as can temporal lobe surgery and electroconvulsive therapy for depression (**C20**), although in this instance it is typically transient.

The best-known type of organic amnesia occurs when a person has problems recalling information from the past, a condition known as a retrograde amnesia. Doctors usually identify the disorder by asking an individual about past events, including personal landmarks (When did you graduate from high school?) and public occurrences he or she is likely to have heard about (Who won the last presidential election?). In most instances, people's abilities to recall different facts vary by time. The information that they learned recently is the most likely to be disrupted, while they often retain knowledge acquired years earlier. Thus, adults with a retrograde amnesia generally remember details about their childhood and early schooling, but they may have great difficulty recalling personal and public events from the last few years.

People can also encounter difficulties in retaining new information. This, too, is a problem of memory, known as an anterograde amnesia. Such individuals have profound difficulty learning anything new. They may acquire information after hearing it repeated many times but then forget it shortly afterward. Doctors generally establish the presence of anterograde amnesia by seeing whether an individual can learn new information—either verbal, such as a story or a list of words, or nonverbal, such as pictures or geometric designs. Often the individual can learn some of this new information after much effort, but he or she retains little after a brief time elapses.

Amnesias of either kind can also be designated as temporary or permanent, depending on the type of brain injury the individual experiences. Permanent amnesia results from destruction of brain tissue. For such damage to disrupt a person's memory but produce no major deficits in other cognitive domains, it must affect only the systems in the brain that are primarily responsible for normal memory. Damage to brain structures in the medial temporal lobe (such as the hippocampus and the entorhinal cortex) is most often the cause of permanent difficulty learning and retaining new information. Such damage can be caused by a variety of mechanisms, including head injury, infection, and stroke.

Temporary amnesia results from processes that disrupt the ability of the brain to function normally for a brief period of time but do not cause permanent brain damage. A blow to the head, as in a sports injury or an automobile accident, is the most common cause (C61). A brief disruption of the blood supply to the brain—for example, from a narrowing of the blood vessels in the brain (C59)—can have the same effect. If these processes do not cause permanent injury, then the person will regain the ability to learn and retain new information, and to recall information from the past. The individual's memory will also function normally in the future. However, memory for the period just preceding and following the damage will usually be lost. This is because it takes time for the brain to consolidate new information, and if this process is disrupted, even briefly, the new information that the individual should have acquired is lost forever.

Often brain damage, whether temporary or permanent, produces both anterograde and retrograde amnesia. However, the severity of the two need not be equal. For example, an individual can have a permanent and profound inability to learn new information but have a retrograde amnesia that goes back only a short period. Similarly, when an individual recovers from a temporary amnesia, the problems with learning may improve before the problems with remembering past events, or the reverse.

Organic Amnesia and the Brain

Studies of people with amnesia have provided surprising insights into how memory normally works. One remarkable finding is that even in severe amnesias, not all memory and learning abilities are impaired. Rather, only memories that are explicit and accessible are affected. These are sometimes called declarative memories, since we can bring them to mind as propositions or images. Declarative memory includes the facts, events, faces, and routes of everyday life. Nondeclarative, or implicit, memories can be expressed only in performance. These include motor skills and perceptual skills and are not affected by amnesia. Thus, a person with severe amnesia still knows how to tie a pair of shoes, even if he or she cannot remember buying those shoes the day before. In contrast, some people retain their memories of most things, but not how to perform certain tasks (apraxia; **C71**) or recognize certain things (agnosia; **C72**). This has led researchers to conclude that the brain has organized its memory functions around fundamentally different information-storage systems, some of which are impaired in amnesia and some of which are not.

Amnesia appears to result from damage to the medial temporal lobe (including the hippocampus and the entorhinal cortex) and the diencephalic midline. Studies have determined that damage to the hippocampus alone is sufficient to cause amnesia, but it appears that when several of these structures are damaged together, the severity of amnesia is worse than when only the hippocampus is damaged.

Functional Amnesia

Problems with memory can also occur for psychological reasons. This is functional amnesia, also known as dissociative, or psychogenic, amnesia. The cause is usually an emotionally traumatic event. The pattern of memory loss in such cases is less systematic and predictable than in the amnesias described above. For example, individuals may not recall their names (which they learned as infants) but may retain a wide variety of skills or facts about the world that they learned as adults.

There are several types of functional amnesia. In dissociative amnesia, a person loses the memory of some important personal experience. This gap, or series of gaps, in memory is usually related to traumatic or extremely stressful situations. For example, a rape victim may lose his or her memory of the event, or a soldier may not be able to recall a battle.

Another type of functional amnesia, called a dissociative fugue, usually begins when a person suddenly, unexpectedly wanders away from home or work. This type of amnesia is also usually related to a stressful event. People with this disorder forget much more extensively; their whole past can become obscure, and they commonly lose all their memories of personal identity. The fugue state may last from a few hours to months or more. Often after recovery, the individual fails to remember anything that occurred during the fugue state.

Dissociative identity disorder is a type of amnesia in which a person appears to have two or more distinct personal identities that alternate control of his or her behavior. Such an individual may not only lose memory of periods from the past but also forget all personal information concerning some extended period of childhood. People with this disorder frequently have histories of severe physical and sexual abuse, especially during childhood.

Although functional amnesias are a popular theme in soap operas and movies, there are relatively few well-documented cases in the scientific literature. Most experts believe that these conditions do exist but that they are exceedingly rare.

Diagnosing and Treating Amnesia

The diagnosis of amnesia usually begins with a complete medical history. Doctors will ask questions to determine the extent and type of a person's memory loss, and whether there are any aggravating or triggering factors, including head injury, emotionally traumatic events, recent surgery, use of drugs, or excessive use of alcohol. A physical examination may include a detailed neurological examination. Doctors test recent, intermediate, and long-term memory.

Treatment varies according to the type of amnesia and the suspected cause. One drug, donepezil, has been found to improve thinking and memory in patients with Alzheimer's disease.

Researchers are still exploring how memory is organized and what structures and connections are involved. We hope that better understanding of the neurology of memory will lead to better diagnosis, treatments, and prevention of amnesia and other neurological diseases that affect memory.

Dementia

Dementia is a group of symptoms involving the progressive impairment of many aspects of brain function at once, particularly in those parts of the cerebrum known as the association areas, which integrate perception, thought, and purposeful action. Doctors make the diagnosis of dementia when a person displays impairment of two or more brain functions, one of which must be memory. Other cognitive impairments can include deterioration in language (aphasia; **C70**), voluntary movement (apraxia; **C71**), the ability to recognize or identify objects (agnosia; **C72**), and the ability to think abstractly and perform complex behaviors.

The causes and symptoms of dementia are many, varied, and often multiple. The most common causes involve impairment to the vascular (blood vessel) or neurological structures of the brain. Some of this damage is progressive and irreversible, while other problems can be stopped or reversed. Dementia can occur at all ages but is most likely to arise among older age groups, especially in people over 75.

Dementia usually appears first as memory loss. Individuals with dementia become impaired in their ability to learn new material, or they may forget previously learned material. They might leave the stove on, lose their keys repeatedly, or forget their own phone numbers. They may have difficulty remembering the names of objects or people, or find it difficult to speak coherently or understand what others say. Some are unable even to pantomime common actions, such as waving good-bye.

Loss of functioning progresses slowly, from decreased problem solving and language skills, to difficulty with ordinary daily activities, and on to severe memory loss and complete disorientation with withdrawal from social interaction. A person may not be aware of his or her dementia, however. Hallucinations, delusions, and paranoid behavior may occur.

All too often the signs of dementia, including types that can be treated, are dismissed as a normal result of aging. While we do undergo some cognitive changes as we age, dementia is a symptom of disease and must be diagnosed and treated as such.

Arrestable or Reversible Causes of Dementia

Causes of dementia that can be stopped or reversed include reactions to drugs, including those used as medications (**C66**). Neuroactive and psychoactive agents, the opiate analgesics, the adrenocortical steroids, and anticholinergic preparations used for movement disorders have all been known to produce dementia. Some individuals have allergic reactions to certain drugs or combinations of them. In addition, alcohol (**C30**) and almost all other drugs that people abuse (**C29**), ranging from heroin to glue, can cause dementia.

Brain infections can also cause dementia, including forms of meningitis (**C37**), encephalitis (**C38**), and syphilis, if untreated. Certain chronic viral illnesses, such as AIDS (**C35**), can produce the symptom. For most of these illnesses, we have treatments. But the infectious prion responsible for the rare Creutzfeldt-Jakob disease (**C39**) can produce extreme dementia that is untreatable.

Metabolic causes of dementia (**C6**) are often treatable. Diseases of the thyroid, parathyroid, adrenals, and pituitary are often easy to identify and treat. When dementia is the result of kidney and liver failure, or the complications of diabetes, addressing the underlying cause often relieves the problem. Dehydration is another common, and easily treated, metabolic cause. Nutritional disorders (**C65**), including thiamine deficiency, pernicious anemia, and folate deficiency, are usually preventable and sometimes reversible if recognized early.

Hypertension, or chronic high blood pressure, is one of the most frequent causes of dementia. Other vascular and cardiac diseases can also produce dementia by obstructing the blood supply to the brain (**C59**). Treating the underlying problem can stop and sometimes reverse these dementias.

Tumors of the brain (**C64**), both benign and malignant, frequently produce dementia. Surgical treatment depends on the size and location of the tumor. Normal pressure hydrocephalus (**C8**), which is a rare cause of dementia, can often be relieved with a shunt.

Head injuries (**C61**) can result in dementia. When the trauma occurs once, as in a car accident or bad fall, the dementia can usually be stopped, but repeated head injury (such as a boxer might experience) can lead to progressive dementia.

Severe depression (**C20**) can also produce dementia. Treating the emotional disorder usually reverses the cognitive problems as well.

Progressive and Nonreversible Causes of Dementia

There are also progressive and nonreversible causes of dementia. We can divide these into two categories: those that have dementia as the primary symptom, and those that have other neurological signs.

Alzheimer's, the most common of all dementing diseases, is discussed in section **C67**. Pick's disease, or frontotemporal dementia (FTD), is the other condition in this category, but it is far less common than Alzheimer's. (For every person with Pick's disease, there are probably 20 or 30 with Alzheimer's.)

The initial symptoms of Pick's disease are not thought to include memory losses, but some recent studies say that memory may be variably affected. More often the disorder appears in personality changes, which can differ from person to person. Some people exhibit apathy, while others lose their inhibitions and become overactive.

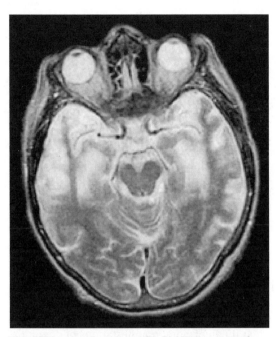

This **MRI scan** of a patient with Pick's disease, or frontotemporal dementia, shows the degeneration of brain tissue in the frontal lobes. The cause of Pick's disease is unknown. SCAN COURTESY OF KEITH JOHNSON, *THE WHOLE BRAIN ATLAS*, WWW.MED.HARVARD.EDU/AANLIB/HOME.HTML

Many develop eating disorders and gain weight, but some display ritualistic behavior (grunting, hand rubbing, foot tapping) and compulsions. Language impairment is the other common sign of FTD. Some people can speak only with great effort, and not fluently; for others, speech is fluent but lacks content. There is also a change in social conduct. Individuals lack insight and lose some of their sense of responsibility. In many cases, psychiatrists are the first doctors to see people with FTD because they are thought to be suffering from depression or psychosis.

Pick's disease involves atrophy of the frontal and temporal lobes of the brain. The neurons in the affected areas come to contain abnormal material, called Pick's bodies. Unlike Alzheimer's,

there are no plaques or intracellular fibers. We do not know the exact cause of this condition.

Pick's disease typically begins between the ages of 35 and 75 and affects men and women equally. No treatments influence its progressive nature, and no surgical procedures are useful. The average course of illness spans ten years from first symptoms until death, but this period is quite variable.

The second category of progressive and nonreversible dementias includes a multitude of diseases of the nervous system in which dementia may or may not occur alongside other symptoms. These include Parkinson's disease (**C41**) and Huntington's disease (**C47**), among other diseases affecting the basal ganglia, the cerebellum, and the motor neurons. Even taken all together, these other causes of dementia do not compare to the very great frequency of Alzheimer's disease.

Diagnosing and Treating Dementia

Since the causes of dementia are many and varied, and some types can be stopped or reversed, the diagnosis must be careful and accurate. Diagnosis is complicated, however, because many dementia-causing diseases, such as Alzheimer's, can only be confirmed or ruled out with certainty at autopsy.

Since people with dementia may not know that they are experiencing cognitive difficulties, family members are sometimes the first to notice such symptoms as minor forgetfulness, restlessness or apathy, a tendency to misplace things, or changes in personality and to bring them to the attention of a doctor. A physician with knowledge of dementia and dementia-causing diseases should perform a careful clinical evaluation. This should include a family history and a chronological account of the person's illness that emphasizes the onset, duration, and specific cognitive, memory, and behavioral changes.

Physicians can use physical, neurological, and psychological evaluations to ascertain not only the primary cause (or causes) of a person's dementia, but also possible coexisting abnormalities that might make the condition worse. These tests might include:

- complete blood count
- electrolyte measurements
- screening metabolic panel
- thyroid function tests
- checks for vitamin B_{12} and folate levels
- tests for syphilis and HIV antibodies
- urinalysis
- electrocardiogram
- chest X ray
- brain imaging

These tests can reveal most of the readily reversible causes of dementia, such as metabolic problems, nutritional deficiencies, and infections. Brain imaging (computed tomography, magnetic resonance imaging, or positron-emission tomography may also be appropriate. Neuroimaging may detect atrophy and perhaps characteristic patterns of decreased blood flow or metabolism in crucial regions.

In treating dementia, a doctor's goal is to control the symptoms. Because they arise from different causes, that treatment varies with the specific disorder. If at all possible, physicians try to identify and treat the underlying causes, not just the symptom. Stopping or changing medications that worsen a person's confusion and are not essential may improve his or her cognitive function. Addressing coexisting medical and psychiatric disorders—for example, treating hypothyroidism with replacement therapy, or treating depression—often greatly improves mental functioning. However, the clinical response to the commonly used anticholinesterase drugs (used for Alzheimer's disease) is modest in terms of improving memory function.

People with dementia may have to take medications to control behaviors that are dangerous to themselves or others. Antipsychotic drugs, antianxiety drugs, and antidepressants are all used to treat the behavioral manifestations of dementia. These are usually given in very low doses and are adjusted as required.

Individuals with progressive dementia may be helped by visiting nurses, volunteer services, support groups, adult protective services, and other community resources. As the disease progresses, a person may require monitoring and assistance in the home or in an institutionalized setting. This may include in-home care, boarding homes, adult day care, or convalescent homes.

Research into the diagnosis and treatment of dementia continues. Advances in genetics and molecular biology may prove helpful in identifying potential biological markers. The most promising paths of research into Pick's disease focus on its genetic bases, and in particular on the mutated tau gene.

Trouble with Speech and Language

To have trouble communicating can be one of the most frustrating neurological symptoms a person may suffer. Such difficulty threatens our ability to express our needs, desires, and thoughts and to maintain relationships with the people we love. Problems with speech and language arise in many disorders, affecting people in different degrees.

Language being a complex function, there are many ways a person can develop a problem speaking, so it is useful to break down the process. By *language,* we refer to the way we use symbols, spoken or written, to communicate. There are many languages (English, Spanish, Chinese, and so on) and many types of language (spoken, written, and signed, plus musical notation, mathematical symbols, and other specialized forms). But most language processing and disorders that impair it are all similarly situated in the brain. *Speech* refers to the mechanics of how we usually produce language: controlling our breathing, voice box, tongue, and lips to form sounds. We can further divide that communication into four steps:

- semantics—the meaning
- syntax—the organization of words into sentences
- phonology—the mechanical and sound aspects of spoken language
- pragmatics—the social aspects of conversation, such as taking turns

Each of these stages can be disturbed by brain disorders and neuropsychiatric diseases that prevent someone from carrying on a normal conversation.

The term *aphasia* refers to the disruption of a person's ability to communicate with language after developing a brain disease. *Dysarthria* refers to abnormalities in articulating that disturb a person's speech as a result of impairment of the motor function.

Mechanisms of Aphasia

Language is mediated primarily by the left hemisphere of the brain. The rear part is responsible for processing the meaning of language (semantics), and the front part for the syntactical elements of speech (grammar, arrangements of words into sentences, and so on).

The most common cause of aphasia is a stroke (**C59, C60**). Strokes involving the rear, or posterior, part of the brain where language meaning is handled thus produce a "fluent aphasia," characterized by many words strung together in long sentences but communicating little meaning. Strokes involving the front part of the brain produce a "nonfluent aphasia," in which a person tends to give short, grammatically simple replies. Patients with fluent aphasia (posterior) typically have difficulty understanding other people's language, whereas patients with nonfluent aphasia can often understand what they hear. If a large stroke involves both the posterior and anterior parts of the left hemisphere, however, the person will have both nonfluent output and difficulty understanding others. When aphasia is due to a single brain lesion such as a stroke, the person generally knows what he or she wants to say but has difficulty formulating the words (nonfluent aphasia) or formulates them incorrectly (fluent aphasia). In general, large brain injuries produce more severe aphasia from which it is more difficult to recover. Brain imaging such as computed tomography (CT) and magnetic resonance imag-

STUTTERING

Stuttering is a communication disorder involving disruptions in the forward flow of speech. The word *stuttering* can be used to refer either to the specific speech disfluencies that are commonly seen in people who stutter or to the overall communication difficulty that people who stutter may experience. There are perhaps as many different patterns of stuttering as there are people who stutter. And there are many different degrees of stuttering, from mild to severe. There is no single cause, but current research is exploring the connections between stuttering and the neurological coordination of speech. Developmental stuttering normally begins between the ages of 2 and 5, tends to run in families, and affects more males than females. Neurogenic stuttering may be caused by brain damage resulting from strokes or blows to the head.

Here are some tips for parents to help a stuttering child:

■ The goal is to keep the child's stuttering at its present level, prevent its further development, and keep the child talking.

■ Don't let the child know you are upset about his or her speech.

■ Keep your child healthy, getting adequate sleep and proper nutrition, and follow a general routine schedule.

■ Look at your child when he or she speaks and show by your expression that you are interested in what the child is saying, not how he or she is saying it.

■ Don't force the child to speak or recite to strangers. However, encourage the child to speak as often as he or she wants.

ing (MRI) demonstrates the lesion and shows its size.

Risk factors for strokes include hypertension, obesity, cigarette smoking, and high levels of blood cholesterol or fat. Controlling your blood pressure, diet, and weight and not smoking will therefore reduce your likelihood of ever developing aphasia. It is much easier to avoid a stroke than to try to recover from one.

Alzheimer's disease (C67) also commonly produces aphasia. The aphasia of Alzheimer's disease is of the fluent type. In most cases, it is mild in the early stages of the disease and progresses slowly as the illness worsens. In a few cases, aphasia is very severe. Do not assume, however, that *any* difficulty remembering words or otherwise using language is a sign of incipient Alzheimer's. Such events are normal as we age.

Brain injury in automobile accidents or other types of trauma (C61) and brain cancers (C64) can produce aphasia if they affect particular parts of the left side of the brain. In rare cases, such brain infections as encephalitis (C38) cause the problem as well.

Aphasia is commonly accompanied by alexia (difficulty reading) and agraphia (difficulty writing). The features of the alexia are similar to those of the aphasia (fluent or nonfluent) because

- **Don't let your child avoid normal responsibilities. Use the same discipline as with any other child.**

- **Don't supply words. Let your child get his or her own words out. Don't interrupt.**

- **Look for emotional tension at home or school when stuttering is more severe.**

- **Praise your child when he or she speaks well. This should not be taken as praise for not stuttering—praise what he or she says, not how he or she says it.**

- **Don't hurry your child when he or she is speaking.**

- **Avoid such suggestions as "Think before you speak," "Talk slower [or faster]," "Wait until you can say it," and so on.**

- **Don't ask the child to substitute an easy word for a hard one, as this will only increase the fear of certain words and phrases.**

- **Encourage speaking at home and in school.**

- **Nothing can ever take the place of love, understanding, and patience when dealing with any children.**

Adapted from www.nsastutter.org (National Stuttering Association); additional sites: www.stutteringrecovery.com (Stuttering Therapy); www.stutteringhomepage.com (Stuttering Homepage)

speaking and reading depend on the same basic language regions of the brain. Alexia occurs more often with lesions in the back part of the left hemisphere than in the front part. Some children with dyslexia (**C1**) have had brain injury at a young age, producing an aphasic syndrome. In most cases, however, dyslexia is a developmental disorder involving reading and writing only.

Mechanisms of Dysarthria

Dysarthrias can be produced by any disturbance of the complex motor apparatus we use to produce sounds: the tongue, lips, vocal cords, and muscles that push air out through our mouths. We can see a temporary form of this difficulty in intoxicated individuals; their speech is slurred because they cannot coordinate their lip and tongue movements. Strokes and tumors that affect the parts of the brain responsible for motor function can produce a more long-lasting dysarthria, as can amyotrophic lateral sclerosis (**C53**) and similar motor neuron disorders. Such brain diseases as Parkinson's (**C41**) reduce voice volume, leading to soft-spoken speech. People with dysarthria are usually able to understand language well and can sometimes communicate by other means.

Naturally, people who express themselves through sign language develop the equivalent of dysarthrias if they cannot use their hands to form words. This condition might arise due to strokes, peripheral neuropathy (**C48**), apraxias (**C71**), and other muscle disorders. Signers can also experience aphasia in sign if they sustain injury to the language-related areas of the left hemisphere.

Brain trauma (**C61**) and cancers (**C64**) can produce dysarthria or other conditions that interfere with communication if they affect the movement and coordination regions of the brain. Usually a person with these conditions experiences other symptoms as well.

Diagnosis and Treatment

Someone having a stroke often notices paralysis of an arm and leg on the same side, or difficulties with vision. Because language is mediated by the left hemisphere of the brain, which controls the right side of the body, the onset of aphasia is frequently accompanied by paralysis of the right arm or leg or both. Any possible stroke is an *emergency,* and the person must be taken to a hospital immediately. There, doctors will diagnose the type of stroke with a brain scan and may administer clot-dissolving chemicals, blood-thinning agents, or other treatments.

A short-lived aphasia, especially in conjunction with right-sided weakness, may be due to a transient ischemic attack (TIA), which temporarily reduces the flow of blood to part of the brain. This, too, is a medical *emergency.* It is also a warning of the possibility of serious strokes unless one takes preventive steps.

Speech therapists often help people who have aphasia after a stroke recover as much of their language function as possible through the optimal use of uninjured brain areas. Fluent and nonfluent aphasia respond to different therapeutic approaches; music and singing often helps a person with nonfluent aphasia speak more freely. Speech therapy maximizes the recovery of injured brain regions and recruits brain areas not typically devoted to language. The prognosis for recovering language after a stroke varies. People with severe aphasia tend to have limited recovery, but those with a mild condition have a better prognosis. Most people exhibit some degree of spontaneous recovery, and speech therapy may help them regain more linguistic skills. Most of the restoration likely to occur is evident within six months of the stroke, and it is nearly complete within two years. After that, if they have not regained speech, people may be able to gesture in order to communicate simple needs but will never return to their previous language skills. Medications are typically of little use.

When an older person slowly develops aphasia along with abnormalities of memory, it is frequently a sign of a degenerative brain disease such as Alzheimer's **(C67)**. Individuals experiencing such a condition should be assessed by a neurologist. There are treatments that can help improve the symptoms of Alzheimer's disease or slow the loss of function, though there is no cure.

If aphasia is due to Alzheimer's disease, then treatment will be directed at the underlying illness. Speech therapy is usually of little value for people with this disorder because Alzheimer's is progressive, meaning the aphasia and other symptoms will get worse.

Speech therapy may be useful in reducing some aspects of dysarthria. Therapists can teach people how to articulate best with the abilities they still have and help them and their families develop alternate means of communication that work well.

Apraxias

"What a piece of work is a man," Shakespeare wrote, "in form and moving how express and admirable." Our brains and bodies can perform an almost infinite variety of movements, from pounding a heavy hammer on a narrow spike, to graceful high dives through the air, to picking up and turning one thin page of a book without tearing it. Through our motor systems, we interact with and change our environment. But the corticospinal, or pyramidal, motor system, from the brain to the nerves to the muscles, needs instructions to work well.

The directions for the pyramidal system reside in the brain in what we call praxis programs. You can also think of these as your "how to" system. They provide such instructions to your motor system as:

- How to select the tools and actions you need to solve a mechanical problem.

- How to position your hands to hold and use the tools.

- How to move your limbs and body in or through space; these movements require both

knowing where you are (egocentric information) and where your target is (allocentric information).

- How rapidly to move.

- How much force to apply.

- How to order certain movements to achieve a goal.

We develop these programs largely through practice on small tasks, especially in the early months and years of life, until we no longer have to think about them except when faced with a very new challenge. But when areas of the brain suffer damage, the programs may be lost. Disorders of this "how to" system are called apraxias.

We use our arms and legs most often to carry out tasks, so apraxias are most apparent when they interfere with limb movement. There are two major groupings of limb apraxias: general problems, and those interfering with specific tasks. Of the five major forms of general limb apraxia, each is defined by the nature of errors that a person makes, and each has a different neuropsychological mechanism. They are:

- limb-kinetic: the person suffers a loss of deftness

- ideomotor: the person makes errors involving space and time

- dissociative: the person can correctly imitate actions, but cannot correctly perform them as described verbally

- ideational: the person cannot perform a series of acts leading to a goal

- conceptual: the person makes content errors and loses mechanical knowledge such that he or she may be unable to use alternative tools or solve novel problems

Three other forms of limb apraxia are task-specific. People with apraxic agraphia have problems printing or writing letters, but as long as they have no other language disturbances (**C70**) they may still be able to spell aloud correctly and type. People with constructional apraxia have problems with drawing or copying pictures. Those with dressing apraxia have trouble dressing themselves. The specificity of these problems indicates that each task—writing, drawing pictures, dressing—is coordinated by a particular area of the brain.

Mechanisms

In general, performing any skilled action requires at least four levels of processing:

- conceptual-semantic knowledge—basically, knowing what you want to accomplish, and how it might be done

- spatial-temporal information—knowing how to hold tools or objects you need to work with and move these tools to accomplish their desired action

- development of motor or innervatory programs—being able to coordinate your bodily movements through nervous system signals

- motor activation—being able to start and control those movements

Each of the apraxic disorders discussed above is related to dysfunction at one or more of these levels of action programming.

The most common disorders that cause apraxia are strokes (**C59, C60**) and such degenerative diseases as Alzheimer's (**C67**) or corticobasal degeneration. However, any disease that produces cortical dysfunction, including brain tumors (**C64**) and trauma (**C61**), may cause apraxia.

Different apraxias are associated with damage to different parts of the brain. Limb-kinetic apraxia, for example, is usually associated with dysfunction of the motor or premotor cortex.

Ideomotor apraxia may be associated with injury to either the parietal lobe or the premotor cortex. People with parietal lesions may be impaired not only at gesturing, pantomiming, and working with tools but also at discriminating and comprehending *other* people's gestures.

Individuals with dissociative apraxia have dysfunctions in the posterior hemisphere. Those with ideational apraxia often have widespread dysfunction, but when the problems are localized they are most likely to be in the frontal lobes. The locus of lesions that cause conceptual apraxia has not been fully determined.

Dressing apraxia is associated with right parietal lesions, apraxic agraphia with left frontal or parietal lesions, and constructional apraxia with left or right parietal lesions.

For right-handed people, most of these apraxias are likely to be associated with dysfunctions in the left hemisphere of the brain. However, dressing apraxia is more likely to arise from problems in the right hemisphere, and constructional apraxia may stem from dysfunction in either half.

Diagnosis and Treatment

Apraxia is not a disease in itself but rather a sign of some other, underlying disease causing damage to the brain. Therefore, when people develop the symptoms of apraxia, neurologists must evaluate them, diagnose the underlying diseases, and, when possible, start treatment. Those treatments are discussed in the relevant sections of this book.

People with apraxia from static deficits—meaning problems that are not getting worse—can often be retrained to perform the same tasks using undamaged areas of their brains. Unfortunately, this type of rehabilitation program is not widely available.

Many activities of daily living, such as cooking, building, and fixing things, require people to perform skilled acts. An apraxic disorder can therefore be terribly disabling. Furthermore, in order to compensate for a disability or avoid problems caused by it, a person must know that he or she is disabled, and often people with apraxia do not recognize their limitations. Caregivers must therefore be certain that patients with apraxia do not attempt tasks that may cause them to injure themselves or others.

Agnosias

Agnosia is a relatively rare disorder involving recognition. An agnosic person can see and hear normally, and seems to think and speak adequately, but cannot recognize someone or something he or she once knew. Careful testing cannot attribute that inability to any problems with sensing the world, general thinking, language, or attention. As one scientist has described agnosia, a normal part of the person's life "has somehow been stripped of its meaning." Agnosia is most commonly seen in patients with dementia or stroke.

For the vast majority of people with agnosia, the problem affects only one information pathway in the brain. For example, an individual may be shown a picture of a harmonica and be unable to name it or demonstrate how to use it. But that same individual can recognize a harmonica immediately on the basis of touch, sound, or hearing a description of its appearance or function. Another person may be unable to recognize a fork by means of touch, but can name the object when he or she sees it.

Based on these differences in how we take in information, we identify three major types of agnosia:

- visual (seeing)
- auditory (hearing)
- tactile (touching)

Perhaps because the human brain devotes more processing resources to vision than to any other sense, visual agnosia is the most common type.

Visual Agnosias

We classify visual agnosias according to the level of processing at which the problems seem to arise. H. Lissauer came up with this system more than a century ago when he distinguished between apperceptive and associative agnosias. He theorized that recognizing something is a two-stage process: first our minds assemble all the incoming information into an image, and then we link that image to what we know from the past to understand its meaning.

People with apperceptive agnosia, Lissauer suggested, are impaired at the first stage. They have such obvious difficulties with visual perception that some are assumed to be blind—but they still manage to avoid bumping into things. Individuals with apperceptive agnosia typically have a lesion in the occipital lobe or the posterior temporal lobes on both sides of the brain. This condition often affects people who are recovering from cortical blindness, which has caused them to lose their sight not because of damage to their eyes or optic nerves but because of damage to the brain regions that process visual information.

Associative agnosia, in contrast, is a disorder characterized by relatively well preserved perception but an inability to access the meaning of what one perceives. Distinguishing between apperceptive and associative agnosias is classically based on a person's ability to copy a figure or draw an object. Apperceptive agnosics typically cannot perform that task at all. In contrast, associative agnosics may be capable of producing an elaborate and accurate copy of a picture—but they cannot identify the object they have drawn. Associative agnosics do not produce their drawings normally: they typically draw (or write) in a laborious and piecemeal fashion, as if they were seeing only one small component of the object at a time.

We can also classify visual agnosics on the basis of the specific things they do not recognize. In prosopagnosia, for example, the problem is relatively specific: people cannot identify faces. These agnosics may recognize cars, words, cups, and other objects quite normally yet cannot recognize their family members or even themselves. People with this disorder have even been seen to speak to their own reflections in mirrors. Prosopagnosics often identify others by means of their clothes or voices, showing that they have not lost their knowledge of the person in question. What is missing is the connection between the face and the person they know. This disorder is associated with a lesion involving the posterior, inferior temporal lobe (fusiform gyrus) in the right hemisphere.

Other visual agnosics may be particularly impaired in the recognition of words (agnosic alexia), objects, or colors. Some visual agnosics may be impaired in recognizing *all* of these things. Explanations for why people can identify one type of thing and not another are controversial. One proposal is that our brains process different stimuli in different ways. We process faces holistically, as one object rather than a collection of features. Words, in contrast, are made up of a finite set of distinct components (letters), each of which must be identified correctly; thus, our brains must break down a word rather than processing it as a unit. Because the processing of these sights is so different, a lesion in a part of the brain that affects one ability may have no effect on another.

Another form of visual agnosia is called simultanagnosia. People with this disorder can recognize objects when seeing them alone but cannot process those same objects when they appear together or in the context of a scene. Studies have shown that some simultanagnosics have "implicit" knowledge that several things are present but are unable to identify them on a conscious level. This may imply that there is not simply one but multiple pathways for recognition.

Auditory and Tactile Agnosias

People with auditory agnosia still have the ability to detect and make simple judgments about sounds, but they cannot identify the sound sources. On hearing an airplane, for instance, people with this disorder may describe the noise as loud and low-pitched but be unable to name its source. In some instances the agnosia may be restricted to speech, a condition termed "pure word deafness." In this condition, people can identify sounds such as a car horn but can't understand spoken language. However, they can read and write. Auditory agnosics typically have bilateral lesions in the superior temporal lobes. Pure word deafness may be associated with bilateral lesions or with a lesion of the left temporal lobe involving the auditory cortex, which prevents information from the right hemisphere from reaching the language cortex in the left hemisphere.

Tactile agnosia is characterized by an inability to identify an object by touch despite being able to manipulate and feel the object. Often individuals with this disorder are able to identify objects by vision, so they can get by in most circumstances. That may be one reason tactile agnosia is so rarely identified.

Diagnosis and Treatment

Although agnosics are rare, they are nonetheless probably underdiagnosed. Many people with agnosia are initially thought to be "confused." They or their loved ones may assume the problem is a form of dementia: Alzheimer's disease (**C67**) or a lesser-known condition (**C68, C69**). Or the problem may appear to be aphasia—a disorder of language (**C70**) rather than recognition.

To diagnose agnosia, physicians must first exclude other potential causes of an individual's problems recognizing people or things. This requires careful testing of the person's mental status and general cognitive abilities so as to exclude dementia or aphasia. Additionally, the doctor must carefully evaluate the person's ability to perceive visual or other stimuli. In the case of visual agnosias, this process should include assessment of the person's visual fields, visual acuity, color perception, reading, facial recognition, drawing, and recognition of line drawings and real objects. A person with poor vision who cannot construct an adequate mental picture of an object does not have an agnosia. Similarly, someone who has forgotten the function and other properties of everyday objects is most likely to be suffering from a progressive degenerative disorder of the brain, such as Alzheimer's disease.

Agnosia is a symptom of brain disorder rather than a disease in itself. The damage to the brain that produces the problem may be vascular, meaning a stroke (**C59, C60**); toxic (**C66**); degenerative; or otherwise. Treating agnosias should start with treating the underlying disorder. Often the damage is reversible, but in some patients it is not. Many patients with agnosia benefit from physical and occupational therapy to manage the practical difficulties of daily life.

Glossary

(Terms in *italics* also appear in this Glossary.)

Action potential a brief change in a neuron's charge that results when ions are exchanged

A-delta fibers fibers that conduct pain rapidly from the peripheral nervous system into the brain

Adrenocorticotrophic hormone (ACTH) a hormone secreted by the pituitary gland that stimulates enlargement of the adrenal gland

Affective having to do with feelings or emotions

Agonists drugs that combine with a receptor to start a reaction in the brain

Akinesia difficulty in starting movement

Alien limb phenomenon movements of a limb that seem intentional but are not

Allodynia extreme sensitivity to touch

Alogia decreased ability to speak

Alpha-2 agonists drugs used to treat attention deficit/ hyperactivity disorder

Amino acids naturally occurring compounds that are the chief components of proteins

Amyloid a kind of protein

Aneurysm an abnormal widening of an artery

Anhedonia loss of interest or pleasure

Antagonist a drug that blocks the action of another

Anticholinergic drugs drugs used to treat Parkinson's disease

Antigen the structure that an antibody attacks

Antineuronal antibodies antibodies that react against nerve cells in the brain

Apoptosis the process of genetically programmed cell death

Atrophy decrease in size of a cell or tissue

Auditory-visual association linking a sound with an image

Autonomic not under voluntary control

Autosomal recessive refers to an inheritance pattern in which both parents must have the trait to pass it on to their child

Avolition lack of goal-oriented behavior

Axon the long fiber of a neuron, which sends out signals

Barbiturate drug that is a depressant for the central nervous system

Behavioral therapy a treatment plan, usually worked out with a doctor, to stop or change a negative behavior

Beta-amyloid peptide a particular protein fragment, implicated in Alzheimer's disease, that results from the breakdown of the protein *amyloid*

Blood-brain barrier normal mechanism in blood vessel wall cells that keeps many toxic substances in the blood from harming the brain

Bradykinesia slowness of movement

Brain-derived neurotrophic factor (BDNF) protein that maintains the function and survival of many kinds of neurons

Brain wave electrical activity of the brain

Candidate gene a gene that is studied in an effort to

understand the source of an inheritable disorder

Central pattern generator neural center in the spinal cord that controls movement

Cerebrospinal fluid (CSF) liquid that keeps the pressure in the brain and spinal cord the same

C-fibers fibers that conduct pain slowly from the peripheral nervous system into the brain

Chelation therapy therapy that removes various heavy metals from the body

Chemotrophic factors chemicals that encourage an *axon* to grow and attract it in the desired direction

Chromosomal marker an identifiable physical location on a chromosome whose inheritance can be monitored

Chromosome the substance that carries genetic information

Circadian rhythms daily patterns of the brain and body hormonal systems regulating basic functions such as waking and sleeping

Cognitive behavioral therapy (CBT) a form of psychotherapy that identifies and treats difficulties arising from a person's irrational thinking, misperceptions, dysfunctional thoughts, and faulty learning

Comorbidity situation in which two diseases exist at the same time in the same patient

Computed tomography (CT) scan a method of creating three-dimensional images of sections of the body

Conditioning a way of changing behavior by repeating an activity

Cortisol the primary stress hormone

Critical periods times when certain parts of the brain are developed and strengthened

Cyclosporin A a drug that helps suppress the immune system

Deep brain stimulation a probing procedure that is similar to surgery but that does not destroy brain tissue

Dermatome an area that gets its sensation from the root of a single nerve

Dialectical behavioral therapy form of behavioral therapy that seeks to change behavior and attitudes

Diplegic paralysis on both sides of the body, mainly affecting the legs

Diplopia double vision

Discrimination ability to detect differences

Distal located away from a point, as opposed to *proximal*

Dominant refers to a gene that is always expressed

Double-blind study a study in which neither the subjects nor the experimenters know which of two drugs is being given

Dura the tough membrane that surrounds the brain

Edema process in which fluid from the blood leaks into the surrounding tissue

Electroencephalogram (EEG) measurement of a person's brain waves

Electrolyte substance that can break up into ions and conduct electricity in solution

Electron microscope microscope in which an electron beam replaces light to form the image

ELISA (enzyme-linked immunosorbent assay) a test that measures the level of antibodies in a person's blood

Embryonic cells cells in the early stages of development

Endoscopic having to do with an endoscope, a small fiber-optic instrument used to see the inside of a hollow organ

Enkephalins natural substances in the brain that have sedating or pain-relieving qualities, similar to endorphins

Enteric nervous system system of nerves in the walls of the intestine

Epidemiologist scientist who studies the prevalence of diseases in a population of people, as well as the characteristic factors of the diseases

Epinephrine hormone that makes the heart beat faster, the blood pressure soar, the muscles tense, and the pupils open wider; also called adrenaline

Event-related potentials (ERPs) electrical brain responses time-locked to a stimulus or lack of a stimulus

Excitotoxicity condition with the potential to damage or kill brain cells by overstimulation; usually involves excess amounts of the amino acid *glutamate* to overexcite the cells

Family-focused therapy a form of group psychotherapy that treats or involves more than one family member in a therapy session

Fasciculation bunching or cramping of a small group of muscle fibers

Freezing behavior sudden immobility caused by fear; also sometimes a symptom in a disorder such as Parkinson's disease

Functional magnetic resonance imaging (fMRI) a type of imaging technique, using radio waves, that can track and create images of brain activity

Glutamate a neurotransmitter that excites brain cells

Gray matter the portion of the brain's nerve tissue that consists primarily of neuronal cell bodies; see also *white matter*

Habituation the brain's gradual familiarity with new stimuli

Hemiplegia paralysis on one side of the body

Hippocampus part of the brain involved in short-term and, especially, long-term memory

Histamine a chemical released from cells during an allergic reaction

Histology the study of cells and tissues

Homonymous having the same name or category, but with a different meaning or relationship

Hypalgesia decreased sensitivity to pain

Hypertonia increased tension and spasm in skeletal muscles, which indicate possible nerve disorder; its opposite, hypotonia, describes decreased tone in skeletal muscles

Hyperventilation increasing amounts of air entering the lung tissue, resulting in dizziness or fainting

Hypervigilance overly acute sensitivity to surroundings

Hypnotics drugs that induce drowsiness or sleepiness and reduce excitement

Hypothalamic-pituitary-adrenal (HPA) axis interactive connection between the brain and the adrenal glands

Immunoglobulin (IG) specific protein involved in fighting infections

Immunologic refers to the science of immunology, the study of how the body fights disease

Infarct tissue that has died from lack of blood supply

Inhibitory neurons neurons that act to slow or repress stimuli or behavior

Innervate to supply with nerves

Interpersonal and social rhythm therapy psychotherapy that combines *interpersonal therapy* with behavioral techniques

Interpersonal therapy a form of psychotherapy that focuses on a patient's relationships

Intrathecally a method of drug delivery in which the medication is injected into the *cerebrospinal fluid* to reach the spinal cord and brain

Kinase an enzyme that catalyzes the transfer of phosphate

Kinesthesis the (brain's) sense of movement and position

Lesion site of any damage to living tissue caused by injury or disease

Long-term memory the part of the memory that stores information for more than a few minutes

Lymphocyte type of white blood cell

Macrocephaly a condition in which the head is abnormally large

Macrophage a cell that attacks and eats invading germs

Magnetic resonance imaging (MRI) method of creating computerized images of internal body tissues using radio waves

Melatonin hormone produced by the pineal gland in the brain that regulates sleep and the *circadian rhythms*

Mitochondria part of a cell responsible for energy production

Mononuclear having a single nucleus

Monoplegic suffering from paralysis affecting a single limb

Morphology the study of the structure or form of organisms

Motoneuron a neuron that connects to a muscle fiber

Motor cortex front part of the brain, which controls movement

Motor function physical activity of the body

Motor nerves carriers of electrical impulses, as opposed to sensory nerves

MtDNA DNA that is contained in the *mitochondria* of the cell

Multipotent cell a cell that is capable of becoming diverse types of cells within a body system

Mutation a change in genes or chromosomes that affects characteristics of the body

Myelin white protective covering (sheath) that insulates nerve fibers

Myelination formation of the *myelin* sheath

Myoglobin protein in red blood cells that stores oxygen

Necrosis death of cells or a portion of living tissue

Negative symptoms fundamental, less obvious symptoms

Neocortex highly developed part of the cerebral cortex that is unique to mammals

Nerve conduction transfer of electrical, heat, and nerve impulses throughout the nervous system

Nerve tract bundle of nerve fibers forming a common pathway

Neuralgia severe, lingering pain along a nerve pathway

Neurofilaments filaments found in the *axon* of a nerve cell

Neurogenesis growth and separation of the components of the nervous system in a fetus

Neurogenic claudication a condition of lower vertebral damage, with symptoms such as limping and lameness

Neuroleptics powerful tranquilizers used to treat psychosis

Neuropeptides peptides (made of two or more *amino acids*) released by neurons, and presumed to act as neurotransmitters

Neurotoxicology study of the effects of poisonous substances on the nervous system

Neurotransplantation transplantation of brain tissue

Nociceptors outer body nerve endings that act as pain receptors sensitive to external stimuli

Non-REM (slow-wave) stages deepest sleep stages, measured in delta brain waves

Norepinephrine a hormone present in small amounts in the brain; also called noradrenaline

Occipital lobe the part of the brain located at the back of the head on both sides

Olfactory having to do with the sense of smell

Oligodendrocytes one of three types of glial cells that make up the central nervous system

Oligodendroglial having to do with *oligodendrocytes*

Oncogenes viral genes that can transform the host cell into a tumorous cell

Oncologic having to do with the study of tumors

Oxytocin a hormone that causes contractions of the uterus and release of milk by the breasts

Paraneoplastic antibodies antibodies produced by a patient's immune system that end up attacking healthy cells as well as cancer cells

Parasympathetic nervous system a part of the *autonomic* nervous system

Paroxysms sharp spasms or convulsions

Perceptual deficits lack or malfunction of the ability to experience or interpret physical sensation

Phobia illogical fear of a particular object or situation

Phonological processing the brain's interpretation of speech sounds as language

Photophobia abnormal sensitivity to light

Phototherapy treatment of disease by using light

Placebo a substance that looks exactly like a drug being tested, so that the patient and physician may not know which is which

Pluripotent stem cells cells that have the ability to develop into any kind of cell in the human body (except placental cells)

Polymorphism occurrence in more than one form

Polyneuropathies disease processes involving a number of peripheral nerves

Polysomnography an all-night sleep recording

Positive symptoms symptoms that are apparent, as opposed to *negative symptoms*

Positron-emission tomography (PET) a type of imaging technique that can track brain activity

Preconscious happening before the conscious mind is aware of it

Prevalence the number of existing cases of a disease in a certain population at a specific time

Primary visual cortex the part of the brain to which the eyes and optic nerves send visual information

Priming the memory function that improves the brain's ability to detect, identify, or respond to a recently processed stimulus

Prion an abnormal protein that causes prion diseases

Proprioception the reception of stimuli produced within the organism

Proximal the closer of two or more items; as opposed to *distal*

Psychopharmacology the use of drugs to influence the mind and behavior

Psychosocial interventions treatments that have both psychological and social aspects

Psychostimulant a drug with antidepressant or mood-elevating properties

Ptosis a drooping of the upper eyelid

Quadriplegia paralysis of both arms and both legs

Recessive a gene whose characteristics do not appear in the person who has a single copy of the gene rather than a pair

Recombinant DNA DNA resulting from experimentally inserting new DNA into a cell; also occurs naturally when cells go through cell division

Rhizotomy cutting spinal nerve roots to relieve pain or paralysis

Satiety factors digestive hormones that are released when the stomach fills; they signal the brain that it is time to stop eating

Schwann cells cells that produce the myelin (the fatty covering) that sheathes the nerves

Second messengers messenger molecules that take the cell's response to the first messenger, amplify it, and direct the response to the appropriate site in the cell

Selective serotonin reuptake inhibitors (SSRIs) a group of antidepressants that increase the levels of serotonin in the brain

Sensory perception experiencing one's environment through physical sensation

Sensory transduction the conversion of signals from the external world into nerve signals

Short-term memory the working memory where the brain temporarily stores information needed at the moment

Single-photon-emission computed tomography (SPECT) test in which a radioactive compound is injected into the body and its photon emissions are traced

Sleep apnea the repeated obstruction of breathing during sleep

Somatosensory relating to sensory activity originating elsewhere than in the special sense organs

Somatosensory cortex part of the brain, located in the parietal lobe, that contains neurons that register the sense of touch

Spasms involuntary muscle contractions

Spinal reflexes body movements directed by the spine without input from the brain

Spongiform having little holes, thus resembling a sponge

Stereotaxic surgery surgery that involves locating deep brain structures by using three-dimensional coordi-nates; for example, guiding surgical instruments a precise number of millimeters below the surface at a point x millimeters from the midline and y millimeters from the front of the brain

Stereotyped showing constant repetition of certain meaningless gestures or movements

Stimulants agents that temporarily increase the activity or efficiency of an organism or any of its parts

Susceptibility genes inherited factors that predispose a person to a certain disease

Sympathetic nerves nerves that make up the sympa-thetic nervous system and activate other tissues

Synapse gap between the *axon* of one neuron and the dendrite or cell body of the next neuron

Tangles fibrous clumps of an abnormal form of the pro-tein *tau*, found inside nerve cells

Tardive dyskinesia disorder of the central nervous sys-tem resulting in twitching of the face and tongue and involuntary movements of the body

Tau a protein that, when dysfunctional, may be linked to such diseases as Alzheimer's

T cells white blood cells that fight infections, tumors, and other diseases

Temporal having to do with the area of the brain behind the eye sockets

Tics involuntary repeated contractions of a part of the body; also, some kinds of involuntary repeated be-havior

Tolerance the ability to become less responsive to a stimulus, especially over a period of continued expo-sure

Tolerate to take a drug without injurious effects

Tomography the taking of sectional X-ray photographs

Totipotent cell a cell that is capable of developing into a complete organism

Transcranial Doppler ultrasonography a kind of ultra-sound that measures changes in blood flow through the brain

Transcranial magnetic stimulation (TMS) a method of studying the brain by using a pair of electromagnets to briefly inactivate specific brain areas

Transporter gene a gene that moves biochemical sub-stances in biological systems

Transporter molecules molecules that help the neu-rons take in neurotransmitter molecules and break them down for reuse

Tremors rhythmic, involuntary, oscillatory movements of muscles around a joint

Tricyclic antidepressants medications used to treat attention deficit/hyperactivity disorder and depression

Triplegic suffering from paralysis affecting three of the four limbs; usually one arm is controllable

Ultradian relating to biological cycles shorter than 24 hours

Urokinase an enzyme found in human urine that is used to dissolve blood clots

Vagus nerve a nerve that gives the brain information about the stomach, heart, lungs, and other internal organs

Vasopressin a hormone that increases blood pressure and decreases urine flow

Ventricles fluid-filled spaces in the brain

Viscera internal organs of the body, such as heart, liver, and intestines, located in the large cavity of the trunk

Visual acuity ability of the eyes to discriminate fine details

Visual-spatial reasoning the ability to solve problems that involve manipulating visual representations or understanding the space around oneself

Walking reflex the tendency of a newborn baby, if held upright under the arms, to dangle the legs down and push against a hard surface with the feet, as if walking

Western blot a test that identifies the specific proteins of the bacteria against which antibodies are directed

White matter the structures in the brain that support the *gray matter*

Appendix A

DRUGS USED TO TREAT THE BRAIN AND NERVOUS SYSTEM

GENERIC NAMES	BRAND NAMES	CLASS	PRESCRIBED TREATMENT
acetazolamide	Diamox	carbonic anhydrase inhibitors	epileptic seizures
acyclovir	Zovirax	antivirals	chicken pox, shingles, herpes
adrenocorticosteroids (prednisone)	Deltasone, Orasone	adrenals	rheumatic conditions, certain cancers, blood disease
alprazolam	Xanax, Alprazolam	benzodiazepines	anxiety disorders, panic disorders
alteplase-recombinant	Activase	thrombolytic agents	stroke (by dissolving blood clots)
amantadine	Symmetrel	unclassified therapeutic agents	influenza A, Parkinsons' disease, and "Parkinsonlike" symptoms
amitriptyline	Elavil, Endep	tricyclic antidepressants	depression, certain types of pain
amobarbital	Amytal, Amytal Sodium	barbiturates	seizures, anxiety or tension, insomnia on a short-term basis
amoxapine	Asendin	tricyclic antidepressants	depression
amphetamine, dextroamphetamine	Adderall, Dexedrine	amphetamines	attention deficit/hyperactivity disorder (ADHD)
atenolol	Tenormin	beta-blockers	high blood pressure

GENERIC NAMES	BRAND NAMES	CLASS	PRESCRIBED TREATMENT
baclofen	Lioresal	skeletal muscle relaxants	multiple sclerosis, cerebral palsy
benztropine mesylate	Benztrop Mes, Cogentin	antiparkinsonian agents	symptoms of Parkinson's disease
bethanechol chloride	Urecholine	parasympatho-mimetic (cholinergic agents)	bladder conditions
botulinun toxin Type A	Botox	toxoids	dystonia, tremor, hemifacial spasms
bromocriptine mesylate	Ergoset, Parlodel	unclassified therapeutic agents	Parkinson's disease
bupropion hydrochloride	Wellbutrin	antidepressants	depression and anxiety
buspirone	BuSpar	miscellaneous anxiolytics–sedatives and hypnotics	anxiety
carbamazepine	Epitol, Tegretol, Carbatrol	miscellaneous anticonvulsants	seizures, nerve pain, trigeminal neuralgia
celecoxib	Celebrex	nonsteroidal anti-inflammatory agents/ specific cox-2 inhibitors	osteoarthritis, rheumatoid arthritis
chlorpromazine	Thorazine	phenothiazines	psychotic disorders, nausea and vomiting, chronic hiccups
cisapride	Propulsid	miscellaneous gastrointestinal drugs	gastric reflux; available in the U.S. only to patients who meet eligibility criteria from the manufacturer; doctor must enroll in a special program to prescribe this medicine
clomipramine	Anafranil	tricyclic antidepressants	obsessive-compulsive disorder
clonazepam	Klonopin	benzodiazepines	seizures, panic and anxiety disorders
clonidine	Catapres, Catapres Tts, Combipres, Clorpres	antihypertensive agents	hypertension
clopidogrel	Plavix		prevention of heart attack, stroke, and blood clots in some patients with artery disease
clozapine	Clozaril	antipsychotic	schizophrenia

GENERIC NAMES	BRAND NAMES	CLASS	PRESCRIBED TREATMENT
cyclophosphamide	Cytoxan, Cytoxan Lyophilized, Neosar	antineoplastic agents	cancer, rheumatoid arthritis, and "minimal change" nephrotic syndrome
cyclosporine	Gengraf, Sandimmune, SangCya, Neoral	antineoplastic agents	immunosuppressant, rheumatoid arthritis
cyproheptadine	Cyprohept, Periactin	antihistamine drugs	allergies, common cold
desipramine	Norpramin	tricyclic antidepressants	depression
dextroamphetamine sulfate	DextroStat, Dexedrine	respiratory and cerebral stimulants	narcolepsy, attention deficit/hyperactivity disorder
diazepam	Valium	benzodiazepines	anxiety disorders
dicyclomine	Bentyl	antimuscarinics/antispasmodics	spasms of the gastrointestinal tract (stomach and intestines), by blocking the actions of spasm-causing chemicals in the body
dihydroergotamine mesylate	Migranal, D.H.E. 45	vasoconstrictor	migraine, cluster headaches
diphenhydramine	Benophen, Belix, Benadryl, Diphen AF	antihistamine drugs	allergies, mild Parkinson's symptoms
donepezil	Aricept	acetylcholinesterase inhibitor	Alzheimer's disease
doxepin	Adapin, Sinequan	tricyclic antidepressants	depression
erythromycin	Eryc, Ery-Tab, PCE 333	antibiotics	bacterial infections, Legionnaires' disease
famciclovir	Famvir	antivirals	herpes, shingles, and cold sores (in people with HIV)
fluoxetine	Prozac, Prozac Weekly, Sarafem	antidepressants (selective serotonin reuptake inhibitors)	depression, obsessive-compulsive disorder, bulimia (binge eating and purging), premenstrual dysphoric disorder
fluphenazine	Prolixin	phenothiazines (tranquilizing agents)	tics
gabapentin	Neurontin	miscellaneous anticonvulsants	seizures
galantamine	Reminyl	acetylcholinesterase inhibitor	Alzheimer's disease

GENERIC NAMES	BRAND NAMES	CLASS	PRESCRIBED TREATMENT
gentamicin	Garamycin, Genoptic, Gentacidin	antibiotics	bacterial infections
glatiramer	Copaxone	acid polymer	relapsing-remitting multiple sclerosis
guanfacine	Tenex	antihypertensive	hypertension
haloperidol	Haldol	antipsychotics	psychotic symptoms, including hallucinations, delusions, and confusion; Tourette's syndrome; behavioral and hyperactive conditions in children
ibuprofen	Advil, Motrin, Motrin-IB, Nuprin	nonsteriodal anti-inflammatory drugs (NSAIDs)	pain relief, primarily for arthritis
imipramine	Tofranil	tricyclic antidepressants	depression
indomethacin	Novo-Methacin, Indocin, Indometacin	nonsteroidal anti-inflammatory drugs (NSAIDs)	pain caused by arthritis, gout, bursitis, and other problems
interferon beta-1a	Avonex, Rebif	multiple sclerosis therapy agents	multiple sclerosis
interferon beta-1b	Betaseron	multiple sclerosis therapy agents	multiple sclerosis
kanamycin	Kantrex	aminoglycoside antibiotic	serious infections in various parts of the body
ketorolac tromethamine	Toradol	nonsteriodal anti-inflammatory drugs (NSAIDs)	pain
levodopa	Larodopa	antidyskinetics	Parkinson's disease
levodopa and carbidopa	Atamet, Sinemet, Sinemet CR	antidyskinetics	Parkinson's disease
lidocaine	Xylocaine, Lidoderm	local anesthetics	herpes zoster (shingles)
lithium	Eskalith, Eskalith CR, Lithobid, Lithonate, Lithotabs	antimanic agents	manic episodes of manic-depressive illness
loratadine	Claritin	antihistamines	allergies
meclizine	Antivert, Bonine	antihistamines	motion sickness and dizziness
methylphenidate	Ritalin, Ritalin-SR, Concerta	stimulants	attention deficit/hyperactivity disorder (ADHD)

GENERIC NAMES	BRAND NAMES	CLASS	PRESCRIBED TREATMENT
methysergide maleate	Sansert	sympatholytic adrenergic blocking agents	prevention of vascular headaches (e.g., migraines) and reduction of their severity.
metoclopramide	Reglan, Octamide, Metoclopramide Intensol	dopaminergic blocking agents	esophageal reflux, gastroparesis, and prevention of side effects associated with some anticancer medications
metoprolol tartrate	Lopressor, Toprol-XL	beta-blockers	hypertension, angina
midodrine	ProAmatine	alpha-1 agonists	the type of low blood pressure that can cause severe dizziness or fainting (neurogenic orthostatic hypotension)
mitoxantrone	Novantrone	antineoplastics	disability or frequency of clinical relapses (attacks) in multiple sclerosis
naltrexone	ReVia, Depade	opioid antagonists	alcoholism and addiction, by blocking receptors for certain chemicals in the brain
naproxen	Naprosyn, Aleve, Anaprox	nonsteroidal anti-inflammatory drugs (NSAIDs)	rheumatoid arthritis, pain
nefazodone hydrochloride	Serzone	antidepressants	depression
nortriptyline	Aventyl HCl, Allegron, Pamelor, Nortrilen	tricyclic antidepressants	depression
olanzapine	Zyprexa, Zyprexa Zydis	antipsychotics	psychotic conditions and hallucinations, delusions, and confusion of schizophrenia, mania
oxazepam	Serax	benzodiazepines	anxiety, nervousness, and tension associated with anxiety disorders, and symptoms associated with alcohol withdrawal
oxybutynin	Ditropan, Ditropan XL, Urotrol	genitourinary smooth muscle relaxants	bladder muscle spasms; may be used to treat bed-wetting
oxycodone	M-Oxy, OxyContin, OxyIR, Percolone, Roxicodone	narcotic analgesics	moderate-to-severe pain, such as after surgery, after an injury, and for some types of headaches
oxytocin	Pitocin	hormones	to induce labor
paroxetine	Paxil	antidepressants (selective serotonin reuptake inhibitors)	major depression

GENERIC NAMES	BRAND NAMES	CLASS	PRESCRIBED TREATMENT
pemoline	Cylert	stimulant	attention deficit/hyperactivity disorder (ADHD)
phenelzine	Nardil	antidepressants (monoamine) oxidase inhibitors [MAOIs]	depression
phenobarbital	Solfoton	barbiturates	seizures; insomnia on a short-term basis
phenytoin sodium	Dilantin Infatabs, Dilantin Kapseals, Dilantin-125	anticonvulsants (hydantoins)	seizures; trigeminal neuralgia
physostigmine	Physostigmine salicylate injection	anticholinesterase	memory loss
pimozide	Orap	antipsychotic/ neuroleptic	tics associated with Tourette's syndrome
pleconaril	Picovir	antivirals	viral meningitis, encephalitis, chronic meningoencephalitis
prednisone (adrenocorticosteroids)	Deltasone, Liquid Pred, Meticorten, Orasone, Prednicen-M, Sterapred, Sterapred DS	steroids (glucocorticoid)	endocrine (hormonal) disorders in which the body does not produce enough of its own steroids; also for arthritis, lupus, severe psoriasis, severe asthma, ulcerative colitis, and Crohn's disease
primidone	Mysoline	barbiturates	seizures; sometimes for tremors
propantheline	Pro-Banthine	antispasmodics/ anticholinergics	cramps or spasms of the stomach, intestines, and bladder (in multiple sclerosis)
propranolol	Inderal, Inderal LA	beta-blockers	hypertension (high blood pressure), chest pain, irregular heartbeats, migraines, tremor, and risk of a recurrent heart attack
protriptyline	Vivactil	tricyclic antidepressants	depression
quetiapine	Seroquel	antipsychotic	psychosis
raloxifene	Evista	benzothiophenes	to prevent and treat osteoporosis (thinning of bones)
riluzole	Rilutek	benzothiazoles	amyotrophic lateral sclerosis (ALS), or Lou Gehrig's disease

GENERIC NAMES	BRAND NAMES	CLASS	PRESCRIBED TREATMENT
risperidone	Risperdal	antipsychotics (tranquilizers)	symptoms of psychotic disorders such as schizophrenia
rivastigmine	Exelon	acetylcholinesterase inhibitors	Alzheimer's disease
selegiline	Carbex, Eldepryl	antidyskinetics	in combination with levodopa, or levodopa and carbidopa, to treat Parkinson's disease
sertraline	Zoloft	antidepressants (selective serotonin reuptake inhibitors)	depression, obsessive-compulsive disorder, panic disorder, and post-traumatic stress disorder (PTSD)
sildenafil	Viagra	selective inhibitor of cyclic guanosine monophosphate	erectile dysfunction (impotence)
statins	Lescol (fluvastatin), Lipitor (atorvastatin), Zocor (simvastatin), Pravachol (pravastatin), Mevacor (lovastatin)	cholesterol-lowering agents	high cholesterol—which increases risk of stroke, heart attack, and dementia
sumatriptan	Imitrex	unclassified	cluster headaches, migraine
tacrine	Cognex	cholinesterase inhibitors	Alzheimer's disease
ticlopidine	Ticlid	platelet aggregation inhibitors	prevention of strokes in patients who have had a stroke or who have experienced transient ischemic attacks (TIAs), or "ministrokes"
tolterodine	Detrol, Detrol LA	Urinary antispasmodic	spasms or overactive bladder
trimipramine	Surmontil	tricyclic antidepressants	depression
valacyclovir	Valtrex	antivirals	shingles, genital herpes
valproate (sodium valproate, valproic acid, divalproex)	Depakene, Depakote, Depakote ER, Depakote Sprinkle	anticonvulsants	seizures, manic symptoms in bipolar disorder, prevention of migraine
vasopressin	Pitressin	hormones (anitdiuretics)	diabetes insipidus, bed-wetting

GENERIC NAMES	BRAND NAMES	CLASS	PRESCRIBED TREATMENT
venlafaxine	Effexor, Effexor XR	antidepressants	depression, generalized anxiety disorder
verapamil	Calan, Calan SR, Covera-HS, Isoptin, Isoptin SR, Verelan, Verelan PM	calcium channel blockers	hypertension, chest pain, and the control of some types of irregular heartbeats
warfarin sodium	Coumadin	anticoagulants	prevent stroke, blockage of major veins and arteries from formation of blood clots
zaleplon	Sonata	sedatives/hypnotics	insomnia
ziprasidone	Geodon	antipsychotics	psychotic disorders such as schizophrenia
zolpidem	Ambien	sedatives/hypnotics	insomnia

Appendix B

SUGGESTED READING

General

Discovering the Brain. Sandra Ackerman. National Academy Press, 1992.

Brain, Mind, and Behavior. Floyd E. Bloom, Charles A. Nelson, and Arlyne Lazerson. W. H. Freeman, 2000.

The Myth of the First Three Years: A New Understanding of Early Brain Development and Lifelong Learning. John T. Bruer. Free Press, 1999.

States of Mind: New Discoveries About How Our Brains Make Us Who We Are. Roberta Conlan, ed. Dana Press/John Wiley and Sons, 1999.

What's Going On in There? How the Brain and Mind Develop in the First Five Years of Life. Lise Eliot. Bantam Doubleday Dell, 1999.

The Essential Guide to Mental Health: The Most Comprehensive Guide to Psychiatry for Popular Family Use. Jack Matthew Gorman. Griffin Trade Paperback, 1998.

The Human Brain: A Guided Tour. Susan Adele Greenfield. Basic Books, 1998.

The Private Life of the Brain: Emotions, Consciousness, and the Secret of Self. Susan Adele Greenfield. John Wiley and Sons, 2000.

Brain Power: Working Out the Human Mind. Susan Adele Greenfield. Element, 2000.

Wild Minds: What Animals Really Think. Marc D. Hauser. Henry Holt, 2000.

A Good Start in Life: Understanding Your Child's Brain and Behavior. Norbert Herschkowitz and Elinore Herschkowitz. Dana Press/Joseph Henry Press, 2002.

Is It Just a Phase? How to Tell Common Childhood Phases from More Serious Problems. Henrietta L. Leonard and Susan Anderson Swedo. Broadway Books, 1999.

The Longevity Strategy: How to Live to 100 Using the Brain-Body Connection. David Mahoney and Richard Restak. Dana Press/John Wiley and Sons, 1998.

Keep Your Brain Young: The Complete Guide to Physical and Emotional Health and Longevity. Guy McKhann and Marilyn S. Albert. Dana Press/John Wiley and Sons, 2002.

Images of Mind. Michael I. Posner and Marcus E. Raichle. Scientific American Library (W. H. Freeman), 1997.

The Mind. Richard Restak. Bantam Books, 1988.

The Secret Life of the Brain. Richard Restak. Dana Press/Joseph Henry Press, 2001.

The Scientific American Book of the Brain (special collaborative issue). Editors of *Scientific American.* Lyons Press, 1999.

The Balance Within: The Science Connecting Health and Emotion. Esther M. Sternberg. W. H. Freeman, 2001.

The Science Times Book of the Brain. Nicholas Wade, ed. The New York Times (Lyons Press), 1998.

Mapping Fate: A Memoir of Family, Risk, and Genetic Research. Alice Wexler. University of California Press, 1996.

A Vision of the Brain. Semir Zeki. Blackwell Science, 1993.

Brain Functions

Evolving Brains. John Morgan Allman. Scientific American Library (W. H. Freeman), 1999.

The Dying of Enoch Wallace: Life, Death, and the Changing Brain. Ira B. Black. McGraw-Hill Companies, 2001.

If a Lion Could Talk: Animal Intelligence and the Evolution of Consciousness. Stephen Budiansky. Free Press, 1998.

Descartes' Error: Emotion, Reason, and the Human Brain. Antonio R. Damasio. Avon Books, 1995.

The Feeling of What Happens: Body and Emotion in the Making of Consciousness. Antonio R. Damasio. Harvest Books, 2000.

The Executive Brain: Frontal Lobes and the Civilized Mind. Elkhonon Goldberg. Oxford University Press, 2001.

Memory: Remembering and Forgetting in Everyday Life. Barry Gordon. Mastermedia Limited, 1995.

Eye and Brain: The Psychology of Seeing. Richard Gregory. Princeton University Press, 1997.

Sleep. J. Allan Hobson. W. H. Freeman, 1995.

Consciousness. J. Allan Hobson. Scientific American Library (W. H. Freeman), 1998.

The Dream Drugstore: Chemically Altered States of Consciousness. J. Allan Hobson. MIT Press, 2001.

Galen's Prophecy: Temperament in Human Nature. Jerome Kagan. Harvard University Press, 1998.

Three Seductive Ideas. Jerome Kagan. Harvard University Press, 1998.

The Emotional Brain: The Mysterious Underpinning of Emotional Life. Joseph LeDoux. Simon and Schuster, 1996.

How the Mind Works. Steven Pinker. W. W. Norton, 1997.

Eminent Creativity, Everyday Creativity, and Health. Mark A. Runco and Ruth Richards. Ablex, 1997.

Searching for Memory: The Brain, the Mind, and the Past. Daniel L. Schacter. Basic Books, 1996.

The Seven Sins of Memory. Daniel L. Schacter. Houghton Mifflin, 2001.

Memory, Brain, and Belief. David L. Schacter and Elaine Scarry. Harvard University Press, 2000.

Memory and Brain. Larry Ryan Squire. Oxford University Press, 1987.

Memory: From Mind to Molecules. Larry R. Squire and Eric R. Kandel. Scientific American Library (W. H. Freeman), 1999.

Brain Disorders

The Broken Brain: The Biological Revolution in Psychiatry. Nancy C. Andreasen. Harper & Row Perennial Library, 1984.

Mood Genes: Hunting for Origins of Mania and Depression. Samuel H. Barondes. W. H. Freeman, 1998.

Molecules and Mental Illness. Samuel H. Barondes. Scientific American Library (W. H. Freeman), 1999.

American Heart Association Family Guide to Stroke: Treatment, Recovery, and Prevention. Louis R. Caplan, Mark L. Dyken, and J. Donald Easton. Times Books, 1994. Out of print.

How to Cope with Depression: A Complete Guide for You and Your Family. J. Raymond DePaulo, Jr. Ballantine Books, 1996.

Understanding Depression: What We Know and What You Can Do About It. J. Raymond DePaulo, Jr. Dana Press/John Wiley and Sons, 2002.

New Hope for People with Bipolar Disorder: A Guide for Patients and Those Who Journey with Them. Jan Fawcett, Bernard Golden, Nancy Rosenfeld, and Frederick K. Goodwin. Prima Publishing, 2000.

Thinking in Pictures: And Other Reports from My Life with Autism. Temple Grandin. Vintage Books, 1996.

An Unquiet Mind: A Memoir of Moods and Madness. Kay Redfield Jamison. Alfred A. Knopf, 1995.

Night Falls Fast: Understanding Suicide. Kay Redfield Jamison. Alfred A. Knopf, 1999.

Buzzed: The Straight Facts About the Most Used and Abused Drugs from Alcohol to Ecstasy. Cynthia Kuhn, Scott Swartzwelder, and Wilkie Wilson. W. W. Norton, 1998.

A Cursing Brain? The Histories of Tourette Syndrome. Howard I. Kushner. Harvard University Press, 1999.

Migraine and Other Headaches: A Practical Guide to Understanding, Preventing, and Treating Headaches. James W. Lance. Simon and Schuster International, 1999.

Guarded Prognosis: A Doctor and His Patients Talk About Chronic Disease and How to Cope with It. Michael D. Lockshin. Hill and Wang, 1998. Out of print.

Stop Walking on Eggshells: Coping When Someone You Care About Has Borderline Personality Disorder. Paul T. Mason, Randi Kreger, and Larry J. Siever. New Harbinger, 1998.

The End of Stress As We Know It. Bruce McEwen. Dana Press/Joseph Henry Press, 2002.

The Hostage Brain. Bruce S. McEwen and Harold M. Schmeck, Jr. Rockefeller University Press, 1994.

Under the Influence: Drugs and the American Workforce. Jacques Normand, Richard O. Lempert, and Charles P. O'Brien. National Academy Press, 1993.

The Man Who Mistook His Wife for a Hat and Other Clinical Tales. Oliver Sacks. Touchstone, 1998.

Why Zebras Don't Get Ulcers: A Guide to Stress, Stress Related Diseases, and Coping. Robert M. Sapolsky. W. H. Freeman, 1998.

Learning Disabilities Spectrum: ADD, ADHD, and LD. Bruce K. Shapiro. York Press, 1998.

Specific Reading Disability: A View of the Spectrum. Bruce K. Shapiro, Pasquale J. Accardo, and Arnold J. Capute. York Press, 1994.

Drugs and the Brain. Solomon H. Snyder. Scientific American Library (W. H. Freeman), 1987.

Decoding Darkness: The Search for Genetic Causes of Alzheimer's Disease. Rudolph E. Tanzi and Ann B. Parson. Perseus Publishing, 2000.

Depression: A Guide for Patients. Michael Edward Thase. Health Information Network, 1997.

Dizziness (The Most Common Complaints Series). B. Todd Troost. Butterworth-Heinemann Medical, 2001.

Why We Hurt: The Natural History of Pain. Frank T. Vertosick, Jr. Harcourt Brace, 2000.

In Search of the Lost Cord: Solving the Mystery of Spinal Cord Regeneration. Luba Vikhanski. Dana Press/Joseph Henry Press, 2001.

Parkinson's Disease: A Complete Guide for Patients and Families. William J. Weiner, Lisa M. Shulman, and Anthony E. Lang. The Johns Hopkins University Press, 2001.

A Mood Apart: The Thinker's Guide to Emotion and Its Disorders. Peter C. Whybrow. HarperPerennial, 1997.

Malignant Sadness: The Anatomy of Depression. Lewis Wolpert. Free Press, 1999.

Appendix C

RESOURCE GROUPS

This appendix lists more than 100 organizations that assist people with brain-related disorders or diseases, their families, and caregivers.

Key

Support groups: **Supp**

Referrals to doctors: **RDocs**

Referrals to other information: **RInfo**

Regional chapters: **Chap**

Literature: **Lit**

Speakers available: **Speak**

Volunteer opportunities: **Vol**

C1 Dyslexia

The International Dyslexia Association
8600 LaSalle Rd., Suite 382
Baltimore, MD 21286-2044
Tel: (800) 222-3123
Fax: (410) 321-5069
Web site: www.interdys.org
E-mail: (Use web site form)
Supp, RDocs, RInfo, Chap, Lit, Speak, Vol

Learning Disabilities Association of America

4156 Library Rd.
Pittsburg, PA 15234-1349
Tel: (412) 341-1515
Fax: (412) 334-0224
Web site: www.ldanatl.org
E-mail: (Use web site form)
Supp, RDocs, Chap, Lit, Speak, Vol

National Center for Learning Disabilities
381 Park Ave. South, Suite 1401
New York, NY 10016
Tel: (888) 575-7373
Fax: (212) 545-9665
Web site: www.ld.org
RInfo, Lit, Vol

C2 Attention Deficit/ Hyperactivity Disorder

Attention Deficit Disorder Association
P.O. Box 543
Pottstown, PA 19464
Tel: (484) 945-2101
Fax: (610) 970-7520
Web site: www.add.org
E-mail: (Use web site form)
Supp, RDocs, Chap, Lit, Speak

C3 Mental Retardation

The Arc of the United States

1010 Wayne Ave., Suite 650
Silver Spring, MD 20910
Tel: (301) 565-3842
Fax: (301) 565-5342
Web site: www.thearc.org
E-mail: info@thearc.org
Supp, RInfo, Chap, Lit, Vol

Nation Down Syndrome Society
666 Broadway
New York, NY 10012-2317
Tel: (800) 221-4602
Fax: (212) 979-2873
Web site: www.ndss.org
E-mail: (Use web site form)
Supp, RDocs, Chap, Lit, Speak, Vol

C4 Cerebral Palsy

United Cerebral Palsy/United Cerebral Palsy Research
    and Education Foundation
1660 L St., NW, Suite 700
Washington, DC 20036
Tel: (800) 872-5827
TTY (202) 973-7197
Fax: (202) 776-0414
Web site: www.ucp.org
E-mail: (Use web site form)
RInfo, Lit, Chap, Vol

C5 Autism

Autism Society of America
7910 Woodmont Ave., Suite 300
Bethesda, MD 20814-3067
Tel: (800) 328-8476
Web site: www.autism-society.org
E-mail: (Use web site form)
Supp, Chap, Lit, Vol

Autism Genetic Resource Exchange
5455 Wilshire Blvd., Suite 2250
Los Angeles, CA 90036-4234
Tel: (323) 931-6577
Fax: (323) 549-0547
Web site: www.agre.org

E-mail: (Use web site form)
RDocs, Chap, Lit, Vol

National Alliance for Autism Research/Autism Speaks
2 Park Ave., 11th Floor
New York, NY 10016
Tel: (212) 525-8584
Fax: (212) 525-8676
Web site: www.autismspeaks.org
E-mail: contactus@autismspeaks.org
Lit, Vol

C7 Neurofibromatosis

Children's Tumor Foundation
95 Pine St., 16th Fl.
New York, NY 10005
Tel: (800) 323-7938
Fax: (212) 747-0004
Web site: www.ctf.org
E-mail: info@ctf.org
Supp, RDocs, Chap, Lit, Speak, Vol

Neurofibromatosis, Inc.
P.O. Box 18246
Minneapolis, MN 55418
Tel: (800) 942-6825
Web site: www.nfinc.org
E-mail: (Use web site form)
Supp, RDocs, RInfo, Chap, Lit, Speak, Vol

C8 Hydrocephalus

Guardians of Hydrocephalus Research Foundation
2618 Ave. Z
Brooklyn, NY 11235-2023
Tel: (718) 743-4473
Fax: (718) 743-1171
Web site: www.ghrf.homestead.com
E-mail: ghrf618@aol.com
Supp, RDocs, RInfo, Lit, Vol

Hydrocephalus Association
870 Market, Suite 705
San Francisco, CA 94102
Tel: (800) 598-3789

Fax: (415) 732-7044
Web site: www.hydroassoc.org
E-mail: info@hydroassoc.org
Supp, RDocs, Lit, Vol

National Hydrocephalus Foundation
12413 Centralia Rd.
Lakewood, CA 90715-1653
Tel: (888) 857-3434
Fax: (562) 924-6666
Web site: www.nhfonline.org
E-mail: hydrobrat@earthlink.net
Supp, RDocs, Lit, Speak, Vol

C9 Spina Bifida
Spina Bifida Association of America
4590 MacArthur Blvd., NW, Suite 250
Washington, DC 20007-4226
Tel: (800) 621-3141
Fax: (202) 944-3295
Web site: www.sbaa.org
E-mail: sbaaa@sbaa.org
Supp, RDocs, RInfo, Chap, Lit, Speak, Vol

C10 Tumors of Childhood
Brain Tumor Foundation for Children
6065 Roswell Rd., NE, Suite 505
Atlanta, GA 30328
Tel: (404) 252-4107
Web site: www.braintumorkids.org
E-mail: btfc@bellsouth.net
Supp, RDocs, RInfo, Lit, Speak, Vol

The Childhood Brain Tumor Foundation
20312 Watkins Meadow Dr.
Germantown, MD 20876
Tel: (877) 217-4166
Local Tel: (301) 515-2900
Web site: www.childhoodbraintumor.org
E-mail: cbtf@childhoodbraintumor.org
Chap, Lit, Speak, Vol

Children's Brain Tumor Foundation
274 Madison Ave., Suite 1004
New York, NY 10016
Tel: (866) 228-4673

Fax: (212) 448-1022
Website: www.cbtf.org
E-mail: info@cbtf.org
Supp, RDocs, Lit, Speak, Vol

Pediatric Brain Tumor Foundation
302 Ridgefield Ct.
Asheville, NC 28806
Tel: (800) 253-6530
Fax: (828) 665-6894
Web site: www.pbtfus.org
E-mail: pbtfus@ pbtfus.org
Supp, RInfo, Chap, Vol

C11 Sleep Disorders
American Sleep Apnea Association
1424 K St., NW, Suite 302
Washington, DC 20005
Tel: (202) 293-3650
Tax: (202) 293-3656
Web sit: www.sleepapnea.org
E-mail: (Use web site form)
Supp, RDocs, Lit, Speak, Vol

National Sleep Foundation
1522 K St., NW, Suite 500
Washington, DC 20005
Tel: (202) 347-3471
Fax: (202) 347-3472
Web sit: www.sleepfoundation.org
E-mail: nsf@sleepfoundation.org
Supp, RDocs, Lit, Speak

Restless Legs Syndrome Foundation
819 Second St., SW
Rochester, MN 55902-2985
Tel: 507-287-6465
Fax: 507-287-6312
Web address: www.rls.org
Email address: rlsfoundation@rls.org
Supp, Chap, Lit, Speak

C12 Narcolepsy
Narcolepsy Network, Inc.
P.O. Box 294
Pleasantville, NY 10570

Tel: (401) 667-2523
Fax: (401) 633-6567
Web site: www.narcolepsynetwork.org
E-mail: Narnet@narcolepsynetwork.org
Supp, RDocs, Lit, Speak, Vol

C13 Epilepsy and Seizures

Epilepsy Foundation
4351 Garden City Dr.
Landover, MD 20785-7223
Tel: (800) 332-1000
Web site: www.efa.org
E-mail: (Use web site form)
Supp, RInfo, Chap, Lit, Vol

C14 Dizziness and Vertigo

Vestibular Disorders Association
P.O. Box 13305
Portland, OR 97213-0305
Tel: (800) 837-8428
Fax: (503) 229-8064
Web site: www.vestibular.org
E-mail: (Use web site form)
Supp, RDocs, Lit, Vol, RInfo

C15 Seeing Problems

Helen Keller National Center for Deaf/Blind Youth
    and Adults
141 Middle Neck Rd.
Sands Point, NY 11050
Tel: (516) 944-8900 Ext. 253
Web site: www.hknc.org
E-mail: hkcinfo@hknc.org
RInfo, Chap, Lit, Speak, Vol

Lighthouse International Headquarters
The Sol and Lilian Goldman Building
111 E. 59th St.
New York, NY 10022-1202
Tel: (800) 829-0500
TTY: (212) 821-9713
Fax: (212) 821-9707
Web site: www.lighthouse.org
E-mail: education@lighthouse.org
Supp, RInfo, Lit, Vol, Chap

Prevent Blindness America
211 W. Wacker Dr., Suite 1700
Chicago, IL 60606
Tel: (800) 331-2020
Web site: www.preventblindness.org
E-mail: info@preventblindness.org
RInfo, Chap, Lit

C16 Hearing Problems

Alexander Graham Bell Association for the Deaf
3417 Volta Pl., NW
Washington, DC 20007
Tel: (202) 337-5220
TTY: (202) 337-5221
Fax: (202) 337-8314
Web site: www.agbell.org
E-mail: info@agbell.org
Supp, RDocs, Chap, Lit, Speak, Vol

American Society of Deaf Children Headquarters
3820 Hartzdale Dr.
Camp Hill, PA 17011
Tel: (800) 942-2732
Fax: (717) 909-5599
Web site: www.deafchildren.org
E-mail: asdc@deafchildren.org
RInfo, Lit, Speak, Vol

Better Hearing Institute
515 King St., Suite 420
Alexandria, VA 22314-3137
Tel: (800) 327-9355
Web site: www.betterhearing.org
E-mail: mail@betterhearing.org
RDocs, RInfo, Lit, Speak

Boys Town National Research Hospital
555 N. 30th St.
Omaha, NE 68131
Tel: (402) 498-6511
Web site: www.boystownhospital.org
RInfo, Lit

National Cued Speech Association
23970 Hermitage Rd.
Cleveland OH 44122-4008
Tel: (800) 459-3529
Web site: www.cuedspeech.org

E-mail: (Use web site form)
RInfo, Lit

National Institute on Deafness and Other
    Communication Disorders
National Institutes of Health
31 Center Dr., MSC 2320
Bethesda, MD 20892-2320
Tel: (800) 241-1044
TTY: (800) 241-1055
Fax: (301) 402-0018
Web site: www.nidcd.nih.gov
E-mail: nidcdinfo@nidcd.nih.gov
RInfo, Lit

Hearing Loss Association of America
7910 Woodmont Ave., Suite 1200
Bethesda, MD 20814
Tel: (301) 657-2248
Fax: (301) 913-9413
Web site: www.hearingloss.org
E-mail: info@hearingloss.org
Supp, Chap, Lit, Speak, Vol

Acoustic Neuroma Association
600 Peachtree Pkwy., Suite 108
Cumming, GA 30041-6899
Phone: (770) 205-8211
Fax: (770) 205-0239
Web site: www.anausa.org
E-mail: info@anausa.org
Supp, RInfo, Chap, Lit, Vol

American Tinnitus Association
P.O. Box 5
Portland, OR 97207-0005
Tel: (800) 634-8978
Fax: (503) 248-0024
Web site: www.ata.org
E-mail: tinnitus@ata.org
Supp, Lit, Vol, RInfo

C17 Smelling and Tasting Problems
Hospital of the University of Pennsylvania
The Smell and Taste Center
5 Ravdin Pavilion
Philadelphia, PA 19104

Phone: (215) 662-6580
Fax: (215) 349-5266
Web site: www.med.upenn.edu/stc/
Email: Tiffany.Bellamy@uphs.upenn.edu
RInfo, Lit

C18 Autonomic Disorders
Dysautonomia Foundation Inc.
315 West 39th St., Suite 701
New York, NY 10018
Tel: (212) 279-1066
Fax: (212) 279-2066
Web site: www.familialdysautonomia.org
E-mail: info@familialdysautonomia.org
RInfo, Lit, Vol

C20 Depression
National Institute of Mental Health
Public Information and Communications Branch
6001 Executive Blvd., Room 8184, MSC 9663
Bethesda, MD 20892-9663
Tel: (866) 615-6464
TTY: (866) 415-8051
Fax: (301) 443-4279
Web site: www.nimh.nih.gov
E-mail: nimhinfo@nih.gov
RInfo, Lit

Depression and Related Affective Disorders Association
8201 Greensboro Dr., Suite 300
McLean, VA 22102
Tel: (888) 288-1104
Web site: www.drada.org
E-mail: info@drada.org
Supp, RDocs, Chap, Lit, Speak, Vol

NARSAD: The Mental Health Research Association
60 Cutter Mill Rd., Suite 404,
Great Neck, New York 11021
Tel: (800) 829-8289
Fax: (516) 487-6930
Web site: www.narsad.org
E-mail: info@narsad.org
Supp, Lit, Speak, Vol

Depression and Bipolar Support Alliance (DBSA)
730 N. Franklin St., Suite 501

Chicago, IL 60610-7224
Tel: (800) 826 -3632
Fax: (312) 642-7243
Web site: www.dbsalliance.org
E-mail: questions@dbsalliance.org
Supp, RInfo, Chap, Lit, Speak, Vol

Postpartum Support International
927 N. Kellogg Ave.
Santa Barbara, CA 93111
Tel: (805) 967-7636
Fax: (805) 967-0608
Web site: www.postpartum.net
E-mail: (Use web site form)
Supp, RDocs, Lit, Speak, Vol

C21 Anxiety and Panic and
C22 Social Phobia
National Institute of Mental Health
Public Information and Communications Branch
6001 Executive Blvd., Room 8184, MSC 9663
Bethesda, MD 20892-9663
Tel: (866) 615-6464
TTY: (866) 415-8051
Fax: (301) 443-4279
Web site: www.nimh.nih.gov
E-mail: nimhinfo@nih.gov

Anxiety Disorders Association of America
8730 Georgia Ave., Suite 600
Silver Spring, MD 20910
Tel: (240) 485-1001
Fax: (240) 485-1035
Web site: www.adaa.org
Supp, RDocs, RInfo, Lit

Freedom from Fear
308 Seaview Ave.
Staten Island, NY 10305
Tel: (718) 351-1717
Fax: (718) 980-5022
Web site: www.freedomfromfear.org
E-mail: help@freedomfromfear.org
Supp, RDocs, Lit, Speak, Vol

National Ataxia Foundation
2600 Fernbrook Ln., Suite 119

Minneapolis, MN 55447
Tel: (763) 553-0020
Fax: (763) 553-0167
Web site: www.ataxia.org
E-mail: (Use web site form)
RInfo, Lit, Speak, Supp

C23 Obsessive-Compulsive Disorder
Obsessive-Compulsive Foundation
676 State St.
New Haven, CT 06511
Tel: (203) 401-2070
Fax: (203) 401-2076
Web site: www.ocfoundation.org
E-mail: info@ocfoundation
Supp, RDocs, Chap, Lit, Speak, Vol

Trichotillomania Learning Center
303 Potrero #51
Santa Cruz, CA 95060
Tel: (831) 457-1004
Fax: (831) 426-4383
Web site: www.trich.org
E-mail: info@trich.org
Supp, RDocs, Lit, Speak, Vol

C24 Bipolar Disorder (Manic-Depressive Illness)
See C20, Depression

C25 Schizophrenia
Nation Alliance on Mental Illness
Colonial Place Three
2107 Wilson Blvd., Suite 300
Arlington, VA 22201-3042
Tel: (888) 999-6264
TDD: (703) 516-7227
Fax: (703) 524-9094
Web site: www.nami.org
E-mail: (Use web site form)
Supp, Chap, Lit, Speak, Vol

NARSAD: The Mental Health Research Association
60 Cutter Mill Rd., Suite 404
Great Neck, NY 11021
Tel: (800) 829-8289
Fax: (516) 487-6930
Web site: www.narsad.org

E-mail: info@narsad.org

Supp, Lit, Speak, Vol

C26 Borderline Personality Disorder

Treatment and Research Advancements Association for
  Personality Disorders

23 Greene St.

New York, NY 10013

Tel: (212) 966-6514

Web site: www.tara4bpd.org

E-mail: (Use web site form)

RDocs, Lit, Speak, Vol

C27 Eating Disorders

National Association of Anorexia Nervosa and
  Associated Disorders

P.O. Box 7

Highland Park, IL 60035

Tel: (847) 831-3438

Web site: www.anad.org

E-mail: (Use web site form)

Supp, RDocs, Chap, Lit, Speak, Vol

C28 Post-Traumatic Stress Disorder

National Center for Post-Traumatic Stress Disorder

215 N. Main St.

White River Junction, VT 05009

Tel: (802) 296-5132

Fax: (802) 296-5135

Web site: www.ncptsd.org

E-mail: ncptsd@ncptsd.org

RInfo, Lit

C29 Substance Abuse and Addiction

American Society of Addiction Medicine

4601 N. Park Ave., Arcade Suite 101

Chevy Chase, MD 20815

Tel: (301) 656-3920

Fax: (301) 656-3815

Web site: www.asam.org

E-mail: email@asam.org

RDocs, Chap, Lit

National Clearinghouse for Alcohol and
  Drug Information

P.O. Box 2345, 11420 Rockville Pike

Rockville, MD 20852

Tel: (800) 729-6686

TDD: (800) 487-4889

Espanola: (877) 767-8432

Web site: www.health.org

E-mail: (Use web site form)

RInfo, Lit, Vol, RDocs, RInfo

National Council on Alcoholism and Drug
  Dependence, Inc.

22 Cortland St., Suite 801

New York, NY 10007-3128

Tel: (212) 269-7797

Fax: (212) 269-7510

Web site: www.ncadd.org

E-mail: national@ncadd.org

RDocs, RInfo, Chap, Lit, Vol

Do It Now Foundation

Box 27568

Tempe, AZ 85285-7568

Tel: (480) 736-0599

Fax: (480) 736-0771

Web site: www.doitnow.org

E-mail: e-mail@doitnow.org

RInfo, Lit, Vol

National Families in Action

2957 Clairmont Rd. NE, Suite 150

Atlanta, GA 30329

Tel: (404) 248-9676

Fax: (404) 248-1312

Web site: www.nationalfamilies.org

E-mail: nfia@nationalfamilies.org

RInfo, Lit, Vol

Operation PAR

2000 4th St. South

St. Petersburg, FL 33705

Tel: (888) PAR-NEXT

Web site: www.operationpar.org

E-mail: (Use web site form)

Supp, RDocs, Lit, Speak, Vol, Rinfo

Phoenix House

164 W. 74th St.

New York, NY 10023

Tel: (212) 595-5810

Fax: (212) 496-6035
Web sit: www.phoenixhouse.org
Email: (Use web site form)
Supp, RDocs, Chap, Lit, Vol

C30 Alcoholism
Al-Anon Family Group
1600 Corporate Landing Pkwy.
Virginia Beach, VA 23456
Tel: (800) 356-9996
Fax: (757) 563-1655
Web site: www.al-anon.alateen.org
E-mail: wso@al-anon.org
Supp, Chap, Lit, Speak, Vol

Alcoholics Anonymous
A.A. World Services, Inc.
P.O. Box 459
New York, NY 10163
Tel: (212) 870-3400
Web site: www.alcoholics-anonymous.org
Supp, Chap, Lit, Speak, Vol

Recovery, Inc.
802 N. Dearborn St.
Chicago, IL 60610
Tel: (312) 337-5661
Fax: (312) 337-5756
Web site: www.recovery-inc.org
Email: inquiries@recovery-inc.org
Supp, Chap, Lit, Vol

C32 Suicidal Feelings
American Association of Suicidology
5221 Wisconsin Ave., NW
Washington, DC 20015
Phone: (202) 237-2280
Fax: (202) 237-2282
Web site: www.suicidology.org
E-mail: info@suicidology.org
RDocs, RInfo, Lit, Speak

C33 Multiple Sclerosis
Multiple Sclerosis Foundation
6350 North Andrews Ave.
Fort Lauderdale, FL 33309-2130

Tel: (888) MSF-OCUS
Fax: (954) 351-0630
Web site: www.msfocus.org
E-mail: support@msfocus.org
Supp, RDocs, Chap, Lit, Speak, Vol

The National Multiple Sclerosis Society
733 Third Ave.
New York, NY 10017
Tel: (800) 344-4867
Web site: www.nationalmssociety.org
Email: (Use web site form)
Supp, Chap, Lit, Vol

C35 Neurological Complications of AIDS
CDC National Prevention Information Network
P.O. Box 6003
Rockville, MD 20849-6003
Tel: (800) 458-5231
TTY: (800) 243-7012
Fax: (888) 282-7681
Web site: www.cdcnpin.org
E-mail: info@cdcnpin.org
RInfo, Lit

C40 Systemic Lupus Erythematosus
American Autoimmune Related Diseases Association
22100 Gratiot Ave.
E. Detroit, MI 48021
Tel: (586)776-3900
Web site: www.aarda.org
E-mail: aarda@aol.com
RDocs, RInfo, Chap, Lit, Vol

American Behçet's Disease Association
PO Box 19952
Amarillo, TX 79114
Tel: (800) 7BEHCETS
Fax: (480) 247-5377
Web site: www.behcets.com
E-mail: (Use web site form)
Supp, RDocs, Lit

Sjögren's Syndrome Foundation, Inc.
8120 Woodmont Ave., Suite 530
Bethesda, MD 20814-2771

Tel: (800) 475-6473
Fax: (301) 718-0322
Web site: www.sjogrens.org
E-mail: tms@sjogrens.org
Supp, Lit, Speak, Vol

C41 Parkinson's Disease and
C42 Parkinsonism Plus
American Parkinson Disease Association
135 Parkinson Ave.
Staten Island, NY 10305
Tel: (800) 223-2732
Fax: (718) 981-4399
Web site: www.apdaparkinson.org
E-Mail: apda@apdaparkinson.org
Supp, RDocs, RInfo, Chap, Lit, Speak, Vol

Muhammad Ali Parkinson Research Center
Barrow Neurological Institute
500 W. Thomas Rd., Suite 720
Phoenix, AZ 85013
Tel: (602) 406-4931
Web site: www.maprc.com
E-mail: info@maprc.com
Supp, RDocs, Lit, Speak, Vol, RInfo

National Parkinson Foundation, Inc
1501 NW 9th Ave., Bob Hope Rd.
Miami, FL 33136-1494
Tel: (800) 327-4545
Fax: (305) 243-5595
Web site: www.parkinson.org
E-mail: contact@parkinson.org
Supp, RDocs, RInfo, Chap, Lit, Speak, Vol

Parkinson's Action Network
1025 Vermont Ave., NW, Suite 1120
Washington, DC 20005
Tel: (800) 850-4726
Fax: (202) 638-7257
Web site: www.parkinsonsaction.org
E-mail: info@parkinsonsaction.org
Supp, RDocs, Lit, Speak, Vol

The Parkinson's Disease Foundation
1359 Broadway, Suite 1509
New York, NY 10018

Tel: (800) 457-6676
Web site: www.pdf.org
E-mail: info@pdf.org
Supp, RDocs, Lit, Speak, Vol

The Parkinson's Institute
1170 Morse Ave.
Sunnyvale, CA 94089
Tel: (800) 786-2958
Web site: www.thepi.org
E-mail: (Use web site form)
Supp, RDocs, RInfo, Lit, Speak, Vol

C43 Tremors
International Essential Tremor Foundation
P.O. Box 14005
Lenexa, KS 66285-4005
Tel: (888) 387-3667
FAX: (913) 341-1296
Web site: www.essentialtremor.org
E-mail: staff@essentialtremor.org
Supp, RDocs, Chap, Lit, Vol

C44 Dystonia, Spasms, and Cramps
National Spasmodic Dysphonia Association
300 Park Boulevard, Suite 350
Itasca, IL 60143
Tel: (800) 795-6732
Fax: (630) 250-4505
Web site: www.dysphonia.org
E-mail: NSDA@dysphonia.org
Supp, RDocs, Chap, Lit

National Spasmodic Torticollis Association
9920 Talbert Ave.
Fountain Valley, CA 92708
Tel: (714) 378-7837
Fax: (714) 378-7830
Web site: www.torticollis.org
E-mail: nstamail@aol.com
Supp, RDocs, RInfo, Chap, Lit, Speak, Vol

C45 Tourette's Syndrome and Tics
Tourette Syndrome Association, Inc.
42-40 Bell Blvd.
Bayside, NY 11361
Tel: (718) 224-2999

Fax: (718) 279-9596
Web site: www.tsa-usa.org
(Use web site form)
Supp, RDocs, Chap, Lit, Speak, Vol

C46 Ataxia
A-T Children's Project
668 S. Military Trail
Deerfield Beach, FL 33442-3023
Tel: (800) 543-5728
Fax: (954) 725-1153
Web site: www.atcp.org
E-mail: info@atcp.org
RDocs, RInfo, Lit, Speak, Vol

National Ataxia Foundation
2600 Fernbrook Ln., Suite 119
Minneapolis, MN 55447
Tel: (763) 553-0020
Fax: (763) 553-0167
Web site: www.ataxia.org
E-mail: naf@ataxia.org
Supp, RDocs, Chap, Lit, Vol

C47 Huntington's Disease
Hereditary Disease Foundation
3960 Broadway, 6th Floor
New York, NY 10032
Tel: (212) 928-2121
Fax: (212) 928-2172
Web site: www.hdfoundation.org
E-mail: cures@hdfoundation.org
RDocs, RInfo, Lit, Vol

Huntington's Disease Society of America
505 Eighth Ave., Suite 902
New York, NY 10018
Tel: (800) 345- 4372
Fax: (212) 239-3430
Web site: hdsainfo@hdsa.org
E-mail: www.hdsa.org
Supp, RInfo, Chap, Lit, Speak, Vol

C49 Guillain-Barré Syndrome
Guillain-Barré Syndrome Foundation International
The Holly Building, 104 ^{1}/$_2$ Forrest Ave.

Narberth, PA 19072
Tel: (610) 667-0131
Fax: (610) 667-7036
Web site: www.gbsfi.com
E-mail: info@gbsfi.com
Supp, RDocs, Chap, Lit, Speak, Vol

C51 Myopathies
Muscular Dystrophy Association
National Headquarters
3300 E. Sunrise Dr.
Tucson, AZ 85718
Tel: (800) 344-4863
Web site: www.mdausa.org
E-mail: mda@mdausa.org
Supp, RDocs, RInfo, Chap, Lit, Speak, Vol

C52 Myasthenia Gravis
Myasthenia Gravis Foundation of America
1821 University Ave. W., Suite S256
St. Paul, MN 55104
Tel: (800) 541-5454
Fax: (651) 917-1835
Web site: www.myasthenia.org
Email: mgfa@myasthenia.org
Supp, RDocs, Chap, Lit, Vol

C53 Amyotrophic Lateral Sclerosis
The ALS Association
27001 Agoura Rd., Suite 150
Calabasas Hills, CA 91301
Tel: (818) 880-9007
Fax: (818) 880-9006
Web site: www.alsa.org
E-mail: (Use web site form)
Supp, RDocs, Lit, Vol

Les Turner ALS Foundation
8142 North Lawndale Ave.
Skokie, IL 60076-3322
Tel: (888) ALS-1107
Fax: (847) 679-9109
Web site: www.lesturnerals.org
E-mail: info@lesturnerals.org
Supp, RInfo, Lit

C54 Headache and
C55 Migraines

American Council for Headache Education
19 Mantua Rd.
Mt. Royal, NJ 08061
Tel: (856)423-0258
Fax: (856)423-0082
Web site: www.achenet.org
E-mail: achehq@talley.com
Supp, RDocs, Lit, Speak

Association for Applied Psychophysiology
   and Biofeedback
10200 West 44th Ave., Suite 304
Wheat Ridge, CO 80033
Tel: (800) 477-8892
Web site: www.aapb.org
E-mail: (Use web site form)
Chap, Lit, RInfo

National Headache Foundation
820 N. Orleans, Suite 217
Chicago, IL 60610
Tel: (888) NHF-5552
Fax: (773) 525-7357
We site: www.headaches.org
E-mail: info@headaches.org
Supp, RInfo, Lit, Speak, Vol

C56 Back Pain and Disk Disease

North American Spine Society
22 Calendar Court, 2nd Floor
La Grange, IL USA 60525
Tel: (877) 774-6337
Web site: www.spine.org
E-mail: info@spine.org
RDocs, RInfo, Lit

C57 Chronic Pain

The American Chronic Pain Association
P.O. Box 850
Rocklin, CA 95677
Tel: (800) 533-3231
Fax: (916) 632-3208
Web site: www.theacpa.org
E-mail: ACPA@pacbell.net
Supp, Chap, Lit, Vol

C58 Trigeminal Neuralgia

Trigeminal Neuralgia Association
925 Northwest 56th Ter., Suite C
Gainesville, FL 32605-6402
Tel: (800) 923-3608
Fax: (352) 331-7078
Web site: www.tna-support.org
E-mail: tnanational@tna-support.org
Supp, RDocs, Chap, Lit, Speak, Vol

C59 Ischemic Stroke and
C60 Hemorrhagic Stroke

American Stroke Association
National Center
7272 Greenville Ave.
Dallas, TX 75231
Tel: (888) 478-7653
Web site: www.strokeassociation.org
Supp, Chap, Lit, Speak, Vol

National Stroke Association
9707 E. Easter Ln.
Englewood, CO 80112
Tel: (800) 787-6537
Fax: (303) 649-1329
web site: www.stroke.org
Supp, Chap, Lit

National Institute of Neurological Disorders
and Stroke Office of Scientific and Health Reports
P.O. Box 5801
Bethesda, MD 20824
Tel: (800) 352-9424
TTY: (301) 468-5981
Web site: www.ninds.nih.gov

Brain Injury Association of America
8201 Greensboro Dr., Suite 611
McLean, VA 22102
Tel: (800) 444-6443
Web site: www.biausa.org
Supp, RDocs, Chap, Lit, Speak, Vol

C61 Brain Trauma, Concussion, and Coma

Brain Injury Association of America
8201 Greensboro Dr., Suite 611
McLean, VA 22102

Tel: (800) 444-6443

Web site: www.biausa.org

Supp, RDocs, Chap, Lit, Speak, Vol

Brain Injury Services

8136 Old Keene Mill Rd., Suite B102

Springfield, VA 22152

Tel: (703) 451-8881

Fax: (703) 451-8820

Web site: www.braininjurysvcs.org

E-mail: kbrown@braininjurysvcs.org

Supp, RDocs, Chap, Lit, Speak, Vol

ThinkFirst Foundation

26 South La Grange Rd., Suite 103

La Grange, IL 60525

Tel: (800) 844-6556

Fax: (708) 588-2002

Web site: www.thinkfirst.org

E-mail: thinkfirst@thinkfirst.org

Chap, Lit, Speak, Vol

Head Injury Hotline

212 Pioneer Bldg

Seattle, WA 98104-2221

Tel: (206) 621-8558

Web site: www.headinjury.com

E-mail: brain@headinjury.com

RDocs, Lit, Speak, Vol, RInfo

Rehabilitation Research Center for TBI & SCI

Santa Clara Valley Medical Center

751 South Bascom Ave.

San Jose, CA 95128

Tel: (408) 793-6433

Fax: (408) 793-6434

Web site: www.tbi-sci.org

E-mail: kimberly.emley@hhs.co.santa-clara.ca.us

Supp, RDocs, Lit, Speak

Coma Recovery Association, Inc.

8300 Republic Airport, Suite 106

Farmingdale, NY 11735

Tel: (631) 756-1826

Fax: (631) 756-1827

Web site: www.comarecovery.org

E-mail: inquiry@comarecovery.org

Supp, RInfo, Chap, Lit

C62 Spinal Cord Injury

National Spinal Cord Injury Association

6701 Democracy Blvd., Suite 300-9

Bethesda, MD 20817

Tel: (800) 962-9629

Fax: (301) 990-0445

Web sit: www.spinalcord.org

Email: info@spinalcord.org

Supp, RInfo, Chap, Lit, Vol

C64 Brain Tumors

American Brain Tumor Association

2720 River Rd.

Des Plaines, IL 60018

Tel: (800) 886-2282

Fax: (847) 827-9918

Web site: www.abta.org

E-mail: info@abta.org

RInfo, Lit, Speak, Vol

Brain Tumor Society

124 Watertown St., Suite 3H

Watertown, MA 02472

Tel: (800) 770-8287

Fax: (617) 924-9998

Web site: www.tbts.org

E-mail: (Use web site form)

Supp, RInfo, Lit, Speak, Vol

The Healing Exchange BRAIN TRUST

186 Hampshire St.

Cambridge, MA 02139-1320

Tel: (617) 876-2002

Fax: (617) 876-2332

Web site: www.braintrust.org

E-mail: info@ braintrust.org

Supp, Lit, Speak, Vol

National Brain Tumor Foundation

22 Battery St., Suite 612

San Francisco, CA 94111-5520

Tel: (800) 934-2873

Fax: (415) 834-9980

Web site: www.braintumor.org

E-mail: nbtf@braintumor.org

Supp, Lit, Vol

C67 Alzheimer's Disease

Alzheimer's Association
225 N. Michigan Ave., 17th Floor
Chicago, IL 60601
Tel: (800) 272-3900
Fax: (312) 335-1110
Web site: www.alz.org
E-mail: info@alz.org
Supp, Chap, Lit, Vol

Alzheimer's Disease Education and Referral Center
P.O. Box 8250
Silver Spring, MD 20907
Tel: (800) 438-4380
Fax: (301) 495-3334
Web site: www.alzheimers.org
E-mail: (Use web site form)
RInfo, Lit

C70 Trouble with Speech and Language

National Aphasia Association
7 Dey St., Suite 600
New York, NY 10007
Tel: (800) 922-4622
Fax: (212) 267-2812
Web site: www.aphasia.org
E-mail: naa@aphasia.org
Supp, RDocs, Lit, Vol

The Dana Alliance for
Brain Initiatives

Bernard W. Agranoff, M.D.
UNIVERSITY OF MICHIGAN

Albert J. Aguayo, M.D.
MCGILL UNIVERSITY

Huda Akil, Ph.D.
UNIVERSITY OF MICHIGAN

Marilyn S. Albert, Ph.D.
JOHNS HOPKINS MEDICAL INSTITUTIONS

Duane F. Alexander, M.D.
NATIONAL INSTITUTE OF CHILD HEALTH
AND HUMAN DEVELOPMENT

Susan G. Amara, Ph.D.
UNIVERSITY OF PITTSBURGH SCHOOL OF MEDICINE

Nancy C. Andreasen, M.D., Ph.D.
UNIVERSITY OF IOWA CARVER COLLEGE OF MEDICINE

Arthur K. Asbury, M.D.
UNIVERSITY OF PENNSYLVANIA SCHOOL OF MEDICINE

Jack D. Barchas, M.D.
WEILL MEDICAL COLLEGE OF CORNELL UNIVERSITY

Robert L. Barchi, M.D., Ph.D.
THOMAS JEFFERSON UNIVERSITY

Yves-Alain Barde
FRIEDRICH MIESCHER INSTITUTE FOR BIOMEDICAL RESEARCH

J. Richard Baringer, M.D.
UNIVERSITY OF UTAH HEALTH SCIENCES CENTER

Carol A. Barnes, Ph.D.
UNIVERSITY OF ARIZONA

Allan I. Basbaum, Ph.D.
UNIVERSITY OF CALIFORNIA, SAN FRANCISCO

Nicolas G. Bazan, M.D., Ph.D.
LOUISIANA STATE UNIVERSITY HEALTH SCIENCES CENTER

M. Flint Beal, M.D.
WEILL MEDICAL COLLEGE OF CORNELL UNIVERSITY

Mark F. Bear, Ph.D.
MASSACHUSETTS INSTITUTE OF TECHNOLOGY

Ursula Bellugi, Ed.D.
THE SALK INSTITUTE FOR BIOLOGICAL STUDIES

James L. Bernat, M.D.
DARTMOUTH MEDICAL SCHOOL

Katherine L. Bick, Ph.D.
WILMINGTON, NC

Anders Björklund, M.D., Ph.D.
UNIVERSITY OF LUND

Peter M. Black, M.D., Ph.D.
BRIGHAM AND WOMEN'S HOSPITAL

Colin Blakemore, Ph.D., ScD, FRS
MEDICAL RESEARCH COUNCIL, UNITED KINGDOM

Floyd E. Bloom, M.D.
NEUROME, INC.

Walter G. Bradley, D.M., F.R.C.P.
UNIVERSITY OF MIAMI MILLER SCHOOL OF MEDICINE

Xandra O. Breakefield, Ph.D.
MASSACHUSETTS GENERAL HOSPITAL

Monte S. Buchsbaum, M.D.
MOUNT SINAI SCHOOL OF MEDICINE

Mary Bartlett Bunge, Ph.D.
UNIVERSITY OF MIAMI SCHOOL OF MEDICINE

Rosalie A. Burns, M.D.
FORMERLY THOMAS JEFFERSON MEDICAL COLLEGE

John H. Byrne, Ph.D.
UNIVERSITY OF TEXAS HEALTH SCIENCE CENTER

Judy L. Cameron, Ph.D.
OREGON NATIONAL PRIMATE RESEARCH CENTER

Louis R. Caplan, M.D.
BETH ISRAEL DEACONESS MEDICAL CENTER

Benjamin S. Carson, Sr., M.D.
JOHNS HOPKINS MEDICAL INSTITUTIONS

William A. Catterall, Ph.D.
UNIVERSITY OF WASHINGTON

Nicholas G. Cavarocchi
CAVAROCCHI RUSCIO DENNIS ASSOCIATES

Verne S. Caviness, M.D., D.Phil.
MASSACHUSETTS GENERAL HOSPITAL

Connie L. Cepko, Ph.D.
HARVARD MEDICAL SCHOOL

Dennis W. Choi, M.D., Ph.D.
FORMERLY MERCK RESEARCH LABORATORIES

Harry T. Chugani, M.D.
WAYNE STATE UNIVERSITY

Patricia S. Churchland, Ph.D.
UNIVERSITY OF CALIFORNIA, SAN DIEGO

David E. Clapham, M.D., Ph.D.
BOSTON CHILDREN'S HOSPITAL

Don W. Cleveland, Ph.D.
UNIVERSITY OF CALIFORNIA, SAN DIEGO

Robert C. Collins, M.D.
FORMERLY UCLA SCHOOL OF MEDICINE

Martha Constantine-Paton, Ph.D.
MASSACHUSETTS INSTITUTE OF TECHNOLOGY

Robert M. Cook-Deegan, M.D.
DUKE UNIVERSITY

Leon N. Cooper, Ph.D.
BROWN UNIVERSITY

Jody Corey-Bloom, M.D., Ph.D.
UNIVERSITY OF CALIFORNIA, SAN DIEGO SCHOOL OF MEDICINE

Carl W. Cotman, Ph.D.
UNIVERSITY OF CALIFORNIA, IRVINE

Joseph T. Coyle, M.D.
HARVARD MEDICAL SCHOOL

Patricia K. Coyle, M.D.
SUNY AT STONY BROOK

Antonio R. Damasio, M.D., Ph.D.
UNIVERSITY OF SOUTHERN CALIFORNIA

Hanna F. Damasio, M.D.
UNIVERSITY OF SOUTHERN CALIFORNIA

Robert B. Daroff, M.D.
CASE WESTERN RESERVE UNIVERSITY SCHOOL OF MEDICINE

William C. de Groat, Ph.D.
UNIVERSITY OF PITTSBURGH SCHOOL OF MEDICINE

Mahlon R. DeLong, M.D.
EMORY UNIVERSITY SCHOOL OF MEDICINE

Martha Bridge Denckla, M.D.
KENNEDY KRIEGER INSTITUTE

J. Raymond DePaulo, Jr., M.D.
THE JOHNS HOPKINS UNIVERSITY SCHOOL OF MEDICINE

Ivan Diamond, M.D., Ph.D.
CV THERAPEUTICS

Marc A. Dichter, M.D., Ph.D.
UNIVERSITY OF PENNSYLVANIA MEDICAL CENTER

David A. Drachman, M.D.
UNIVERSITY OF MASSACHUSETTS MEMORIAL MEDICAL CENTER

Felton Earls, M.D.
HARVARD MEDICAL SCHOOL

Gerald M. Edelman, M.D., Ph.D.
THE SCRIPPS RESEARCH INSTITUTE

Robert H. Edwards, M.D.
UNIVERSITY OF CALIFORNIA, SAN FRANCISCO

Salvatore J. Enna, Ph.D.
UNIVERSITY OF KANSAS MEDICAL CENTER

Eva L. Feldman, M.D., Ph.D.
UNIVERSITY OF MICHIGAN

James A. Ferrendelli, M.D.
UNIVERSITY OF TEXAS-HOUSTON MEDICAL CENTER

Howard L. Fields, M.D., Ph.D.
UNIVERSITY OF CALIFORNIA, SAN FRANCISCO

Gerald D. Fischbach, M.D.
COLUMBIA UNIVERSITY COLLEGE OF
PHYSICIANS AND SURGEONS

Kathleen M. Foley, M.D.
MEMORIAL SLOAN-KETTERING CANCER CENTER

Ellen Frank, Ph.D.
UNIVERSITY OF PITTSBURGH SCHOOL OF MEDICINE

Michael J. Friedlander, Ph.D.
BAYLOR COLLEGE OF MEDICINE

Stanley C. Froehner, Ph.D.
UNIVERSITY OF WASHINGTON

Fred H. Gage, Ph.D.
THE SALK INSTITUTE FOR BIOLOGICAL STUDIES

Michael S. Gazzaniga, Ph.D.
UNIVERSITY OF CALIFORNIA, SANTA BARBARA

Apostolos P. Georgopoulos, M.D., Ph.D.
UNIVERSITY OF MINNESOTA

Alfred G. Gilman, M.D., Ph.D.
UNIVERSITY OF TEXAS SOUTHWESTERN MEDICAL CENTER

Sid Gilman, M.D., F.R.C.P.
UNIVERSITY OF MICHIGAN MEDICAL CENTER

Gary Goldstein, M.D.
KENNEDY KRIEGER INSTITUTE

Murray Goldstein, D.O., M.P.H.
FORMERLY UNITED CEREBRAL PALSY RESEARCH
AND EDUCATIONAL FOUNDATION

Frederick K. Goodwin, M.D.
GEORGE WASHINGTON UNIVERSITY MEDICAL CENTER

Enoch Gordis, M.D.
FORMERLY NATIONAL INSTITUTE ON
ALCOHOL ABUSE AND ALCOHOLISM

Barry Gordon, M.D., Ph.D.
THE JOHNS HOPKINS MEDICAL INSTITUTIONS

Gary L. Gottlieb, M.D., M.B.A.
BRIGHAM AND WOMEN'S HOSPITAL

Jordan Grafman, Ph.D.
NATIONAL INSITUTE OF NEUROLOGICAL DISORDERS AND STROKE

Bernice Grafstein, Ph.D.
WEILL MEDICAL COLLEGE OF CORNELL UNIVERSITY

Ann M. Graybiel, Ph.D.
MASSACHUSETTS INSTITUTE OF TECHNOLOGY

Michael E. Greenberg, Ph.D.
CHILDREN'S HOSPITAL BOSTON

Paul Greengard, Ph.D.
THE ROCKEFELLER UNIVERSITY

William T. Greenough, Ph.D.
UNIVERSITY OF ILLINOIS AT URBANA-CHAMPAIGN

Diane E. Griffin, M.D., Ph.D.
JOHNS HOPKINS BLOOMBERG SCHOOL OF PUBLIC HEALTH

Murray Grossman, M.D.
UNIVERSITY OF PENNSYLVANIA SCHOOL OF MEDICINE

Robert G. Grossman, M.D.

THE METHODIST HOSPITAL

Robert J. Gumnit, M.D.
MINCEP EPILEPSY CARE

James F. Gusella, Ph.D.
MASSACHUSETTS GENERAL HOSPITAL

Zach W. Hall, Ph.D.
CALIFORNIA INSTITUTE FOR REGENERATIVE MEDICINE

Mary E. Hatten, Ph.D.
THE ROCKEFELLER UNIVERSITY

Stephen L. Hauser, M.D.
UNIVERSITY OF CALIFORNIA, SAN FRANCISCO

Kenneth M. Heilman, M.D.
UNIVERSITY OF FLORIDA COLLEGE OF MEDICINE

Stephen F. Heinemann, Ph.D.
THE SALK INSTITUTE FOR BIOLOGICAL STUDIES

John G. Hildebrand, Ph.D.
UNIVERSITY OF ARIZONA

J. Allan Hobson, M.D.
MASSACHUSETTS MENTAL HEALTH CENTER

Susan Hockfield, Ph.D.
MASSACHUSETTS INSTITUTE OF TECHNOLOGY

Richard J. Hodes, M.D.
NATIONAL INSTITUTE ON AGING

H. Robert Horvitz, Ph.D.
MASSACHUSETTS INSTITUTE OF TECHNOLOGY

David H. Hubel, M.D.
HARVARD MEDICAL SCHOOL

A. James Hudspeth, M.D., Ph.D.
THE ROCKEFELLER UNIVERSITY

Richard L. Huganir, Ph.D.
THE JOHNS HOPKINS UNIVERSITY SCHOOL OF MEDICINE

Steven E. Hyman, M.D.
HARVARD UNIVERSITY

Judy Illes, Ph.D.
STANFORD UNIVERSITY SCHOOL OF MEDICINE

Thomas R. Insel, M.D.

NATIONAL INSTITUTE OF MENTAL HEALTH

Kay Redfield Jamison, Ph.D.
THE JOHNS HOPKINS UNIVERSITY SCHOOL OF MEDICINE

Richard T. Johnson, M.D.
THE JOHNS HOPKINS UNIVERSITY SCHOOL OF MEDICINE

Edward G. Jones, M.D., Ph.D.
UNIVERSITY OF CALIFORNIA, DAVIS

Robert J. Joynt, M.D., Ph.D.
UNIVERSITY OF ROCHESTER

Lewis L. Judd, M.D.
UNIVERSITY OF CALIFORNIA, SAN DIEGO SCHOOL OF MEDICINE

Jerome Kagan, Ph.D.
HARVARD UNIVERSITY

Ned H. Kalin, M.D.
UNIVERSITY OF WISCONSIN SCHOOL OF MEDICINE

Eric R. Kandel, M.D.
COLUMBIA UNIVERSITY COLLEGE OF
PHYSICIANS AND SURGEONS

Stanley B. Kater, Ph.D.
UNIVERSITY OF UTAH

Robert Katzman, M.D.
UNIVERSITY OF CALIFORNIA, SAN DIEGO SCHOOL OF MEDICINE

Claudia H. Kawas, M.D.
UNIVERSITY OF CALIFORNIA, IRVINE

Zaven S. Khachaturian, Ph.D.
THE RONALD AND NANCY REAGAN RESEARCH INSTITUTE

Masakazu Konishi, Ph.D.
CALIFORNIA INSTITUTE OF TECHNOLOGY

Michael J. Kuhar, Ph.D.
YERKES NATIONAL PRIMATE RESEARCH
CENTER OF EMORY UNIVERSITY

Patricia K. Kuhl, Ph.D.
UNIVERSITY OF WASHINGTON

Anand Kumar, M.D.
UNIVERSITY OF CALIFORNIA, LOS ANGELES

David J. Kupfer, M.D.
UNIVERSITY OF PITTSBURGH SCHOOL OF MEDICINE

Story C. Landis, Ph.D.
NATIONAL INSTITUTE OF NEUROLOGICAL
DISORDERS AND STROKE

Lynn T. Landmesser, Ph.D.
CASE WESTERN RESERVE UNIVERSITY

Anthony E. Lang, M.D., F.R.C.P.C
UNIVERSITY OF TORONTO

Joseph E. LeDoux, Ph.D.
NEW YORK UNIVERSITY

Alan I. Leshner, Ph.D.
AMERICAN ASSOCIATION FOR THE ADVANCEMENT OF SCIENCE

Allan I. Levey, M.D., Ph.D.
EMORY UNIVERSITY

Irwin B. Levitan, Ph.D.
UNIVERSITY OF PENNSYLVANIA SCHOOL OF MEDICINE

Pat R. Levitt, Ph.D.
VANDERBILT UNIVERSITY

Lee E. Limbird, Ph.D.
MEHARRY MEDICAL COLLEGE

Margaret S. Livingstone, Ph.D.
HARVARD MEDICAL SCHOOL

Rodolfo R. Llinas, M.D., Ph.D.
NEW YORK UNIVERSITY SCHOOL OF MEDICINE

Don M. Long, M.D., Ph.D.
THE JOHNS HOPKINS UNIVERSITY SCHOOL OF MEDICINE

Peter R. MacLeish, Ph.D.
MOREHOUSE SCHOOL OF MEDICINE

Robert C. Malenka, M.D., Ph.D.
STANFORD UNIVERSITY MEDICAL CENTER

Eve Marder, Ph.D.
BRANDEIS UNIVERSITY

William R. Markesbery, M.D.
UNIVERSITY OF KENTUCKY

Joseph B. Martin, M.D., Ph.D.
HARVARD MEDICAL SCHOOL

Robert L. Martuza, M.D., F.A.C.S.
MASSACHUSETTS GENERAL HOSPITAL

Richard Mayeux, M.D., M.Sc.
COLUMBIA UNIVERSITY MEDICAL CENTER

Bruce S. McEwen, Ph.D.
THE ROCKEFELLER UNIVERSITY

James L. McGaugh, Ph.D.
UNIVERSITY OF CALIFORNIA, IRVINE

Guy M. McKhann, M.D.
THE JOHNS HOPKINS UNIVERSITY

Lorne M. Mendell, Ph.D.
SUNY AT STONY BROOK

Marek-Marsel Mesulam, M.D.
NORTHWESTERN UNIVERSITY FEINBERG SCHOOL OF MEDICINE

Bradie Metheny
RESEARCH POLICY ALERT

Brenda A. Milner, Sc.D.
MCGILL UNIVERSITY

William C. Mobley, M.D., Ph.D.
STANFORD UNIVERSITY

Richard C. Mohs, Ph.D.
LILLY RESEARCH LABORATORIES

John H. Morrison, Ph.D.
MOUNT SINAI SCHOOL OF MEDICINE

Michael A. Moskowitz, M.D.
MASSACHUSETTS GENERAL HOSPITAL

Vernon B. Mountcastle, M.D.
THE JOHNS HOPKINS UNIVERSITY

Lennart Mucke, M.D.
UNIVERSITY OF CALIFORNIA, SAN FRANCISCO

Richard A. Murphy, Ph.D.
THE SALK INSTITUTE FOR BIOLOGICAL STUDIES

Lynn Nadel, Ph.D.
UNIVERSITY OF ARIZONA

Karin B. Nelson, M.D.
NATIONAL INSTITUTE OF NEUROLOGICAL
DISORDERS AND STROKE

Eric J. Nestler, M.D., Ph.D.
THE UNIVERSITY OF TEXAS SOUTHWESTERN MEDICAL CENTER

Charles P. O'Brien, M.D., Ph.D.
UNIVERSITY OF PENNSYLVANIA

Edward H. Oldfield, M.D.
NATIONAL INSTITUTE OF NEUROLOGICAL
DISORDERS AND STROKE

John W. Olney, M.D.
WASHINGTON UNIVERSITY SCHOOL OF MEDICINE

Luis F. Parada, Ph.D.
UNIVERSITY OF TEXAS SOUTHWESTERN MEDICAL CENTER

Herbert Pardes, M.D.
NEW YORK-PRESBYTERIAN HOSPITAL

Steven M. Paul, M.D.
LILLY RESEARCH LABORATORIES

Audrey S. Penn, M.D.
NATIONAL INSTITUTE OF NEUROLOGICAL DISORDERS

Edward R. Perl, M.D., M.S.
UNIVERSITY OF NORTH CAROLINA AT CHAPEL HILL

Michael E. Phelps, Ph.D.
DAVID GEFFEN SCHOOL OF MEDICINE AT UCLA

Jonathan H. Pincus, M.D.
GEORGETOWN UNIVERSITY MEDICAL CENTER

Fred Plum, M.D.
WEILL MEDICAL COLLEGE OF CORNELL UNIVERSITY

Jerome B. Posner, M.D.
MEMORIAL SLOAN-KETTERING CANCER CENTER

Michael I. Posner, M.S., Ph.D.
UNIVERSITY OF OREGON

Robert M. Post, M.D.
NATIONAL INSTITUTE OF MENTAL HEALTH

Donald L. Price, M.D.
THE JOHNS HOPKINS UNIVERSITY SCHOOL OF MEDICINE

Stanley B. Prusiner, M.D.
UNIVERSITY OF CALIFORNIA, SAN FRANCISCO

Dominick P. Purpura, M.D.
ALBERT EINSTEIN COLLEGE OF MEDICINE

Dale Purves, M.D.
DUKE UNIVERSITY MEDICAL CENTER

Remi Quirion, Ph.D., F.R.S.C, C.Q.
CIHR INSTITUTE OF NEUROSCIENCES,
MENTAL HEALTH, AND ADDICTION

Marcus E. Raichle, M.D.
WASHINGTON UNIVERSITY SCHOOL OF MEDICINE

Pasko Rakic, M.D., Ph.D.
YALE UNIVERSITY SCHOOL OF MEDICINE

Judith L. Rapoport, M.D.
NATIONAL INSTITUTE OF MENTAL HEALTH

Allan L. Reiss, M.D.
STANFORD UNIVERSITY SCHOOL OF MEDICINE

Richard M. Restak, M.D.
NEUROLOGY ASSOCIATES

James T. Robertson, M.D.
UNIVERSITY OF TENNESSEE, MEMPHIS

Robert G. Robinson, M.D.
UNIVERSITY OF IOWA COLLEGE OF MEDICINE

Robert M. Rose, M.D.
MIND, BRAIN, AND BODY HEALTH INITIATIVE

Roger N. Rosenberg, M.D.
UNIVERSITY OF TEXAS SOUTHWESTERN MEDICAL CENTER

Allen D. Roses, M.D.
GLAXOSMITHKLINE

Edward F. Rover
THE DANA FOUNDATION

Lewis P. Rowland, M.D.
COLUMBIA UNIVERSITY MEDICAL CENTER

Gerald M. Rubin, Ph.D.
UNIVERSITY OF CALIFORNIA, BERKELEY

Stephen J. Ryan, M.D.
DOHENY EYE INSTITUTE

Murray B. Sachs, Ph.D.
THE JOHNS HOPKINS UNIVERSITY SCHOOL OF MEDICINE

William Safire
THE DANA FOUNDATION

Martin A. Samuels, M.D., F.A.A.N, M.A.C.P.
BRIGHAM AND WOMEN'S HOSPITAL

Joshua R. Sanes, Ph.D.
HARVARD UNIVERSITY

Clifford B. Saper, M.D., Ph.D.
HARVARD MEDICAL SCHOOL

Daniel L. Schacter, Ph.D.
HARVARD UNIVERSITY

John L. Schwartz, M.D.
PSYCHIATRIC TIMES AND GERIATRIC TIMES

Philip Seeman, M.D., Ph.D.
UNIVERSITY OF TORONTO

Terrence J. Sejnowski, Ph.D.
THE SALK INSTITUTE FOR BIOLOGICAL STUDIES

Dennis J. Selkoe, M.D.
BRIGHAM AND WOMEN'S HOSPITAL

Carla J. Shatz, Ph.D.
HARVARD MEDICAL SCHOOL

Bennett A. Shaywitz, M.D.
YALE UNIVERSITY SCHOOL OF MEDICINE

Sally E. Shaywitz, M.D.
YALE UNIVERSITY SCHOOL OF MEDICINE

Gordon M. Shepherd, M.D., D.Phil.
YALE MEDICAL SCHOOL

Eric M. Shooter, Ph.D., Sc.D.
STANFORD UNIVERSITY SCHOOL OF MEDICINE

Ira Shoulson, M.D.
UNIVERSITY OF ROCHESTER

Donald H. Silberberg, M.D.
UNIVERSITY OF PENNSYLVANIA MEDICAL CENTER

Sangram S. Sisodia, Ph.D.
UNIVERSITY OF CHICAGO

Solomon H. Snyder, M.D.
THE JOHNS HOPKINS UNIVERSITY SCHOOL OF MEDICINE

Larry R. Squire, Ph.D.
UNIVERSITY OF CALIFORNIA, SAN DIEGO

Peter H. St. George-Hyslop, M.D.
UNIVERSITY OF TORONTO

Charles F. Stevens, M.D., Ph.D.
THE SALK INSTITUTE FOR BIOLOGICAL STUDIES

Oswald Steward, Ph.D.
UNIVERSITY OF CALIFORNIA AT IRVINE COLLEGE OF MEDICINE

Thomas C. Südhof, M.D.
UT SOUTHWESTERN MEDICAL CENTER

Larry W. Swanson, Ph.D.
UNIVERSITY OF SOUTHERN CALIFORNIA

Paula Tallal, Ph.D.
RUTGERS UNIVERSITY AT NEWARK

Carol A. Tamminga, M.D.
THE UNIVERSITY OF TEXAS SOUTHWESTERN MEDICAL CENTER

Robert D. Terry, M.D.
FORMERLY UNIVERSITY OF CALIFORNIA, SAN DIEGO

Hans F. Thoenen
MAX-PLANCK INSTITUTE FOR PSYCHIATRY

Allan J. Tobin, Ph.D.
HIGH Q FOUNDATION

James F. Toole, M.D.
WAKE FOREST UNIVERSITY SCHOOL OF MEDICINE

Daniel C. Tosteson, M.D.
HARVARD MEDICAL SCHOOL

John Q. Trojanowski, M.D., Ph.D.
UNIVERSITY OF PENNSYLVANIA SCHOOL OF MEDICINE

Richard W. Tsien, Ph.D.
STANFORD UNIVERSITY SCHOOL OF MEDICINE

Leslie Ungerleider, Ph.D.
NATIONAL INSTITUTE OF MENTAL HEALTH

David C. Van Essen, Ph.D.
WASHINGTON UNIVERSITY SCHOOL OF MEDICINE

Nora D. Volkow, M.D.
NATIONAL INSTITUTE ON DRUG ABUSE

Christopher A. Walsh, M.D., Ph.D.
BETH ISRAEL DEACONESS MEDICAL CENTER

James D. Watson, Ph.D.
COLD SPRING HARBOR LABORATORY

The European Dana Alliance for the Brain

Yves Agid
HÔPITAL DE LA SALPÊTRIÈRE, PARIS, FRANCE

Adriano Aguzzi
UNIVERSITY OF ZURICH, SWITZERLAND

Per Andersen
UNIVERSITY OF OSLO, NORWAY

João Lobo Atunes
UNIVERSITY OF LISBON, PORTUGAL

Dominque Aunis
INSERM STRASBOURG, FRANCE

Carlos Avendaño
UNIVERSITY OF MADRID, SPAIN

Alan Baddeley
UNIVERSITY OF YORK, UNITED KINGDOM

Yves-Alain Barde
UNIVERSITY OF BASEL, SWITZERLAND

Carlos Belmonte
INSTITUTO DE NEUROSCIENCIAS, ALICANTE, SPAIN

Alim-Louis Benabid
INSERM AND JOSEPH FOURIER UNIVERSTIY
OF GRENOBLE, FRANCE

Yehezkel Ben-Ari
INSERM-INMED, MARSEILLE, FRANCE

Fabio Benefenati
UNIVERSITY OF GENOVA, ITALY

Michael Berger
UNIVERSITY OF VIENNA, AUSTRIA

Giovanni Berlucchi
UNIVERSITÀ DEGLI STUDI DI VERONA, ITALY

Giorgio Bernardi
UNIVERSITY TOR VERGATA-ROMA, ITALY

Alain Berthoz
COLLÈGE DE FRANCE, PARIS, FRANCE

Konrad Beyreuther
UNIVERSITY OF HEIDELBERG, GERMANY

Anders Björklund
LUND UNIVERSITY, SWEDEN

Colin Blakemore
MEDICAL RESEARCH COUNCIL, UNITED KINGDOM

Joel Bockaert
CNRS, MONTPELLIER, FRANCE

Alexander Borbély
UNIVERSITY OF ZURICH, SWITZERLAND

Thomas Brandt
UNIVERSITY OF MUNICH, GERMANY

Patrik Brundin
LUND UNIVERSITY, SWEDEN

Herbert Budka
UNIVERSITY OF VIENNA, AUSTRIA

Jan Bureš
ACADEMY OF SCIENCES, PRAGUE, CZECH REPUBLIC

Irina Bystron
UNIVERSITY OF ST PETERSBURG, RUSSIA

Arvid Carlsson
UNIVERSITY OF GÖTEBORG, SWEDEN

Jean-Pierre Changeux
INSTITUT PASTEUR, PARIS, FRANCE

Marina Chernisheva
UNIVERSITY OF ST PETERSBURG, RUSSIA

Alexandr Chvatal
INSTITUTE OF EXPERIMENTAL MEDICINE
ASCR, PRAGUE, CZECH REPUBLIC

François Clarac
CNRS, MARSEILLE, FRANCE

Francesco Clementi
UNIVERSITY OF MILAN, ITALY

Graham Collingrige
UNIVERSITY OF BRISTOL, UNITED KINGDOM

Michel Cuénod
UNIVERSITY OF LAUSANNE, SWITZERLAND

Milka Culic
UNIVERSITY OF BELGRADE, YUGOSLAVIA

Kay Davies
UNIVERSITY OF OXFORD, UNITED KINGDOM

Jose Maria Delgado-Garcia
UNIVERSIDAD PABLO DE OLAVIDE, SEVILLE, SPAIN
PRESIDENT OF THE SPANISH NEUROSCIENCE SOCIETY

Johannes Dichgans
UNIVERSITY OF TÜBINGEN, GERMANY

Ray Dolan
UNIVERSITY COLLEGE LONDON, UNITED KINGDOM

Yadin Dudai
WEIZMANN INSTITUTE OF SCIENCE, REHOVOT, ISRAEL

Károly Elekes
HUNGARIAN ACADEMY OF SCIENCES, TIHANY, HUNGARY
PRESIDENT OF THE HUNGARIAN NEUROSCIENCE SOCIETY

Ferhan Esen
OSMANGAZI UNIVERSITY, ESKISEHIR, TURKEY

Ulf Eysel
RUHR-UNIVERSITÄT BOCHUM, GERMANY

Alberto Ferrus
INSTITUTO CAJAL, MADRID, SPAIN

Cesare Fieschi
UNIVERSITY OF ROME, ITALY

Russell Foster
UNIVERSITY OF OXFORD, UNITED KINGDOM

Richard Frackowiak
UNIVERSITY COLLEGE LONDON, UNITED KINGDOM
PRESIDENT OF THE BRITISH NEUROSCIENCE ASSOCIATION

Hans-Joachim Freund
UNIVERSITY OF DÜSSELDORF, GERMANY

Tamás Freund
UNIVERSITY OF BUDAPEST, HUNGARY
PRESIDENT OF FEDERATION OF EUROPEAN
NEUROSCIENCE SOCIETIES

Jean-Marc Fritschy
UNIVERSITY OF ZURICH, SWITZERLAND

Luis Garcia-Segura
INSTITUTO CAJAL, MADRID, SPAIN

Willem Gispen
UNIVERSITY OF UTRECHT, THE NETHERLANDS

Albert Gjedde
AARHUS UNIVERSITY HOSPITAL, DENMARK

Jacques Glowinski
COLLÈGE DE FRANCE, PARIS, FRANCE

Lady Susan Greenfield
THE ROYAL INSTITUTION OF GREAT BRITAIN,
LONDON, UNITED KINGDOM

Igor Grigorev
INSTITUTE FOR EXPERIMENTAL MEDICINE,
ST PETERSBURG, RUSSIA

Sten Grillner
KAROLINSKA INSTITUTE, STOCKHOLM, SWEDEN

Riitta Hari
HELSINKI UNIVERSITY OF TECHNOLOGY, ESPOO, FINLAND

Nuran Hariri
UNIVERSITY OF EGE, IZMIR, TURKEY; PRESIDENT
OF THE TURKISH NEUROSCIENCE SOCIETY

Anton Hermann
UNIVERSITY OF SALZBURG, AUSTRIA

Norbert Herschkowitz
UNIVERSITY OF BERN, SWITZERLAND

Etienne Hirsch
HÔPITAL DE LA SALPÊTRIÈRE, PARIS, FRANCE

Florian Holsboer
MAX-PLANCK-INSTITUTE OF PSYCHIATRY, MUNICH, GERMANY

Peter Holzer
UNIVERSITY OF GRAZ, AUSTRIA

Sir Andrew Huxley
UNIVERSITY OF CAMBRIDGE, UNITED KINGDOM

Giorgio Innocenti
KAROLINSKA INSTITUTE, STOCKHOLM, SWEDEN

Leslie Iversen
UNIVERSITY OF OXFORD, UNITED KINGDOM

Susan Iversen
UNIVERSITY OF OXFORD, UNITED KINGDOM

Julian Jack
UNIVERSITY OF OXFORD, UNITED KINGDOM

Marc Jeannerod
INSTITUT DES SCIENCES COGNITIVES, BRON, FRANCE

Barbro Johansson
LUND UNIVERSITY, SWEDEN

Leszek Kaczmarek
NENCKI INSTITUTE OF EXPERIMENTAL
BIOLOGY, WARSAW, POLAND

Markku Kaste
UNIVERSITY OF HELSINKI, FINLAND

Ann Kato
CENTRE MÉDICAL UNIVERSITAIRE, GENEVA, SWITZERLAND

Christopher Kennard
IMPERIAL COLLEGE SCHOOL OF MEDICINE,
LONDON, UNITED KINGDOM

Hubert Kerschbaum
UNIVERSITY OF SALZBURG, AUSTRIA

Helmut Kettenmann
MAX-DELBRÜCK-CENTRE FOR MOLECULAR
MEDICINE, BERLIN, GERMANY

Martin Korte
TECHNICAL UNIVERSITY BRAUNSCHWEIG, GERMANY

Malgorzata Kossut
NENCKI INSTITUTE OF EXPERIMENTAL
BIOLOGY, WARSAW, POLAND.

Elias Kouvelas
UNIVERSITY OF PATRAS, GREECE

Oleg Krishtal
BOGOMOLETZ INSTITUTE OF PHYSIOLOGY, KIEV, UKRAINE

Theodor Landis
UNIVERSITY HOSPITAL GENEVA, SWITZERLAND

Lars Lannfelt
UNIVERSITY OF UPPSALA,SWEDEN

Martin Lauritzen
UNIVERSITY OF COPENHAGEN, DENMARK

Juan Lerma
INSTITUTO DE NEUROCIENCIAS, CSIC-UMH, ALICANTE, SPAIN

Willem Levelt
MAX-PLANCK-INSTITUTE FOR PSYCHOLINGUISTICS,
NIJMEGEN, THE NETHERLANDS

Rita Levi-Montalcini
EUROPEAN BRAIN RESEARCH INSTITUTE, ROME, ITALY

Deolinda Lima
UNIVERSITY OF PORTO, PORTUGAL

José Lopez-Barneo

Menahem Segal
WEIZMANN INSTITUTE OF SCIENCE, REHOVOT, ISRAEL

Idan Segev
HEBREW UNIVERSITY, JERUSALEM, ISRAEL

Tim Shallice
UNIVERSITY COLLEGE LONDON, UNITED KINGDOM

Wolf Singer
MAX-PLANCK-INSTITUTE FOR BRAIN
RESEARCH, FRANKFURT, GERMANY

David Smth
UNIVERSITY OF OXFORD, UNITED KINGDOM

Henk Spekreijse
UNIVERSITY OF AMSTERDAM, THE NETHERLANDS

Günther Sperk
UNIVERSITY OF INNSBRUCK, AUSTRIA

Michael Stewart
THE OPEN UNIVERSITY, MILTON KEYNES, UNITED KINGDOM

Petra Stoerig
HEINRICH-HEINE UNIVERSITY, DÜSSELDORF, GERMANY

Piergiorgio Strata
UNIVERSITY OF TURIN, ITALY

Eva Sykova
INSTITUTE OF EXPERIMENTAL MEDICINE
ASCR, PRAGUE, CZECH REPUBLIC

Hans Thoenen
MAX-PLANCK-INSTITUTE FOR PSYCHIATRY,
MARTINSRIED, GERMANY

József Toldi
UNIVERSITY OF SZEGED, HUNGARY

Eduardo Tolosa
UNIVERSITY OF BARCELONA, SPAIN

Merab Tsagareli
BERITASHVILI INSTITUTE OF PHYSIOLOGY,
TBLISI, REPUBLIC OF GEORGIA

Jerzy Vetulani
INSTITUTE OF PHARMACOLOGY, KRAKOW, POLAND

Sylvester Vizi
HUNGARIAN ACADEMY OF SCIENCES, BUDAPEST, HUNGARY

Lord Walton of Detchant
UNIVERSITY OF OXFORD, UNITED KINGDOM

Hans Winkler
AUSTRIAN ACADEMY OF SCIENCES, AUSTRIA

Zvi Wollberg
HEBREW UNIVERSITY, SCHOOL OF MEDICINE, ISRAEL

Semir Zeki
UNIVERSITY COLLEGE LONDON, UNITED KINGDOM

Karl Zilles
HEINRICH-HEINE-UNIVERSITY, DÜSSELDORF, GERMANY

TERM MEMBERS

Francesc Artigas
SPANISH SOCIETY OF NEUROSCIENCE
UNIVERSITY OF BARCELONA, SPAIN

Friedrich G. Barth
AUSTRIAN ACADEMY OF SCIENCES, AUSTRIA

Gerard Boer
DUTCH NEUROFEDERATION, NETHERLANDS INSTITUTE
FOR BRAIN RESEARCH, THE NETHERLANDS

Marja Bresjanac
SLOVENIAN NEUROSCIENCE ASSOCIATION
(SINAPSA), LJUBLJANA, SLOVENIA

Eero Castrén
BRAIN RESEARCH SOCIETY OF FINLAND,
UNIVERSITY OF HELSINKI, FINLAND

Erik De Schutter
BELGIAN SOCIETY FOR NEUROSCIENCE,
UNIVERSITY OF ANTWERP, BELGIUM

Gaetano Di Chiara
UNIVERSITY OF CAGLIARI, ITALY

Aase Frandsen
DANISH SOCIETY FOR NEUROSCIENCE, COPENHAGEN
UNIVERSITY HOSPITAL, DENMARK

Dieter Heiss
EUROPEAN FEDERATION OF NEUROLOGICAL
SOCIETIES, UNIVERSITY OF KÖLN, GERMANY

Klaus-Peter Hoffmann
GERMAN NEUROSCIENCE SOCIETY, RUHR-
UNIVERSITÄT BOCHUM, GERMANY

Ferdinand Hucho
EUROPEAN SOCIETY FOR NEUROCHEMISTRY,
FREIE UNIVERSITÄT BERLIN, GERMANY

Simon Khechinashvili
GEORGIAN NEUROSCIENCE ASSOCIATION, BERITSASHVILI
INSTITUTE OF PHYSIOLOGY, TBLISI, REPUBLIC OF GEORGIA

Ivica Kostovic
INSTITUTE FOR BRAIN RESEARCH, ZAGREB, CROATIA

Julien Mendlewicz
EUROPEAN COLLEGE OF NEUROPSYCOPHARMACOLOGY,
ULB ERASME HOSPITAL, BRUSSELS, BELGIUM

Ryszard Przewlocki
POLISH NEUROSCIENCE SOCIETY, POLISH
ACADEMY OF SCIENCES, KRAKOW,POLAND

Geneviéve Rougon
INSTITUT DE BIOLOGIE DU DEVELOPPEMENT
DE MARSEILLE CNRS, FRANCE

Eric M. Rouiller
SWISS SOCIETY OF NEUROSCIENCE, UNIVERSITY
OF FRIBOURG, SWITZERLAND

Terje Sagvolden
UNIVERSITY OF OSLO, NORWAY
NORWEGIAN NEUROSCIENCE SOCIETY

Ana Sebastião
PORTUGUESE SOCIETY FOR NEUROSCIENCE,
UNIVERSITY OF LISBON, PORTUGAL

Fotini Stylianopoulou
HELLENIC SOCIETY FOR NEUROSCIENCE,
UNIVERSITY OF ATHENS, GREECE

Josef Syka
CZECH NEUROSCIENCE SOCIETY, ACADEMY OF
SCIENCES, PRAGUE, CZECH REPUBLIC

Zvi Wollberg
ISRAEL SOCIETY FOR NEUROSCIENCE,
TEL AVIV UNIVERSITY, ISRAEL

Leon Zagrean
NATIONAL NEUROSCIENCE SOCIETY OF ROMANIA, CAROL
DAVILA UNIVERSITY OF MEDICINE, BUCHAREST, ROMANIA

About the Editors

Floyd E. Bloom, M.D., Professor Emeritus in the Molecular and Integrative Neuroscience Department, was formerly the Chairman of the Department of Neuropharmacology at The Scripps Research Institute in California. Bloom is one of the major architects of modern brain science. He was the first to appreciate the need for in-depth study of neurotransmitter systems and was one of the first neurobiologists to use modern molecular biological techniques to explore brain function. His work has contributed to the development of treatments for numerous disorders, including addiction, dementia, and major psychoses. His past positions include Director of Behavioral Neurobiology at The Salk Institute and Chief of the Laboratory of Neuropharmacology of the National Institute of Mental Health. He is a member of the National Academy of Sciences and the Institute of Medicine, a past-president of the American Association for the Advancement of Science, of the Society for Neuroscience, and of the American College on Neuropsychopharmacology, and recipient of numerous awards and honors. From May 1995 through June 2000, he was editor in chief of *Science*, the world's leading peer-reviewed scientific journal, and in 2000 was co-founder of a biotech startup, Neurome, Inc., serving as its chief executive for two years. Dr. Bloom lives in San Diego with his wife, Jody Corey-Bloom, M.D., Ph.D., Professor of Neuroscience at the University of California, San Diego.

M. Flint Beal, M.D., an internationally recognized authority on neurodegenerative disorders, is Neurologist in Chief of the New York and Presbyterian Hospital and Anne Parrish Titzell Professor and Chairman of Neurology at the Weill Medical College of Cornell University in New York City. Author or co-author of more than 300 scientific articles and more than 100 books, book chapters, and book reviews, he was named in 2000 one of the Institute of Scientific Information's Most Highly Cited Researchers. He serves on the editorial boards of seven journals, including *Annals of Neurology, Journal of Molecular Neuroscience, Experimental Neurology*, and *Neurobiology of Disease*. He is listed in the second edition of *America's Top Doctors*. His own research focuses on the mechanisms of neural degeneration in Alzheimer's, Huntington's, and Parkinson's diseases, and in amyotrophic lateral sclerosis (ALS, or Lou Gehrig's disease). Before moving to Cornell, Dr. Beal was Professor of Neurology at Harvard Medical School and chief of the neurochemistry laboratory at Massachusetts General Hospital. He is a member of the Alpha Omega Alpha Medical Honorary Society and recipient of the Derek Denny-Brown Neurological Scholar Award of the American Neurological Association. He serves on the Council of the American Neurological Association and is on the science advisory committees of several disease organizations. He is vice president of the American Neurological Association. He is a member of the Institute of Medicine of the National Academy of Sciences. He lives in New York City with his wife, Judy Beal, Ph.D., Dean for Nursing at Simmons College in Boston, Massachusetts.

David J. Kupfer, M.D., is Thomas Detre Professor and Chairman of the Department of Psychiatry at the University of Pittsburgh School of Medicine and Director of Research at the Western Psychiatric Institute and Clinic. Elected to the Institute of Medicine of the National Academy of Sciences in 1990, he has written more than 915 articles, books, and book chapters on the use of medication in depression, the causes of depression, and the relationship between biological rhythms, sleep, and depression. He is a past president of the American College of Neuropsychopharmacology and the Society of Biological Psychiatry and has received numerous awards and honors, including the A. E. Bennett Research Award in Clinical Science, the Institute of Medicine's 1998 Rhoda and Bernard Sarnat International Prize in Mental Health, and the Twenty-sixth Annual Award of the Institute of Pennsylvania Hospital in Memory of Edward A. Strecker. He and his wife, Dr. Ellen Frank, Professor of Psychiatry and Psychology at the University of Pittsburgh School of Medicine, live in Pittsburgh, Pennsylvania.

Index

(Page numbers in *italics* refer to illustrations. Page numbers in **boldface** refer to main discussions of conditions, diseases, and disorders.)

abscesses, ataxia and, 501–2, 503

absence (petit mal) seizures, 176, 320, *321*

abstinence, addiction and, 424

abstract thinking, 107, 131, 172, 272, 639

abuse, in early life, 93, 99, 365, 372, 395, 396, 637

acamprosate, 425

acetaminophen, 168, 446, 543, 563, 629

acetazolamide, 661

acetylcholine, 43, 144, 366, 602; Alzheimer's disease and, 627, 629; myasthenia gravis and, 531–32, 533

acetylcholinesterase, 618

acoustic neuroma, 305, 343

acrylamide monomer, 618

action potentials, 9–10

action tremor, 490

acupuncture, 369, 370, 546

acute disseminated encephalomyelitis (ADEM), 436, 438, 462

acyclovir, 446, 447, 464, 521, 661

addiction, 11, 26, 111, 184, 365, **411–18;** adolescent substance

abuse and, 111; brain mechanisms and, 413–14, 415; contributing factors to, 413; definition and recognition of, 411–12; prevalence of, 413; prognosis for, 416–18; resource groups for, 680; signs of, 412; tolerance and, 412, 414–16; treatment of, 415–16; withdrawal and, 176–77, 319, 354, 412, 414–16, 419, 424, 425. *See also* alcoholism

A-delta fibers, 166

adjustment disorder with depressed mood, 364

adolescence, 102–15; brain maturation in, 104–9, *106, 196,* 197; brain trauma in, 110–11; cognitive development in, 104–7; mental disorders in, 112–14 *(see also* childhood, conditions that appear in); myelination in, 105, 107, 108, 114; puberty and, 103–4, 107–9, 113, 152; risk taking in, 109–12; sports in, 109–10; substance abuse in, 103, 110, 111–12; suicide in, 110, 114, 431; teenage pregnancy and, 261

adrenal glands, 37, 103, 143, 146, 147–48, 151, 432, 640; stress response and, 48, *49,* 407; tumors in, 285, 303

adrenaline. *See* epinephrine

adrenal medulla, 47, 144

adrenocorticosteroids, 603, 640, 661, 666

adrenocorticotrophic hormone (ACTH), *49,* 145, 147, 149, 432

adrenoleukodystrophy, 281

adult brain, 116–31; continued growth and development of, 120–21; disorders in, 122–23; habits for long-term health and, 129–30; habituation and, *117,* 117–18; memory and, 123–25; myth of older brain and, 130–31; "normality" and, 118–19; plasticity of, 116–17, 119–20, 122. *See also* aging

Advance Directives, 634

advanced sleep-phase syndrome, 312

aerobic exercise, 36–37, 38–39, 52, 121

affect, 183, 184

affective disorders. *See* mood disorders

agensia, 140

age-related macular degeneration (AMD), 338–39, *339*

aggression, 111, 149, 186, 194, 206, 401, **426–28;** borderline personality disorder and, 394, 397; brain mechanisms and, 426–27, *427;* emotion regulation and, 426, 427–28; environmental influence and, 428; impulsive vs. premeditated, 426

aggressive behavior: Alzheimer's disease and, 626, 631

aging, 12, 22, 124–31, *127,* 199, 208, 605, 613, 625; attention and, 127, 197; autonomic disorders and, 354; corpus callosum and, 126–27; dementia and, 12, 39, 130, 639; depression and, 128–29; everyday creativity and, 239; hearing loss and, 341, 344; intelligence and, 212, *213,* 215; language abilities and, 230; memory and, 124–25, *223,* 223–25, 626; movement and, 164; neuron loss and, 126; neurotoxins and, 620; reflexes and, 127–28; senses and, 140, 348–49; sexual function and, 152; sleep patterns and, 128, *128,* 157; stimulation and, 39–40; vision problems and, 338–39, *339;* white matter loss and, 125–26, 127, 128

agitation, 426; suicide and, 429, 431, 432, 433

agnosias, 46, 218, 637, 639, **651–53;** auditory, 652–53; diagnosis and treatment of, 653; tactile, 653; visual, 233, 235, 651–52, 653

agoraphobia, 330, 331, 372

agraphia, 645–46; apraxic, 649

AIDS. *See* HIV/AIDS

AIDS dementia complex (ADC), 451

air travel headache, 544

akinesia, 163, 477, 484

akinetic-rigid syndrome, 484

alcohol, 40, 51, 53, 157, 326, 365, 372, 377, 394, 406, 409, 410, 416, 420, 515, 579, 620, 640; aging and, 129; blood level of, 423; brain function and, 422, 423; prenatal development and, 72, 81, 257, 260–61, 278; sleep disorders and, 308, 309, 314

alcohol abuse: by adolescents, 111–12; altered states of consciousness and, 176, 177; binge drinking and, 420; defined, 420; hangover and, 540, 543; intelligence and, 215, 216; tremors and, 491, 492. *See also* substance abuse

alcoholic neuropathy, 420

Alcoholics Anonymous (AA), 415, 417, 423–24

alcoholism, 122, 163, 176, 184, 365, 377, 412, 413, 414, 417, **419–25,** *421,* 429, 635; causes of, 420–21; damage caused by, 420; diagnosis of, 422–23; intelligence and, 215; nutritional disorders and, 610, 611, 612, 614; resource groups for, 680–81; symptoms of, 419–20; teenage alcohol use and, 111, 112; treatment of, 415, 423–25; withdrawal symptoms and, 176–77, 319, 354, 414, 419, 424, 425. *See also* addiction

alexia, 233, 645–46

alien limb phenomenon, 489

allergic reactions, to medications, 140, 640

all-night sleep recordings, *308,* 309

allodynia, 444

alpha-fetoprotein (AFP), 76, 296

alpha-2 agonists, 500

alprazolam, 375, 661

alteplase-recombinant, 661

altered states of consciousness, 176–77

Alzheimer, Alois, 18, 625

Alzheimer's Association, 631

Alzheimer's disease, 12, 13, 18, 22, 25, 26, 36, 130, 163, 177, 199, 208, 215, 290, 420, 468, 478, 537, 602, 605, 616, **625–34,** 649, 653; aphasia and, 645, 647; brain changes in, *627,* 627–28, *628;* caregivers of people with, 148; considerations for family and friends coping with, 632–33; dementia and, 125, 177, 198, 626, 628, 641, 642; depression and, 365, 626, 628–29, 630; diagnosis of, 626–27; drug treatments for, 629–30; dyslexia and, 251; late stages of, 631–34; memory impairment and, 18, 124–25, 625–26, 627, 629, 630, 635, 638; other treatments for, 630–31; parkinsonism and, 486; resource groups for, 685–86; risk factors for, 628–29; smelling ability and, 350–51; symptoms of, 625–26; wandering away from home and, 631

amantadine, 481, 661

amblyopia, 87

American Association on Mental Retardation (AAMR), 259

American Psychiatric Association, 183–84, 410

American Spinal Injury Association, 592

amino acids, 278

aminoglycoside antibiotics, 343

amiodarone, 515

amitriptyline, 368, 403, 544, 564, 630, 661

amnesias, 176, 218, 224, 225, **635–38;** diagnosis and treatment of, 637–38; functional, 635, 637; organic, 635–37; retrograde and anterograde, 635–36

amniocentesis, 76, 77, 259

amobarbital, 661

amoxapine, 661

amoxicillin, 456

amphetamines, 111, 258, 318, 354, 392, 410, 415, 416, 500, 579, 661

amygdala, 68, 151, 168, 354; decision making and, 204–5, *205;* development of, 106, 108; emotions and, *181,* 181–82, 219, 223; fear network and, 373, *373;* senses and, *137;* temperament and, 96–97, 192; violence and aggression and, 427, *427*, 428

amyloid protein, 627–28, 629

amyotrophic lateral sclerosis (ALS), 130, 162, 523, **535–38**, 557, 599, 646; diagnosis of, 536; mechanisms of, 535–36, *536*; patterns of, 537; resource groups for, 683; treatment and care for, 537–38

anabolic steroids, 410

analgesics. *See* pain relievers

anemia, 312, 330, 613, 640

anencephaly, 64, 76, 615

anesthesia, 168, 177

anesthesia dolorosa, 567

aneurysm, 541, 553, 578, 579, 580

anger, 50, 52–53, 397, 430; violence and aggression and, 426, 427, 428

angiography, 573, 578, 606

angular gyrus, 91, 92

animals, 135, 162, 196; brain of, *4*, 5; narcolepsy in, 316; overeating in, *153*, 153–54; pain-modulating pathway in, 169; parenthood and, 119–20

animal studies, 15, 19–22, 32, 36–37, 45, 62; treatment of animals in, 20

annulus fibrosus, 555

anorexia nervosa, 44, 113, 156, 399–404, *400*, 626; causes of, 401–2; criteria defining, 399–400; diagnosis and treatment of, 402–3; nutritional disorders and, 613, 615, 616; recovery and mortality rates for, 403–4; resource groups for, 679

anosmia, 140, 347, 348, 349, 350–51

anterior cingulate cortex (ACC), 198, 205, *205*, 428

anterior cingulate gyrus, 105, 562

anterior commissure, *78*, 79

anterior fontanel, 289

anterograde amnesia, 636

antibiotics, side effects of, 343, 621

antibodies: lupus and, 472–73, 474; multiple sclerosis and, 438, 439, 441; paraneoplastic, 601, 602

anticancer drugs: neurotoxic diseases and, 617, 619, 621, 623. *See also* chemotherapy

anticholinergic medications, 480, 499, 640

anticholinesterase medications, 492, 533, 629, 642

anticipation phenomenon, 29

anticoagulant medications, 335, 340

anticonvulsant medications, 313, 388, 408, 424, 564, 631

antidepressant medications, 318, 354, 408, 564, 642; Alzheimer's disease and, 630, 631; anxiety and panic and, 374–75; bipolar disorder and, 387; borderline personality disorder and, 397–98; changes associated with psychotherapy compared to, 122, 367, 369; depression and, 367–69, 422; eating disorders and, 403; Huntington's disease and, 509–10; placebo effect and, 55. *See also* selective serotonin reuptake inhibitors; tricyclic antidepressants; *specific antidepressants*

antiepileptic medications, 324, 619, 621

antigens, 602

antigravity system, 162

antioxidants, 129–30, 481, 630

antiphospholipid antibody, 473

antipsychotic medications, 387, 388, 393, 398, 403, 509, 510, 631, 642

antisocial personality disorder, 413

anxiety, 31, 40, 52, 99, 122, 156, 174, 205, 251, 264, 273, 314, 330, 354, 365, **371–75**, 382, 405, 412, 422, 431, 468, 477, 492, 498, 549; brain mechanisms and, 372–73, *373*; chronic fatigue syndrome and, 357, 359; diagnosis of, 373–74; generalized anxiety disorder (GAD), 371, 372–75; headache and, 543, 546; helping someone suffering from, 375;

obsessive-compulsive disorder and, 379, 380; resource groups for, 678–79; social (social phobia), 374, 376–78, 678–79; symptoms of, 371–72; temperament and, 193–94; treatment of, 374–75. *See also* panic attacks; panic disorder

anxiety-management therapy, 374, 408

anxiety-relieving drugs (anxiolytics), 374–75, 378, 398, 413, 415, 417, 642

apathy, 486

Apgar evaluation, 83

aphasia, 6–7, 489, 639, **643–47**, 653; diagnosis and treatment of, 646–47; mechanisms of, 643–46

apolipoprotein E (ApoE) gene, 628, 629

apoptosis, 77–80, 536

appetite, 147, 150, 336, 366; depression and, 363, 364, 385, 430

apraxias, 163, 219, 489, 637, 639, 646, **648–50;** diagnosis and treatment of, 650; limb, five major forms of, 648–49; mechanisms of, 649–50

apraxic agraphia, 649

Armed Services Vocational Aptitude Battery (ASVAB), 211

Arnold Chiari malformation, 294–96, *296*

arousal, 174, 182, 222, 359

arsenic, 515, 620, 621

arteries: blockages of, 571–72; vascular headache and, 542–43

arthritis, 166, 168, 329, 495, 559, 562; lupus and, 471; Lyme disease and, 454, 455, 456

arthropod-borne viruses (arboviruses), 462, 464–66, *465*

ascorbic acid (vitamin C), 611, 615

Asperger's syndrome, 270, 271, 272, 382

aspirin, 147, 168, 335, 343, 475, 543, 563, 564, 573, 574, 629

association areas, 639

associative agnosia, 651, 652
astrocytomas, 301, 302, 304, 606–7
ataxia, 163, 279, 473, 487, **501–4,** *502,* 516; causes of, 502; diagnosis and treatment of, 501, 503–4; medical emergencies and, 501–2; nutritional disorders and, 611, 612, 613, 616; resource groups for, 682; symptoms of, 501
atenolol, 378, 661
atherosclerosis, 164, 571–72, 579
athletics, 109–10. *See also* exercise
atonic seizures, 320–21
atrial fibrillation, 573
atrophy, 525, 641; spinal cord injury and, 591, 595. *See also* multiple system atrophy
attention, 21, 43, 172, 175, 196–99, 256, 308; aging and, 127; brain development and, *91,* 100, 105, 118; deficits in, 172, 175, 176–77, 254, 273, 436, 611; defined, 196–97; disorders of, 198; prefrontal cortex and, 197, 198, *199;* spatial, 234, *234,* 235
attention deficit/hyperactivity disorder (ADHD), 98, 99, 194, 198, 199, 251, **254–58,** 262–63, 271, 383; in adulthood, 255; advice for parents of children with, 257; brain mechanisms and, 255–56; diagnosis of, 256, 257–58; genetic and nongenetic factors in, 256–57; medication strategies for, 255, 256, 258; resource groups for, 673–74; three subtypes of, 254; Tourette's syndrome and, 497, 498, 499, 500
atypical depression, 364
audiograms, 345–46
auditory agnosias, 652–53
auditory cortex, 22, 63, 86, *138, 139, 229,* 653
auditory evoked brain-stem response, 344
auditory nerve, 139, 341, 342, 346; disorders of, 343; tumors on or near, 140, 305, 343

auditory-visual processing disorders, 253
aura, migraine and, 548, 549, 550
autism, 26, 46, 98, 198, 238, 263, 264, **270–77;** causes of, 98, 273–74; diagnosis of, 274–75; manifestations of, 270–73; resource groups for, 674; treatment and teaching for, 98, 275–77
Autism Diagnostic Instrument (ADI), 275
autoantibodies, 474
autoimmune disorders, 472; chronic fatigue syndrome and, 359; encephalomyelitis, 436, 438, 462, 466–67; narcolepsy and, 317. *See also* Guillain-Barré syndrome; multiple sclerosis; myasthenia gravis; systemic lupus erythematosus
autologous bone marrow rescue, 300
automations, 321
autonomic disorders, 148, **352–56;** diagnosis and treatment of, 355–56; problems and their causes, 352–54; resource groups for, 678
autonomic nervous system (ANS), 47, 151, 160, 192, 219, 330, 420, 487, 517; acute pain and, 559; anxiety and, 372, 373; body regulation and, 143–45, 146, 148, 160, 352, 554; eating behavior and, 44; overactivity of, 354; spinal cord injury and, 591
axons, 10, 11–12, 17, *17,* 74–75, 81, 84, 99, 160–61, 222; diffuse axonal injury and, 586; myelination of, *80,* 80–81, *91;* stimulating growth of, 598
azathioprine, 441, 534

Babinski sign, 536, 557
back: normal wear and tear and, 556; spinal anatomy and, 553–54

back pain, 122, **553–58,** 559; cervical spondylotic myelopathy and, 556, 557; disk herniation and, 436, 494, 553–57, *554;* lumbar spinal stenosis and, 556, 557–58; resource groups for, 685; spondylosis and, 555, 556–57
baclofen, 268, 567, 662
bacterial toxins, 617, 622
balance, 45, 94, 136, 158–64, *328*
balance problems, 299, 468, 473, 501, 505, 605; dizziness and, 327–31; multiple sclerosis and, 336, 435; parkinsonism and, 479, 484, 487
barbiturates, 503, 614
Barrington's nucleus, 145
basal ganglia, 68, 94, 174, 192, 229, 255, 381, 386, 391, 577, 641; autonomic disorders and, 352–53; cerebral palsy and, 266, 267, *268,* 269; Huntington's disease and, 507; movement and, 160, 163, 164; parkinsonism and, 479, 480, 483, 486, 488; VZV latent in, 445, 447
basic behaviors, 143, 146–47
basic drives, 150–57; concepts of, 152–53; differences and disorders of, 155–57; recent discoveries about, 153–54
Becker muscular dystrophy, 526
behavioral genetics, 212–13, 238
behavioral intelligence, *173,* 173–74
behavioral therapy, 374. *See also* cognitive behavioral therapy
Behçet's disease, 472
Bell's palsy, **420–22,** 435, 454; diagnosis and treatment of, 520–22; symptoms of, 520, *521*
benign paroxysmal positional vertigo (BPPV), 328–29
benzodiazepines, 329, 330, 373, 374, 375, 378, 398, 413, 424, 493, 622, 631; sleep disorders and, 310, 312, 314
benztropine, 499, 662
beta-adrenergic antagonists, 631

beta-amyloid peptide, 627
beta-blockers, 378, 493, 541
betel nut, 410, 411
bethanechol chloride, 662
bicycle helmets, 31, *32*, 101, 111
bilateral thalamotomy, 493
binge drinking, 420
binge eating, 394, 399, 400, 401, 403. *See also* bulimia nervosa
biofeedback, 546
biological rhythms. *See* circadian rhythms
biological toxins, 617
biopsy, 299, 302, 525–26, 606
biotin, 611, 615
bipolar disorder (manic-depressive illness), 113, 122, 183, 359, 364, 367, 374, **385–89**, *387*, 395, 413; creativity and, 240, *241*, 242–44; diagnosis and treatment of, 387–89; relapse prevention and, 388, 389; resource groups for, 678; searching for cause of, 386–87; suicide and, 243, 364, 385, 386, 429, 433
bipolar spectrum disorder, 386
birth control pills, 365, 370
birth defects, 34, 64, 72, 76, 615. *See also* spina bifida
birth injuries, 267, *268*, 496
bladder, 144, 145, 148, 160, 554
bladder dysfunction, 355, 356, 612; back problems and, 553, 555, 557; multiple sclerosis and, 336, 436, 440, 443; parkinsonism and, 478, 487, 488; spinal cord injury and, 591, 593
blepharospasm, 495
blindness, 86, 233, 283, 435, 461, 467, 524, 541, 601; coping with, 337; visual agnosias and, 651–52. *See also* vision problems
blood-brain barrier, 300, 609, 617, *618*
blood flow in brain, 122, 353, 636, 640; ADHD and, 256; aging and, 125; brain ischemia and ischemic stroke and, 570–75; depression and, 365, 366; exercise

and, 36, 121; injuries involving vessels within skull and, 583–85; PET and MRI technology and, 23, 26; smoking and, 129; vision problems and, 338–40
blood pressure, 52, 166, 176, 355, 487, 517, 591; chronic fatigue syndrome and, 360; doctor's visits and, 56; high *(see* hypertension); orthostatic hypotension and, 329–30, 353, 354, 355; regulation of, 142, 143, 145, 147, 148, 160, 352; stress and, 37, 48, 50, 53; stroke and, 572, 573, 574, 579
bloodstream, monitoring of, 45, 143, 147
blood thinners, 335, 573, 579
blood vessels: in brain, structural abnormalities in, 319; lupus and, 473
body dysmorphic disorder, 381
body function, disorders of, 306–61. *See also* autonomic disorders; chronic fatigue syndrome; dizziness; epilepsy; narcolepsy; seizures; sleep disorders; vertigo
body image, distorted, 400, *400*
body regulation, 142–49, 160, 554; autonomic disorders and, 148, 352–56; basic behaviors and, 143, 146–47; emotions and, 182, 183; endocrine system and, 143, 145–46, 148–49; monitoring of internal organs and, 142–43; neuroimmunology and, 147–48; peripheral nervous system and, *144*, 148; spinal cord injury and, 591
body temperature, 32, 45, 293, 366; brain temperature and, 156; regulation of, 146, *147*, 149; sleep deprivation and, 155; stress and, 97
body weight, 44, 47; overweight, 54, 101, 573. *See also* obesity
bone marrow, 283, 300
bone spurs, 553, 554, 556, 557

borderline personality disorder, **394–98**, 429; causes of, 396; diagnosis and treatment of, 396–98; family members and, 395; manifestations of, 394–95; resource groups for, 679
Borrelia burgdorferi, 453–57. *See also* Lyme disease
botulinum toxin, 268, 489, 493, 499, 662
bovine spongiform encephalopathy, 469–70
bowel, 144, 145, 148, 160
bowel dysfunction, 355, 612; back problems and, 555, 557; multiple sclerosis and, 436, 440, 443; parkinsonism and, 478, 487, 488; spinal cord injury and, 591
bradykinesia, 477, 484, 505
brain, *2, 3*–57; blood flow in *(see* blood flow in brain); bottom-up approach to, 8–11; caring for, 31–40, 101, 120; chemical processes in, 10–11, 14, 15; electrical charges in *(see* electrical charges in brain); gender differences in, *78*, 79; glucose metabolism in *(see* glucose metabolism in brain); human vs. animal, *4*, 5; learning secrets of, 14–30 *(see also* neuroscience); myth that we use only ten percent of, 10; plasticity of *(see* plasticity); regions of, 3–5, 15–16; size and weight of, 3, 84, 119, 126, 213–14; temperature of, 156; top-down approach to, 5–8; variability of, 197–98. *See also specific topics*
brain-body loop, 41–57, *42*; circadian rhythms and, 42–44, *43, 47*; disorders in, 54; eating behavior and, 44, 47; learning and, 46–47; mind-body medicine and, 53–57; mood and emotions and, 41, 51–53; navigating our environment and, 45–46; sexual response and, 45; stress and, 47–51

brain cancer. *See* brain tumors; brain tumors of childhood

brain cells. *See* glial cells; neurons

brain-derived neurotrophic factor (BDNF), 36, 121

brain development, 61–102; in adolescence, 104–9, *106, 196,* 197; in adulthood, 120–21; genes and, 11, 66, 68, 69, 73, 86, 87; nature and nurture and, 11, 64–66, 84, 86–87; stimulation and, 39–40, 66. *See also* adolescence; adult brain; child development; prenatal development

brain-imaging technologies, 23–27, 98; other technologies combined with, 27–28

brain infarct, 570

brain stem, 3, 5, 43, 45, 68, 139, *142,* 150, 161, 166, 198, 341, 349, 432, 435, 479, 521, 540, 588; Arnold Chiari malformation and, 294–96, *296;* ataxia and, 502, *502;* body regulation and, 142, 145, 146; consciousness and, 174, 175; dizziness and, 329, 330, 331; hemorrhage in, 577; movement and, 160, 162, 502; parkinsonism and, 486, 488; tumors in, 299, 301, 304, 345, 354, 606, 607

brain surgery, 19. *See also specific conditions and procedures*

brain swelling: head trauma and, 582, 587–89; tumors and, 604–5, 609. *See also* encephalitis

"brain track" analogy, 188–89

brain trauma. *See* head trauma

brain tumors, 19, 148, 288, 319, 521, 531, 557, 579, **604–9,** 640, 649; ataxia and, 501–2, 503; on or near auditory nerve, 140, 305, 343; benign vs. malignant, 604; in brain stem, 299, 301, 304, 345, 354, 606, 607; causes of, 605; cell phones and, 38, 605; challenges of, to patient and family, 608; diagnosis of, 605–6; gliomas, 301–2, *606,* 606–7, 608, 609;

headache and, 298, 299, 541, 542, 548, 605; memory impairment and, 605, 635; meningiomas, 286, 604, 605, 606, 607, 608; neurofibromatosis and, 285; in pituitary, 336–38, 604, 607; primary central nervous system lymphoma, 450; primary vs. secondary, 604; resource groups for, 685; risk factors for, 605; speech and language difficulties and, 605, 645, 646; symptoms of, 604–5; treatment of, 608–9; trigeminal neuralgia and, 566, 567; types of, 606–8; use of term, 604; vision problems and, 232, 299, 302, 336–38

brain tumors of childhood, 92, **298–305,** 607; common, by location (chart), 304; embryonal tumors, 302–3; emotional impact of, 299; hydrocephalus and, 288, 290, 299, 300, 302; resource groups for, 675; symptoms of, 298–99; treatment of, 299–301

breakfast and the brain, 35

breathing, 145, 160; diaphragmatic, 374, 375, 546; hyperventilation and, 330, 331, 374; sexual response and, 45, 151; stress and, 37, 97

breathing difficulties, 502; Guillain-Barré syndrome and, 516–17, 518; muscular dystrophy and, 527; spinal cord injury and, 591

Broca, Paul, 6, 17–18, 228

Broca's area, 6, 18, 63, 89, 91, 120, 228, *228, 229*

Brodal, Per, 75

bromocriptine, 312, 337, 662

brucellosis, 460

bulimia nervosa, 113, 399–404; causes of, 401–2; criteria defining, 400–401; diagnosis and treatment of, 402–3; recovery and mortality rates for, 404; resource groups for, 679

Bunina bodies, 536

buprenorphine, 416

bupropion, 368, 415, 662

buspirone, 374, 378, 398, 662

B vitamins, 34, 438, 503, 515, 538, 557, 610–14, 615, 640. *See also* folic acid

caffeine, 222, 309, 314, 409, 410, 416, 492–93; headache and, 543

CAGE test, 423

calcium, 71, 146, 494, 550, 616

calcium channel blockers, 564

cAMP (cyclic adenosine monophosphate), 598

cancer, 111, 298, 417, 445, 460, 503, 529, 537, 553, 572, 614; chronic pain and, 559, 560–61, 562, 564; depression and, 55, 605; paraneoplastic syndromes and, 600–603. *See also* brain tumors; brain tumors of childhood

cancer centers, for children, 300

cannabinoids, 410, 413, 415, 416

Cannon, Walter, 47–48, 146

CA1 region, 225

capsulotomy, 384

carbamazepine, 314, 324, 388, 424, 446, 547, 567, 621, 662

carbidopa, 481, 664

cardiovascular system, *42*

carpal tunnel syndrome, 436, 512–13

cars. *See* driving safety; vehicular accidents

catalepsy, 315

cataplexy, 308, 315, 316, 317, 318

cataracts, 21, 122–23

catecholamines, 52

cauda equina, 553, 555, 557, 558

caudate nucleus, 18, 223

CD4 T lymphocyte, 448, 449

cefotaxime, 456

ceftriaxone, 456

celecoxib, 168, 662

cell phones, 38, 605

cell transplant therapy, 595, 598–99

centenarians, study of, 39–40

central nervous system (CNS), 67, 215, 511; injuries to (*see* nervous system injuries); neurotoxic diseases and, 617, 618, 623; pain and, 561, 562, 563. *See also specific topics*

central nervous system infections: HIV/AIDS and, 449–50; Lyme disease and, 455, 456

central nervous system lymphoma, primary, 450

central pattern generator (CPG), 595

central sensitization, 168

central sleep apnea syndrome, 311, 312

CEO analogy, 187

cerebellar tremor, 490, 491

cerebellar vermis, 99

cerebellum, 3, 5, 16, 94, 118, 174, 229, 255, 330, 391, 435, 488, 641; Arnold Chiari malformation and, 294–96, *296;* ataxia and, 502, *502,* 504; cerebral palsy and, 266; degeneration of, 468, 492, 616; hemorrhage in, 577; movement and, 160, *160,* 162, 163, 502; paraneoplastic syndromes and, 601, 602; prenatal development and, 68, 69; tumors in, 301, 302–3, 304, 606, *606*

cerebral palsy (CP), 86, 264, **265–69,** 325; brain MRI scans and, *268;* causes of, 265, 266–67, 278, 283; classifications of, 266; diagnosis of, 267, 269; resource groups for, 674; symptoms of, 265; treatment of, 267–69

cerebral toxoplasmosis, 450

cerebrospinal fluid (CSF), 160, *289,* 582, 585; brain tumors and, 299, 302; 5-HIAA concentration in, 426; hydrocephalus and, 288–92; Lyme disease and, 455; meningitis and, 458, 460–61, *461;* spinal tap and, 460–61, *461,* 541, 553

cervical nerves, *592*

cervical spondylotic myelopathy, 556, 557

C-fibers, 166

change, habituation and, *117,* 117–18

channelopathies, 550–51

Charcot disease, 535. *See also* amyotrophic lateral sclerosis

Charcot-Marie-Tooth neuropathy, 514

chemicals, neurotoxic. *See* neurotoxins and neurotoxic diseases

chemotherapy, 515, 607, 608, 609; childhood tumors and, 299–303

chemotrophic factors, 75

chicken pox, 444–45, 466

child development, 12, 83–101; attachment with parent or primary caretaker and, 93, 95; cognitive development and, 94–95; critical periods and, 21, *85,* 85–90; enhancement of stimulation and, 39, 101; enrichment of environment and, 95–96; extreme deprivation and adversity and, 92–93; gradual building of skills in, 94–96; helping children explore world and, 99–101; language acquisition and, 23, 84, 86, 90–92, 99–100, 227–28, 230; memory and, 91, 94, 95; milestones of, 91; mother's depression and, 100; myelination and, 81, 85, *91,* 95; nature and nurture and, 84, 86–87; neurological impairments and, 97–99; neuronal branching and, 84–87, *85;* newborns and, 83–90, 94 *(see also* infants); nutrition and, 33–34; premature births and, 86; pruning and, 85–87; supportive care and, 92–94; temperament and, 96–97; between toddlerhood and puberty, 99–101; toddler years and, 84, 92–99; vision and, 86, 87, 88–89, 91. *See also* adolescence; prenatal development

childhood, conditions that appear in, 97–99, 112–14, 247–305. *See also* attention deficit/hyperac-

tivity disorder; autism; brain tumors of childhood; cerebral palsy; dyslexia; hydrocephalus; mental retardation; metabolic diseases; neurofibromatosis; spina bifida

childhood disintegrative disorder (CDD), 270

children, 623; air travel and, 544; chicken pox in, 444–45; epilepsy and seizures in, 319, 320, 322, 324; hearing loss in, 344; measles in, 466; meningitis in, 459, 460, 461; narcolepsy in, 316; neurotoxic problems in, 617; nutritional needs of, 33–34, 35; obsessive-compulsive disorder in, 379, 381, 382–83, 384; parkinsonism in, 485; separation anxiety in, *191;* sleepwalking and night terrors in, 313–14; temperament of, 190–91, 192–94, *193;* Tourette's syndrome in, 498, 499. *See also* adolescence; infants

chin tremor, 491

chlorpromazine, 387, 393, 403, 622, 662

cholesterol, 278, 571; blood level of, 35–36, 339, 432, 502, 515, 524, 572, 573, 579, 612, 616; dietary, 35–36; transient ischemic attacks and, 334, 335

cholinesterase inhibitors, 492, 533, 629, 642

chorea, 473, 505, 509

choreo-athetosis, 163

chorionic villus sampling (CVS), 77, 259

choroid plexus, 288

choroid plexus papillomas, 303, 304

chromosomes, 28, 77, 508

chronic fatigue immune dysfunction syndrome (CFIDS), 359

chronic fatigue syndrome (CFS), **357–61;** diagnosis of, 358–59, 360; possible origins of, 359–60; support groups for, 358; symp-

chronic fatigue syndrome (CFS) (*cont.*)
  toms of, 357–58; treatment of, 360–61
chronic inflammatory demyelinating polyneuropathy (CIDP), 518
chronic pain. *See* pain, chronic
chronic wasting disease (CWD), 470
chronological ordering of events, 172
cingulotomy, 384, 564
circadian rhythms, 143, 147, *147*, 360; brain-body loop and, 42–44, *43*, 47; disorders of, 311, 388–89
cisapride, 662
citalopram, 368
clomipramine, 383, 662
clonazepam, 314, 375, 378, 489, 499, 662
clonidine, 499, 500, 662
clopidogrel, 662, 674
clots, 52, 53, 572, 573, 579
clozapine, 393, 398, 662
clumsiness, 330, 516; amyotrophic lateral sclerosis and, 535, 536; parkinsonism and, 477, 484, 486
cluster headache, 27, *542*, 542–43, *545*
cobalamin (vitamin B$_{12}$), 438, 503, 538, 557, 610, 611, 613–14, 615
cocaine, 72, 354, 410, 411, 413–14, *414*, 415, 416, 417, 422, 579, 620
cochlear implants, 140, 344, 346
codeine, 446, 564
Cogan's syndrome, 343
cognitive behavioral therapy (CBT): addiction and, 415; anxiety and panic and, 374, 375; borderline personality disorder and, 397; chronic fatigue syndrome and, 359, 360; eating disorders and, 403; obsessive-compulsive disorder and, 381, 383–84; post-traumatic stress disorder and, 408; social phobia and, 377, 378
cognitive development, 94–95, 104–7, 300. *See also* language acquisition

cognitive function, 200–44; creativity, talents, and skills and, 236–44; decision making and planning and, 201–9; visualization and navigation and, 232–35. *See also* intelligence; language; learning; memory; speech; thinking
cognitive impairment, 537, 614–15, 617; Huntington's disease and, 505–6; parkinsonism and, 478, 481, 486, 488–89; public misunderstanding of, 198–99. *See also* language difficulties; memory impairment; speech problems; thinking, disorders of
cognitive tests, 210–12, *211*
cognitive therapy, 367, 389. *See also* cognitive behavioral therapy
cold, common, 50, 148
cold exposure, headache and, 547
cold sores, 463
color blindness, 233, 235
color discrimination, 138, 232, 233
coma, 177, 279, 459, 588, 616; encephalitis and, 463, 464; Glasgow coma scale and, 587–89; head trauma and, 584, 588, 589; hemorrhagic stroke and, 577; lupus and, 472, 473, 474; neurotoxic diseases and, 617, 618; nutritional disorders and, 611, 612; persistent vegetative state and, 177, 588, 589; resource groups for, 684–85
communication skills: autism and, 270, 272, 276–77. *See also* language; speech
comorbidity, 429
compensation, 125, 127
competence, intelligence vs., 212
complex partial seizures, 176, 321
compound skull fractures, 583
compulsions, 44, 380–81, 641. *See also* obsessive-compulsive disorder
computed tomography angiography (CTA), 573

computed tomography (CT) scans, 23, 25, 573, 582
computers, 187, 202, *203*, 203–4, 206, 231; neuroscience and, 26–27
concentration impairments, 308, 311
conceptual apraxia, 649
concussion, 176, 585, 587–89; resource groups for, 684–85
conditioning, 19–20, *218*, 219, 220, 223
conduct disorders, 413, 426, 498
conductive hearing loss, 342–43
confusion, 176, 468, 474, 581, 617; stroke and, 571, 576
congophilic amyloid angiopathy, 579
consciousness, 63, 171–78, 290; altered states of, 176–77; disturbances of, 581; encephalitis and, 462, 466; meaning of, 171–72; neurological underpinnings of, 174–76; psychological dimensions of, 172–74
constructional apraxia, 649, 650
context, in language, 227
continuous positive airway pressure (CPAP) device, *310*, 311
control. *See* inhibition and control
control disorders. *See* emotional and control disorders
contusion, 585–86, 587
coordination, 158–64, 175, 279
coordination problems, 299, 468, 505; ataxia and, 501–4; paraneoplastic syndromes and, 601, 603; parkinsonism and, 486, 487
coprolalia, 497, 498
corpus callosum: aging and, 126–27; brain development and, 99, 106–7, 274, 325; gender differences in, *78*, 79
cortex, *2*, *9*, 18, *18*, 22, 45, 46, 146, 174, 177, 336, 354, 386; correlation of body areas to sections of, 6, 19; dyslexia and, 250; headache and, 550; of humans vs. animals, 5; intelligence and,

214; language and, 229; learning and, 24; memory and, 223; myelination of, 81; pain messages and, 561–62; parkinsonism and, *478*, 486, 488; prenatal development and, 62, 63, 68, 71–74, 77; senses and, 6, 107, *137, 139;* sleep-wake cycle and, 43–44; stroke and, 339; top-down approach and, 5–8; tumors in, 301, 304; vertical organization of, 21; wrinkled surface of, 5, 73, 74, 119. *See also specific cortical areas*
corticobasal degeneration (CBD), 486, 488–89, 649
corticosteroids, 473, 475, 518, 524, 528, 533
corticotrophin-releasing hormone (CRH), *49,* 147, 192, 365, 373, 432
cortisol, 37, *43, 49,* 93, 97, 100, 108, 147–48, 366; post-traumatic stress disorder and, 407, 408
Costen's syndrome, 540
cough headache, 542
Coumadin, 335, 475, 573, 574, 668
coup and contrecoup, 586, *586*
cramps, 354, 406, **494,** 524–25, 535; resource groups for, 682
cranial sutures, hydrocephalus and, 288, 289, 299
craniopharyngiomas, 304
creatine kinase (CK), 525
creative advantage, 242–43, 244
creativity, 236, 239–44; eminent, 238, 239–40; everyday, 238–39, 244; mood disorders and, 240–44, *241;* schizophrenia and, 243, 244
Creutzfeldt-Jakob disease (CJD), **468–70,** 620, 640; causes of, 468–70; diagnosis and treatment of, 470
critical periods, 21, *85,* 85–90
crossed extension, 162
cryptococcus, 461
Cushing's syndrome, 37
cyclooxygenase, 168, 563–64

cyclophosphamide, 441, 475, 663
cyclosporine, 533, 663
cyproheptadine, 403, 663
cytomegalovirus, 517

Damasio, Antonio, 204
Dana Alliance for Brain Initiatives: American participants in, 687–93; European associates of, 695–99
Darwin, Charles, 180
Dawson, Geraldine, 100
daydreaming, 174
deafness, 86, 263, 615; "sudden," 344. *See also* hearing problems
decision making, 201–7, 208; brain mechanisms and, 201–2, 204–5, *205;* higher-level reasoning and, 206; less-than-optimal, 202–4; moral reasoning and, 206, 207
declarative memory, 124, 217–18, *218,* 219, 220, 223, 224, 636
Deep Blue, *203,* 203–4
deep brain stimulation (DBS), 384, *482,* 483, 493, 496
deep dyslexia, 251
degenerative disorders. *See* neurodegenerative disorders
degenerative joint disease (spondylosis), 555, 556–57
dehydration, 640
dehydroeplandrosterone (DHEA), 103
delayed sleep-phase syndrome, 312
delirium, 176–77
delusions, 363, 386, 390, 391, 612, 617, 626, 630–31, 639
dementia, 176, 177, 215, 290, 390, 467, 468, 473, 537, 612, 629, **639–42,** *641;* aging and, 12, 39, 130, 639; agnosias and, 651, 653; Alzheimer's disease and, 125, 177, 198, 626, 628, 641, 642; arrestable or reversible causes of, 640; attention and motivation deficits and, 198; Cushingold, 37; diagnosis of, 639, 641–42; parkinsonism and, 478, 483, 486, 488–89, 641; prevention of,

39, 40; progressive or nonreversible causes of, 640–41; symptoms of, 639; treatment of, 642; use of term, 130
demerol, 564
demyelinating optic neuritis, 336
dendrites, 12, 17, 34, 39, 74, 75, 84, *85,* 99
dengue, 464
dental pain, 436, 565–66
dentate gyrus, 224
dentistry, 349, 605; trigeminal neuralgia and, 565–66
dependence. *See* addiction
depressed skull fractures, 583
depression, 7, 26, 27, 31, 38, 53, 99, 111, 122, 129, 183, 194, 198, 205, 208, 251, 264, 330, **363–70,** 382, 390, 393, 406, 412, 468, 473, 478, 614, 616, 623, 635, 640; in adolescence, 112–13; aging and, 128–29; alcohol and, 422; Alzheimer's disease and, 365, 626, 628–29, 630; anxiety and, 365, 371, 372, 373, 374; bipolar disorder and, 364, 367, 385, 386, *387;* borderline personality disorder and, 395; cancer and, 55, 605; chronic fatigue syndrome and, 357, 359, 360, 361; chronic pain and, 559; coping with, 369; creativity and, 239, 240, 242; diabetes and, 54, 364; dystonia and, 495; eating disorders and, 399, 402; forms of, 364–65; headache and, 543, 544, 546, 549, 551; heart health and, 51–52, 128; Huntington's disease and, 506, 509–10; major depressive disorder, 364, 365, 367, 371, 377, 394; multiple sclerosis and, 436, 440, 441, 443; Parkinson's disease and, 477; postpartum, 100; resource groups for, 678; risk factors and causes of, 365–67; seasonal, 364, 369–70; serotonin and, 365, 366, 367–68, *368;* sleep disorders and, 315, 363, 364, 365, 366, 367, 385, 430;

depression (*cont.*)
smelling ability and, 350–51; stroke and, 52, 54, 364; suicide and, 364, 367, 372, 385, 429–33; symptoms of, 363–64, *366,* 430; treatment of, 367–70, *368*

dermatomyositis, 474, 528–29

desipramine, 403, 515, 663

detoxification, 424; withdrawal and, 176–77, 319, 354, 412, 414–16, 419, 424, 425

development, 155, 281; cognitive, 94–95, 104–7; motor, 158, 159, 162, 260. *See also* adolescence; brain development; child development; prenatal development

developmental disorders, 74; dyslexia and, 248, 250–51; metabolic diseases and, 279. *See also* autism

dexamethasone, 609

dextroamphetamine, 500, 661, 663

diabetes insipidus, 148

diabetes mellitus, 101, 156, 157, 312, 319, 329, 339, 364, 460, 473, 502, 518, 572, 615; autonomic failure and, 355, 356; brain-body loop and, 54; depression and, 54, 364; treatment of, 356

diabetic peripheral neuropathy, 515

dialectical behavioral therapy, 397

diaphragmatic breathing, 546

diarrhea, 53, 354, 517; nutritional disorders and, 612, 613, 615

diazepam, 663

dicyclomine, 663

diencephalic midline, 637

diencephalon, 68, 223

diet. *See* nutrition

dieting, 151, 156. *See also* anorexia nervosa; eating disorders

diffuse axonal injury (DAI), 586

diffuse demyelinating diseases, 619

digestion, 44, 53, 144, 145, 148; stress response and, 47–48, 143

dihydroergotamine mesylate, 551, 663

diphenhydramine, 499, 663

diphenylhydantoin, 503

diplegia, 266

diplopia. *See* double vision

dipyridamole, 574

discourse, 226, 227

disequilibrium, 327

disk disease, 436, 494, **553–57,** *554;* resource groups for, 685. *See also* back pain

dissection techniques, 16–18

disseminated zoster, 446

dissociative amnesia, 637

dissociative apraxia, 649

dissociative fugue, 637

dissociative identity disorder, 637

distal sensory polyneuropathy, 451–52

distractibility, 127, 174, 186, 192, 254, 273

diuretics, 343

divalproex, 388

dizziness, **327–31,** *328,* 353, 487, 502, 570; causes of, 328–31, 435; diagnosis of, 331; resource groups for, 676; symptoms of, 327–28

Dizziness Simulation Battery, 331

DNA (deoxyribonucleic acid), 28, 68, 508, 525; mitochondrial (mtDNA), 126, 281–82

dogs: narcolepsy in, 316; stress response in, 47–48

donepezil, 630, 638, 663

dopamine, 44, 192, 312, 408; ADHD and, 194, 255–56; alcohol and, 422; drug use and, 204, 413–14, *414;* eating and, 53, 401; emotional and control disorders and, 366, 377, 381, 401; inhibition and control and, 188; parkinsonism and, 27, 163, 479, *479,* 480, 481, 485, 487; reward pathways and, 109, 110, 422; Tourette's syndrome and, 497, 499

dopamine-blocking drugs (neuroleptics), 387, 393, 485, 499, 509, 631

Doppler ultrasonography, 578

dorsal column stimulators, 564

dorsal root ganglion, 601

dorsolateral frontal cortex, 214

dorsomedial thalamic nucleus, 198

dose-response effect, 620

dothiepin, 544

double-blind studies, 55–56

double depression, 365

double vision (diplopia), 336, 435, 454, 516, 523, 531, 570, 577, 615

Down's syndrome, 76, 77, 215, 259–60, 262, 264, 628

doxepin, 368, 663

dreams, 155, 175, 307, 314, 317, 478

dressing apraxia, 649–50

drives. *See* basic drives

driving safety, 31, 38, 101, 111, 208. *See also* vehicular accidents

drop attacks, 320–21

drugs, 12, 53, 72; neurotransmitters and, 10–11. *See also* addiction; medications; substance abuse; *specific drugs*

drug testing, 412

Duchenne muscular dystrophy, 524, 525, 526, 528

dura, 160, 583

dysarthria, 643, 646, 647

dyscalculia, 253

dysexecutive syndrome, 186

dysgerminomas, 304

dysgraphia, 253

dyskinesias, 479, 481, 483, 488

dyskinetic cerebral palsy, 266, 267, *268,* 269

dyslexia, 26, 46, 230, 238, **248–53,** 646; diagnosing of, 248–49; forms of, 250–51; helping child with, 249–50, 251–53; misconceptions and realities about, 249–50; resource groups for, 673; visual deficits and, 252

dysphonia, 495

dysthymia, 364–65

dystonia, 164, 489, 493, **494–96,** 505; resource groups for, 682

ears, 62, *138,* 139; air travel and, 544; anatomy of, 341–42; sensory cells in, 136, 138. *See also* hearing; hearing problems

eating, 51, 101, 129–30, 146, 347; as basic drive, 150–51, *153,* 153–54, 155; binge, 394, 399, 400, 401, 403; brain-body loop and, 44, 47; brain care and, 31, 33–36, *35. See also* nutrition

eating disorders, 44, 110, 112, 113, 156, 157, 382, **399–404,** 406, 641; causes of, 401–2; confronting person with, 404; criteria defining, 399–401; diagnosis and treatment of, 402–3; recovery and mortality rates for, 403–4; resource groups for, 679

echolalia, 497, 498

echopraxia, 497

Ecstasy, 111

Edelman, Gerald, 172

edema, 605, 609

edrophonium, 532

education, intelligence and, 215

Einstein, Albert, 236

electrical charges in brain, 8–10, 14, 15, 74–75, 80–81; action potentials and, 9–10; EEGs and, 10, 23, *90, 320, 323;* epileptic seizures and, 19, 319–26, *320–23;* research on, 18–19, 20–21

electrical stimulation, 19; spinal cord regeneration and, 598

electroconvulsive therapy (ECT), 367, 369, 635

electrode recording, 20–21

electroencephalography (EEG), 10, 23, *90, 320,* 323

electromyography (EMG), 525, 555

electron microscopy, *9,* 15, 526

ELISA test, 455

embolism, 335, 340, 572, 573

embryonal tumors, 302–3

embryonic growth, 66–67. *See also* prenatal development

embryonic stem cells, 481, 598–99

emotional and control disorders, 183–84, 249, 362–433. *See also* addiction; aggression; alcoholism; anxiety; bipolar disorder; borderline personality disorder; depression; eating disorders; obsessive-compulsive disorder; panic disorder; posttraumatic stress disorder; schizophrenia; social phobia; substance abuse; suicidal feelings; violence

emotional memory, 219, 223

emotions, 100, 136, 172, 175, 180–84, 229; brain-body loop and, 41, 51–53; brain development and, 87, 93, 106, 108–9; communication of, 182–83; consciousness and, 172, 173, 174; decision making and, 203–8; individual differences in, 182; language and, 227, 229, 230; memory and, 181, 182, 183, 219, 223; neurological impairments and, 98, 99; pain and, 168, 169; regulation of, violence and aggression and, 426, 427–28; strong, loss of muscle strength triggered by, 308, 315, 316, 317, 318; temperament and mood vs., 182–83

encephalitis, 176, 261, 447, 455, 496, 635, 640, 645; arthropodborne viruses, 462, 464–66, *465;* herpes simplex virus, 462, *463,* 463–64; meaning of word, 462; seizures and, 319, 324, 462, 465; symptoms of, 462; viral, **462–67**

encephalitis lethargica, 485

encephalomyelitis, 462, 601; autoimmune, 436, 438, 462, 466–67

encephalomyelitis associated with cancer, 600

endocrine system, *42,* 143, 145–46, 151, 166, 278, 359; problems with, 148–49

end-of-life decision, 634

endorphins, 56, 169, 562, 564

enkephalin, 11, 169

enriched environments, 95–96, 121, 222

enteric nervous system, 144–45

entorhinal cortex, 26, 223, 225, *627,* 636, 637

environmental spatial impairment, 234–35

environmental toxins, 215, 257, 486, 617, 618–19. *See also* neurotoxins and neurotoxic diseases

enzyme-replacement therapy, 283

enzyme tests, 525

ependymomas, 302, 304, 607

epidural hematomas, 584, *584*

epilepsy, 23, 26, 74, 159, 174, 224, 251, 315, **319–26,** 548, 580, 614, 617; abnormal tastes and smells and, 321, 347, 350; antiepileptic medications and, 324, 619, 621; causes of, 319; diagnosis and treatment of, 323–25; living with, 325–26; resource groups for, 676; safety measures for, 325; special diet for, 36; statistics on, 319; types of, 322. *See also* seizures

epinephrine (adrenaline), 48, *49,* 50, 52, 53, 143, 408, 493

episodic memory, 217–18, *218,* 224

Epley canalith repositioning maneuver, 329

Epstein-Barr virus, 360, 450, 517

Erasistratus, 16

ergotamine, 543, 551

erythema migrans, 454, 456

erythrocyte sedimentation rate (ESR), 524

erythromycin, 343, 663

escitalopram, 368

essential tremor (ET), 490–91, 492, 493

estrogen, 45, 103–4, 125, 146, 151, 549

estrogen replacement therapy, 629

ethnicity, IQ scores and, 214

Evarts, Edward, 21

event-related potentials (ERPs), 249

evoked response test, 439

evolution, 203

Ewing, John, 423
excitotoxicity, 537
executive functions, 197
exercise, 208; brain-body loop and, 52, 53, 54; brain care and, 31, 36–37, 38–39, 40, 121, 128, 129, 130, 164, 573; headache and, 540, 541, 543; sleep disorders and, 309, 314
exertional headache, 540, 541, 543
expertise, 240
expert memory, 123
exposure therapy, 374, 408
exposure with response prevention (ERP), 383
extrapyramidal cerebral palsy, 266, 267, *268*, 269
eye discomfort, while reading, 252
eyelid drooping. *See* ptosis
eye movements: abnormal, 486, 501, 611, 612, 615, 616; intentional, 175
eye pain, 435, 436
eyes, 48, *138*, 139, 144; hydrocephalus and, 289, 290; prenatal development and, 62, 63; sensory cells in, 123, 136, 137, 138. *See also* retinas; vision; vision problems

Fabry disease, 281
face agnosia, 233, 235, 652
facet joints, 553
facial expressions, emotions and, 180, 182
facial numbness, 330, 454
facial pain, 336, 436, 454; trigeminal neuralgia and, 565–68
facial spasms, 494
facial weakness, 299, 330, 454, 516, 527; Bell's palsy and, 520–22
facioscapulohumeral muscular dystrophy, 527–28
fainting, 176, 327, 353, 487
famciclovir, 446, 663
familial hemiplegic migraine, 550
family-focused treatment (FFT), 389
fascicles, 75

fasting, 547, 549
fat (body), 108, 150, 153–54
fat consumption, 33–34, 35–36
fatigue, 57, 353, 406, 430, 473; chronic fatigue syndrome and, 357–61; multiple sclerosis and, 435, 436, 440; muscular, 524, 530; parkinsonism and, 477, 484; sleep disorders and, 308, 309, 311, 315
fear, 97, 174, 426, 427; amygdala and, 373, *373*; brain mechanisms and, 181, 372–73, *373*; obsessive-compulsive disorder and, 380, 383; phobias and, 219, 372, 373, 374; post-traumatic stress disorder and, 406–8; sleep terrors and, 313–14
feelings. *See* emotions
feet, peripheral neuropathy and, 514–15
female hormones: migraine and, 549. *See also specific hormones*
fetal alcohol syndrome, 72, 215, 260–61
fetal development. *See* prenatal development
fever, 176, 319, 471, 615; encephalitis and, 462, 465, 466, 467
fibrillary astrocytomas, 301
fibromyalgia, 357, 524
fight or flight response. *See* stress response
filopodia, 75
Fischer, Kurt, 100
fitness, 54; brain care and, 31, 36–37, 38–39, 40. *See also* exercise
5-hydroxy-indoleacetic acid (5-HIAA), 426
fixation of gaze, 498
flow, 242
fludrocortisone, 355
fluent aphasia, 644, 645, 646
fluorohydrocortisone, 330
fluoxetine, 368, 383, 403, 663
fluphenazine, 499, 663
fluvoxamine, 383
focal cortical resection, 325

focal dystonia, 495
focal seizures, 319, 321, 325
focal unconsciousness, 176
folic acid (folate), 22, 34, 64, 261, 611, 613, 614–15, 640; birth defects and, 64, 293, 296, 297, 615
follicle-stimulating hormone, 145, 149
food additives, 257, 547, 549, 605
food allergens, 257
Food and Drug Administration, U.S. (FDA), 56
foods, 605; headache and, 547, 549. *See also* eating; nutrition
foot drop, 524, 529
forced-use therapy, 46, 593, 594, 595–97
forebrain, 67, 68, 146, 168
forgetting, 222. *See also* memory
4-aminopyridine (4-AP), 597
Fowler, Lorenzo N., 15
fractures, 555, 583
fragile X syndrome, 274
free radicals, 537
Freud, Sigmund, 152–53, 240, 267
Fritsch, Gustav, 19, 159
frontal cortex. *See* prefrontal cortex
frontal lobes, 111, 118, 168, 181, 386; of children with depressed mothers, 100; development of, *91*, 104–5, *106*, 107, 108; disturbances of, 198, 199, 330, 347, 386, 486, 586, 641, 649; functions of, 173–74, 175, 201; memory and, 223
frontal lobotomy, modified, 169
frontal release signs, 185
frontotemporal dementia (FTD), 215, 537, 640–41, *641*, 642
functional amnesia, 635, 637
functional neuroimaging, 26–27, 50, 197
fusiform gyrus, 652
future: intentionality and, 196; planning for, 207–9

gabapentin, 388, 446, 452, 515, 564, 567, 663

gadolinium, 439
Gage, Phineas, 7, *8*, 186, 197, 201–2, 396
galantamine, 630, 663
Galen, 16, 191
Gall, Franz Joseph, 15–16
Galton, Francis, 212, 213
Galvani, Luigi, 19
gamma-aminobutyric acid (GABA), 168, 192, 373, 422, 425
ganglia. *See* basal ganglia
gangliogliomas, 302, 304
ganglioneurons, 607
Garrod, Archibald, 279
gastroenteritis, 466
gastrointestinal disease, 610
Gaucher's disease, 281, 283
gender differences, *78*, 79, 97, 103–4, 108, 119, 229; cultural or societal expectations and, 194; sensory systems and, 140
gender identity, 152
generalized anxiety disorder (GAD), 371, 372–75
generalized seizures, 319, 320–21, 324
generalized tonic-clonic seizures, 320, 324
genes: brain development and, 11, 66, 68, 69, 73, 86, 87; interplay of environment and, 86–87, 93; neuroscience research and, 28–29; predispositions and, 111, 130
gene-splicing techniques, 28
gene therapy, 283
gentamicin, 329, 343, 664
Georgopoulos, Apostolos, 21
germ cell tumors, 304–5
giant cell arteritis, 343
gifted children, 237
ginkgo biloba, 125, 630
Glasgow coma scale (GCS), 587–89
glatiramer, 439–41, 664
glia, 507
glial cells, 8, 80, 301, 386, 598; prenatal development and, 68–69, *73*, 74
glioblastomas, 301, 304, 607

gliomas, 301–2, 304, *606*, 606–7, 608, 609
globus pallidus internal (GPi), 483
glucocorticoids, 37–38, 147, 609; multiple sclerosis and, 439, 441, 442
glucose, 23–24, 147, 610; diabetes and, 54
glucose metabolism in brain, 122, 365, 366; aging and, 126; in childhood, 84, 99; violence and aggression and, 427
glutamate, 28, 373, 537, 538
glutaric aciduria, 265, 279
glycerol, 568
Golgi, Camillo, 14, 17, *17*
gonadotropin-releasing hormone, 103
gonadotropins, 103
gonads, 146, 149
Gowers' sign, 524
grand mal seizures, 320, 324
granulomatous arteritis, 447
grasp reflex, 185–86
gravity, 158, 162, 327
gray matter, 71, 126
Greenfield, Susan, 13
grief, 365
growth factors, 36, 80, 481, 609
growth hormone, *43*, 145, 149, 155, 336, 337, 366, 469
guanfacine, 499, 664
guided imagery, 546
Guillain-Barré syndrome (GBS), 81, 148, 511, **516–19**, 521; causes of, 517; resource groups for, 683; treatment of, 517–19
gunshot wounds to head, 586, 589

habituation, *117*, 117–18
Haemophilus influenzae type b (Hib), 459, 461
hair cells, 136, 139, 140, *328*, 341, 342, 343, 346
Hallervorden-Spatz syndrome, 496
hallucinations, 114, 177, 308, 363, 390, 391, 417, 473, 488, 612, 616, 626, 639; hypnagogic, 315, 317, 318

hallucinogens, 410
haloperidol, 387, 393, 499, 631, 664
hand tremor, 490, 491
hangover, 540, 543
Harvard Medical School, 146
HD gene, 506–7, 508
headache, 27, 122, 168, 170, 290, 406, **540–47**, 559, 571, 581, 615; arising from structures in face and neck, 540, 544–45; brain tumors and, 298, 299, 541, 542, *548*, 605; causes of, 454; encephalitis and, 462, 465; morning, sleep disorders and, 308, 311; resource groups for, 683–84; serious, "thunderclaps" and, 541–42, 576, 577; stroke and, 541, 576, 577, 578; tension, 53, 540, 542, 543–44, *545*, 551; treatment of, 546; vascular, 542–43; when to become concerned about, 540–42. *See also* migraine
head trauma, 31, 46, 101, 140, 143, 157, 176, 177, 230, 232, 281, 288, 319, 354, 460, 496, 541, **581–90**, 595, 629, 649; ADHD and, 257; in adolescence, 110–11; attention and motivation deficits and, 198; concussion and, 176, 585, 587–89; coup and contrecoup in, 586, *586;* dementia and, 640; diagnosis of, 581–83; dyslexia and, 248, 251; injury involving blood vessels within skull and, 583–85; injury to brain tissue and, 585–89, *586;* injury to skull and, 583; intellectual deficits and, 215, 216; memory impairment and, 221, 635, 636; mental retardation and, 260, 261, 263; olfactory loss and, 347, 349; predicting long-term outcome of, 587–89; prevention of, 31, *32*, 34; rehabilitation after, 589–90; resource groups for, 684–85; speech and language difficulties and, 645,

head trauma (*cont.*)
646; suggestions for family members after, 590; symptoms of, 581, 582
health care, 22, 101
health insurance, 57
hearing, 22, 87, 136–40, 142, 175, 327; auditory pathway and, *138, 139, 139, 141,* 341–42, *342;* development of, 76–77, 81, 86, 91, 92; differences in acuity of, 140; ear anatomy and, 341–42; screening newborns for, 344; sensory cells and, 136, 138, 139, 140
hearing aids, 344, *345,* 346
hearing problems, 140, 224, 230, 264, 286, 329, **341–46,** 454, 567, 605, 615; agnosias and, 652–53; central auditory system disorders and, 342, 344–45; conductive hearing loss, 342–43; coping with, 346; diagnosis and treatment of, 345–46; inner ear or auditory nerve disorders and, 343–44, 346; meningitis and, 459, 461; resource groups for, 676–77; sensorineural hearing loss and, 342–46; smoking and, 129; tinnitus and, 343, 344, 345. *See also* cochlear implants
heart, 144, 146, 554
heart attack, 51–53, 504, 574, 615; anger and, 52–53; depression and, 51–52
heart disease, 129, 364, 460; depression and, 51–52, 128
heart rate, 160, 166, 355, 372, 407; atrial fibrillation and, 573; depression and, 52, 100; irregular, 111, 311, 330, 340, 454, 580; regulation of, 143, 144, 145; sexual response and, 45, 151; stress and, 37, 48, 53, 97
heat stroke, 176, 319
heavy metals, 619, 620, 621
helmets, brain care and, 31, *32,* 101, 111
helplessness, 239

hemangioblastoma, 608
hematomas, 576; head trauma and, 583–85, *584*
hemiballismus, 164
hemifacial spasms, 493, 494
hemiplegia, 163, 266
hemisomatopagnosia, 46
hemispatial neglect, 234, *234,* 235
hemispheric structure of brain, *2, 3, 5,* 228–29
Hemophilus influenzae, 261
hemorrhage, 86, 129, 288; ataxia and, 501, 502, 503, 504; headache and, 540, 541, 576, 577, 578; hemorrhagic stroke and, 576–80, *577;* intracerebral, 354, 576–78, 579; intraventricular, 576, 577, 578, 579; subarachnoid, 576, 577, 578, 579, 580, 585
hemorrhagic stroke, 339, 541, 570, **576–80,** *577,* 583; causes of, 577–78, 579; diagnosis and treatment of, 578–80; ischemic stroke vs., 572–73, 578, 580; resource groups for, 685; risk factors for, 579; symptoms of, 576–77, 578
heparin, 340, 475, 574
hepatitis, 464, 517
herbal teas and supplements, 71, 72
herniated disk. *See* back pain; disk disease
heroin, 11, 72, 410, 411, 413, 414–15, 416, 417, 422, 564, 617, 620
Herophilus, 16
herpes simplex, 460, 521; encephalitis and, 462, *463,* 463–64
herpes virus, human (HHV), 359
herpes zoster. *See* shingles
Hib, 459, 461
high blood pressure. *See* hypertension
hindbrain, 67, 68, 166
hippocampus, 18, 20, 26, 28, 177, 373, 407, 427, *627;* amnesias and, 636, 637; depression and, 38; development of, 68, 94, 108; emotions and, 181, *181;* exercise

and, 36, 37; intelligence and, 214; memory and, 123–24, *205,* 223, 225; planning ahead and, 207–9; stress and, 37–38
Hiroshima bombing, 74
histamine, 43
histochemistry, 526
histology, 17
Hitzig, Eduard, 19, 159
HIV/AIDS, 370, 417, 438, **448–52,** 460, 517, 640; AIDS dementia complex and, 451; anti-HIV drugs and, 448–49, 450, 451, 452, 619, 621; ataxia and, 503; central nervous system infections and, 449–50; neuropathies and, 451–52; research on, 452; resource groups for, 681; shingles and, 445–46
Hoffman's sign, 536
holoprosencephaly, 267
Holter, John, 290–91
homocysteine, 572, 613, 615
homosexuality, 431
hopelessness, suicide and, 429, 430, 431, 432
hormones, 45, 143, 150, 359; in adolescence, 103–4, 107–9, 113; brain-body loop and, 42, 43, 44; child development and, 93; eating behavior and, 44; endocrine system and, 143, 145–46, 148–49; female, migraine and, 549; parenthood and, 119–20; postpartum depression and, 100; sex, 79, 151; sleep-wake cycle and, 43; stress, 48, *49,* 166 *(see also* cortisol; epinephrine; norepinephrine)
Horner's syndrome, 303
HTLV-1, 438
Hubel, David, 21
human genome, 260
human herpes virus (HHV), 359
human leukocyte antigen (HLA), 318, 438
hunger, 150
Huntington's disease (HD), 18, 27, *28, 29,* 130, 468, 492, 496,

505–10, *507,* 641; diagnosis of, 507–9; genetics of, 28–29, 506–7, 508; nutrition and, 509; resource groups for, 683; symptoms of, 505–6; treatment of, 509–10

hydralazine, 613

hydrocephalus, 76, **288–92,** 459, 487, 580, 585; in adults, 288, 290; Arnold Chiari malformation and, 294–96, *296;* brain tumors and, 288, 290, 299, 300, 302; communicating, 288; diagnosis and treatment of, 290–92, *291;* normal-pressure, 289, 290, 640; obstructive, 288, 290, 292; resource groups for, 675; spina bifida and, 294; symptoms of, 288–90

hypalgesia, 444

hyperactivity, 192, 254, 273, 431; agitation and, 429, 431, 432, 433. *See also* attention deficit/hyperactivity disorder

hyperbaric oxygen therapy, 269

hypersomnia, 412

hypertension, 101, 311, 334, 339, 353, 354, 356, 640; ataxia and, 502, 504; doctor's visits and, 56; idiopathic intracranial, 541; lupus and, 472, 473; stroke and, 572, 579

hypertonia, 265, 266, 283

hyperventilation, 330, 331, 374

hypervitaminosis, 610, 619

hypnagogic hallucinations, 315, 317, 318

hypnotics, 308, 310, 410, 417

hypocretin, 317, *317,* 318

hypomania, 364, 386

hypothalamic-pituitary-adrenal (HPA) axis, 147–48, 359, 407

hypothalamus, 27, 45, 68, 119, *142,* 168, 192, 336; adolescent development and, 103, 108; autonomic disorders and, 352–53; basic drives and, 150, 151, *152,* 153, 154; body regulation and, 142–49; circadian rhythms and, 43, 543; eating behavior and, 44,

401; emotions and, *181,* 182; injuries to, 149; narcolepsy and, 317, *317;* sexual response and, 45; stress response and, *49,* 97; tumors in, 301, 354

hypothermia, paroxysmal, 149

hypothyroidism, 330, 365, 503, 615, 626

hypotonia, 279, 283

ibuprofen, 168, 563, 664

ice-cream headache, *545,* 547

ideational apraxia, 649

ideomotor apraxia, 649

idiopathic hypogonadotropic hypogonadism, 79

idiopathic intracranial hypertension, 541

imagery abilities, 235

imaginative play, 272–73

imipramine, 368, 403, 544, 664

immune staining, 526

immune system, *42,* 63, 143, 147–48, 239, 353, 383, 473, 561, 614; chronic fatigue syndrome and, 359; disorders of, 140, 148, 343 *(see also* autoimmune disorders); meningitis and, 458, 460; narcolepsy and, 317; paraneoplastic syndromes and, 600–601, 603; shingles and, 445–46, 447; sleep deprivation and, 155; spinal cord regeneration and, 598; stress and, 148

immunoglobulin, intravenous infusions of (IVIG), 441, 518, 529, 533, 603

immunosuppressants, 515

immunotherapy, 533–34

implicit memory. *See* nondeclarative memory

impotence, 330, 356, 436, 440, 488

impulsive aggression, 426, 427–28

impulsivity, 107, 111, 273, 401, 404; ADHD and, 254–55; borderline personality disorder and, 394, 395, 396, 397; suicide and, 114, 429, 430, 431, 432; Tourette's syndrome and, 497, 498, 500

inclusion body myositis (IBM), 529

indomethacin, 664

induction, 66

infants, 83–90, 94, 181; cranial sutures unfused in, 288, 289, 299; critical periods and, 21, *85,* 85–90; language acquisition in, 23, 227–28, 230; meningitis in, 459, 460, 461; motor skills of, 158, 159; newborn, examination and evaluation of, 83–84; newborn, screening tests for, 261, 282, 344; nutritional needs of, 33–34; premature, 72, 86, 261, 266, 267; sensory systems of, 136; temperament of, 190–91, 192–93, *193;* vision of, 21. *See also* child development

infection, 143, 168, 267, 319, 572, 579; congenital, 261; immune system and, 147, 155

infectious disorders, 143, 444–70. *See also* Creutzfeldt-Jakob disease; encephalitis; HIV/AIDS; Lyme disease; meningitis; shingles

inferior temporal gyrus, 98

inflammation, 148, 168

inflammatory myopathies, 523, 528–29

influenza, 517

inhalants, 410, 417

inhibition, temperament and, 192–95

inhibition and control, 185–89, *186,* 201; "brain track" analogy, 188–89; CEO analogy and, 187; defined, 185; referee analogy and, 189; Stroop task and, 188–89

injury: pain and, 165, 166–68. *See also* head trauma; spinal cord injury

inner ear, 136, 138, 139, 140, 327, 341–42; disorders of, 343–44, 346; dizziness and, *328,* 329, 330, 331

innervation, 146

insomnia, 157, 307–12, 405, 412, 626; causes of, 309; CJD and, 468; depression and, 363, 364, 430; narcolepsy and, 315, 316, 318; treatment of, 309–10
insulin, 146, 150
intelligence, 119, 210–16; aging and, 212, *213*, 215; behavioral, *173*, 173–74; biology of, 212–14; creativity and, 240; dynamic nature of, 215–16; general, 210, 212; general, autism and, 271–72; general, talent and, 238; intellectual, 173, 174; use of term, 210
intelligence quotient (IQ), 210; ethnicity and, 214; IQ tests and, 210–12, *211*, 214; mental retardation and, 259, 262
intentionality, 196
intention tremor, 490
interferons, 336, 439–41, 664
interleukins, 147
International Classification of Disease, 409
interpersonal and social rhythm therapy (IPSRT), 388–89
interpersonal therapy, 367
intestinal cramps, 494
intestines, 144, 145, 146, 554
intonation, 227
intoxication, 423
intracerebral hematomas, 585
intracerebral hemorrhage, 354, 576–78, 579
intrathecal baclofen, 268, 269
intravenous immunoglobulin (IVIG), 441, 518, 529, 533, 603
intraventricular hemorrhage, 576, 577, 578, 579
iodine, 34
iron, 34, 71
irregular words, 251
irritable bowel syndrome, 371, 372
ischemia, 51, 225, 570–75, *574*, 587; causes of, 571–72; diagnosis and treatment of, 572–75; symptoms of, 570–71; transient ischemic attacks (TIAs) and, 140, 330, 334–35, *335*, 340, 570–71, 646
ischemic stroke, 143, 334, 339, 473, **570–75,** *574*, 576, 577, 579, 583–84; causes of, 571–72; diagnosis and treatment of, 572–75; hemorrhagic stroke vs., 572–73, 578, 580; recovery from, 575; resource groups for, 685; symptoms of, 570, 571; transient ischemic attacks (TIAs) and, 140, 330, 334–35, *335*, 340, 570–71, 646; warning signs of, 571
isoniazid, 613
Ixodes ticks, 453, 456

Jackson, John Hughlings, 159
James, William, 171
Janusian theory, 242
Japanese encephalitis virus, 465, 466
jargon aphasia, 7
JC, 450
jet lag, 311
Jung, Karl, 242

Kagan, Jerome, 96–97
Kahneman, Daniel, 202
kanamycin, 343, 664
Kandel, Eric, 20
Kasparov, Garry, *203*, 203–4
kernicterus, 267
ketogenic diet, 36
ketorolac tromethamine, 664
kidneys, 144, 460, 591, 615, 619, 640; lupus and, 471, 472, 473, 475
kinesthesia, 45, 136
kinetic tremor, 490, 491
Kingsolver, Barbara, 48
knowledge, 174, 175
Korsakoff syndrome, 612

LAAM, 416
labor and delivery, 267, *268*
lacerations, 586
LaCrosse encephalitis virus, 464, 465

lactate, 612
lactic acid, 278
Lake Maracaibo, Venezuela, *28, 29,* 506, *506*
Lambert-Eaton myasthenic syndrome (LEMS), 602
lamotrigine, 324, 388
language, 5, 124, 172, 175, 226–31; brain regions involved in, 6–7, *228*, 228–29, *229*, 643–44, 646; defined, 643; forms of, 226–27; reading and, 92, *228*, 230, 233; as special kind of code, 226, 227; writing and, 92, 228, 229. *See also* speech
language acquisition, 23, 63, 84, 86, 90–92, 99–100, 227–28, 230; delays in, 260, 274
language difficulties, 230–31, 238, 489, 576, 605, 639, 641, **643–47;** Alzheimer's disease and, 230, 625, 627; autism and, 272, 276–77; resource groups for, 686. *See also* aphasia; dyslexia; speech problems
lateral geniculate nucleus, 139, 338
lateralization, 228–29
L-dopa, 312
lead, 215, 257, 261, 515, 620, 621, 623
learned helplessness, 365
learned nonuse, 593, 595–97
learning, 18, 24–25, 217–25; brain-body loop and, 46–47; brain plasticity and, 12, 46–47, 116; child development and, 91, 96, 99–100; conscious mental and behavioral capacities and, 172; modes of memory and, 217–19, *218*; sleep and, 32–33, 155; stages of, 219–21; structural changes in brain and, 221–23, *237*
learning impairments, 72, 86, 274, 284, 290, 461; anterograde amnesia and, 636; dyslexia and, 248–53
Leborgne, Monsieur (Tan), 6

left hemisphere, language and, 92, 643–44, 646
left-temporal-lobe seizures, *322*
leg movements, sleep disturbances and, 157, 309, 311–13, 478
leg pain, 467
leg weakness, 330, 336, 535, 555; brain tumors and, 299, 303; Guillain-Barré syndrome and, 516; myopathies and, 523–24; peripheral neuropathy and, 513, 514, 515
leptin, 44, 108, *153*, 153–54
lesion studies, 17–18, 153
leukemia, 298, 300, 344, 445
leukodystrophy, 282, 283, 619
levetiracetam, 324
levodopa, 480–81, 485, 487, 488, 664
Lewy bodies, *478*; dementia with, 198, 215, 486
Lhermitte's sign, 436
lidocaine, 447, 664
life support, 634
light-headedness, 328, 331, 353, 487
light sensitivity, 459, 475
light therapy: for circadian rhythm disorders, 311; for depression, 369–70
limb-girdle muscular dystrophy (LGMD), 527, 528
limbic system, 98, 99, 150, 153, 234, 391, 396; emotions and, *181*, 181–82, 183, 184; stress response and, 406–7
limb-kinetic apraxia, 649
Lincoln, Abraham, 432
linear skull fractures, 583
lipid levels, 502
Lissauer, H., 651
lissencephaly, 74, 267, *268*
listening: language acquisition and, 90–92; to music, 120
Listeria monocytogenes, 460
lithium, 367, 387, 388, 398, 433, 503, 631, 664
Little, Sir William, 266–67
liver, 111, 144, 418, 424, 613, 615, 640

liver disease, 278, 610, 614, 615, 616
locomotion: after spinal cord injury, 593, 595–97. *See also* movement; walking
logical principles, decision making and, 202–4
long-term potentiation, 20
loratadine, 664
Lou Gehrig's disease, 535. *See also* amyotrophic lateral sclerosis
lumbar nerves, *592*
lumbar puncture (spinal tap), 460–61, *461*, 541, 553
lumbar spinal stenosis, 556, 557–558
lung disease, 460
lungs, 144, 554, 615
lupus. *See* systemic lupus erythematosus
luteinizing hormone, 145, 149
Lyme disease, 438, **453–57**, 460; areas of risk for, *453*; avoiding, 457; diagnosis and treatment of, 455–56; *Ixodes* ticks and, 453, 456; symptoms of, 453–55, *454*
lymphoma, 445, 450, 609
lysosomal storage diseases, 279

macular degeneration, 338–39, *339*
mad cow disease, 469–70
magnetic resonance angiography (MRA), 573
magnetic resonance imaging (MRI), *25*, 25–27, 153, 163; functional (fMRI), 26–27, 50
magnetoencephalography (MEG), 27
magnocellular pathway, 252
malnutrition, 610, 614, 615, 616
manganese, 34
mania, 183, 184, 364, 367, 385–86, *387. See also* bipolar disorder
manic-depressive illness. *See* bipolar disorder
marijuana, 72, 410, 411, 413, 415, 416; headache and, 543
marine toxins, 617, 622
massage therapy, 546
massa intermedia, *78*, 79

mathematics, dyscalculia and, 253
Mazziotta, John, 24
measles, 261; encephalomyelitis and, 462, 466–67
meclizine, 329, 664
medial temporal lobe, 223, 224
medications: allergic reactions to, 140, 640; pregnancy and, 72; used to treat brain and nervous system (chart), 661–68. *See also specific medications*
medications, side effects of, 157, 319, 331, 343, 365, 478, 496, 515, 626, 635; autonomic disorders and, 354; dementia and, 640, 642; neurotoxic diseases and, 503, 617, 619, 621, 622; smelling or tasting problems and, 349, 351; tremors and, 490, 492
medulla oblongata, 44, 45, 68, *142*, 154, 353; body regulation and, 145; tumors in area of, 301–2
medulloblastomas, 302–3, 304
melancholia, 183, 184
MELAS (mitochondrial encephalopathy, lactic acidosis, and stroke), 281
melatonin, 43, 103, 108
memory, 19, 25, 26, 36, 111, 118, 123–25, 176, 177, 217–25; aging and, 124–25, *223*, 223–25, 626; brain development and, 63, 91, 94, 95, 96, 106; brain regions and structures involved in, 219, *220*, 223; consciousness and, 172, 174, 175, 176; creativity and, 240; declarative, 124, 217–18, *218*, 219, 220, 223, 224, 636; dementia and, 639, 642; emotional, 219, 223; emotions and, 181, 182, 183; episodic, 217–18, *218*, 224; expert, 123; H.M. case and, 224; long-term, 18, 123–24, 207–9, 212, 214, 221, 222–23, 224, 235; making most of, 222; modes of, 217–19, *218*; nondeclarative or implicit, 124, 174, *218*, 218–19, 220, 224, 636–37; organization and struc-

memory (*cont.*)

ture of, 221, 223, 636–37; pain and, 168; planning ahead and, 207–9; post-traumatic stress disorder and, 408; procedural, *218,* 218–19, 223, 224; research on, 20; semantic, 217–18, *218,* 224; sensory, 220; short-term or working, 104, 107, 112, 124, 212, 220–21, 222, 224; skills and, *218,* 218–19, 223, 224, 236–37; sleep and, 32–33; smoking and, 129; stages of, 219–21; stress and, 37; structural changes in brain and, 221–23; visual, 235

memory impairment, 39, 40, 124, 198, 218–19, 420, 436, 455, 478, 505, 537, 570, 605; agnosias and, 46, 218, 233, 235, 637, 639, 651–53; Alzheimer's disease and, 18, 124–25, 625–26, 627, 629, 630, 635, 638; amnesias and, 176, 218, 224, 225, 635–38; nutritional disorders and, 611, 612, 613, 616; paraneoplastic syndromes and, 601

Ménière's disease, 329, 344

meninges, *458*

meningiomas, 286, 604, 605, 606, 607, 608

meningitis, 288, **458–61,** 467, 504, 640; bacterial, 176, 458, 459–60, 461; causes of, 458, 472; diagnosis and treatment of, 460–61, *461;* headache and, 540, 541; Lyme disease and, 454, 456, 460; mental retardation and, 260, 261, 461; seizures and, 319, 324, 459, 461; spina bifida and, 294–97, *295;* symptoms of, 458–59; viral or fungal, 458, 460, 461

meningocele, 294, *295,* 297

meningococcus, 459

meningovascular neurosyphilis, 467

menopause, 128, 549, 629

menstrual cycle, 43, 61, 140, 149, 549

mental retardation, 72, 74, 86, 238, **259–64,** 325; apparent at different ages, 261; autism and, 271–72, 273, 274; causes of, 260, 262, 263, 274, 278, 283, 461; definitions of, 259; diagnosis of, 259–60, 262–64; integration into larger society and, 261–62; lowering risk of, 260–61; muscular dystrophy and, 526, 527; resource groups for, 674; treatment of, 264. *See also* Down's syndrome

mercury, 618, 620, 621, 623

merlin, 286

mesencephalon, 198

metabolic diseases, 278–83; cerebral palsy and, 265, 267, 278, 283; classes and examples of, 280; dementia and, 640; diagnosis and treatment of, 282–83; mechanisms and causal factors in, 279–81; mental retardation and, 260, 261, 263, 274, 278, 283; phenylketonuria (PKU) and, 261, 274, 278, 282; resource groups for, 674; symptoms of, 278–79

metabolism, 37, 44, 146, 151, 278; sleep deprivation and, 155. *See also* glucose metabolism in brain

methadone, 416

methamphetamine, 111, 411

methotrexate, 441, 614

methyl ethyl ketone, 619

methylmalonic acid, 613

methylmalonic acidemia, *268*

methylphenidate (Ritalin), 329, 330, 403, 500, 664; ADHD and, 255, 256, 258

methylprednisolone, 336, 439, 441, 442, 592–93, 597

methysergide, 543, 665

metoclopramide, 355, 665

metoprolol tartrate, 665

microsmia, 349

microvascular decompression, 567

midbrain, 44, 154, 192, 427, 540, 617; pain and, 168, 169; parkinsonism and, 486, 487; prenatal development and, 67, 68

midbrain periaqueductal gray, 168

midodrine, 330, 355, 665

Mignot, Emmanuel, 316

migraine, 122, 170, 334, 344, 372, 436, 498, 540, 542, 543, *545,* 547, **548–52;** aura and, 548, 549, 550; diagnosis and treatment of, 551–52; factors in, 548–51; female hormones and, 549; resource groups for, 683–84; stages in, 550; symptoms of, 548; treatment of, 546; vision problems and, 334

Miller Fisher syndrome, 516

Milner, Brenda, 224

mimicry phenomenon, 438

mind, 13

mind-body connection. *See* brain-body loop

mind-body medicine, 53–57; challenges ahead for, 57; placebo effect and, 55–56

minerals, 34

mirtazapine, 368

mistakes, brain activity and, 25, 205

mitochondria, 278, *281;* metabolic diseases and, 281–82

mitochondrial DNA (mtDNA), 126, 281–82

mitochondrial myopathies, 524

mitoxantrone, 441, 665

mixed state, 386

modafinil, 318

molecular biology, 27

M1, 597

monitoring of internal organs, 142–43

monoamine oxidase inhibitors (MAOs), 369, 377–78, 387

mononeuritis multiplex, 473

mononucleosis, 450, 517

monosodium glutamate (MSG), 547

mood, 111, 172, 412; in adolescence, 108, 109; brain-body loop and, 41, 51–53; creativity and, 240–44, *241;* eating and, 151; multiple sclerosis and, 436, 440; sleep disorders and, 308, 309; use of term, 183

mood disorders, 183–84, 273, 390, 406, 414, 474, 498. *See also* bipolar disorder; depression

mood stabilizers, 367, 387, 396, 398

morality, 198

moral reasoning, 206, 207

morphine, 11, 169, 170, 410, 564

mosquitoes, encephalitis and, 464–66, *465*

motivation, 196–99; defined, 196; disorders of, 198; dopamine-based reward system and, 109, 110; prefrontal cortex and, 197, 198, *199*

motor, 158–59, 636–37

motor cortex, 21, 47, 94, 159, *160,* 162, 163, 266, 649; language and, *228,* 229, *229;* skills and, 237, *237*

motor development, 84, 94, 95, 260

motor neurons, 77, 81, 160–61, *161,* 162, 502, 511, 535, 641, 646; amyotrophic lateral sclerosis and, 535–37, *536;* cerebral palsy and, 265, 266; spinal cord injury and, 591

motor skills: coordination and, 158; learning of, 158–59; nondeclarative or implicit memory and, 636–37

motor tics, 497, 498

Mountcastle, Vernon, 21

mouth, 62. *See also* taste

movement, 21, 87, 158–64, 175; aging and, 164; brain-body loop and, 45–46; brain mechanisms and, 159–63, *160, 161,* 502, 511, 531, 554, 648; cerebral palsy and, 265–69; child development and, 84, 94, 95; dizziness and, 327–31; perception of, 27, 232, 233, 327; preconscious behavior and, 172, *173,* 173–74, 175; prenatal development and, 62, 63, 70, 75; spinal "brain" and, 594–95; spinal cord and, 160–61; spinal reflexes and, 161, 162; starting, 162–63, 164

movement and muscle disorders, 160, 163–64, 476–538, 501, 640, 646. *See also* amyotrophic lateral sclerosis; apraxias; ataxia; Bell's palsy; cramps; dystonia; Guillain-Barré syndrome; Huntington's disease; myasthenia gravis; myopathies; parkinsonism plus; Parkinson's disease; peripheral neuropathy; spasms; tics; Tourette's syndrome; tremors

MPTP, 617

multiple chemical sensitivity (MCS), 623

multiple sclerosis (MS), 81, 122, 351, 355, **435–43,** 472, 521, 557; ataxia and, 501, 503, 504; clinical patterns of, 436; diagnosis of, 336, *438,* 438–39; dizziness and, 330, 331, 435; hearing problems and, 345; mechanisms and factors in, 436–38, *437;* prognosis for, 441–43; reducing complications of, 443; resource groups for, 681; symptoms of, 435–36, 437, 440; treatment of, 439–41; tremors and, 440, 490, 491, 492; trigeminal neuralgia and, 566, 567; vision problems and, 335–36, 435, 442

multiple sleep latency test, 317–18

multiple system atrophy (MSA; Shy-Drager syndrome), 148, 329–30, 354, 486, 487–88

multisensory dizziness, 329, 331

mumps, 460

muscle pain, 524

muscles, 37, 48, 94, 108, 119, 525; aches in, sleep disorders and, 308, 309; biopsy of, 525–26; cramps in, 494, 524–25, 535; disorders of (*see* movement and

muscle disorders); motor regulatory system and, 159–63, *161,* 502, 511, 531, 554; paraneoplastic syndromes and, 601; spasms of (*see* spasms); spinal cord injury and, 591, 593; weakness of, 523–24, 530–31, 601, 602

muscular dystrophy, 523, 524, 526–28; Becker, 526; Duchenne, 524, 525, 526, 528; facioscapulohumeral, 527–28; limb-girdle (LGMD), 527, 528; myotonic, 527; treatment of, 528

muscular stiffness (rigidity), 163, 266, 615, 626; parkinsonism and, 477, 483, 484

music, 276; brain development and, 46–47, 118, 237, *237;* listening to, 120

musician's cramp, 495

myalgia, 524

myasthenia gravis, 472, 473, 523, 524, 525, **530–34,** *532,* 623; conserving energy in, 534; diagnosis and treatment of, 532–34; mechanism behind, 531–32; resource groups for, 683; symptoms of, *530,* 530–31

mycophenolate, 534

myelin, 34, 166, 278, 466, 517; adolescent development and, 105, 107, 108, 114; child development and, 81, 85, *91,* 95; HIV/AIDS and, 450; multiple sclerosis and, 81, 336, 437, *437,* 438, 441, 443; prenatal development and, 63, 77, *80,* 80–81; spinal cord injury and, 597, 598; trigeminal neuralgia and, 566, 568

myelitis, 447

myelography, 555

myelomeningocele, 294–96, *295,* 297

myocionus, 468

myoclonic seizures, 320

myoclonus, stimulus-sensitive, 489

myoglobin, 523

myopathies, **523–29;** inflammatory, 523, 528–29; resource groups for, 683; symptoms of, 523–25; testing and diagnosis of, 525–26. *See also* muscular dystrophy

myositis, 473

myotonia, 524–25

myotonic muscular dystrophy, 527

Nagasaki bombing, 74

nalmefene, 415

naltrexone, 415, 424, 665

naprosyn, 563

naproxen, 665

narcolepsy, 149, 157, 309, 312–13, **314–18;** causes and brain mechanisms of, 316–17, *317;* diagnosis and treatment of, 317–18; resource groups for, 676

National Acute Spinal Cord Injury Study (NASCIS), 592–93

National Collaborative Perinatal Project, 267

National Comorbidity Survey, 413

National Health and Nutrition Examination Survey (NHANES I), 51–52

National Institute of Mental Health, 389

National Institutes of Health (NIH), 267, 595–96; office of Complementary and Alternative Medicine of, 54, 57

National Longitudinal Study on Adolescent Health, 110

Native Americans, 431

nature-nurture debate, 111, 237, 238

nausea, 576, 577, 581, 605; nutritional disorders and, 612, 615, 616

navigation through space, 232, 233–35

neck disorders, headache and, 540, 544–45

neck pain, 553, 555, 556

neck stiffness, 541, 576, 577; encephalitis and, 462, 465, 467

neck-tongue syndrome, 545

nefazodone, 368, 397, 665

negative affect, 426

neglect, in early years, 99

Neisseria meningitidis, 459

neocortex, *627;* development of, 136; senses and, 136, 139–40

Neonatal Behavioral Assessment Scale (NBAS), 83

neostriatum, 198

nerve cells. *See* neurons

nerve conduction studies, 525

nerve deafness, 342–46

nerve growth factors, 564

nerve root compression, 616

nerve roots, 160, 553–54

nerves, 42; early research on, 16–17

nervous system injuries, 569–623. *See also* brain tumors; head trauma; neurotoxins and neurotoxic diseases; paraneoplastic syndromes; spinal cord injury; stroke; vitamin deficiencies

neural crest, 67

neuralgia, *545,* 545–47

neural stem cells, 598

neural tube, 62, 64, 66–67, *67,* 68

neural tube defects, 296, 297, 615

neuritis, 511. *See also* peripheral neuropathy

neuroblastomas, 303

neurodegenerative disorders, 12, 130, 215, 485–86, 496, 557, 601–2, 635, 649, 653; speech and language difficulties and, 230, 645, 647. *See also* Alzheimer's disease; Lewy body dementia; parkinsonism plus; Parkinson's disease

neuroepithelial cells, 67

neurofibrillary tangles, 627, 628, *628*

neurofibromas, 284, 285

neurofibromatosis, **284–87,** 305, 343, 605, 607; resource groups for, 674

neurofibromin, 284, 285–86

neurofilaments, 537

neurogenesis, 68

neurogenic claudication, 558

neurogenic pain, 591, 593

neuroimmunology, 147–48

neurokinins, 366

neuroleptics, 387, 393, 485, 499, 509, 631

neuromeres, 67

neuromuscular disorders, 260

neuronal cell adhesion molecules (N-CAMs), 75

neurons, 8–10, *9,* 11, 14, 93; adolescent development and, 104, 105; aging and loss of, 126, 164; Alzheimer's disease and, 627, *628;* axons and dendrites of, 10, 11–12, 17, *17 (see also* axons; dendrites); cerebral palsy and, 265, 266; chemical processes and, 10–11, 14, 15; child development and, 84–87, *85,* chromosomes and DNA in, 28; connections among, 11–13, 39, 46–47, 74–76, 80, 84–87, *85,* 106, 119, *628 (see also* synapses); death of, in normal development, 11, 77–80, 85–87, 107; differentiation of, 68, 71; early research on, 14–15, 16–17, *17, 18;* electrical charges and, 8–10, 14, 15, 18–19, 20–21, 23, 74–75, 80–81; embryonic, implanting into muscles, 595, 597; exercise and, 36, 121; memory and, 221–23; motor *(see* motor neurons); myelination of, 34, 63, 77, *80,* 80–81, 85, *91,* 95, 105, 107, 108, 114; pain transmission and, 166, 168–69; prenatal development and, 63, 66–81; specialization of, 21

neuro-oncology, 606

neuropathic pain, 560, 562

neuropathic tumor, 491–92

neuropathy. *See* peripheral neuropathy

neuropeptides, 148

neuroprotective therapies, 592–95, 597

neuroscience, 14–30; animal studies in, 15, 19–22, 119–20; brain-imaging technologies in, 23–27; combining technologies in, 27–28; early developments in, 14–18; electrical studies in, 18–19, 20–21; frontiers of, 29–30; gene studies in, 28–29; "normality" and, 118–19; Nun Study in, 22; postmortem studies in, 16–18; staining techniques in, 14, 17, *17, 18*

neurosyphilis, 462, 467

neurotoxicology, 617

neurotoxins and neurotoxic diseases, 215, 257, 278, 392, 486, 496, 503, **617–23**, 653; ataxia and, 503; blood-brain barrier and, 617, *618;* common, and their effects (chart), 621–22; diagnosis and treatment of, 619–23; dose-response effect and, 620; many types of, 617–19; peripheral neuropathy and, 515, 617, 618, 619; pseudoneurotoxicity and, 623; tremors and, 490, 492

neurotransmitters, 10–11, 15, 27, 34, 42, 66, 74, 104, 222, 278, 359, 540, 550; depression-heart disease link and, 52; eating and, 44, 401, 404; substance abuse and, 413–14, *414,* 422. *See also specific neurotransmitters*

newborns, 83–90, 94; examination and evaluation of, 83–84; meningitis in, 459, 460, 461; screening tests for, 261, 282, 344; sensory systems of, 136. *See also* infants

New England Centenarian Study (NECS), 39–40

n-hexane, 618, 619, 621

niacin, 611, 612–13

nicotine, 314, 409, 410, 411, 415, 417, 418, 422; prenatal development and, 257

nicotine dependence, 365

night blindness, 615

nightmares, 314

night terrors, 313–14

nitrites, 547

nitrous oxide, 613

N-methyl-D-aspartate (NMDA), 422

N-methyl-D-aspartate (NMDA) antagonists, 564

Nobel Prize, 14, 17, 20, 21

nocardiosis, 460

nociceptors, 166–69

nocturnal myoclonus, 309, 311–13

nodding off, 308

nodes of Ranvier, 437

nondeclarative (implicit) memory, 124, 174, *218,* 218–19, 220, 224, 636–37

nonfluent aphasia, 644, 646

nonimmune fetal hydrops, 279

nonobstructive sleep apnea, 311, 312

non-REM (NREM) sleep, 23, 152, 155, 307

nonspecific arousal, 174–75

nonsteroidal anti-inflammatory drugs (NSAIDs), 330, 551, 563, 564

nonverbal communication, 272

norepinephrine (noradrenaline), 43, 48, 50, 52, 53, 113, 143, 194, 256, 373, 401, 408, 413, 432, 540, 544; depression and, 365, 366, 368

"normality," 118–19

normal-pressure hydrocephalus, 289, 290, 640

nortriptyline, 368, 515, 665

nose, 62, 137–38, *138,* 347; air travel and, 544; sensory cells in, 137–38. *See also* smell; smelling problems

nuchal translucency scan, 76

nuclear blasts, 74

nucleus accumbens, 151

nucleus pulposus, 555

numbness, 489, 548, 560, 605, 613, 617; back problems and, 554, 555, 558; facial, 330, 454; multiple sclerosis and, 336, 436; neck problems and, 545; painful (anesthesia dolorosa), 567; pe-

ripheral neuropathy and, 511, 512, 513, 514, 515; stroke and, 339, 571, 576, 577; transient ischemic attack and, 334; trigeminal neuralgia and, 565, 567

Nun Study, 22

nutrition, 22, 308; brain care and, 31, 33–36, *35;* diabetes and, 54; during pregnancy, 70–71, 81

nutritional disorders, 278, **610–16,** 626, 640. *See also* vitamin deficiencies; *specific vitamins*

nystagmus, 611

obesity, *153,* 153–54, 156, 157, 311, 541, 572

obsessions, 380, 381

obsessive-compulsive disorder (OCD), 273, 374, **379–84,** 401; brain mechanisms in, 381, *382,* 383; causes of, 381–82; in children, 379, 381, 382–83, 384; diagnosis of, 382–83; helping someone who has, 384; manifestations of, 379–81; resource groups for, 679; Tourette's syndrome and, 381, 382, 497, 498, 499, 500; treatment of, 383–84

obsessive-compulsive (OC) spectrum illnesses, 381

obstructive sleep apnea, 157, 309, *310,* 310–11, 312, 313, 478

occipital cortex, 332

occipital lobes, 233, 235, 652; consciousness and, 174, 175

occupational chemicals, 617, 618–19, 621

occupational counseling, 439

occupational therapy, 599

odors, 549

olanzapine, 387, 388, 393, 398, 403, 665

olfactory ensheathing glia (OEG), 598

olfactory nerve, 139, 598

olfactory pathway, *138,* 139, *139, 141, 348*

oligodendrocytes, 80, *80*

oligodendroglial precursors, 597

oligodendrogliomas, 302, 304, 607
olivopontocerebellar atrophy, 487
omega-3 fatty acids, 36
oncogenes, 609
ophthalmoplegia, 611
opioid agonists, 416
opioid antagonists, 415–16, 422
opioids (opiates), 192, 313, 354; endogenous, alcohol and, 422; as pain relievers, 452, 564, 640; substance abuse and addiction and, 409, 410, 411, 413, 414–16, 417
opposite-limb movement, 162
optic chiasm, 332, *333;* pressure on, 336–38
optic nerve, 139, 303, 332, *333,* 334, 339, 435, 612; damage to, *335,* 335–36; tumors on, 285, 301, 302, 303, 305, 606, 607
optic neuritis, 335–36, 435, 442
orbital frontal cortex (OFC), 204–5, *205;* violence and aggression and, 427, 428
orexin, 317, *317,* 318
organic amnesias, 635–37
organ transplants, 445, 515
orgasm, 151, 157, 541
oromandibular dystonia, 495
orphans, 92–93
orthostatic hypotension, 329–30, 353, 354, 355
orthostatic truncal tremors, 491
Osler, Sir William, 267
osteoarthritis (spondylosis), 555, 556–57
osteophytes (bone spurs), 553, 554, 556, 557
otoacoustic emissions, 344
otoliths, *328,* 329
ovaries, 146, 151
overeating, 53, 54, 153–54; binge eating and, 394, 399, 400, 401, 403
overinclusiveness, 242, 243
overweight, 54, 101, 573. *See also* obesity
oxazepam, 424, 665
oxcarbazepine, 324

oxybutynin, 356, 665
oxycodone, 447
oxytocin, 119, 145, 192, 665

pain, 57, 165–70, 205, 273, **539–68;** acute vs. chronic, 165–66, 559; functions of, 165, 540; multiple sclerosis and, 440; muscle (myalgia), 524; neurogenic, 591, 593; physiology of, 6, 160, 161, 166–68, *167;* placebo effect and, 56; psychology of, 168–69; seeing your doctor about, 562; sensory cells and, 136–37; spasms and, 494; spinal reflexes and, 162; treatment of, 168, 169–70. *See also* back pain; headache; migraine; trigeminal neuralgia
pain, chronic, 165–66, 406, **559–64,** *560;* acute pain vs., 165–66, 559; diagnosis and treatment of, 561, 562–64; effects of, 559–60; physiology of, 561–62; psychological state and, 561, 563; resource groups for, 685; types of, 560–61
pain-intensity scales, 563
pain pathways, lesioning of, 564
pain relievers (analgesics), 168, 169, 446–47, 495, 543, 561, 563–64, 567, 591, 640
paint sniffing, 619
palilaia, 498
pallidotomy, 483
pancreas, 146, 610
PANDAS (pediatric autoimmune neuropsychiatric disorders associated with streptococcal infections), 383
panic attacks, 330, 331, 356, 372, 374, 376; post-traumatic stress disorder and, 405, 406; suicide and, 431, 432, 433
panic disorder (PD), 194, 273, **372–75,** 549, 623; diagnosis and treatment of, 372–75; resource groups for, 678–79; symptoms of, 372
pantothenic acid, 611, 615
parabrachial nucleus, 145

parahippocampal cortex, 26, 223
paralysis, 163, 297, 502, 601, 618, 646; Bell's palsy and, 520–22; Guillain-Barré syndrome and, 516–19; lupus and, 472, 473; during REM sleep, 307, 317; sleep, 308, 315; spinal cord injury and, 591, 593, *594,* 595
paraneoplastic cerebellar degeneration (PCD), 601, 603
paraneoplastic syndromes, 503, **600–603;** antibody-associated, 602; nervous system, examples of (chart), 601; treatment of, 603; underlying causes of, 600–603
paranoid behavior, 639
paraplegia, 591, *594*
parasomnias, 313–14
parasympathetic nervous system, 144, 145, 146, 352, *353;* autonomic disorders and, 352–56; fear response and, 406–7
parathyroid, 146, 640
paraventricular nucleus, 145, 147
parenthood, plasticity and, 119–20
paresthesia ("pins and needles"), 489, 516, 554, 565
paretic neurosyphilis, 467
parietal lobes, 21, *106;* apraxias and, 649; consciousness and, 174, 175–76; visual and spatial processing and, *232,* 234, 235
parkinsonism, use of term, 484
parkinsonism plus, 480, 483, **484–89;** causes of, 485–86; corticobasal degeneration and, 486, 488–89; drug-induced, 485; multiple system atrophy and, 486, 487–88; progressive supranuclear palsy and, 486–87, 488; resource groups for, 681–82; symptoms of, 484–85; use of term, 484
Parkinson's disease (PD), 27, 122, 130, 148, 163, 230, 330, 350, 354, 468, **477–83,** *479,* 496, 537, 602, 616, 617, 619, 641, 646; causes of, *479,* 479–80; course of,

478–79; diagnosis of, 480; other forms of parkinsonism vs., 480, 484–85, 487; resource groups for, 681–82; symptoms of, 477–78, *478*; treatment of, 480–83, *482*, 485, 487, 488; tremors and, 477, 478, *478*, 480, 483, 485, 487, 490, 491, 492

paroxetine, 330, 368, 374, 375, 383, 665

paroxysmal hypothermia, 149

partial (focal) seizures, 319, 321, 325

Pavlov, Ivan, 19–20, 219

pellagra, 612

pemoline, 258, 500, 666

Penfield, Wilder, 19

penicillin, 456, 467

perception, 639; implicit memory and, 636–37; visual and spatial processing and, 232–35. *See also* senses; *specific senses*

perceptive agnosia, 651–52

percutaneous radio-frequency rhizotomy, 567

performance anxiety, 378

periodic limb movement disorder, 309, 311–13

peripheral nervous system, *144*, 148, 437, 511–12, *512*, 516; lupus and, 472, 473; neurotoxic diseases and, 617–18; pain and, 561, 562; paraneoplastic syndromes and, 601

peripheral neuropathy, 329, 330, **511–15**, *512*, 523, 646; carpal tunnel syndrome, 436, 512–13; diabetic, 355, 515; generalized, 513–15; hereditary, 514; HIV/AIDS and, 451–52; Lyme disease and, 454–55; nutritional disorders and, 611, 612, 613, 615, 616; sensory, 514–15; tremors and, 491–92; ulnar neuropathy, 513

perirhinal cortex, 223

periventricular leukomalacia (PVL), 266

persistent vegetative state (PVS), 177, 588, 589

personality, 299, 605; cultural or societal expectations and, 194; differences in, 197–98; experiences and, 191, 193–94; family influence and, 193–94; temperament and, 40, 50, 84, 96–97, 182–83, 190–95

personality disorders, 114, 365, 390, 404, 406, 430

pervasive developmental disorder not otherwise specified (PDD-NOS), 270, 274

pervasive developmental disorders (PDDs), 270, 274; Asperger's syndrome, 270, 271, 272, 382; diagnosis of, 274–75; Rett's disorder, 270, 272, 275. *See also* autism

pesticides, 480, 619, 620, 621, 623

petit mal (absence) seizures, 176, 320, *321*

Phelps, Michael, 24

phencyclidine (PCP), 410, 413, 417, 617

phenelzine, 666

phenobarbital, 615–16, 666

phenylketonuria (PKU), 261, 274, 278, 282

phenytoin, 324, 567, 614, 615–16, 621, 666

phobias, 219, 372, 373, 374

phonemes, 226

phonological dyslexia, 250–51

phonological loop, 221

phonology, 643

photophobia, 459

photopsias, 335

photoreceptors, 123, 136, 137

photosensitivity, 459, 475

phototherapy, 369–70

phrenology, 15–16

physical therapy, 546, 589, 599. *See also* rehabilitative therapy

physiological tremor, 491

physostigmine, 492, 666

Piaget, Jean, 94

Pick's bodies, 641

Pick's disease, 198, 208, 215, 640–41, *641*, 642

pilocytic astrocytomas, 301, 607

pimozide, 499, 666

pineal gland, 43; tumors in or near, 304–5, 607

"pins and needles." *See* paresthesia

pituitary gland, *42*, 43, *49*, *142*, 145–46, 147–48, *152*, 154, 300, 304, 407, 432, 469, 640; adolescent development and, 103, 108; problems with, 148–49; tumors in, 336–38, 604, 607

placebo effect, 55–56

planning ahead, 207–9

plant toxins, 617, 622

planum temporale, *78*, 79

plaques of Alzheimer's disease, 627, *627*, 628

plasma exchange, 441, 518, 603

plasmapheresis, 533

plasticity, 11–13, 21–22, 39, 92, 116–17, 119–20, 122, 231; critical periods and, *85*, 85–90; learning and, 12, 46–47, 116; nature and nurture and, 64–66; parenthood and, 119–20

platelet "stickiness," 52, 53

play, imaginative, 272–73

pleconaril, 461, 666

pneumonia, 460, 466, 484, 487, 488, 503, 517, 626

polio, 525

polyarteritis, 343, 472

polymorphism, 628

polymyalgia rheumatica, 524

polymyositis, 529

polyneuropathy, 472

polysomnography, *308*, 309

pons, 44, 68, *142*, 154; body regulation and, 145; tumors in, 301

position in space, awareness of, 45, 160, 161, 172, 175–76, 327; dizziness and, 327–31

positron-emission tomography (PET), 23–25, *24*, 26, 27, 153, 163

posterior cingulate gyrus, 234–35

postherpetic neuralgia (PHN), 446–47

postmeasles encephalomyelitis, 462, 466–67
postmortem studies, 16–18
postpartum depression, 100
post-traumatic stress disorder (PTSD), 99, 322, 374, **405–8,** 623; borderline personality disorder and, 395; diagnosis and treatment of, 408; fear response and, 406–8; resource groups for, 680; strategies for coping with, 407; symptoms of, 405–6, 408
postural tremor, 490, 491
potassium, 9, 336, 550
Prader-Willi syndrome, 149
pragmatics, 643
praxis programs, 648
preconscious behavior, 172, *173,* 173–74, 175
prednisone, 343, 439, 473, 475, 518, 521, 528, 529, 533, 543, 661, 666
prefrontal cortex (PFC), 198, 255, 373, 391; attention and motivation and, 197, 198, *199;* damage to, 7, *8,* 99, 186, 188, 197, 198, 201–2, 204, 396; decision making and, 201–2, 204, *205;* development of, 85, 91, 94, 105, 107, *196,* 197, 208; inhibition and control and, 185–89, *186;* planning ahead and, 207–9; violence and aggression and, 427, *427,* 428
pregnancy, 61, 67, 69–70; ADHD and complications during, 256–57; depression during, 100; fetal alcohol syndrome and, 72, 215, 260–61; multiple sclerosis and, 442; nutritional needs during, 34, 70–71, 81, 615; substances to avoid or reduce during, 72, 81. *See also* prenatal development
premature birth, 72, 86, 261, 266, 267
premotor cortex, 163, 649
prenatal care, 261
prenatal development, 26, 33, 61–82, *65,* 84, 215; in first month

of pregnancy, 62, 66–67, *67;* in second and third months of pregnancy, 62, 67–69; in second trimester, 62–63, 69–71; in final trimester, 63, 73–82; aggregation of brain cells in, 70, 74; birth defects and, 34, 64, 72, 76, 615 (*see also* spina bifida); cerebral palsy and, 265, 266, 267; connections among neurons formed in, 74–76, 80; cortical cell migration in, 70, *73,* 73–74; gender differences and, *78,* 79; hydrocephalus and, 76, 290; mental retardation and, 259–61; milestones in, 62–63; neuron proliferation in, 66, 68, 71; neurotoxins and, 620; nutrition and, 34, 70–71, 81; origin of brain structures in, 68–69, 70–71; substances to avoid or reduce during pregnancy and, 72, 81
prenatal experiences, 81–82
prenatal tests, 69, *69,* 76–77, 259, 296
presbycusis, 344
pressure: headache and, 547; sensations of, 137, 327. *See also* blood pressure; hypertension
presyncope, 327
primary afferent nociceptors, 166–69
primidone, 493, 666
priming, *218,* 219, 223
primitive neuroectodermal tumors (PNETs), 303, 304, 607
prion diseases, 468–70, *469*
problem solving, 240
procarbazine, 303
procedural memory, *218,* 218–19, 223, 224
progesterone, 45, 151, 549
programmed cell death, 77–80
progressive headache, 541
progressive multifocal leukoencephalopathy (PML), 450
progressive muscle relaxation, 546
progressive supranuclear palsy (PSP), 350, 486–87, 488

prolactin, 145, 149, 337
propantheline, 666
propranolol, 378, 493, 541, 666
proprioception, 45, 327, 613
prosopagnosia, 652
prostaglandins, 147, 168
protease inhibitors, 449
proteins: in diet, 28, 33, 70–71; misfolded, prion diseases and, 468–70, *469;* paraneoplastic syndromes and, 600–601, 603
protomap, 68, 73–74
protriptyline, 666
PrP, prion disease and, 468–70, *469*
pruning, synaptic, 85–87, 107, 111
pseudoephedrine, 544
pseudoneurotoxicity, 623
pseudowords, 250, 251
psychogenic amnesia, 637
psychopathy, 194
psychotherapy, 194, 546; bipolar disorder and, 388–89; borderline personality disorder and, 397; changes associated with antidepressant medications compared to, 122, 367, 369; depression and, 122, 367, 369; eating disorders and, 402–3; post-traumatic stress disorder and, 408
psychotic behavior, Alzheimer's disease and, 630–31
ptosis (eyelid drooping), 523, 542; Bell's palsy and, 520–22; myasthenia gravis and, 530, *530,* 531, 532
puberty, 103–4, 107–9, 113, 152
pulse, 517
pure alexia, 233
pure word deafness, 653
purging behavior, 399, 400–401, 402, 404
putamen, 98, 223
pyridostigmine, 623
pyridoxine (vitamin B₆), 515, 611, 613
pyruvate, 612
pyruvate dehydrogenase deficiency, 267

quadriplegia, 266, 591, *594*

quetiapine, 393, 666

quickening, 70

radiation therapy, 349, 350, 568, 605, 607, 608–9; childhood tumors and, 299–304

radicular (referred) pain, 545, 554

Rakic, Pasko, 68, 73–74

raloxifene, 666

Ramón y Cajal, Santiago, 14, 17, *18*

rapid eye movement (REM) behavior disorder, 314

rapid eye movement (REM) sleep, 23, 152, *152*, 154, 155, 307, 366; learning and memory formation and, 32–33; narcolepsy and, 316–18

rashes: dermatomyositis and, 528–29; lupus and, 471; Lyme disease and, 453–54, *454*, 456; shingles and, 444, *444*, 446

Raven Progressive Matrices Tests, 211, 214

reading, 92, *228*, 230, 233, 570; alexia and, 233, 645–46. *See also* dyslexia

reasoning ability, 202; higher-level, 206

recognition, agnosias and, 46, 233, 235, 637, 639, 651–53

recombinant DNA technology, 283

recombinant tissue plasminogen activator (rt-PA), 574

referee analogy, 189

referred pain, 545, 554

reflexes, 62, 84, 112, 554, 557, 591; aging and, 127–28; body regulation and, 142–49; inhibition and control and, 185–86, 188; spinal, 161, 162

regenerative therapies, 597–99

rehabilitative therapy, 439; head trauma and, 589–90; spinal cord injury and, 593, 599; stroke and, 46, 47, 575

relaxation, 39, 309, 546, 551, 563

remyelination therapies, 597, 598

repetitive behavior, 273

repetitive nerve stimulation, 525

resistance training, 164

resource groups, 673–86

resting tremor, 163

restless legs syndrome, 309, 312–13, 478

retinas, 86, 123, 137, 139, 175, 233, 332, 449, 612, 616; artificial, 339; degeneration disorders in, 338–39, *339*; impaired blood flow to, 334–35; paraneoplastic syndromes and, 601; tumors in, 303–5

retinitis pigmentosa (RP), 338

retinoblastomas, 303–5

retinopathy, 86

retrograde amnesia, 635, 636

Rett's disorder, 270, 272, 275

reverse transcriptase (RT), 448–49

rheumatoid arthritis, 472, 474, 560

riboflavin, 611, 615

rifampin, 459

rigidity. *See* muscular stiffness

riluzole, 538, 666

risk taking, 109–12; healthy risks and, 109–10; unhealthy risks and, 110–12

risperidone, 393, 398, 499, 631, 667

Ritalin. *See* methylphenidate

rivastigmine, 630, 667

Rocky Mountain spotted fever, 460

rofecoxib, 168

RT inhibitors, 448–49

rubella, 261, 466

Sacks, Oliver, 57

sacral nerves, *592*

Safe Return, 631

St. John's wort, 369, 370

sarcoid, 148

sarcoidosis, 438, 521

satiety factors, 44

savants, 237–38, 272

scanning electron micrography (SEM), *9*

schizophrenia, 7, 18, 22, 26, 46, 74, 113–14, 122, 177, 188, 198, 208, 263, 315, 350, 365, 386, **390–93**, 429; brain mechanisms and, 391, *392*; childhood behaviors and, 391–92; creativity and, 243, 244; diagnosis and treatment of, 393; resource groups for, 679; risk factors for, 392; symptoms of, 390, 391

Scholastic Aptitude Test (SAT), 211, 215

School Sisters of Notre Dame, 22

Schumann, Robert, 241

Schwann cells, 597

schwannomas, 286, 607

sciatica, 554

scleroderma, 472, 474

scrapie, 470

scrupulosity, 380

seasonal depression, 364, 369–70

seborrhea, 478

sedatives, 275, 354, 410, 417, 631

seeing. *See* vision; vision problems

seizures, 19, 111, 176, 224, 264, 274, 282, 285, 286, 309, **319–26**, 336, 354, 580, 617; brain tumors and, 299, 302, 319, 605, 608, 609; brain wave recordings of, *320, 321, 322*; causes of, 319; defined, 319; diagnosis and treatment of, 323–25; helping someone with, 323; lupus and, 472, 473; meningitis and, 319, 324, 459, 461; metabolic diseases and, 278, 279, 283; nutritional disorders and, 612, 613; resource groups for, 676; types of, 319, 320–21. *See also* epilepsy

selective dorsal rhizotomy, 268, 269

selective serotonin reuptake inhibitors (SSRIs), 275, 330, 368, *368*, 375, 378, 383, 387, 397, 401, 403, 500, 510, 544, 630

selegiline, 667

selenium, 538

self, 174; consciousness and, *171*, 171–72

self-injurious behavior, 273, 394, 395, 397, 406, 498

self-stimulation, 273

semantic memory, 217–18, *218*, 224

semantics, 643, 644

semicircular canals, *328*, 329

senile dementia, 12

senility, 124, 130

senses, 6, 39, 107, 136–40, *137*, 142, 172, 511; aging and, 140, 348–49; autism and, 273; brain-body loop and, 45–46; conversion of signals from external world into nerve signals and, 137–38, *141*; cortical areas associated with, *139*; differences in, 140; discrimination between different signals and, 138–40; disorders of, 140, 327–51; emotions and, 182; habituation and, *117*, 117–18; pathways of, *138*, 139, *139*, *141*; purpose of, 136

sensitization, 166–68

sensory cells, 136–40, *137*, *141*

sensory cortex, *138*, *139*, 162, 223

sensory memory, 220

sensory peripheral neuropathy, 514–15, 615, 616

sensory problems, 332–51; learned nonuse and, 593, 595–97; multiple sclerosis and, 436; tasting problems, 140, 349, 350, 351, 677. *See also* hearing problems; smelling problems; vision problems

sensory transduction, 137–38, *141*

sentences, 226, 227

separation anxiety, *191*

serotonin, 43, 52, 111, 113, 192, *366*, 373, 413; alcohol and, 422; anorexia nervosa and, 156; borderline personality disorder and, 396, 397; depression and, 365, 366, 367–68, *368*; eating disorders and, 401; headache and, 540, 544; obsessive-compulsive disorder and, 381, 383, 401; suicide and, 366, 432; violence and aggression and, 426, 427, 428. *See also* selective serotonin reuptake inhibitors

sertraline, 368, 375, 383, 667

serum screening, 76–77

setpoints, 44, 47, 147

setting sun sign, 289

sex drive, 150, 151–52, 153, 154, 155, 366

sex headache, 540, 541

sex hormones, 79, 151. *See also specific hormones*

sexual behavior, 110, 151–52, 155

sexual development, 152, 155

sexual dysfunction, 156–57, 355, 356; parkinsonism and, 478, 487–88; spinal cord injury and, 591

sexual intercourse, 151, 155

sexual response, 151, 156–57; brain-body loop and, 45

shingles (herpes zoster), **444–47,** 560; chicken pox in childhood and, 444–45; diagnosis and treatment of, 446–47; immune system and, 445–46, 447; rash in, 444, *444*, 446

shock treatment, 367, 369

shunts, 290–92, *291*

Shy-Drager syndrome. *See* multiple system atrophy

shyness, 96–97, 191, 192; social phobia vs., 376

sickle-cell anemia, 281, 560, 562

side effects. *See* medications, side effects of

sight. *See* vision

sign language, 227, 228, 646

sildenafil, 356, 667

silicones, 290

simple partial seizures, 321

simultanagnosia, 234

sinusitis, 540, 544, *545*

Sjögren's syndrome, 438, 472

skilled action: four levels of processing in, 649. *See also* apraxias

skills, 173, 175, 236–37, *237*, 238, 240; gradual building of, in childhood, 94–96; motor, 158–59, 636–37; procedural memory and, *218*, 218–19, 223, 224

skull, 213, 585, 604; brain swelling and, 582; injuries involving

blood vessels within, 583–85; injuries to, 583; prenatal development and, 73; shape of, 15–16

sleep, 23, 37, 51, 53, 111, 150, 152, 153, 155, 175, 359, 366, 498, 549; age and, *33*, 103, 128, *128*, 157; all-night recordings of, *308*, 309; brain care and, 31, 32–33; chronic pain and, 559; non-REM (NREM), 23, 152, 155, 307; normal, 307; rapid eye movement (REM), 23, 32–33, 152, *152*, 154, 155, 307, 316–18, 366

sleep apnea: nonobstructive, 311, 312; obstructive, 157, 309, *310*, 310–11, 312, 313, 478

sleep deprivation, 32–33, 103, 155, 314, 319, 326

sleep disorders, 129, 157, **307–14,** 412, 414, 631; chronic fatigue syndrome and, 359–60; circadian rhythm disorders, 311; common, 312–13; depression and, 315, 363, 364, 365, 366, 367, 385, 430; eating disorders and, 399, 402; evaluation of, *308*, 308–9; management of, 314; nocturnal myoclonus and restless legs syndrome, 309, 311–13; parasomnias, 313–14; Parkinson's disease and, 478; posttraumatic stress disorder and, 405, 406; resource groups for, 675–76. *See also* insomnia; narcolepsy

sleep drunkenness, 308

sleep hygiene, 309

sleepiness, daytime, 307, 308, 311, 312, 314, 315; nodding off and, 308

sleep medications, 157, 309–10

sleep paralysis, 308, 315

sleep terrors, 313–14

sleep-wake cycles, *43*, 43–44, 143, 149; abnormalities in, 388–89; in adolescence, 103; circadian rhythm disorders and, 311

sleepwalking, 307, 313

smell, 136–40, 142, 347–51; differences in acuity of, 140, 348–49;
olfactory pathway and, *138*, 139,
139, 141, 348; sensory cells and,
136, 137–38, 347
smell identification tests, *141*
smelling problems, 140, **347–51,**
615; diagnosis and treatment of,
351; resource groups for, 677;
seizures and, 321; as sign of
neurological disease, 350–51
Smith-Lemli-Opitz syndrome, 278
smoking, 40, 51, 53, 72, 111, 129,
164, 334, 339, 629; maternal,
261; stroke and, 572, 573, 579
social behavior, 99, 175, 274;
autism and, 270–71
social contact, 131, 215
social phobia (social anxiety disorder), 194, 374, **376–78;** causes
of, 377; diagnosis and treatment
of, 377–78; manifestations of,
376–77; resource groups for,
678–79
sodium, 9, 74, 336, 550
solvents, chemical, 617, 618, 619,
621, 623
somatic pain, 560
somatization disorder, 374
somatosensory cortex, 6, 45, *138,*
139
sound, transformed into electrical
signals, 341–42
spasms, 435, 490, **494,** 555, 556,
561, 616; resource groups for,
682; spinal cord injury and, 591,
593; vasospasm, 580
spastic cerebral palsy, 266, 267,
268–69
spasticity, 163, 268, 279, 283;
multiple sclerosis and, 435,
440, 443
spatial awareness, 160, 161, 172,
175–76
spatial learning, 28
spatial system, 233–35; attention
and, 234, *234,* 235
spatial-visual reasoning, 210, 214,
215

special education, 264; dyslexia
and, 249–50, 251–53
speech, 27, 226–31; auditory agnosias and, 653; brain mechanisms and, 6–7, *228,* 228–29,
229; defined, 643; development
of, 84, 90–92, 227–28, 230, 248,
344. *See also* language
speech problems, 230–31, 454, 501,
505, 531, 535, 603, 605, **643–47;**
brain tumors and, 299;
dysarthria, 643, 646, 647; early
research on, 6–7; metabolic diseases and, 279, 283; multiple
sclerosis and, 435; parkinsonism
and, 477, 478, 484, 487; resource
groups for, 686; stroke and, 18,
570, 576, 577; stuttering, 644–45.
See also language difficulties
speech therapy, 646–47
Spencer, Aiden, 20
spina bifida, 76, 261, **293–97,** *295,*
615; Arnold Chiari malforma-
tion and, 294–96, *296;* causes of,
293; overt, 293–97, *295;* prevention and treatment of, 64,
296–97; resource groups for, 675
spina bifida occulta, 293–94, *295,*
296
spinal "brain," 594–95
spinal canal, 553, 556, 557
spinal cord, 3, 42, 139, 151, 288,
302, *353,* 436, 488, 540, 553, 554,
607, 612, 613, 616; anatomy of,
160–61; autonomic disorders
and, 352–53; back pain and, 555,
557; lupus and, 472, 473; movement and, 160–61, 502, 594–95;
nerves of, divided into five levels, *592;* pain messages and,
160, 161, 166, 168–69, 561, 562;
paraneoplastic syndromes and,
601; peripheral nervous system
and, 511; prenatal development
and, 62, 67; sensory functions
of, 6, 160, 161; spinal "brain"
and, 594–95; VZV in, 447
spinal cord compression, 436,
438

spinal cord injury, 34, 47, 265, 355,
591–99, *594;* diagnosis of, 592;
learned nonuse and, 593,
595–97; medical treatment of,
592–93; muscle atrophy and,
591, 595; recovery after, 593–99,
596; regenerative therapies and,
597–99; remyelination therapies
and, 597, 598; resource groups
for, 685; spinal "brain" and,
594–95
spinal tap (lumbar puncture),
460–61, *461,* 541, 553
spine, 160; anatomy of, 160–61,
553–54
spondylosis, 555, 556–57
spongiform diseases, 469, *470*
sports, 109–10
staining techniques, 14, 17, *17, 18*
starvation, 146, 151
statins, 515, 667
stem cells, 339, 481, 598–99
stereotactic biopsy, 606
stereotactic neurosurgery, 269, 300
steroids, 329, 336, 410, 461, 466,
473, 475, 504, 521, 605, 609, 640.
See also corticosteroids; *specific*
steroids
sticky molecules, 74
stimulants, 255, 256, 258, 308, 318,
410, 500
stimulation, 66, 121, 222; brain care
and, 39–40; of children, 101;
prenatal, 81–82; threshold of, in
infants, 192
stimulus-sensitive myoclonus, 489
stomach, 142, 144, 150. *See also*
eating
streptococcal infection, 383
Streptococcus pneumoniae, 460
stress, 40, 54, 326, 388, 463, 491,
563; brain-body loop and,
47–51; brain care and, 37–39;
common illnesses and, 50–51;
conditions exacerbated by, 491,
495, 498; depression and, 365,
366–67, 368, 430; emotional,
51–53; functional amnesia and,
637; harmful effects of, 37–38;

stress (*cont.*)
   headache and, 168, 544, 546, 549, 551; immune system and, 148; individual responses to, 49–50; management of, 38–39, 50–51; overstimulation and, 39; placebo effect and, 56; post-traumatic stress disorder and, 405–8; sleep disorders and, 309, 314; suicidal feelings and, 429
stress hormones, 48, *49,* 166. *See also* cortisol; epinephrine; norepinephrine
stress patterns, in language, 226–27
stress response (fight or flight response), 37, 47–49, *49,* 93, 97, 143; post-traumatic stress disorder and, 406–8
striatonigral degeneration, 487
striatum, 507
stroke, 17–18, 31, 35, 46, 101, 162, 163, 164, 176, 225, 354, 379, 447, 467, 496, 516, 524, 535, 548, 566, 605, 615, 629, 649; agnosias and, 651, 653; anger and, 53; ataxia and, 501, 502, 503, 504; being prepared in case of, 571; Bell's palsy and, 520, 521; depression and, 52, 54, 364; diagnosis and treatment of, 340, 572–75, 578–80; dizziness and, 330, 331, 570; dyslexia and, 248, 251; hearing loss and, 344, 345; heat, 176; hemorrhagic, 339, 541, 570, 572–73, **576–80,** *577,* 583, 685; ischemic, 143, 334, 339, 473, **570–75,** *574,* 576, 577, 578, 579, 583–84, 685; lupus and, 473; memory impairment and, 570, 635, 636; multiple sclerosis and, 435, 436; parkinsonism and, 485, 487; prevention of, 572; recovery after, 12, 46, 47, 575, 580, 595; resource groups for, 685; risk factors for, 339, 572, 579, 645; speech and language difficulties and, 230, 644–45, 646–47; symptoms of, 570, 571, 576–77, 578; transient ischemic attacks

(TIAs) and, 140, 330, 334–35, *335,* 340, 570–71, 646; vision problems and, 140, 232, 332, 334, 335, 338–40, 570–71, 572, 576, 577
Stroop test, 188–89
strychnine, 617
stupor, 176, 177
stuttering, 644–45
subarachnoid hemorrhage, 576, 577, 578, 579, 580, 585
subcortical dementia, 486
subdural hematomas, *584,* 584–85
subiculum, 224
substance abuse, 40, 157, 204, 216, 255, 314, 326, 394, **409–18,** 579, 617, 620, 640; in adolescence, 103, 110, 111–12; altered states of consciousness and, 174, 176, 177; definitions of abuse and, 409; drug categories and, 409–10; emotional and control disorders and, 365, 372, 374, 377, 394, 406; and mental syndromes caused by different kinds of drugs, 416–17; pregnancy and, 72, 81; prevalence of, 413; resource groups for, 680; schizophrenia and, 390, 392, 393; signs of, 410; suicide and, 429, 430, 431. *See also* addiction; alcohol abuse; alcoholism
substantia nigra, 163, 479
subthalamic nucleus, 483
sudden death, 51, 356
suicidal feelings, 364, 365, **429–33;** case study in, 432; diagnosis and treatment of, 432–33; eating disorders and, 401, 402; psychiatric illnesses and, 429; recognizing, 430–32; resource groups for, 681
suicide, 184, 406, 426, 617; among adolescents and young adults, 110, 114, 431; bipolar disorder and, 243, 364, 385, 386, 429, 433; borderline personality disorder and, 394, 395, 429; depression and, 364, 367, 372, 385, 429–33;

examples of people at risk for, 429–30; serotonin activity and, 366, 432; statistics on, 430, *430*
sumatriptan, 543, 667
sumultanagnosia, 652
sunlight, circadian rhythms and, 43, 143
superoxide dismutase, 537
supportive psychotherapy, 397
suprachiasmatic nucleus (SCN), 43
supraoptic nucleus, 145
suprasellar region, tumors in, 304
surface dyslexia, 251
swallowing difficulties, 443, 454, 484, 502, 505, 516, 530, 535; myopathies and, 523, 527, 529
sweat glands, 554
sweating, 143, 151, 352, 353–54, 355
swelling. *See* brain swelling
sympathetic nervous system, 97, 143, 144, 145, 146, 148, 352, *353;* autonomic disorders and, 352–56; post-traumatic stress disorder and, 406–8; tumors in, 303
synapses, 10, 17, 20, 222; adolescent development and, 106, 107, 111, 114; child development and, 84–87, *85,* 93, 94, 95, 96, 99; prenatal development and, 70, 74–75, 76; pruning of, 85–87, 107, 111
syncope (fainting), 176, 327, 353, 487
syntax, 227, 643, 644
syphilis, 343, 438, 460, 461, 467, 640
systemic lupus erythematosus (SLE), 343, 438, **471–75,** 532; diagnosis of, 474; neurological symptoms of, 471–74; resource groups for, 681; treatment of, 473–75

tabes dorsalis, 467
tabetic neurosyphilis, 467
tacrine, 630, 667
tactile agnosias, 653
talents, 236, 237–38

tardive dyskinesia, 164, 499

taste, 136–40, 142, 347; differences in acuity of, 140; gustatory pathway and, 45, *138,* 139, *139, 141;* sensory cells and, 136, 347

tasting problems, 140, **349, 350,** 615; diagnosis and treatment of, 351; resource groups for, 677

tau protein, 486, 487, 488, 627, 642

Tay-Sachs disease, 281

T cells, multiple sclerosis and, 438, 441, 442–43

teenagers. *See* adolescence

telencephalon, 68

temperament, 40, 50, 84, 96–97, 190–95; brain mechanisms and, 191–92; emotions and, 182–83; finding right fit in life and, 194–95; infant, deviation from, 192–94; psychiatric disorders and, 194. *See also* personality

temperature: sensations of, 6, 160, 161, 166. *See also* body temperature

temporal arteritis, 541

temporal lobes, 19, 26, 168, 229, 336, 341, 347, 386, 391, 463, 586, 635, 641; agnosias and, 652, 653; amnesias and, 635, 636, 637; consciousness and, 174, 175; visual and spatial processing and, *232,* 233, 235

temporomandibular joint (TMJ) dysfunction, 540

tension headache, 53, 540, 542, 543–44, *545,* 551

Ter-pegossian, Michael, 24

testes, 146, 151

testosterone, 79, 103–4, 108, 129, 146, 151

tetrabenazine, 499

tetrahydroaminoacridine, 630

thalamotomy, 483, 493

thalamus, 45, 68, 97, 229, 252, *373,* 391, 427, 483, 493, 577; cerebral palsy and, 266, *268,* 269; consciousness and, 174, 175; emotions and, 181, *181;* senses and, *137, 138,* 139, *348,* 349; sleep-wake cycle and, 43–44; tumors in, 304

thiamine (vitamin B$_1$), 503, 610–12, 640

thinking, 299, 639; abstract, 107, 131, 172, 272, 639; brain development and, 87, 91, 106, 107; emotions and, 181, 183

thinking, disorders of, 473, 605, 611, 624–53. *See also* agnosias; Alzheimer's disease; apraxias; dementia; language difficulties; speech problems

thoracic nerves, *592*

thrombosis, 571

"thunderclaps," 541–42, 576, 577

thymectomy, 533

thymus, 148, 532, *532,* 533

thyroid, 146, 278, 492, 503, 531, 640; hypothyroidism and, 330, 365, 503, 615, 626

thyroiditis, 532

thyroid-stimulating hormone, 145, 149

tic douloureux. *See* trigeminal neuralgia

ticks: encephalitis and, 464, *465,* 466; Lyme disease and, 453, 456

ticlopidine, 667

tics, 163, 381, 382, 490; resource groups for, 682. *See also* Tourette's syndrome

time: consciousness and, 171, 172. *See also* circadian rhythms

time-isolation laboratories, 43

tinnitus, 329, 343, 344, 345

titubation, 491

tobacco, 111, 409, 410, 411, 415, 417, 418

toddlers, 84, 92–99. *See also* child development

tolerance, 412, 414–16, 419, 421, 423

tolterodine, 356, 667

tones, in language, 226

tongue, 62, 136, 139

tongue tremor, 491

topiramate, 324, 388

torticollis, 164, 495

touch, 45, 136–40, 142, 160, 161, 233, 327; agnosias and, 653; allocation of brain territory and, 6; sensory cells and, 136–37; somatosensory pathway and, 6, *138,* 139, *139, 141*

Tourette's syndrome (TS), 198, **497–500;** diagnosis and treatment of, 498–500; obsessive-compulsive disorder and, 381, 382, 497, 498, 499, 500; resource groups for, 682; symptoms of, 497–98

toxicology screening, 412

toxins. *See* neurotoxins and neurotoxic diseases

toxoplasmosis, cerebral, 450

TPA (tissue plasminogen activator), 340

transcranial magnetic stimulation (TMS), 27

transformed migraine, 551

transient ischemic attacks (TIAs), 570–71, 646; dizziness and, 330; vision problems and, 140, 334–35, *335,* 340, 570–71

transketolase, 612

"transporter" molecules, 104

transverse myelitis, 472, 473

trauma, 93, 267, 372, 406; borderline personality disorder and, 395, 396; depression and, 365, 366; post-traumatic stress disorder and, 405–8

trauma, head or brain. *See* head trauma

tremors, 163, **490–93,** 501; cerebellar, 490, 491; defined, 490; diagnosis and treatment of, 492–93; essential (ET), 490–91, 492, 493; factors in, 492; frequencies of, 490–91; multiple sclerosis and, 440, 490, 491, 492; neuropathic, 491–92; parkinsonian, 477, 478, *478,* 480, 483, 485, 487, 490, 491, 492; physiological, 491; resource groups for, 682 trichotillomania, 381

tricyclic antidepressants (TCAs), 368–69, 387, 452, 500, 515, 544, 622, 630

trigeminal nerve, 566, *566*

trigeminal neuralgia (tic douloureux), 436, *545*, 545–47, **565–68;** diagnosis and treatment of, 567–68; mechanisms of, 566–67; resource groups for, 685; symptoms of, 565–566

trimipramine, 667

triptans, 551

tryptophan, 156, 612–13

tuberculosis, 460, 461

tuberous sclerosis, 274

tumors, 438; neurofibromatosis and, 284–87; in thymus gland, 532, 533. *See also* brain tumors; brain tumors of childhood; cancer

tunnel vision, 336–38

Turner's syndrome, 215

Tversky, Amos, 202

Twain, Mark, 15, 126

12-step programs, 415

ubiquitin, 536

ulcers, 50

ulnar neuropathy, 513

ultrasound, 69, *69*, 76, 578

upright posture, 158, 162

urokinase, 574

"use it or lose it" principle, 39–40, 87, 231, 596

vaccinations, 261, 439; autoimmune encephalomyelitis and, 462; chicken pox and, 445; encephalitis and, 466; Guillain-Barré syndrome and, 517; Lyme disease and, 456; meningitis and, 459, 460

vagus nerve, 142–43, 144

valacyclovir, 446, 667

valium, 268, 422

valproate, 324, 367, 667

valproic acid, 293

varicellazoster virus (VZV), 445, 446, 447

vascular headache, 542–43

vascular tumors, 608

vasculitis, 467, 471, 473, 474

vasopressin, 119, 145, 148–49, 192, 667

vasospasm, 580

vehicular accidents, 110–11, 112, 198, 261, 423, 581, 586, 636, 645. *See also* driving safety

venlafaxine, 368, 374, 397, 668

venoms, 617, 622

ventralis intermedius nucleus, 493

ventral tegmentum, 192, 198

ventricles, 67, 68, 71; tumors in, 304

ventriculoperitoneal shunts, *291*, 291–92

ventriculostomy drain, 582

verapamil, 543, 668

vertebrae, 553–54; spina bifida and, 293–97, *295*

vertebral compression fracture, 553

vertigo, **327–31,** 344; resource groups for, 676. *See also* dizziness

Vesalius, Andreas, *16*

vestibular nuclei, 330

vestibular system, 327, 329, 341

vincristine, 303, 617, 621

violence, 110, **426–28,** *427. See also* aggression

visceral pain, 560

visceral sensory nerves, 142

vision, 22, 96, 136–40, 142, 175, 327; development of, 21, 76–77, 86, 87, 88–89, 91; navigating through space and, 232, 233–35; processing of visual information and, *232*, 232–35; sensory cells and, 123, 136, 137, 138; ultimate goals of, 232; visual pathway and, 27, 87, *138*, 139, *139, 141*, 233, 332, *333, 335*

vision problems, 122–23, 140, 264, 279, 290, 329, **332–40,** 353, 468, 501, 541, 605; agnosias and, 233, 235, 651–52, 653; blindness, 86, 233, 283, 337, 435, 461, 467, 524, 541, 601; color blindness, 233, 235; damage to optic nerve and, *335*, 335–36; diagnosis of, 332; double vision, 336, 435, 454, 516, 523, 531, 570, 577, 615; impaired blood flow in brain and, 338–40; impaired blood flow to retina and, 334–35; macular degeneration and, 338–39, *339*; meningitis and, 459, 461; multiple sclerosis and, 335–36, 435, 442; navigational problems and, 234–35; nutritional disorders and, 612, 613, 615, 616; pressure on optic chiasm and, 336–38; quick medical attention necessary for, 332–33; reading difficulties and, 252; resource groups for, 676; retinitis pigmentosa and, 338; spatial attention and, 234, *234*, 235; stroke and, 140, 232, 332, 334, 335, 338–40, 570–71, 572, 576, 577; symptoms and probable causes of (chart), 334; tumors and, 299, 302, 336–38

visual cortex, 22, 27, 63, 94, *138, 139*, 214, *232*, 233, 235, 332, *333*, 338, *373*; critical period and, 21, 87

visualization, 232–35; brain mechanisms and, *232*, 232–33; navigating through space and, 232, 233–35

visual memory, 235

visual-spatial reasoning, 210, 214, 215

visuospatial loop, 221

vitamin deficiencies, 503, 538, 557, **610–16,** 619, 626, 640

vitamins, 70; excessive intake of, 610, 619; fat-soluble, 611, 615–16; vitamin A, 611, 615; vitamin B_1 (thiamine), 503, 610–12, 640; vitamin B_6 (pyridoxine), 515, 611, 613; vitamin B_{12} (cobalamin), 438, 503, 538,

557, 610, 611, 613–14, 615; vitamin C (ascorbic acid), 611, 615; vitamin D, 71, 611, 615–16; vitamin E, 125, 129–30, 538, 611, 616, 630; vitamin K, 611, 616; water-soluble, 610–15. *See also* folic acid

vitamin supplements, 610

vocal tics, 497–98

voice tremor, 491, 493

Volta, Alessandro, 19

voltage-gated calcium channel (VGCC) antigen, 602

volunteer work, 131

vomiting, 145, 290, 299, 435, 576, 577, 581, 605; nutritional disorders and, 612, 613, 616; as purging behavior, 399, 400, 402

wakefulness, 307

walking, 158–59, 161; child development and, 84, 94; after spinal cord injury, 593, 595–97

walking difficulties, 163, 330, 501, 570; nutritional disorders and, 611, 612, 613; paraneoplastic syndromes and, 601, 603

warfarin (Coumadin), 335, 475, 573, 574, 668

Watson, James, 14

weakness, 459, 473, 605; brain tumors and, 299, 303; facial, 299,

330, 516, 520–22, 527; Guillain-Barré syndrome and, 516–19; multiple sclerosis and, 336, 435, 436; muscle, 523–24, 530–31, 601, 602; nutritional disorders and, 613, 615, 616; paraneoplastic syndromes and, 601; peripheral neuropathy and, 511, 512, 513; stroke and, 339, 570, 571, 576, 577; transient ischemic attack and, 334. *See also* leg weakness

Wechsler Adult Intelligence Scale, 211

Wegener's granulomatosis, 343, 472

weight. *See* body weight; obesity; overweight

Wernicke, Carl, 6–7, 18, 228

Wernicke-Korsakof disease, 420, 611–12

Wernicke's aphasia, 7

Wernicke's area, 18, 90–92, 120, 228, *228, 229*

Western blot test, 455

West Nile virus, 464, 465

Wexler, Nancy, *29*

whiplash, 593

white coat hypertension, 56

white matter, 71, 74; aging and, 125–26, 127, 128. *See also* myelin

white-matter pathways, 265, 266

Wiesel, Torsten, 21

Williams syndrome, 215, 262

Wilson's disease, 492, 496

withdrawal, 319, 354, 414–15, 419; as sign of addiction, 412; treatment of, 415–16, 424, 425; withdrawal delirium and, 176–77

words, 226–27

World Health Organization, 410

writer's cramp, 495

writing, 92, 228, 229

writing difficulties, 501, 570; agraphia and, 645–46; apraxic agraphia and, 649; dysgraphia and, 253

writing tremor, 490, 491

xanthoastrocytomas, 302, 304

X chromosomes, 262, 274, 281

X rays, 23, 605; computed tomography (CT) scans and, 23, 25, 573, 582

Youth Risk Behavior Survey, 431

zalepion, 310, 668

Zellweger's syndrome, 278

zinc, 34, 629

ziprasidone, 393, 668

zolpidem, 310, 668

zonisamide, 324

zoster sine herpete, 446

OTHER DANA PRESS
BOOKS AND PERIODICALS

www.dana.org/books/press

BOOKS FOR GENERAL READERS

Brain and Mind

THE CREATING BRAIN: The Neuroscience of Genius
Nancy C. Andreasen, M.D., Ph.D.

Andreasen, a noted psychiatrist and bestselling author, explores how the brain achieves creative breakthroughs—in art, literature, and science—including questions such as how creative people are different and the difference between genius and intelligence. She also describes how to nurture and develop our creative capacity. 33 illustrations/photos.

Cloth: 225 pp. 1-932594-07-8 • $23.95

THE ETHICAL BRAIN
Michael S. Gazzaniga, Ph.D.

Explores how the lessons of neuroscience help resolve today's ethical dilemmas, ranging from when life begins to "off-label" use of drugs such as Ritalin by students preparing for exams, and other topics, from free will and personal responsibility to public policy and religious belief. The author, a pioneer in cognitive neuroscience, is a member of the President's Council on Bioethics.

Cloth: 225 pp. 1-932594-01-9 • $25.00

A GOOD START IN LIFE: Understanding Your Child's Brain and Behavior from Birth to Age 6
Norbert Herschkowitz, M.D., and Elinore Chapman Herschkowitz

Updated with the latest information and new material, the authors show how young children learn to live together in family and society and how brain development shapes a child's personality and behavior, discussing appropriate rule-setting, the child's moral sense, temperament, language, playing, aggression, impulse control, and empathy.

Cloth: 283 pp. 0-309-07639-0 • $22.95

Paper: (Updated version with 13 illustrations) 312 pp. 0-9723830-5-0 • $13.95

BACK FROM THE BRINK: How Crises Spur Doctors to New Discoveries about the Brain
Edward J. Sylvester

In two academic medical centers, Columbia's New York Presbyterian and Johns Hopkins Medical Institutions, a new breed of doctor, the neurointensivist, saves patients with life-threatening brain injuries. 16 illustrations/photos.

Cloth: 296 pp. 0-9723830-4-2 • $25.00

THE BARD ON THE BRAIN: Understanding the Mind Through the Art of Shakespeare and the Science of Brain Imaging
Paul Matthews, M.D., and Jeffrey McQuain, Ph.D.
Foreword by Diane Ackerman

Explores the beauty and mystery of the human mind and the workings of the brain, following the path the Bard pointed out in 35 of the most famous speeches from his plays. 100 illustrations.

Cloth: 248 pp. 0-9723830-2-6 • $35.00

STRIKING BACK AT STROKE: A Doctor-Patient Journal
Cleo Hutton and Louis R. Caplan, M.D.

A personal account with medical guidance for anyone enduring the changes that a stroke can bring to a life, a family, and a sense of self. 15 illustrations.

Cloth: 240 pp. 0-9723830-1-8 • $27.00

UNDERSTANDING DEPRESSION: What We Know and What You Can Do About It
J. Raymond DePaulo Jr., M.D., and Leslie Alan Horvitz.
Foreword by Kay Redfield Jamison, Ph.D.

What depression is, who gets it and why, what happens in the brain, troubles that come with the illness, and the treatments that work.

Cloth: 304 pp. 0-471-39552-8 • $24.95
Paper: 296 pp. 0-471-43030-7 • $14.95

KEEP YOUR BRAIN YOUNG: The Complete Guide to Physical and Emotional Health and Longevity
Guy McKhann, M.D., and Marilyn Albert, Ph.D.

Every aspect of aging and the brain: changes in memory, nutrition, mood, sleep, and sex, as well as the later problems in alcohol use, vision, hearing, movement, and balance.

Cloth: 304 pp. 0-471-40792-5 • $24.95
Paper: 304 pp. 0-471-43028-5 • $15.95

THE END OF STRESS AS WE KNOW IT
Bruce McEwen, Ph.D., with Elizabeth Norton Lasley
Foreword by Robert Sapolsky

How brain and body work under stress and how it is possible to avoid its debilitating effects.

Cloth: 239 pp. 0-309-07640-4 • $27.95
Paper: 262 pp. 0-309-09121-7 • $19.95

IN SEARCH OF THE LOST CORD: Solving the Mystery of Spinal Cord Regeneration
Luba Vikhanski

The story of the scientists and science involved in the international scientific race to find ways to repair the damaged spinal cord and restore movement. 21 photos; 12 illustrations.

Cloth: 269 pp. 0-309-07437-1 • $27.95

THE SECRET LIFE OF THE BRAIN
Richard Restak, M.D.
Foreword by David Grubin

Companion book to the PBS series of the same name, exploring recent discoveries about the brain from infancy through old age.

Cloth: 201 pp. 0-309-07435-5 • $35.00

THE LONGEVITY STRATEGY: How to Live to 100 Using the Brain-Body Connection
David Mahoney and Richard Restak, M.D.
Foreword by William Safire

Advice on the brain and aging well.

Cloth: 250 pp. 0-471-24867-3 • $22.95
Paper: 272 pp. 0-471-32794-8 • $14.95

STATES OF MIND: New Discoveries about How Our Brains Make Us Who We Are
Roberta Conlan, Editor

Adapted from the Dana/Smithsonian Associates lecture series by eight of the country's top brain scientists, including the 2000 Nobel laureate in medicine, Eric Kandel.

Cloth: 214 pp. 0-471-29963-4 • $24.95
Paper: 224 pp. 0-471-39973-6 • $18.95

The Dana Foundation Series On Neuroethics

HARD SCIENCE, HARD CHOICES: Facts, Ethics, and Policies Guiding Brain Science Today
Sandra Ackerman, Editor

This book, the newest in the Dana Foundation Series on Neuroethics, is based on an invitational meeting co-sponsored by the Library of Congress, the National Institutes of Health, the Columbia University Center for Bioethics, and the Dana Foundation. Top scholars and scientists discuss new and complex medical and social ethics brought about by advances in neuroscience.

Paper: 200 pp. 1-932594-02-7 • $12.95

NEUROSCIENCE AND THE LAW: Brain, Mind, and the Scales of Justice
Brent Garland, Editor.
Foreword by Mark S. Frankel.
With commissioned papers by Michael S. Gazzaniga, Ph.D., and Megan S. Steven; Laurence R. Tancredi, M.D., J.D.; Henry T. Greely, J.D.; and Stephen J. Morse, J.D., Ph.D.

How discoveries in neuroscience influence criminal and civil justice, based on an invitational meeting of 26 top neuroscientists, legal scholars, attorneys, and state and federal judges convened by the Dana Foundation and the American Association for the Advancement of Science.

Paper: 226 pp.1-932594-04-3 • $8.95

BEYOND THERAPY: Biotechnology and the Pursuit of Happiness.
A Report of the President's Council on Bioethics
Special Foreword by Leon R. Kass, M.D., Chairman.
Introduction by William Safire

Can biotechnology satisfy human desires for better children, superior performance, ageless bodies, and happy souls? This report says these possibilities present us with profound ethical challenges and choices. Includes dissenting commentary by scientist members of the Council.

Paper: 376 pp. 1-932594-05-1 • $10.95

NEUROETHICS: Mapping the Field. Conference Proceedings.
Steven J. Marcus, Editor

Proceedings of the landmark 2002 conference organized by Stanford University and the University of California, San Francisco, at which more than 150 neuroscientists, bioethicists, psychiatrists and psychologists, philosophers, and professors of law and public policy debated the implications of neuroscience research findings for individual and societal decision-making. 50 illustrations.

Paper: 367 pp. 0-9723830-0-X • $10.95

Immunology

FATAL SEQUENCE: The Killer Within
Kevin J. Tracey, M.D.

An easily understood account of the spiral of sepsis, a sometimes fatal crisis that most often affects patients fighting off nonfatal illnesses or injury. Tracey puts the scientific and medical story of sepsis in the context of his battle to save a burned baby, a sensitive telling of cutting-edge science.

Cloth: 225 pp. 1-932594-06-X • $23.95
Paper: 225 pp. 1-932594-09-4 • $12.95

Arts Education

A WELL-TEMPERED MIND: Using Music to Help Children Listen and Learn
Peter Perret and Janet Fox
Foreword by Maya Angelou

Five musicians enter elementary school classrooms, helping children learn about music and contributing both to higher enthusiasm and improved academic performance. This charming story gives us a taste of things to come in one of the newest areas of brain research: the effect of music on the brain. 12 illustrations.

Cloth: 225 pp. 1-932594-03-5 • $22.95
Paper: 225 pp. 1-932594-08-6 • $12.00

Free Educational Books

(Information about ordering and downloadable PDFs are available at www.dana.org.)

PARTNERING ARTS EDUCATION: A Working Model from ArtsConnection

This publication illustrates the importance of classroom teachers and artists learning to form partnerships as they build successful residencies in schools. Partnering Arts Education provides insight and concrete steps in the ArtsConnection model. 55 pp.

ACTS OF ACHIEVEMENT: The Role of Performing Arts Centers in Education.

Profiles of more than 60 programs, plus eight extended case studies, from urban and rural communities across the United States, illustrating different approaches to performing arts education programs in school settings. Black-and-white photos throughout. 164 pp.

PLANNING AN ARTS-CENTERED SCHOOL: A Handbook

A practical guide for those interested in creating, maintaining, or upgrading arts-centered schools. Includes curriculum and development, governance, funding, assessment, and community participation. Black-and-white photos throughout. 164 pp.

**THE DANA SOURCEBOOK OF BRAIN SCIENCE: Resources
for Teachers and Students, Fourth Edition**

A basic introduction to brain science, its history, current understanding of the brain, new developments, and future directions. 16 color photos; 29 black-and-white photos; 26 black-and-white illustrations. 160 pp. ISBN: 1-932594-19-1

**THE DANA SOURCEBOOK OF IMMUNOLOGY: Resources for
Secondary and Post-Secondary Teachers and Students**

An introduction to how the immune system protects us, what happens when it breaks down, the diseases that threaten it, and the unique relationship between the immune system and the brain. 5 color photos; 36 black-and-white photos; 11 black-and-white illustrations. 116 pp. ISBN: 1-932594-15-9

Periodicals

Dana Press also offers several periodicals dealing with arts education, immunology, and brain science. These periodicals are available free to subscribers by mail. Please visit www.dana.org.